Deep Learning in Medical Signal and Image Processing

Muhammad Aamir
College of Computer Science and Artificial Intelligence, Huanggang Normal University, China

Uzair Aslam Bhatti
School of Information and Communication Engineering, Hainan University, China

Ziaur Rahman
College of Computer Science and Artificial Intelligence, Huanggang Normal University, China

Jameel Ahmed Bhutto
College of Computer Science and Artificial Intelligence, Huanggang Normal University, China

Waheed Ahmed Abro
Faculty of Sciences Jean Perrin, University of Artois, France

IGI Global
Scientific Publishing
Publishing Tomorrow's Research Today

Vice President of Editorial Melissa Wagner
Director of Acquisitions Mikaela Felty
Director of Book Development Jocelynn Hessler
Production Manager Mike Brehm
Cover Design Phillip Shickler

Published in the United States of America by
IGI Global Scientific Publishing
701 East Chocolate Avenue
Hershey, PA, 17033, USA
Tel: 717-533-8845
Fax: 717-533-7115
Website: https://www.igi-global.com E-mail: cust@igi-global.com

Library of Congress Cataloging-in-Publication Data

Names: Aamir, Muhammad, 1986- editor | Bhatti, Uzair Aslam, 1986- editor | Rahman, Ziaur, 1989- editor | Bhutto, Jameel Ahmed, 1988- editor | Abro, Waheed Ahmed, 1987- editor
Title: Deep learning in medical signal and image processing / edited by Muhammad Aamir, Uzair Aslam Bhatti, Ziaur Rahman, Jameel Ahmed Bhutto, Waheed Ahmed Abro.
Description: Hershey, PA : IGI Global Scientific Publishing, [2025] | Includes bibliographical references and index. | Summary: "The principal objective of this book is to connect AI technology with medical science. The book equips healthcare researchers and professionals with real examples and innovative methods to enhance data analysis in medical imaging and signal processing"-- Provided by publisher.
Identifiers: LCCN 2024055597 (print) | LCCN 2024055598 (ebook) | ISBN 9798369398166 h/c | ISBN 9798369398173 s/c | ISBN 9798369398180 ebook
Subjects: LCSH: Diagnostic imaging--Data processing | Image processing--Data processing | Signal processing--Data processing | Deep learning (Machine learning)--Scientific applications
Classification: LCC RC78.7.D53 D45 2025 (print) | LCC RC78.7.D53 (ebook) | DDC 616.07/540285--dc23/eng/20250403
LC record available at https://lccn.loc.gov/2024055597
LC ebook record available at https://lccn.loc.gov/2024055598

British Cataloguing in Publication Data
A Cataloguing in Publication record for this book is available from the British Library.

Table of Contents

Detailed Table of Contents

Jameel Ahmed Bhutto, College of Computer Science and Artificial Intelligence, Huanggang Normal University, China
Ziaur Rahman, College of Computer Science and Artificial Intelligence, Huanggang Normal University, China
Muhammad Aamir, College of Computer Science and Artificial Intelligence, Huanggang Normal University, China
Aftab Ul Nabi Shahani, South China University of Technology, China
Awais Khan Jumani, South China University of Technology, China
Kamlesh Kamlesh, South China University of Technology, China

Image fusion plays a crucial role in the field of image processing by integrating information from multiple images to produce one output image that incorporates all substantial information. This chapter presents a thorough literature overview of image fusion, organized into six main aspects. It categorizes IF techniques into multiscale decomposition, edge-preserving, subspace-based, sparse representations, deep learning, and hybrid methods by providing an in-depth review of the basic concepts and methodologies of each category. Each category will be studied through its specific sub-techniques, emphasizing its distinctive qualities and fundamental concepts. The chapter further explores the assessment metrics crucial for analyzing the performance and efficacy of IF techniques, emphasizing both quantitative and qualitative evaluations. This literature review presents an essential aid for professionals and researchers aiming at generating and improving IF approaches across numerous applications.

P. Selvakumar, Department of Science and Humanities, Nehru Institute of Technology, Coimbatore, India
S. Anitha, Rajarajeswari College of Engineering, India
Law Kumar Singh, Amity University, Punjab, India
P. V. Sathish Jackson, Sathyabama Institute of Science and Technology, India
Deepika Yadav, SRM University, Sonepat, India
T. C. Manjunath, Rajarajeswari College of Engineering, India

This shift toward AI-driven; it represents a fundamental change in how medical services are delivered and managed. datasets. These technologies can facilitate, making healthcare more efficient and effective. opportunities presented potential processes, AI has shown promise in areas such as radiology, where it can detect tumors in imaging scans with a level of accuracy that rivals that of experienced radiologists. Furthermore, diagnostic capabilities over time as they are exposed to new data considering their unique genetic makeup, lifestyle, and health history. This approach not only enhances treatment efficacy but

Alzheimer's disease (AD) is a disease of the brain that slowly destroys memory and thinking ability. It is one of the most common forms of dementia in people over the age of 65 worldwide. Early detection of Alzheimer's disease helps medical personnel diagnose this disease, which certainly reduces the risk of death. Therefore, early detection of Alzheimer's disease is an important healthcare issue. In order to achieve accurate and timely diagnosis, and for detection of AD in its early stages, many Artificial Intelligence (AI) and Machine learning approaches have been proposed using data from brain imaging. AI and ML are used for many medical and health purposes, such as disease detection. In this chapter, the main focus is on the diagnosis and detection of Alzheimer's disease using CNN model. A Convolutional Neural Network (CNN) is a deep learning model specialized in detecting and classifying patterns in visual data, commonly used for tasks like image recognition, object detection, and classification.

This chapter presents an automated biomedical image classification system, HBDL-FBTA (Hybrid Bio-inspired Deep Learning with Fusion Brain Tumor Analysis), focused on brain tumors—abnormal cell growths in the brain or surrounding tissues that require early, accurate detection for effective treatment. The HBDL-FBTA employs pre-processing to enhance image quality, Swin-UNet-based segmentation for precise region delineation, and fusion-based feature extraction for robust feature acquisition. It uses Humpback Whale Optimization with Simulated Annealing (HSSA) for parameter tuning and a Gated Recurrent Unit (GRU) for reliable classification. Simulations on benchmark datasets, including BraTS2017, demonstrate superior performance, achieving accuracies of 94.51% on ISIC 2017 and 95.38% on ISIC 2020 datasets. Future work will focus on evaluating computational complexity on large-scale datasets, integrating multi-modal imaging data, and developing interpretable deep learning models to enhance clinical adoption and reliability.

Classification of brain tumors has emerged as a major issue medical diagnostics. In this research, we propose a model that integrates both CNN and Vit architectures, combined with an attention-based feature fusion mechanism to improve MRI data classification. The proposed model successfully integrates the capability of Convolutional Neural Networks (CNNs) in capturing localized features and that of Vision Transformers (ViTs) in capturing global contextual information. Multi-scale feature extraction is performed using DenseNet-201, followed by tokenization and embedding transformation for input into ViTs. The attention-based feature fusion enables the proposed network to dynamically integrate

methods. These methods expose the model to more diversity by simulating real-world variations. Thus, data collection and labeling costs are reduced while the model's performance and generalization capacity increase. Data augmentation plays a role in the basis of success, especially in studies where medical images are processed. This study explains the techniques used for image augmentation in detail. It also reveals the performance results of the methods used on data sets and their effects on deep models. The study includes the most frequently used methods and provides a detailed literature review.

The chapter delves into the transformative impact of Convolutional Neural Networks (CNNs) on medical imaging, highlighting their ability to enhance diagnostic accuracy, streamline workflows, and enable real-time image analysis. It provides a comprehensive overview of CNN architectures, their principles, and their integration into diverse medical imaging modalities, such as X-rays, MRIs, and CT scans. Through case studies, the chapter explores CNN applications in detecting brain tumours, pneumonia, and skin cancer, while addressing advanced techniques like transfer learning, GAN-based data augmentation, and hybrid models. The discussion emphasizes the role of Explainable AI (XAI) in overcoming challenges related to model interpretability and ethical considerations, such as patient confidentiality and bias. With a focus on future advancements, including personalized medicine and seamless integration into clinical workflows, the chapter underscores CNNs' potential to redefine diagnostic imaging, improving patient outcomes and revolutionizing healthcare.

Is poised to transform the landscape, personalizing plans, and streamlining efficiencies. Emerges as a powerful ally in addressing these challenges. Quickly far beyond human capabilities presents unprecedented improvement. This brings us to diagnostics. In, have shown remarkable promise, diabetic retinopathy, and. By training on extensive datasets, AI models, and pathologists' abnormalities precision, thus the likelihood of misdiagnosis. For instance, systems experts interpret medical images, allowing for earlier intervention and better patient outcomes. AI also offers substantial advancements alongside, optimizing efficacy and minimizing side systems that can identify specific biomarkers that indicate how might medication, be prescribed. This shift toward personalized treatment not only enhances the effectiveness of therapies but also fosters patient engagement and satisfaction. Operational efficiencies in healthcare systems are. Predictive analytics can optimize scheduling and supply chain. AI systems manage staff resources more effectively.

Emerging trends in medical applications are transforming healthcare by enhancing diagnostic accuracy, personalizing treatment, and improving operational efficiency. Key developments include advanced techniques for medical imaging, predictive analytics for patient outcomes, and the integration of genomic data for tailored therapies. Additionally, decision support systems and administrative automation are streamlining workflows across healthcare settings. Ethical considerations, such as data privacy and algorithmic bias, highlight the need for responsible implementation. Looking ahead, collaboration between technology and healthcare professionals, along with robust regulatory frameworks, will be essential for maximizing the potential of these innovations in transforming patient care.

Emotions play a crucial role in human cognition and influence decision-making, behavior and social interactions. Understanding and predicting emotions based on physiological signals such as brain activity can open new avenues in various fields, including neuroscience, mental health and human-computer interaction. Electroencephalography (EEG) is a non-invasive technique that records electrical activity in the brain and provides insights into the neural processes associated with emotional states. This chapter presents a case study of emotion prediction from EEG data using machine learning techniques for accurate classification. The EEG data, preprocessed for noise reduction and artifact removal, trains a GRU-based neural network to capture temporal patterns. A SoftMax-activated layer predicts emotions with performance evaluated for accuracy. This study shows that EEG data and deep learning models can be powerful tools for emotion recognition, which could be used in the future in personalized mental health care, emotion tracking and better human-computer interaction.

Recurrent Neural Networks (RNNs), particularly Long Short-Term Memory (LSTM) and Gated Recurrent Unit (GRU) architectures, are powerful tools for modeling clinical time-series data where sequential information is essential. This paper explores the effectiveness of RNNs in analyzing patient vital signs, electrocardiogram (ECG) readings, and other time-sensitive health data. The recurrent design of these networks enables the capture of short- and long-term dependencies, vital for predicting patient outcomes, anomaly detection, and aiding in diagnostic decisions. We review recent advancements in

In the recent past medical imaging has emerged as a tool for better diagnosis of patients. The diagnosis mechanism includes Non-invasive methods and further treatment of various diseases viz., pneumonia cancer and other neurological disorders. To address the challenges in the existing methods, this chapter introduces a novel Multi-Stream Attention-Based Convolutional Neural Network (MSA-CNN) technique which is a deep learning architecture. The main component of the proposed architecture is an Attentional mechanism that dynamically assigns prominence to the features of each modality, concentrating on the most relevant regions of the images that are of interest, to improve the models interpretability. Further, a Noise-Aware Loss Function is introduced to handle noise in the images to enhance model performance. Results show that the proposed technique is observed to have an accuracy of 95.7% on the Chest X-ray dataset, outperforming the existing benchmarking techniques to have 89.3% using AlexNet, 92.4% using ResNet-18 respectively.

This chapter proposes a novel hybrid approach that combines the strengths of wavelet transform with the powerful learning capabilities of autoencoder networks to achieve superior denoising performance. By leveraging wavelet decomposition to process images at multiple scales and feeding these decomposed signals into a deep autoencoder network, we effectively suppress noise while maintaining high-frequency details. Extensive experiments demonstrate that our method outperforms existing techniques, yielding significant improvements in both peak signal-to-noise ratio (PSNR) and structural similarity index (SSIM). The results suggest that the integration of wavelet transform and autoencoder networks offers a promising solution for robust image denoising, especially in scenarios with complex noise patterns.

Artificial Intelligence (AI) is rapidly transforming medical applications, paving the way for innovative solutions in diagnostics, treatment, and healthcare management. This review explores future trends in AI for medical applications, focusing on advancements that promise to redefine patient care and medical research. Natural Language Processing (NLP) is revolutionizing the interpretation of clinical notes, medical literature, and electronic health records (EHRs). The future of AI in medical applications lies in its ability to augment human expertise, enhance decision-making, and enable precision medicine. As

Preface

The rapid advancements in deep learning have significantly transformed the landscape of medical signal and image processing, enabling unprecedented improvements in diagnostic accuracy, treatment planning, and healthcare automation. With the ever-growing volume of medical data, the integration of deep learning techniques has become essential for efficient and reliable medical decision-making. This edited volume, *Deep Learning in Medical Signal and Image Processing*, aims to provide a comprehensive exploration of the latest developments, challenges, and applications of deep learning in the field of medical imaging and signal processing.

The book brings together a diverse group of experts who have contributed state-of-the-art research findings and practical insights into the implementation of deep learning techniques across various medical domains. The chapters cover a wide spectrum of topics, including image fusion, biomedical signal processing, AI-driven healthcare ethics, deep learning-based transformers, and convolutional neural networks (CNNs) for disease detection and classification. The book also delves into innovative approaches for tumor detection, attention-driven feature fusion, and data augmentation techniques, showcasing how artificial intelligence is revolutionizing modern medical imaging.

Through this collection of research contributions, we aim to bridge the gap between theoretical advancements and practical applications, providing valuable resources for researchers, practitioners, and students interested in the field of deep learning for medical imaging. The book serves as a guide for understanding emerging trends, evaluating the effectiveness of different methodologies, and exploring future research directions in the realm of artificial intelligence-driven healthcare solutions.

CHAPTER OVERVIEWS

Chapter 1: Emerging Trends in Image Fusion for Real-World Applications

This chapter provides a comprehensive review of image fusion (IF) techniques, categorizing them into multiscale decomposition, edge-preserving, subspace-based, sparse representation, deep learning, and hybrid methods. It examines the methodologies, sub-techniques, and unique characteristics of each category, highlighting their significance in various applications. Additionally, the chapter discusses key assessment metrics for evaluating IF techniques, ensuring a thorough understanding of both qualitative and quantitative performance measures. This analysis serves as a valuable resource for researchers and professionals looking to advance IF methodologies.

Chapter 2: Ethical and Regulatory Challenges in AI-Driven Healthcare

AI is transforming healthcare, offering advanced capabilities in diagnostics, personalized medicine, and predictive analytics. This chapter explores the ethical and regulatory concerns associated with AI integration in healthcare, addressing issues such as data privacy, algorithmic bias, and the risk of misuse. It also discusses AI's potential to revolutionize medical services, particularly in fields like radiology, where it enhances accuracy and efficiency. The chapter highlights the need for robust ethical frameworks and regulatory policies to ensure responsible AI implementation in healthcare.

Chapter 3: Biomedical Signal Processing for Real-Time Health Monitoring

Biomedical signal processing plays a crucial role in modern healthcare, enabling accurate real-time health monitoring. This chapter examines key signal acquisition and preprocessing techniques used to improve the reliability of physiological signals such as ECG, EEG, and EMG. It explores challenges in noise reduction and the role of advanced filtering techniques in enhancing signal clarity, particularly in wearable medical devices. The chapter emphasizes how technological advancements are driving the development of more efficient and effective health monitoring systems.

Chapter 4: Deep Learning-Based Transformers for Medical Image Processing

Deep learning has transformed medical image processing, with U-Net and Transformer-based models emerging as powerful tools for segmentation tasks. This chapter explores the limitations of traditional Convolutional Neural Networks (CNNs) in handling long-distance dependencies and how transformer modules address these challenges. It presents an in-depth analysis of U-Net and Transformer-based architectures, categorizing models based on the integration of transformer modules. The discussion highlights their impact on improving segmentation accuracy in medical imaging applications.

Chapter 5: Detecting Alzheimer's Disease with CNN Models

Alzheimer's disease is a progressive neurodegenerative disorder requiring early and accurate detection for effective treatment. This chapter examines the role of Convolutional Neural Networks (CNNs) in diagnosing Alzheimer's using brain imaging data. It explores the application of deep learning in pattern recognition and classification, demonstrating CNNs' potential to enhance diagnostic accuracy. The chapter discusses how AI-driven techniques support medical professionals in early disease detection, improving patient outcomes and healthcare efficiency.

Chapter 6: Deep Learning for Tumor Detection in Brain MRI Scans

This chapter introduces an end-to-end deep learning framework for brain tumor detection and segmentation in MRI scans. The proposed system, HBDL-FBTA, utilizes Swin-UNet-based segmentation, fusion-based feature extraction, and an optimization algorithm for parameter tuning. By leveraging Gated Recurrent Units (GRU), the system achieves high classification accuracy on benchmark datasets. The chapter also explores future directions, including large-scale dataset analysis and multi-modal imaging integration, to enhance clinical adoption and reliability.

Chapter 7: Attention-Driven Feature Fusion for Brain Tumor Classification

Brain tumor classification remains a significant challenge in medical imaging. This chapter presents a hybrid model combining CNNs and Vision Transformers (ViTs) with attention-driven feature fusion. The integration of CNNs for localized feature extraction and ViTs for global contextual analysis enhances MRI-based tumor classification. Experimental results showcase superior accuracy, sensitivity, and specificity in classifying High-Grade Gliomas (HGG), Low-Grade Gliomas (LGG), and non-tumor regions, reinforcing the model's effectiveness in automated diagnosis.

Chapter 8: CNNs for Enhanced Decision-Making in Medical Imaging

Convolutional Neural Networks (CNNs) have revolutionized medical imaging by improving diagnostic accuracy and decision-making processes. This chapter explores CNN applications in multi-modal imaging data integration, disease detection, and image segmentation. It discusses CNNs' role in assisting clinicians with early diagnosis, emergency medical interventions, and robotic surgery. The chapter highlights how deep learning models can capture subtle patterns that may be overlooked by human specialists, leading to more reliable and efficient medical diagnoses.

Chapter 9: Transforming Medical Imaging with CNNs for Diagnosis and Treatment

CNNs are reshaping the landscape of medical imaging, enhancing diagnostic precision and treatment planning. This chapter delves into CNN architectures such as ResNet and U-Net, discussing their applications in radiology, pathology, and ophthalmology. It examines the impact of deep learning in reducing diagnostic errors and enhancing real-time imaging systems. Ethical considerations, including data security and AI transparency, are also addressed, emphasizing the need for responsible AI deployment in medical practice.

Chapter 10: Data Augmentation in Deep Image Processing

Data augmentation is a critical technique for enhancing deep learning model performance, especially in medical image processing. This chapter explores various augmentation strategies, including geometric transformations, color adjustments, noise addition, and optical distortions. It highlights how these techniques improve model generalization, reduce overfitting, and lower data collection costs. The chapter provides a detailed review of augmentation methods and their impact on deep learning applications in healthcare.

Chapter 11: CNNs in Medical Imaging for Improved Diagnosis and Treatment

Convolutional Neural Networks (CNNs) are playing a pivotal role in modern medical imaging, enabling accurate disease detection and treatment planning. This chapter reviews CNN architectures and their applications across diverse imaging modalities such as X-rays, MRIs, and CT scans. Case studies highlight CNN-based diagnosis of brain tumors, pneumonia, and skin cancer. The chapter also explores advanced techniques like transfer learning and GAN-based augmentation, emphasizing their potential to enhance diagnostic workflows and patient care.

Chapter 12: Emerging Trends in AI for Medical Applications

Artificial Intelligence (AI) is revolutionizing healthcare by improving diagnostics, treatment personalization, and operational efficiency. This chapter discusses AI-driven advancements in medical imaging, predictive analytics, and decision support systems. It highlights AI's role in optimizing resource management, reducing diagnostic errors, and enhancing patient care. Ethical concerns such as data privacy and algorithmic bias are also addressed, underscoring the importance of responsible AI deployment in healthcare.

Chapter 13: AI Innovations in Healthcare Applications

AI is transforming healthcare by enabling advanced diagnostic capabilities, personalized treatment strategies, and workflow automation. This chapter explores the latest trends in AI for medical applications, including predictive analytics for disease progression and genomic data integration for precision medicine. Ethical considerations, such as bias mitigation and regulatory compliance, are discussed. The chapter emphasizes the importance of collaboration between AI researchers and healthcare professionals for the effective implementation of AI solutions.

Chapter 14: Emotion Prediction Using EEG Signals

Understanding human emotions through physiological signals is an emerging field with applications in mental health and human-computer interaction. This chapter presents a case study on emotion prediction using EEG data and machine learning techniques. It details the preprocessing steps, noise reduction methods, and the GRU-based neural network model used for classification. The chapter highlights the potential of EEG-based emotion recognition for personalized healthcare, emotion tracking, and improving human-computer interactions.

Chapter 15: Enhancing Clinical Diagnostics and Patient Monitoring with Recurrent Neural Networks: A Comparative Study of LSTM and GRU Architectures

Recurrent Neural Networks (RNNs), particularly Long Short-Term Memory (LSTM) and Gated Recurrent Unit (GRU) architectures, are essential for analyzing clinical time-series data such as patient vital signs and electrocardiogram (ECG) readings. This chapter explores how these models capture short- and long-term dependencies, aiding in patient outcome prediction, anomaly detection, and diagnostic decision-making. By leveraging real-world clinical datasets, the chapter demonstrates the superiority of RNNs over traditional machine learning models in healthcare applications, addressing challenges like irregular sampling, missing data, and interpretability.

Chapter 16: Enhancing Model Accuracy in Diabetes Prediction through Hybrid Feature Selection

Diabetes mellitus remains a major global health concern, necessitating early and accurate detection. This chapter introduces a hybrid feature selection method that combines filter, wrapper, and embedded techniques to optimize diabetes prediction models. The approach effectively removes irrelevant features, selects optimal subsets, and refines the model during training. Using patient data including age, BMI, blood pressure, and glucose levels, various machine learning models—such as logistic regression, random forests, and XGBoost—are evaluated using performance metrics like accuracy, precision, recall, and AUC-ROC.

Chapter 17: Integrating Artificial Intelligence into Healthcare Workflows

AI is revolutionizing healthcare by enabling large-scale data analysis, predictive insights, and automation of complex processes. This chapter focuses on AI-driven diagnostics, particularly leukemia classification, utilizing deep learning models such as EfficientNetB3 and InceptionV3. By incorporating explainability techniques like LIME, the chapter enhances model transparency, fostering trust among medical professionals. The integration of AI in diagnostic workflows demonstrates its potential to improve accuracy, expedite leukemia subtype identification, and overcome challenges in healthcare systems.

Chapter 18: Multi-Stream Attention-Based Convolutional Neural Network for Medical Imaging

Medical imaging has advanced significantly in diagnosing diseases such as pneumonia and cancer. This chapter introduces a novel Multi-Stream Attention-Based Convolutional Neural Network (MSA-CNN) designed to enhance diagnostic accuracy. The model employs an attention mechanism to prioritize relevant image regions and a Noise-Aware Loss Function to handle image distortions. Performance evaluation on the Chest X-ray dataset shows a remarkable 95.7% accuracy, surpassing benchmark models like AlexNet and ResNet-18, demonstrating the effectiveness of the proposed approach.

Chapter 19: Wavelet-Autoencoder Hybrid Model for Enhanced Image Denoising in Medical Imaging

Medical image denoising is essential for improving diagnostic accuracy. This chapter proposes a hybrid model that integrates wavelet decomposition with autoencoder networks to enhance noise suppression while preserving image details. By processing images at multiple scales and leveraging deep learning capabilities, the model achieves superior performance in terms of peak signal-to-noise ratio (PSNR) and structural similarity index (SSIM). Experimental results confirm the model's effectiveness in handling complex noise patterns, making it a valuable tool in medical imaging.

Chapter 20: Future Trends in Artificial Intelligence for Medical Applications

AI continues to reshape healthcare through innovations in diagnostics, treatment planning, and patient management. This chapter explores emerging AI trends, such as Natural Language Processing (NLP) for clinical notes analysis, predictive modeling for personalized medicine, and AI-driven decision support systems. Ethical considerations, cost reduction, and improved patient outcomes are also discussed, emphasizing the need for continued research, validation, and regulatory oversight to maximize AI's potential in healthcare.

Chapter 21: Brain Tumor Level Detection in 3D MRI Images: An Advanced Approach for Analyzing and Classifying Tumor Severity Using Volumetric MRI Data

This chapter presents an advanced framework for brain tumor detection and classification using 3D MRI images. The proposed system utilizes Support Vector Machine (SVM) and Adaptive Neuro-Fuzzy Inference System (ANFIS) classifiers for precise tumor identification. Preprocessing techniques such as grayscale conversion, noise removal, and contrast enhancement improve image quality, followed by segmentation and feature extraction to classify tumor severity levels. The approach enables early detection and accurate diagnosis, offering a promising solution for neuroradiology applications.

OVERVIEW OF THE BOOK

The first chapter, *A Comprehensive Survey on Emerging Trends in Image Fusion with Real-World Applications*, discusses various image fusion techniques and their significance in enhancing medical imaging accuracy. This is followed by *Addressing Ethical and Regulatory Challenges in AI-Driven Healthcare*, which explores the ethical implications and governance of AI applications in medical settings.

Subsequent chapters delve into advanced biomedical signal processing, deep learning-based transformers, and CNN-based methodologies for disease detection, such as Alzheimer's and brain tumors. The book further examines how convolutional neural networks can enhance decision-making in medical imaging, offering insights into multi-modal data integration, segmentation, and real-time diagnostics. The final chapters address data augmentation strategies and the transformative potential of AI in medical imaging, emphasizing its role in improving diagnostic accuracy and personalized treatment planning.

We express our sincere gratitude to all the contributing authors who have shared their valuable research and expertise in this book. Their dedication and commitment to advancing the field of deep learning in medical imaging have made this volume possible. We are also thankful to our respective institutions for their continuous support in fostering research and innovation in artificial intelligence and healthcare.

A special note of appreciation goes to our reviewers, whose critical evaluations and insightful feedback have helped refine the quality of this book. Their contributions have ensured that the work presented here meets the highest academic and scientific standards.

Finally, we extend our appreciation to the readers who will engage with this book. We hope that this volume serves as a valuable reference and inspires further research and innovation in the field of deep learning for medical signal and image processing. We believe that the future of AI-driven healthcare holds immense potential, and we are honored to contribute to this transformative journey.

Chapter 1

A Comprehensive Survey on Emerging Trends in Image Fusion With Real World Applications

Jameel Ahmed Bhutto
https://orcid.org/0000-0003-4896-7205
College of Computer Science and Artificial Intelligence, Huanggang Normal University, China

Muhammad Aamir
https://orcid.org/0000-0002-7679-0980
College of Computer Science and Artificial Intelligence, Huanggang Normal University, China

Ziaur Rahman
College of Computer Science and Artificial Intelligence, Huanggang Normal University, China

Aftab Ul Nabi Shahani
South China University of Technology, China

Awais Khan Jumani
South China University of Technology, China

Kamlesh Kamlesh
South China University of Technology, China

ABSTRACT

Image fusion plays a crucial role in the field of image processing by integrating information from multiple images to produce one output image that incorporates all substantial information. This chapter presents a thorough literature overview of image fusion, organized into six main aspects. It categorizes IF techniques into multiscale decomposition, edge-preserving, subspace-based, sparse representations, deep learning, and hybrid methods by providing an in-depth review of the basic concepts and methodologies of each category. Each category will be studied through its specific sub-techniques, emphasizing its distinctive qualities and fundamental concepts. The chapter further explores the assessment metrics crucial for analyzing the performance and efficacy of IF techniques, emphasizing both quantitative and qualitative evaluations. This literature review presents an essential aid for professionals and researchers aiming at generating and improving IF approaches across numerous applications.

DOI: 10.4018/979-8-3693-9816-6.ch001

1. INTRODUCTION

Image fusion (IF) is a process of merging multiple images to generate one output image that produces substantial information than any individual images (Bhutto, Guosong, et al., 2024). The prime motive of any IF method is to generate all useful information from input photos to enhance the quality such as spatial resolution, spectral information, contrast and all detailed features. IF is essential in domains where superior, enhanced visual data is vital for further investigation, including remote sensing, surveillance, medical imaging (Rahman et al., 2022), and computer vision. In multimodal medical image fusion (MMIF), the amalgamation of pictures from many imaging modalities, including magnetic resonance imaging (MRI), computed tomography (CT), positron emission tomography (PET), and Ultrasound, is essential. Every imaging modality possesses distinct advantages and drawbacks for the provision of information genres. The MRI is superior in soft tissue contrast, whereas CT offers detailed structural information. By integrating pictures from multiple modalities, healthcare providers can achieve a more holistic understanding of the patient's anatomy (Wang et al., 2022). Therefore, it helps in facilitating precise diagnosis, treatment planning, and disease monitoring, especially in intricate circumstances like tumor detection and neurological investigations. Infrared (IR) and visible image (VI) fusion (IRVI-IF) integrate thermal infrared data with visible light images to yield a more comprehensive and informative representation of the scene. This is essential in applications such as surveillance, security, and remote sensing, where temperature fluctuations must be analyzed in conjunction with visual information (Zhang et al., 2022). Ultimately, multi-focus image fusion (MFIF) integrates several photos captured at varying focal lengths to provide an image that has precise focus through a wider depth of field, commonly utilized in fields such as microscopy, photography, and robotics (Li et al., 2020).

Most IF techniques adhere to a methodical three-phase procedure that is present in Figure 1.

Figure 1. Basic diagram of image fusion

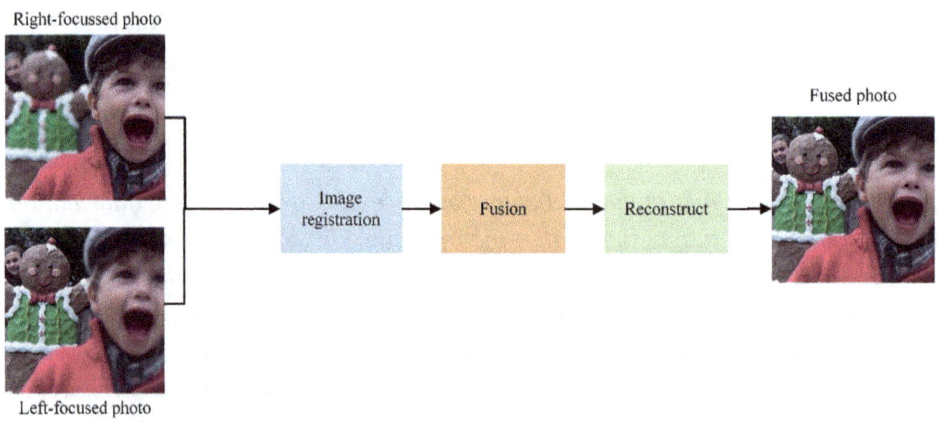

Initially, the source pictures are projected into a designated transform domain to facilitate effective feature analysis. The modified coefficients reflecting various attributes of the photos are amalgamated employing suitable fusion techniques to guarantee the retention of critical information from all source images. Ultimately, an inverse transformation is employed on the amalgamated coefficients for restoring the fused photo in the spatial domain.

Image fusion methods can be categorized into three fundamental categories that are pixel-level, feature-level, and decision-level fusion. Each level possesses distinct advantages and is appropriate for specific applications, depending on the characteristics of the input photos and the specified fusion objectives.

Pixel-level fusion is the fundamental simple method of fusion, wherein pixel values from various images are amalgamated to generate a new image (Li et al., 2017). This approach is typically employed to retain intricate information from each image, including edges, textures, and intensities. Methods of this type are generally computationally less complex but may have difficulties in handling noise and may not consistently maintain semantic features properly. Feature-level fusion involves initially processing images to extract significant features, such edges, textures, or important details, which are subsequently merged (Dogra et al., 2017). Feature-level fusion is especially advantageous when the objective is to emphasize characteristics within images, such as anatomical structures in medical imaging or object boundaries in surveillance film. This approach generally yields superior outcomes compared to pixel-level fusion in applications where structure information is critical (Sarwar et al., 2024). Decision-level fusion relies on the outcomes of classifications generated by each image rather than integrating the raw data (Ma et al., 2019). This fusion method is commonly employed in diagnostic systems, wherein various classifiers evaluate distinct information sources, and their outcomes are amalgamated to render a final decision.

The prime objective of this chapter is to understand the overall idea of IF such as its working phenomena, categories and sub-categories of IF, and their assessment quality parameters to evaluate the effectiveness of each fusion approach. In addition, this chapter will also present application of IF. Besides, this chapter also addresses the challenges experienced in the IF approaches and provides solutions to overcome these challenges. Finally, the detailed conclusion is discussed. Therefore, this chapter is designed on six building blocks as presented in Figure 2.

Figure 2. Overall organization of whole chapter

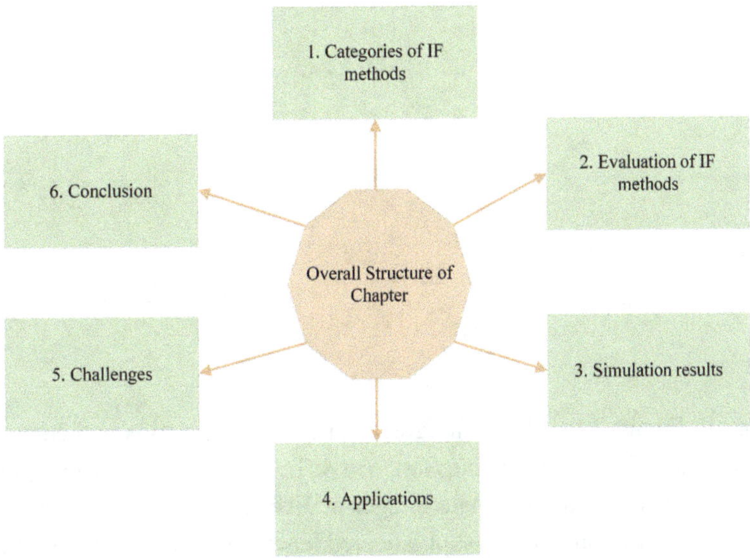

The remainder of this chapter is arranged as follows. Section 2 discusses the categories of IF methods and their sub-categories. The evaluation metrics will be elaborated in section 3. The Simulation results are carried out in section 4. Section 5 presents the application of IF while section 6 highlights the challenges in the field of IF. Finally, the chapter will be concluded in section 7 that gives the overall conclusion of this work.

2. CATEGORIES OF IF

IF has garnered considerable interest because of its rising needs across different sectors. In the past two decades, numerous scholars have attempted to develop IF approaches that produce all pertinent information while eliminating noise and artifacts. The IF techniques are broadly categorized into six main categories that are presented in Figure 3.

Figure 3. Categorization of image fusion methods

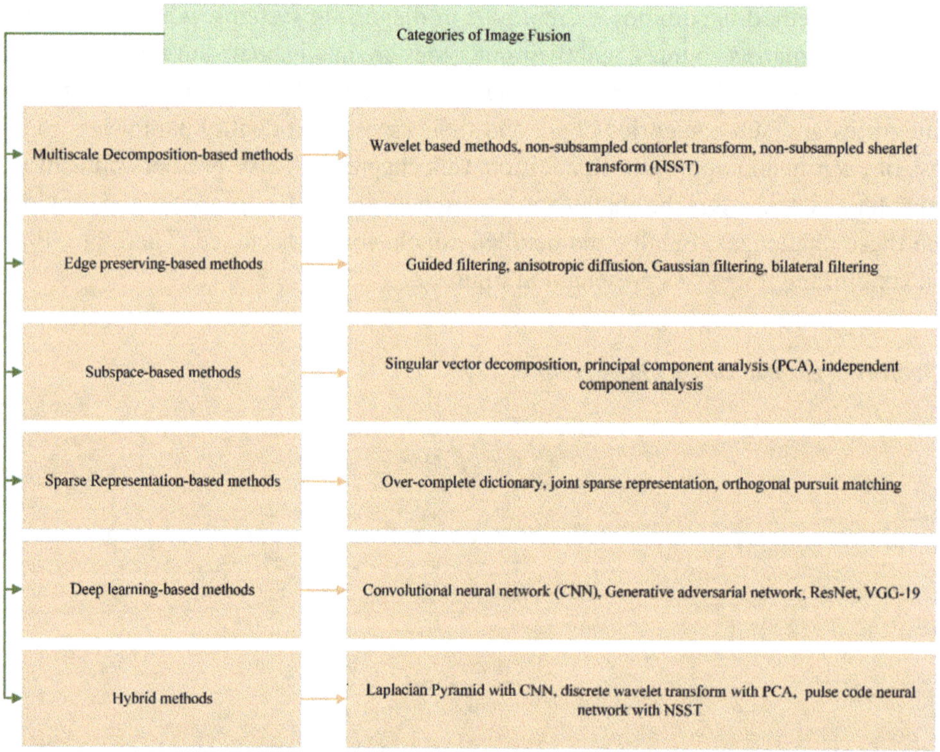

It can be depicted in Figure 3 that IF is categorized into six categories and each category is further divided into sub-categories (Bhutto, Tian, Du, Sun, Yu, & Tahir, 2022). These categories emphasize the variety of techniques employed to amalgamate images at different levels of processing intricacy, which vary from basic pixel-based fusion to more sophisticated learning-based methods. We will discuss each category along with its sub-categories.

2.1 Multi-Scale Decomposition (MSD) Based Methods

MSD methods have demonstrated efficacy in IRVI-IF, MFIF, and MMIF throughout the past few decades. The MSD approaches split the original photos into components of varying scales. Each component signifies the sub-image at various scales, while real-world objects generally consist of components at differing scales (Rahman et al., 2021). Numerous research has shown that MSD approaches comply with human visual features, allowing merged pictures to provide an optimal visual impression (Bhutto, Tian, Du, Sun, Yu, & Soomro, 2022). Typically, IF schemes depend on MSD consist of three phases, as presented in Figure 4.

Figure 4. Block diagram of MSD approach

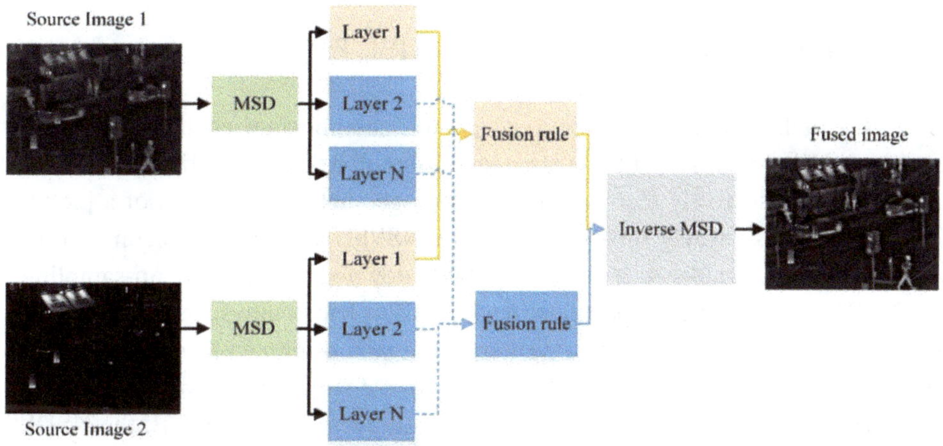

Initially, each source picture is segmented into a sequence of multi-scale representations (MSR). The MSR of the source pictures are amalgamated in accordance with a specified fusion rule. The fused image is obtained through equivalent inverse multi-scale transformations applied to the fused representations. The essence of multi-scale transformation-based fusion methodologies resides in the choice of transforms and fusion criteria.

Now, we will discuss the commonly used sub-categories.

2.1.1 Discrete Wavelet Transform (DWT)

It provides a concise representation of a frequency elements of signal, enhancing frequency information and temporal resolution (Aamir et al., 2019). It splits the picture into frequency sub-bands at many scales by partitioning it into high-frequency (HF) and low-frequency (LF) sub-bands (Bhutto et al., 2020). The LF encompasses the mean intensity of images, while the HF comprises information regarding the edges of images. In DWT, down-sampling decreases computational time and accelerates the process. The DWT technique decomposes several images into distinct LF and HF sub-bands. Unlike the pixel-based method, this approach mitigates spectral distortion in the fused images by delivering a high signal-to-noise ratio at a reduced spatial resolution. Wavelet fusion surpasses spatial domain fusion in reducing color distortions. Nonetheless, the DWT has issues of oscillation, shift variance, aliasing, and a deficiency in directionality.

2.1.2 Discrete Stationary Wavelet Transform (DSWT)

Down-sampling in discrete wavelet transform (DWT) induces a deficiency in shift-invariance, leading to distortion, artifacts, and blurring effects that culminate in suboptimal output photo quality. These challenges can be addressed by removing the down-sampling in DSWT (Aamir et al., 2019; Lianfang et al., 2018). Consequently, it maintains superior quality and provides a more informative output photo. The source pictures are divided into horizontal and vertical approximations using LF and HF filters in both column and row directions. The identical filtration is applied to the split components both row-wise and column-wise to acquire approximate vertical, horizontal, and diagonal details. Authors have employed DSWT to split the source photos into one LF sub-band and three HF sub-bands (low-high, high-low, and high-high sub-band) without utilizing down-sampling. The resulting photo enhances spectral information but inadequately captures spatial characteristics.

2.1.3 Non-Subsampled Contourlet Transform (NSCT)

The NSCT is a multi-scale, multi-directional photo decomposing technique that integrates non-subsampled pyramid filter banks (NSPFB) with non-subsampled directional filter banks (NSDFB). This splitting technique can effectively recreate the authentic geometrical structure of a picture, including edges and contours, and is entirely shift-invariant. The NSPFB analyses the picture with two-channel non-subsampled 2D filter banks, circumventing both down-sampling and up-sampling processes. Additionally, NSDFB is employed to partition band-pass sub-bands into several orientations. The non-subsampled pyramids are constructed utilizing iterative non-subsampled filter banks to achieve MSD. Subsequently, all filters are up sampled by a factor of 2 for the subsequent level, so fulfilling the perfect reconstructing criteria. Following the application of decomposition via NSPFB, the NSDFB, which is shift-invariant, is implemented. It is a two-channel non-subsampled filter bank iterative approach that attains superior directional decomposition (Ibrahim et al., 2023). The identical procedure will be employed for the intended higher-level decomposition. The NSCT has been extensively utilized in applications including IRVI-IF, MF-IF, and MMIF because of its potential to mitigate the pseudo-Gibbs phenomena and the impact of misregistration.

2.1.4 Non-Subsampled Shearlet Transform (NSST)

The NSST is a multi-scale, multi-directional picture segmentation technique that proficiently retains prominent characteristics across many scales and orientations. The NSST technique consists of two primary stages which are MSD and directional localization. The MSD is derived via the use of NSPF, whereas the directional localization is attained using small-scale shearing filters (SFs). This approach employs shearing transforms to augment the efficacy of decomposition (Sharma et al., 2024). Simultaneously, it demonstrates efficiency in convolution computations within the temporal domain. These local SFs can eliminate obstructive effects and mitigate Gibbs' phenomenon.

2.2 Edge Preserving Filtering Based Fusion Methods

Numerous scholars have developed edge-preserving filtering-based MSD techniques that yield superior outcomes. Edge-preserving filtering techniques have emerged as a prominent tool for research for numerous picture fusion applications over the past two decades. The required photos are segmented using filtering into a base layer and detailed layers. The base layer is obtained by an edge-preserving filter that precisely captures the primary variations in intensity. Conversely, the detail layers comprise a series of distinct photos that achieve coarse resolution at fine sizes. These filtering methods preserve spatial coherence and mitigate halo effects surrounding textures and edges (Li et al., 2023).

In numerous practical image fusion contexts, including MMIF, MF-IF and IRVI-IF, precise boundaries (edges) are essential for accurate analysis. Consequently, edge-preserving filters are frequently employed to amalgamate source pictures, ensuring the retention of detailed information, especially at object boundaries, while mitigating undesirable noise or blurring in other areas of the photos. An author applies in (Shreyamsha Kumar, 2015) the cross bilateral filtering (CBF) approach. This method determines the weights by assessing the picture strength by the subtraction of the CBF from the source pictures. Subsequently, these weights are directly multiplied with the source pictures using weight normalization. This direct multiplication results in the introduction of artefacts and noise. There are various methods in edge preserving based fusion approach such as bilateral filtering, Gaussian filtering (Rahman et al., 2019), guided filtering, anisotropic diffusion, non-local means filtering, and so on.

2.3 Subspace Based Methods

Subspace-based techniques seek to map high-dimensional input photos into low-dimensional subspace. Natural photos typically contain redundant information, and low-dimensional subspaces can effectively encapsulate the intrinsic structures of the original photos. Furthermore, processing low-dimensional subspace data requires less time and memory compared to high-dimensional input photos (Mitianoudis et al., 2013). Furthermore, low-dimensional subspace representation can enhance generalization. Several scholars have employed subspace approaches in image fusion, yielding superior spatial information. Furthermore, these strategies are time-efficient owing to the advantages of dimensionality reduction. The most often employed subspace approaches are principal component analysis (PCA) (Bhutto, He, et al., 2024), independent component analysis (ICA), non-negative matrix factorization (NMF) (Kong, Lei, & Zhao, 2014), singular vector decomposition (SVD), and intensity hue saturation (IHS). Subspace methods are more computationally efficient as they reduce the dimensionality of data leading to faster processing time. Besides, these methods helps to capture significant energy information in the images.

2.4 Spare Representation (SR) Based Methods

SR techniques have been effectively employed across several domains, such as image analysis, computer vision, pattern recognition, and machine learning, to elucidate the human visual system (Zhang et al., 2018). In contrast to IRVI-IF, MMIF, and MFIF techniques utilizing MSD with predetermined basis functions, SR image fusion approaches seek to acquire an over-complete dictionary from a substantial collection of high-quality natural photos (Adnan et al., 2020). Subsequently, the source photos may be represented sparsely by the acquired dictionary, hence potentially improving the representation of significant and stable photos (Bhutto, Khan, & Rahman, 2023). Furthermore, misregistration or noise can introduce bias into the fused multi-scale representation coefficients, resulting in visual artifacts in the fused photo. To mitigate visual artifacts and enhance resilience to misregistration, SR-based techniques employ a sliding window approach to partition source photos into many overlapping patches (Liu et al., 2015). The SR-based image fusion approaches typically consist of four stages, as shown in Figure 5.

Figure 5. The fundamental diagram of SR-based image fusion

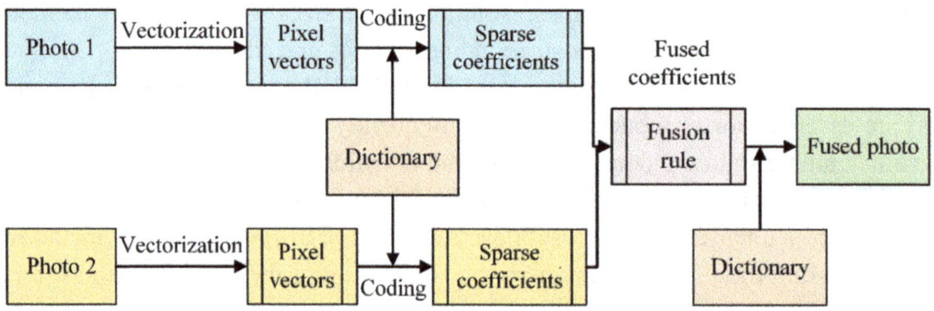

Initially, each source picture is segmented into many overlapping patches with a sliding window technique. Secondly, an over-complete dictionary (OCD) is derived from numerous high-quality photos, and sparse coding is carried out on each patch to acquire the sparse representation coefficients utilizing the learnt OCD. The sparse representation coefficients are amalgamated in accordance with a specified fusion rule. The fused photo is ultimately reconstructed utilizing the fused coefficients derived from the learnt OCD (Bin et al., 2016). The essence of sparse representation-based fusion methodologies resides in the formulation of an OCD and the implementation of sparse coding.

There are several sub-categories of SR approaches such as over-complete dictionary (OCD), orthogonal matching pursuit (OMP), k-means singular vector decomposition, joint sparse representation and so on.

2.6 Deep Learning (DL) Based Methods

The growing importance of deep learning (DL) has garnered substantial focus over the past ten years (Rahman et al., 2024; Rahman, Zhang, & Bhutto, 2023; Sarwar et al., 2024). Recent advancements in DL have led to the development of many fusion techniques utilizing convolutional neural networks (CNN) in the domain of image fusion, including MMIF, IRVI-IF, and MF-IF. CNN is a multistage feedforward artificial neural network utilizing trainable supervised learning, and the convolution operation is multi-dimensional (Aamir et al., 2019). In a convolutional network, the initial parameter is typically referred to as the input. The second parameter is referred to as a kernel function, while the result is referred to as a feature map. The fundamental CNN model for IF typically has four stages, as highlighted in Figure 6.

Figure 6. Basic diagram of IF by CNN

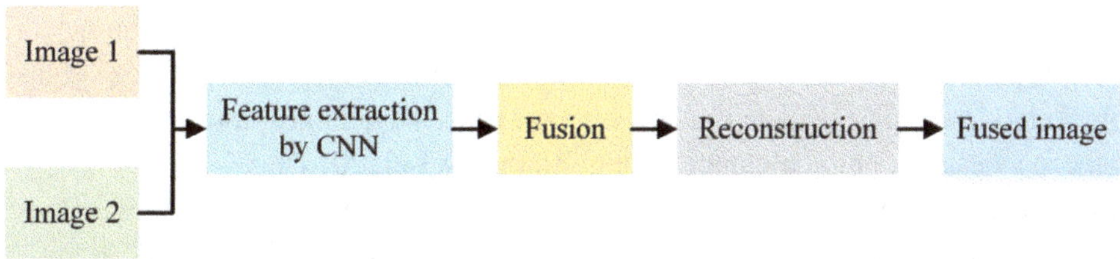

The input images are initially processed by a CNN for feature extraction, followed by the application of fusion methods to the recovered features. The reconstruction is ultimately employed to provide a final fused image. Sparse weights, isomorphic representations, and parameter sharing are fundamental principles in CNN design. Matrix multiplication is employed in CNNs to regulate connect interactions. The connection between input and output units necessitates substantial storage capacity. Consequently, storage needs are diminished, and computational efficiency is enhanced by carrying out a local convolution operation on a limited number of neurons that are directly next to the preceding stage. Feature extraction in computer vision predominantly depends on convolutional layers, which generally provide more pertinent data than conventional manual techniques (Bhutto, Siddique, et al., 2024).

There are numerous sub-categories of DL that have taken noteworthy attention due to their outstanding performance such as Siamese CNN, VGG-19, ResNet, generative adversarial network and autoencoders (Bhutto, Sunkari, et al., 2023; Bhutto, Zhang, & Rahman, 2023; Nabi et al., 2024).

2.7 Hybrid Fusion Methods

Despite the development of numerous MSDs, subspace, SRs, and DL techniques, the integration of methods from other fields has demonstrated significant efficacy in IF. Various transformations include distinct advantages with certain limitations (Bhutto, Mubashir, et al., 2023). The MSD fusion can extract spatial features of varying scales within the image. Nevertheless, they cannot represent the LF component in a sparse manner. In this scenario, integrating the LF coefficients by basic fusion methods like averaging or choose-max may compromise fusion performance, as the LF coefficients encapsulate the primary energy of the image (Sun, Tian, Du, et al., 2023). The fusion based on SR can yield more significant representations of the original photos through dictionary learning, which are more precisely suited to the data. Nonetheless, reconstructing the intricate details of the original images is challenging due to the finite quantity of atoms in a dictionary. Other transformations, including the IHS and PCA transforms, are efficient and rapid for the fusion of remote sensing, according to the relevant fusion protocols (Zhou et al., 2016). Nonetheless, these methods are not immediately applicable to additional image fusion applications such as MF-IF, MMIF. The CNN and DL-based fusion techniques have garnered significant interest during the past ten years. CNN and DL yield superior outcomes compared to previous single domain fusion techniques (Yu et al., 2023). However, these methods are not immediately applicable to spatial domain approaches, leading to the loss of significant features.

The hybrid approaches leverage the characteristics and benefits of various techniques (Sun, Tian, Du, & Bhutto, 2023). Consequently, numerous fusion algorithms integrating diverse transformations have been presented in the past decade to fully leverage these advantages, minimize errors, and ensure the utilized approaches are complementary (Kong, Zhang, & Lei, 2014).

The authors in the paper (Lianfang et al., 2018) have used amalgamated approaches that use combined median and average filter, DSWT, and PCA which is depicted in Figure 7.

Figure 7. The block diagram of hybrid method

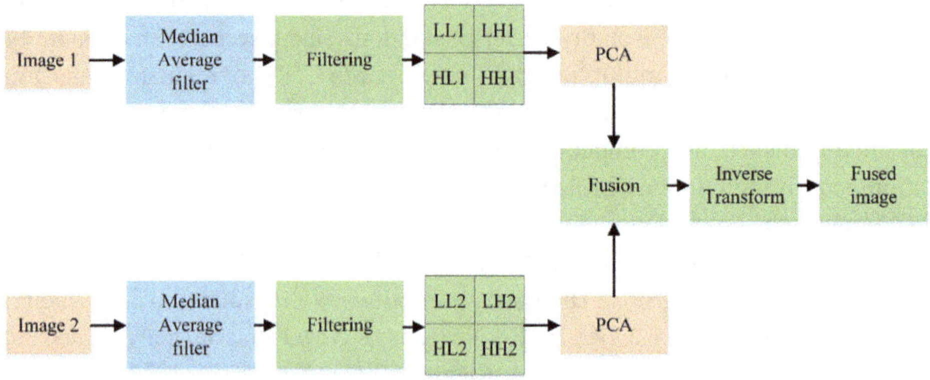

The amalgamated median and average filter at the pre-processing stage is deployed that uses a statistical histogram to efficiently eliminate noise. This technique employs an adaptive filter mask to effectively diminish noise with rapid computing. Then DSWT is used to process images because of its shift-invariance quality that restore smooth edges and contours. Additionally, this approach uses the Haar wavelet, which has appealing properties including orthogonality, compact support, and limitless support in the frequency domain. After that, PCA is utilized to fuse the decomposed images in order to remove unnecessary information while maintaining robust operation. The final fused image that contains improved spatial and spectral information with minimal noise is then obtained by applying inverse DSWT.

Another hybrid method is presented in paper (Bhutto et al., 2020). An amalgamated histogram equalization fast gray level grouping (HE-FGLG) technique is developed that automatically improves contrast of photo. Photos collected from HE-FGLG are fed to NSCT. The actual geometrical structure can be well captured by this decomposition technique. For LF photos that retain energy information, a local energy-based fusion technique is used by selecting either the averaging or selection mode. For HF photos, the mean-gradient fusion technique is used to preserve the smooth contours, edges, borders, and texture. After that, gray-PCA is employed that helps in dimension reduction while preserving all rich features in photos.

Numerous scholars have designed hybrid methods, and these methods produce better results than any individual IF method (Sun et al., 2022).

3. EVALUATION OF IF METHODS

Assessing the performance of IF approaches is a crucial challenge. The evaluation process is categorized into qualitative and quantitative evaluation (Zhang et al., 2014). We will discuss both in detail.

3.1 Qualitative Evaluation

Qualitative assessment is employed for assessing the quality of the final fused image based on human visual perception, including factors such as brightness, contrast, edges, contours, and noise. Consequently, researchers in IF assess qualitative evaluations based on the human visual system. It is the most used and favored method for visually comparing differences in images as perceived by the human eye (Yu et al., 2022).

3.2 Quantitative Evaluation

Quantitative assessment is conducted to further substantiate the quality of the fused image. Quantitative assessment is employed to determine the variance based on mathematical computations (Liu et al., 2017; Zhu et al., 2021). There are various parameters that are used to determine the quantitative evaluation, and we will present a few of them here.

3.2.1 Quality transfer ratio from input photos to fused photo (Q_F^{XY})

The Q_F^{XY} is employed to monitor the transfer of intricate details, including edges, textures, and boundaries, from source images to a final output image (Z. Liu et al., 2018). A higher value of Q_F^{XY} indicates that more detail is transmitted from the source images to the produced image.

3.2.2 Feature Mutual Information (FMI)

The FMI is calculated to analyze the alteration of photo attributes, such as contrast, textures, and edges, from individual source photos to a final output photo (Jin et al., 2017). A larger FMI value will result in more transformation of information from source photos to generated photos. Therefore, higher value of FMI reflects that output photo contains more information from source photos.

3.2.3 Structural Similarity Index (SSIM)

The SSIM denotes the structural similarity between the input photos and the output photo. A higher SSIM score indicates that a significant amount of comparable information is derived from the input images to the fused images (Y. Liu et al., 2018).

3.2.4 Noise in the Fused Photo (N_F^{XY})

The N_F^{XY} is calculated to determine the level of noise and artifacts present in the resulting image. An elevated N_F^{XY} value signifies the occurrence of substantial noise or artifacts (Yan et al., 2020).

4. SIMULATION RESULTS FOR EXISTING METHODS

This section presents the implementation of four image fusion methods and their quality is assessed by four quality parameters. The methods used in this chapter are principal component analysis (PCA) (Kumar & Muttan, 2006), discrete wavelet transform (DWT) (Tawade et al., 2014), non-subsampled shearlet transform with pulse code neural network (NSST-PCNN) (Kong, Zhang, & Lei, 2014), and convolutional neural network with anisotropic diffusion (CNN-AD) (Bhutto, Guosong, et al., 2024). We have evaluated their performance based on qualitative and quantitative evaluation parameters. We have used the Q_F^{XY}, FMI, SSIM, and N_F^{XY}.

Figure 8. (a) center focused, (b) corner focused, (c) PCA, (d) DWT, (e) NSST-PCNN, (f) CNN-AD

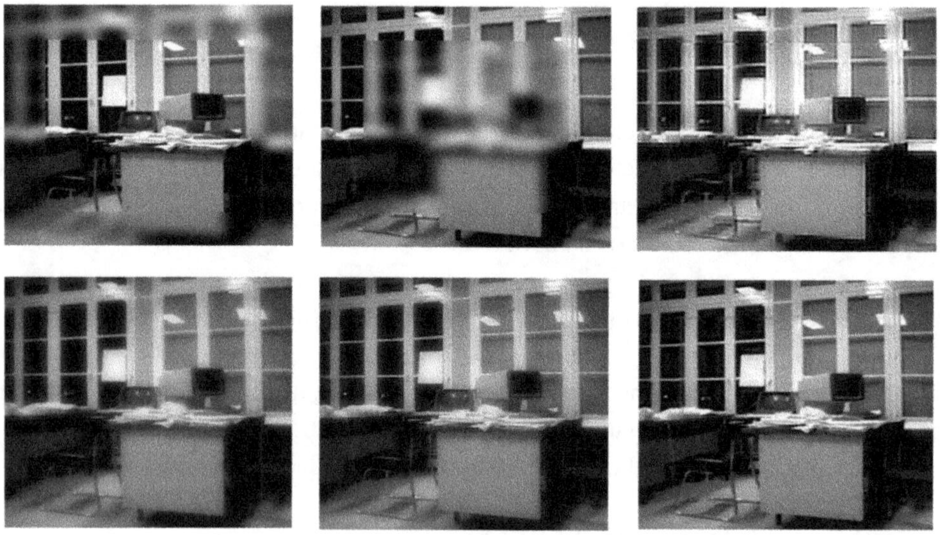

Figure 9. (a) center focused, (b) corner focused, (c) PCA, (d) DWT, (e) NSST-PCNN, (f) CNN-AD

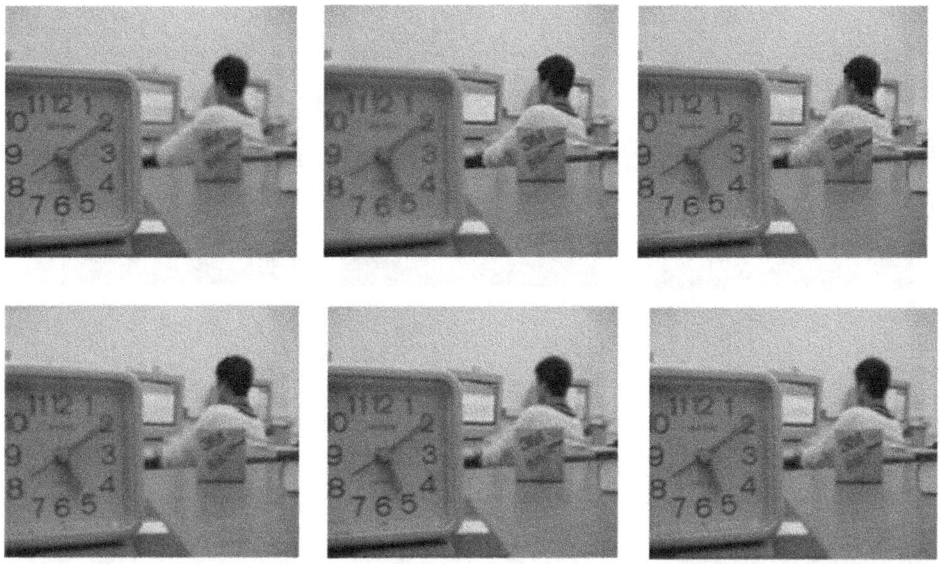

Figure 10. (a) CT image, (b) MRI image, (c) PCA, (d) DWT, (e) NSST-PCNN, (f) CNN-AD

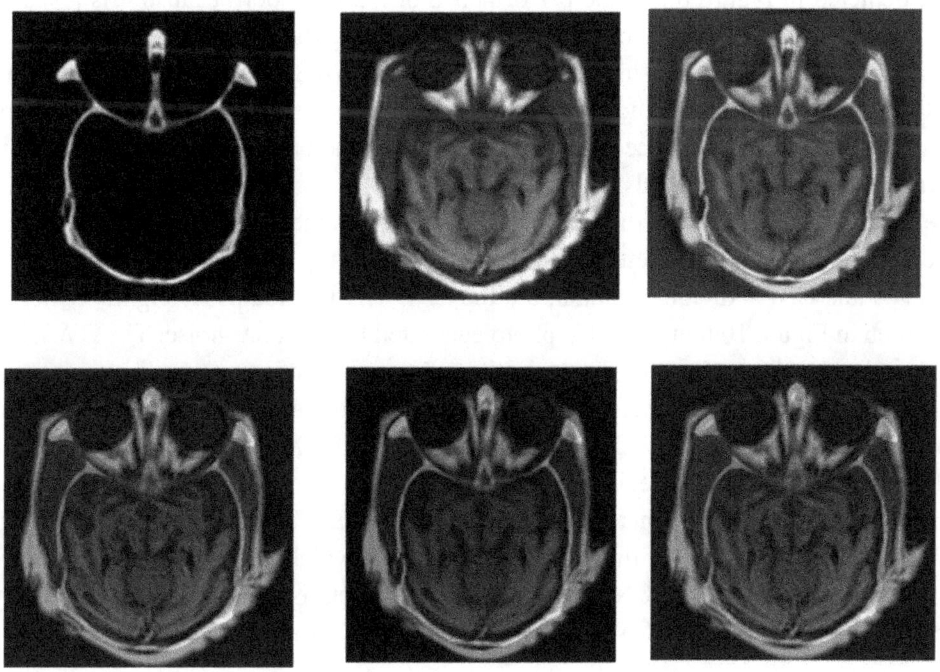

Figure 11. (a) CT image, (b) MRI image, (c) PCA, (d) DWT, (e) NSST-PCNN, (f) CNN-AD

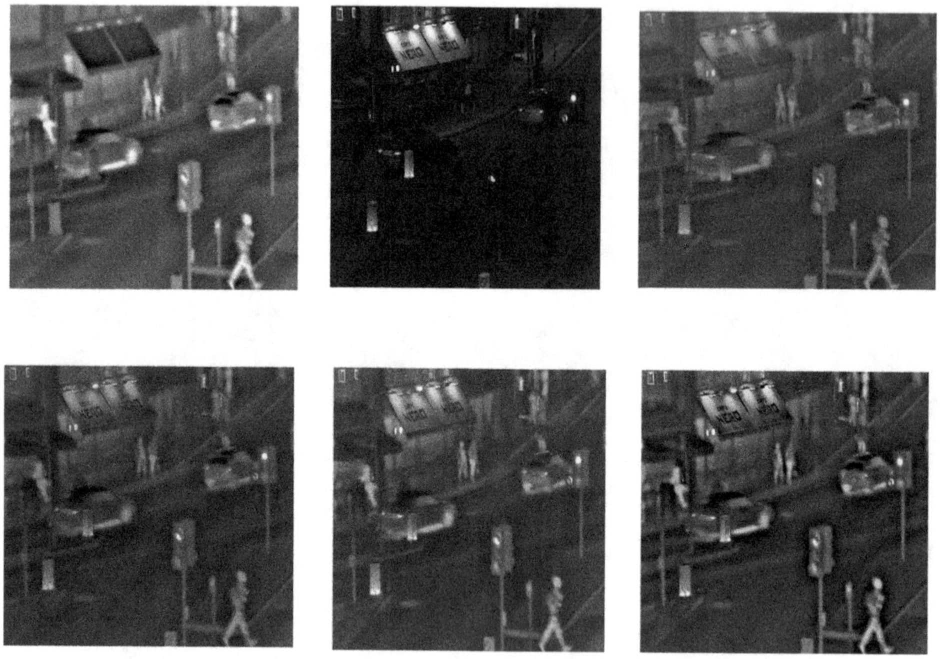

It can be depicted in Figure 8 that the performance of PCA is poor because it is a spatial method technique so it cannot capture spectral information. DWT produces better results than PCA, but its quality isn't satisfactory because DWT uses shift-invariant that results in degradation in fused photo. The quality of NSST-PCNN is better than PCA and DWT since it uses the hybrid method that helps to capture more information. The fused image produced by CNN-AD is vivid and has less noise. In addition, it contains richer information than other methods.

It can be observed in Figure 9 that the performance of the PCA method is poor, and noise is introduced in the fused image. The DWT has better results than PCA, but the fused image is blurred. The quality of NSST-PCNN and CNN-AD looks similar, but the CNN-AD method has a slightly better contrast.

It can be seen in Figure 10 that the fused photo generated by PCA has noise. The DWT method also has artifacts and pixel discontinuities due to limited directional information. The image obtained by CNN-AD has better visual effects, but it has uneven illumination, and due to that, the fused image lost some vital information. The NSST-PCNN has vivid contrast and high resolution. Besides, it captures smooth edges and contours more precisely.

It can be observed in Figure 11 that the quality of PCA and DWT looks resemble and the results are satisfactory. However, the contrast of fused images is not vivid, which results in loss of some information. The fusion performance of NSST-PCNN is weaker since the details are not clear and it lost most of the information. The fusion result of the CNN-AD is better, and the contrast and texture information are better.

Table 1. The average values of quantitative parameters for all IF methods

Method	PCA	DWT	NSST-PCNN	CNN-AD
Q_F^{XY}	0.6736	0.7043	0.8193	0.8794
FMI	0.5336	0.5692	0.6225	0.6113
SSIM	3.8501	4.5213	6.7895	6.7937
N_F^{XY}	0.3397	0.2993	0.2337	0.1209

The quality of fused photos is further analyzed by quantitative parameters in Table 1. It can be seen that NSST-PCNN and CNN-AD produces better values than PCA and DWT. Since it can be concluded that hybrid methods achieve satisfactory results than single domain methods.

5. APPLICATIONS FOR IF

IF has played a significant role in the field of computer vision and it has been employed in a variety of applications such as medical diagnosis and treatment, remote sensing, surveillance and photography applications. We will discuss some of its applications in sub-sections of this chapter.

5.1 Medical Diagnosis

The predominant number of medical diagnostics are conducted by computers or physicians evaluating medical imagery. The imaging methods of medical modalities vary, as these focuses on depicting bodily information (Huang et al., 2020). Computed tomography (CT), magnetic resonance imaging (MRI), positron emission tomography (PET), single-photon emission computed tomography (SPECT), and ultrasound are among the most prevalent medical modalities. Some modalities concentrate on delineating the anatomy of organs and tissues, whilst others emphasize the characterization of regional metabolic intensity. In this context, integrating medical photos from several modalities can significantly enhance diagnostic accuracy and efficiency, while minimizing redundant information and boosting photo quality.

Figure 10 illustrates the integration of CT and MRI imaging for the diagnosis of a medical issue. Certain disorders not only alter the physical structure of tissues but also enhance the intensity of local metabolism. The integration of functional and structural medical imaging can enhance diagnostic accuracy for various disorders. Therefore, MMIF can be utilized in numerous applications such as Alzheimer's disease (AD), COVID-19 detection, brain tumor disease (Aamir et al., 2023; Aamir et al., 2022; Guan et al., 2021), coronary artery disease (Rahman, Bhutto, et al., 2023), and so on.

5.2 Remote Sensing (RS)

RS applications depend on acquiring images from a distance to derive critical information about the Earth's surface. The objective of RS fusion technique is to integrate inconsistencies in information from identical or different scenes into a singular image that is spatially, and temporally coherent. RS systems analyze image pixels throughout various segments of the electromagnetic spectrum, resulting in variations in spatial, spectral, and temporal resolution (Yang et al., 2016). These data sets comprise multispectral images (MS) characterized by high spectral resolution and decreased spatial resolution, as well as panchromatic images (PAN) featuring broad spectral bandwidth and elevated spatial resolution.

The fusion of PAN photos with MS photos is referred to as pan sharpening. The spectral range of PAN and MS photos is similar, while the spectral distribution of hyperspectral (HS) photos is considerably larger. The fusion of PAN and MS images is simpler than that of PAN and HS images. The amalgamation of these types of photos integrates the geometrical characteristics of a scene into a singular image, resulting in a composite that conveys a greater amount of consolidated information than any individual image. It is additionally employed for remote sensing monitoring. Therefore, RS can be applied in various applications such as land cover cataloguing, mineral examination, vegetation recognition, and so on.

5.3 Photography

Due to the restricted depth of field in cameras, it is unfeasible to get a sharp focus on all objects located at varying distances from the camera in a single shot. To address this issue, multi-focus image fusion integrates several photographs of the identical scene, each with varying focus points, to produce a uniformly focused fused image (Yang et al., 2019). The fused image effectively retains pertinent information from the source data. Figure 8 and Figure 9 are common examples of multi-focus image fusion. Recently, MFIF has been employed in several applications, including object detection, recognition, and tracking.

5.4 Surveillance and Navigation

Surveillance and navigation require clear, resilient, and articulate images or videos. The complementary attributes of infrared and visible pictures render effective fusion sources for this purpose. Infrared and visible images provide object information through distinct imaging characteristics. Infrared photographs record the heat radiation of objects, unaffected by variations in illumination, weather, and other disturbances. Nonetheless, infrared images possess insufficient spatial resolution, rendering them inadequate for distinguishing details. In contrast, visible images possess high spatial resolution and vibrant colors, rendering objects inside them distinct and immediately recognizable. The fusion of these two photos markedly enhances visibility and facilitates various practical applications (Xu et al., 2021). Figure 11 is the practical fusion of infrared and visible photos. The IRVI-IF has been employed in a variety of real time applications including pedestrian recognition, fruit recognition, object detection, and so on.

6. CHALLENGES IN IF

Various IF methods have been implemented, but there are still a lot of open-ended problems in many different areas. This section focusses on challenges and future trends in a number of application areas, including monitoring, medical diagnosis, remote sensing, and photography.

In the realm of photography, as source photos are invariably captured at varying intervals, moving objects could appear in disparate positions throughout the capturing process, thus resulting in ghost artifacts in the fused photo. Designing methods that are insensitive to mis-registration presents a significant challenge in addressing this problem. Additionally, another research path involves the application of IF algorithms in integrated consumer camera systems for practical photographic purposes.

The primary challenge in remote sensing is reducing visual distortions during the fusion of multispectral, hyperspectral, and panchromatic images. Moreover, although the input photos are often obtained using the same platform, varying imaging sensors may not properly align in focus, and their acquisition timings are not similar. In this scenario, accurate registration is difficult due to the substantial resolution and spectral disparity across the source photos. Ultimately, the rapid advancement of remote sensing sensors will render the development of innovative algorithms for the integration of images obtained from new aircraft or satellite sensors a prominent research focus.

In the field of medical diagnostics, accurate registration poses a significant challenge due to the diverse acquisition methods of medical photos. Furthermore, implementing procedures aimed at certain clinical issues constitutes a complex and nontrivial aspect of medical diagnosis. The idea is that the design of fusion approaches necessitates both medical domain expertise and algorithmic ability. Furthermore, as the required fusion outcomes may differ from those of conventional image fusion, the quantitative assessment of medical image fusion techniques presents a significant challenge.

In surveillance applications, two primary needs should be addressed. Fusion approaches are anticipated to be computationally efficient, enabling their implementation in real-time surveillance. Conversely, due to the significant variability of image capture conditions in outdoor environments, developing fusion algorithms that are resilient to suboptimal conditions such as noise and under- or over-exposure is a critical issue.

7. CONCLUSION

Image Fusion (IF) represents a powerful technique in the field of image processing, combining multiple images to produce a fused photo that has significant spatial information with enriched detailed features. The various categories of IF methods, such as MSD, edge preserving filtering, subspace-based methods, SR, Deep Learning (DL), and hybrid Fusion approaches have been discussed in detail that present the advantages, disadvantages, and their usages in specific applications. In addition, each category is further discussed in sub-categories from traditional approaches like PCA and DWT to most advanced techniques such as CNN-AD. The evaluation of IF methods through both qualitative and quantitative metrics, including quality transfer ratio, feature mutual information, structural similarity index, and noise in the fused photos provide a quantitative evaluation for assessing the effectiveness of fusion methods. These metrics not only facilitate the comparison of different fusion techniques but also guide future improvements in fusion quality. Simulation results on existing methods, such as PCA, DWT, NSST-PCNN, and CNN-AD have been designed that underline the performance capabilities of these models across various application domains. The applications of IF in critical fields such as medical imaging, remote sensing, photography, and surveillance underscore its significant impact on real-world challenges.

However, despite the progress made, challenges remain in terms of real-time processing, computational cost, and fusion quality under varying conditions. Future research must focus on overcoming these challenges while refining existing methods and exploring new innovations in deep learning and hybrid fusion techniques. Ultimately, Image Fusion will continue to play a critical role in the development of next-generation imaging systems across diverse sectors, enhancing the ability to extract meaningful insights from complex image data.

REFERENCES

Aamir, M., Pu, Y. F., Rahman, Z., Tahir, M., Naeem, H., & Dai, Q. (2019). A Framework for Automatic Building Detection from Low-Contrast Satellite Images. Symmetry (20738994), 11(1).

Aamir, M., Rahman, Z., Abro, W. A., Bhatti, U. A., Dayo, Z. A., & Ishfaq, M. (2023). Brain tumor classification utilizing deep features derived from high-quality regions in MRI images. *Biomedical Signal Processing and Control*, *85*, 104988. DOI: 10.1016/j.bspc.2023.104988

Aamir, M., Rahman, Z., Abro, W. A., Tahir, M., & Ahmed, S. M. (2019). An optimized architecture of image classification using convolutional neural network. *International Journal of Image. Graphics and Signal Processing*, *11*(10), 30–39. DOI: 10.5815/ijigsp.2019.10.05

Aamir, M., Rahman, Z., Dayo, Z. A., Abro, W. A., Uddin, M. I., Khan, I., Imran, A. S., Ali, Z., Ishfaq, M., Guan, Y., & Hu, Z. (2022). A deep learning approach for brain tumor classification using MRI images. *Computers & Electrical Engineering*, *101*, 108105. DOI: 10.1016/j.compeleceng.2022.108105

Aamir, M., Rahman, Z., Pu, Y. F., Abro, W. A., & Gulzar, K. (2019). Satellite image enhancement using wavelet-domain based on singular value decomposition. *International Journal of Advanced Computer Science and Applications*, *10*(6). Advance online publication. DOI: 10.14569/IJACSA.2019.0100667

Adnan, S., Fu, Y., Bhutto, J. A., Rehman, J. N. U., Wagan, R. A., & Ghulam, A. (2020). An improved CoSaMP multiuser detection for uplink grant free NOMA system. *International Journal of Advanced Computer Science and Applications*, *11*(4). Advance online publication. DOI: 10.14569/IJACSA.2020.01104108

Bhutto, J. A., Guosong, J., Rahman, Z., Ishfaq, M., Sun, Z., & Soomro, T. A. (2024). Feature extraction of multimodal medical image fusion using novel deep learning and contrast enhancement method. *Applied Intelligence*, *54*(7), 1–24. DOI: 10.1007/s10489-024-05431-z

Bhutto, J. A., He, Z., Najeeb, J., Naeem, S., Mahmoud, E. A., & Elansary, H. O. (2024). Data driven analysis of aromatase inhibitors through machine learning, database mining and library generation. *Chemical Physics*, *577*, 112143. DOI: 10.1016/j.chemphys.2023.112143

Bhutto, J. A., Khan, A., & Rahman, Z. (2023). Image restoration with fractional-order total variation regularization and group sparsity. *Mathematics*, *11*(15), 3302. DOI: 10.3390/math11153302

Bhutto, J. A., Lianfang, T., Du, Q., Soomro, T. A., Lubin, Y., & Tahir, M. F. (2020). An enhanced image fusion algorithm by combined histogram equalization and fast gray level grouping using multi-scale decomposition and gray-PCA. *IEEE Access : Practical Innovations, Open Solutions*, *8*, 157005–157021. DOI: 10.1109/ACCESS.2020.3018264

Bhutto, J. A., Mubashir, T., Tahir, M. H., Ahmad, F., Sayed, S. R., El-ansary, H. O., & Ishfaq, M. (2023). Virtual screening and library enumeration of new hydroxycinnamates based antioxidant compounds: A complete framework. *Journal of Saudi Chemical Society*, *27*(4), 101670. DOI: 10.1016/j.jscs.2023.101670

Bhutto, J. A., Siddique, B., Moussa, I. M., El-Sheikh, M. A., Hu, Z., & Yurong, G. (2024). Machine learning assisted designing of non-fullerene electron acceptors: A quest for lower exciton binding energy. *Heliyon*, *10*(9), e30473. DOI: 10.1016/j.heliyon.2024.e30473 PMID: 38711638

Bhutto, J. A., Sunkari, V., Patil, A. M., Vanathi, D., Loganayagi, S., & Nayak, M. (2023). Detection and Analysis of Gene Functioning and Manipulation using Deep Learning. 2023 4th International Conference on Smart Electronics and Communication (ICOSEC)

Bhutto, J. A., Tian, L., Du, Q., Sun, Z., Yu, L., & Soomro, T. A. (2022). An improved infrared and visible image fusion using an adaptive contrast enhancement method and deep learning network with transfer learning. *Remote Sensing (Basel)*, *14*(4), 939. DOI: 10.3390/rs14040939

Bhutto, J. A., Tian, L., Du, Q., Sun, Z., Yu, L., & Tahir, M. F. (2022). CT and MRI medical image fusion using noise-removal and contrast enhancement scheme with convolutional neural network. *Entropy (Basel, Switzerland)*, *24*(3), 393. DOI: 10.3390/e24030393 PMID: 35327904

Bhutto, J. A., Zhang, R., & Rahman, Z. (2023). Symmetric Enhancement of Visual Clarity through a Multi-Scale Dilated Residual Recurrent Network Approach for Image Deraining. *Symmetry*, *15*(8), 1571. DOI: 10.3390/sym15081571

Bin, Y., Chao, Y., & Guoyu, H. (2016). Efficient image fusion with approximate sparse representation. *International Journal of Wavelets, Multresolution, and Information Processing*, *14*(04), 1650024. DOI: 10.1142/S0219691316500247

Dogra, A., Goyal, B., & Agrawal, S. (2017). From multi-scale decomposition to non-multi-scale decomposition methods: A comprehensive survey of image fusion techniques and its applications. *IEEE Access : Practical Innovations, Open Solutions*, *5*, 16040–16067. DOI: 10.1109/ACCESS.2017.2735865

Guan, Y., Aamir, M., Rahman, Z., Ali, A., Abro, W. A., Dayo, Z. A., ... & Hu, Z. (2021). A framework for efficient brain tumor classification using MRI images.

Huang, B., Yang, F., Yin, M., Mo, X., & Zhong, C. (2020). A review of multimodal medical image fusion techniques. *Computational and Mathematical Methods in Medicine*, *2020*(1), 8279342. DOI: 10.1155/2020/8279342 PMID: 32377226

Ibrahim, S. I., Makhlouf, M., & El-Tawel, G. S. (2023). Multimodal medical image fusion algorithm based on pulse coupled neural networks and nonsubsampled contourlet transform. *Medical & Biological Engineering & Computing*, *61*(1), 155–177. DOI: 10.1007/s11517-022-02697-8 PMID: 36342598

Jin, X., Jiang, Q., Yao, S., Zhou, D., Nie, R., Hai, J., & He, K. (2017). A survey of infrared and visual image fusion methods. *Infrared Physics & Technology*, *85*, 478–501. DOI: 10.1016/j.infrared.2017.07.010

Kong, W., Lei, Y., & Zhao, H. (2014). Adaptive fusion method of visible light and infrared images based on non-subsampled shearlet transform and fast non-negative matrix factorization. *Infrared Physics & Technology*, *67*, 161–172. DOI: 10.1016/j.infrared.2014.07.019

Kong, W., Zhang, L., & Lei, Y. (2014). Novel fusion method for visible light and infrared images based on NSST–SF–PCNN. *Infrared Physics & Technology*, *65*, 103–112. DOI: 10.1016/j.infrared.2014.04.003

Kumar, S. S., & Muttan, S. (2006). PCA-based image fusion. Algorithms and Technologies for Multispectral, Hyperspectral, and Ultraspectral Imagery XII, Li, J., Guo, X., Lu, G., Zhang, B., Xu, Y., Wu, F., & Zhang, D. (2020). DRPL: Deep regression pair learning for multi-focus image fusion. *IEEE Transactions on Image Processing*, *29*, 4816–4831.

Li, J., Han, D., Wang, X., Yi, P., Yan, L., & Li, X. (2023). Multi-sensor medical-image fusion technique based on embedding bilateral filter in least squares and salient detection. *Sensors (Basel), 23*(7), 3490. DOI: 10.3390/s23073490 PMID: 37050552

Li, S., Kang, X., Fang, L., Hu, J., & Yin, H. (2017). Pixel-level image fusion: A survey of the state of the art. *information Fusion, 33*, 100-112.

Lianfang, T., Ahmed, J., Qiliang, D., Shankar, B., & Adnan, S. (2018). Multi focus image fusion using combined median and average filter based hybrid stationary wavelet transform and principal component analysis. *International Journal of Advanced Computer Science and Applications, 9*(6), 34–41. DOI: 10.14569/IJACSA.2018.090605

Liu, C., Qi, Y., & Ding, W. (2017). Infrared and visible image fusion method based on saliency detection in sparse domain. *Infrared Physics & Technology, 83*, 94–102. DOI: 10.1016/j.infrared.2017.04.018

Liu, Y., Chen, X., Wang, Z., Wang, Z. J., Ward, R. K., & Wang, X. (2018). Deep learning for pixel-level image fusion: Recent advances and future prospects. *information Fusion, 42*, 158-173.

Liu, Y., Liu, S., & Wang, Z. (2015). A general framework for image fusion based on multi-scale transform and sparse representation. *information Fusion, 24*, 147-164.

Liu, Z., Blasch, E., Bhatnagar, G., John, V., Wu, W., & Blum, R. S. (2018). Fusing synergistic information from multi-sensor images: an overview from implementation to performance assessment. *information Fusion, 42*, 127-145.

Ma, J., Ma, Y., & Li, C. (2019). Infrared and visible image fusion methods and applications: A survey. *information Fusion, 45*, 153-178.

Mitianoudis, N., Antonopoulos, S.-A., & Stathaki, T. (2013). Region-based ICA image fusion using textural information. 2013 18th International Conference on Digital Signal Processing (DSP)

Nabi, A. U., Shi, J., Jumani, A. K., & Bhutto, J. A. (2024). Hybrid Transformer-EfficientNet Model for Robust Human Activity Recognition: The BiTransAct Approach. *IEEE Access : Practical Innovations, Open Solutions*.

Rahman, Z., Aamir, M., Gulzar, K., Bhutto, J. A., Ishfaq, M., Dayo, Z. A., & Mohammadani, K. H. (2024). A Non-Reference Low-Light Image Enhancement Approach Using Deep Convolutional Neural Networks. In *Deep Learning for Multimedia Processing Applications* (pp. 146–159). CRC Press.

Rahman, Z., Ali, Z., Khan, I., Uddin, M. I., Guan, Y., & Hu, Z. (2022). Diverse image enhancer for complex underexposed image. *Journal of Electronic Imaging, 31*(4), 041213–041213. DOI: 10.1117/1.JEI.31.4.041213

Rahman, Z., Bhutto, J. A., Aamir, M., Dayo, Z. A., & Guan, Y. (2023). Exploring a radically new exponential retinex model for multi-task environments. *Journal of King Saud University. Computer and Information Sciences, 35*(7), 101635. DOI: 10.1016/j.jksuci.2023.101635

Rahman, Z., Pu, Y.-F., Aamir, M., & Ullah, F. (2019). A framework for fast automatic image cropping based on deep saliency map detection and gaussian filter. *International Journal of Computers and Applications, 41*(3), 207–217. DOI: 10.1080/1206212X.2017.1422358

Rahman, Z., Pu, Y.-F., Aamir, M., & Wali, S. (2021). Structure revealing of low-light images using wavelet transform based on fractional-order denoising and multiscale decomposition. *The Visual Computer*, *37*(5), 865–880. DOI: 10.1007/s00371-020-01838-0

Rahman, Z., Zhang, R., & Bhutto, J. A. (2023). A symmetrical approach to brain tumor segmentation in MRI using deep learning and threefold attention mechanism. *Symmetry*, *15*(10), 1912. DOI: 10.3390/sym15101912

Sarwar, U., Bhasin, N. K., Bordoloi, D., Kadyan, S., Kezia, S., & Muthuperumal, S. (2024). Revolutionizing Business Intelligence with AI Insights and Strategies. 2024 8th International Conference on I-SMAC (IoT in Social, Mobile, Analytics and Cloud)(I-SMAC)

Sharma, D. K., Sachdeva, J., Ahuja, C. K., & Singh, A. (2024). A Novel Hybrid Multimodal Medical Image Fusion Scheme Based on Non-subsampled Shearlet Transform. *Circuits, Systems, and Signal Processing*, •••, 1–22.

Shreyamsha Kumar, B. (2015). Image fusion based on pixel significance using cross bilateral filter. *Signal, Image and Video Processing*, *9*(5), 1193–1204. DOI: 10.1007/s11760-013-0556-9

Sun, Z., Tian, L., Du, Q., & Bhutto, J. A. (2023). Sample hardness guided softmax loss for face recognition. *Applied Intelligence*, *53*(3), 2640–2655. DOI: 10.1007/s10489-022-03504-5

Sun, Z., Tian, L., Du, Q., Bhutto, J. A., & Wang, Z. (2022). Feature learning via multi-action forms supervising force for face recognition. *Neural Computing & Applications*, *34*(6), 1–12. DOI: 10.1007/s00521-021-06598-z

Sun, Z., Tian, L., Du, Q., Bhutto, J. A., & Wang, Z. (2023). Facial mask attention network for identity-aware face super-resolution. *Neural Computing & Applications*, *35*(11), 8243–8257. DOI: 10.1007/s00521-022-08098-0

Tawade, L., Aboobacker, A. B., & Ghante, F. (2014). Image fusion based on wavelet transforms. *International Journal of Bio-Science and Bio-Technology*, *6*(3), 149–162. DOI: 10.14257/ijbsbt.2014.6.3.18

Wang, R., Fang, N., He, Y., Li, Y., Cao, W., & Wang, H. (2022). Multi-modal medical image fusion based on geometric algebra discrete cosine transform. *Advances in Applied Clifford Algebras*, *32*(2), 19. DOI: 10.1007/s00006-021-01197-6

Xu, H., Wang, X., & Ma, J. (2021). DRF: Disentangled representation for visible and infrared image fusion. *IEEE Transactions on Instrumentation and Measurement*, *70*, 1–13. DOI: 10.1109/TIM.2021.3056645

Yan, X., Gilani, S. Z., Qin, H., & Mian, A. (2020). Structural similarity loss for learning to fuse multi-focus images. *Sensors (Basel)*, *20*(22), 6647. DOI: 10.3390/s20226647 PMID: 33233568

Yang, Y., Nie, Z., Huang, S., Lin, P., & Wu, J. (2019). Multilevel features convolutional neural network for multifocus image fusion. *IEEE Transactions on Computational Imaging*, *5*(2), 262–273. DOI: 10.1109/TCI.2018.2889959

Yang, Y., Wan, W., Huang, S., Yuan, F., Yang, S., & Que, Y. (2016). Remote sensing image fusion based on adaptive IHS and multiscale guided filter. *IEEE Access : Practical Innovations, Open Solutions*, *4*, 4573–4582. DOI: 10.1109/ACCESS.2016.2599403

Yu, L., Tian, L., Du, Q., & Bhutto, J. A. (2022). Multi-stream adaptive spatial-temporal attention graph convolutional network for skeleton-based action recognition. *IET Computer Vision*, *16*(2), 143–158. DOI: 10.1049/cvi2.12075

Yu, L., Tian, L., Du, Q., & Bhutto, J. A. (2023). Multi-stream adaptive 3d attention graph convolution network for skeleton-based action recognition. *Applied Intelligence*, *53*(12), 14838–14854. DOI: 10.1007/s10489-022-04179-8

Zhang, L., Li, H., Zhu, R., & Du, P. (2022). An infrared and visible image fusion algorithm based on ResNet-152. *Multimedia Tools and Applications*, *81*(7), 9277–9287. DOI: 10.1007/s11042-021-11549-w

Zhang, Q., Liu, Y., Blum, R. S., Han, J., & Tao, D. (2018). Sparse representation based multi-sensor image fusion for multi-focus and multi-modality images: A review. *information Fusion, 40*, 57-75.

Zhang, Y., Chen, L., Zhao, Z., Jia, J., & Liu, J. (2014). Multi-focus image fusion based on robust principal component analysis and pulse-coupled neural network. *Optik (Stuttgart)*, *125*(17), 5002–5006. DOI: 10.1016/j.ijleo.2014.04.002

Zhou, Z., Wang, B., Li, S., & Dong, M. (2016). Perceptual fusion of infrared and visible images through a hybrid multi-scale decomposition with Gaussian and bilateral filters. *information Fusion, 30*, 15-26.

Zhu, B., Wang, Z., Tian, L., Guo, J., Wang, L., & Bhutto, J. (2021). An Improved Fractional-Order Variational Optical Flow Model Combining Structure Tensor. *Mathematical Problems in Engineering*, *2021*(1), 9960784. DOI: 10.1155/2021/9960784

Chapter 2
Addressing Ethical and Regulatory Challenges in AI-Driven Healthcare

P. Selvakumar
https://orcid.org/0000-0002-3650-4548
Department of Science and Humanities, Nehru Institute of Technology, Coimbatore, India

S. Anitha
Rajarajeswari College of Engineering, India

Law Kumar Singh
https://orcid.org/0000-0002-7073-6852
Amity University, Punjab, India

P. V. Sathish Jackson
https://orcid.org/0009-0008-7489-8841
Sathyabama Institute of Science and Technology, India

Deepika Yadav
https://orcid.org/0000-0001-8978-6107
SRM University, Sonepat, India

T. C. Manjunath
https://orcid.org/0000-0003-2545-9160
Rajarajeswari College of Engineering, India

ABSTRACT

This shift toward AI-driven; it represents a fundamental change in how medical services are delivered and managed. datasets. These technologies can facilitate, making healthcare more efficient and effective. opportunities presented potential processes, AI has shown promise in areas such as radiology, where it can detect tumors in imaging scans with a level of accuracy that rivals that of experienced radiologists. Furthermore, diagnostic capabilities over time as they are exposed to new data considering their unique genetic makeup, lifestyle, and health history. This approach not only enhances treatment efficacy but also minimizes adverse effects, as therapies can be customized to fit the specific needs of each patient. Predictive analytics, powered by AI, can also forecast disease progression and treatment responses, healthcare providers to intervene early and optimize care strategies.Despite these opportunities, the integration of AI into healthcare misuse.

DOI: 10.4018/979-8-3693-9816-6.ch002

INTRODUCTION TO AI-DRIVEN HEALTHCARE: OPPORTUNITIES AND CHALLENGES

This shift toward AI-driven; it represents a fundamental change in how medical services are delivered and managed. datasets. These technologies can facilitate, making healthcare more efficient and effective. opportunities presented potential processes, AI has shown promise in areas such as radiology, where it can detect tumors in imaging scans with a level of accuracy that rivals that of experienced radiologists (Aamir et al., 2023; Aamir et al. 2022; Guan et al., 2021). Furthermore, diagnostic capabilities over time as they are exposed to new data considering their unique genetic makeup, lifestyle, and health history. This approach not only enhances treatment efficacy but also minimizes adverse effects, as therapies can be customized to fit the specific needs of each patient. Predictive analytics, powered by AI, can also forecast disease progression and treatment responses, healthcare providers to intervene early and optimize care strategies.Despite these opportunities, the integration of AI into healthcare misuse. Healthcare organizations must navigate complex regulations, such as the Health Insurance Portability and Accountability Act (HIPAA) in the United States, to ensure that patient information is safeguarded while still leveraging AI for insights.populations they serve, the AI's outputs may perpetuate existing disparities in healthcare. others, leading to unequal treatment outcomes. Addressing this issue requires a commitment to diversity in data collection and rigorous testing of AI systems across various populations addition, the workforce implications in healthcare augment healthcare professionals' capabilities, there are re-skilling. As AI takes over routine tasks, healthcare workers may need to adapt to new roles that emphasize interpersonal skills and complex decision-making, rather than solely technical proficiency.

ETHICAL FOUNDATIONS OF AI IN HEALTHCARE: PRINCIPLES, VALUES, AND RESPONSIBILITIES

Central to this discussion are the foundational values of beneficence, non-maleficence, autonomy, and justice, which guide healthcare practices and decision-making. Understanding how these principles interact with AI technologies is crucial for establishing a robust ethical framework that fosters trust among patients, healthcare providers, and the technology itself (Aamir et al., 2023).Beneficence and Non-maleficence are foundational principles in healthcare ethics that emphasize the obligation to promote good and prevent harm. AI systems, by their nature, are designed to enhance patient care—improving diagnostic accuracy, streamlining workflows, and personalizing treatment plans. However, the deployment of these technologies must be approached with caution. healthcare providers. This could inadvertently result in harm if the AI system produces erroneous recommendations. Therefore, it is essential to implement rigorous validation and continuous monitoring interest of patients.Autonomy, another critical ethical principle, relates to respecting patients' rights to make informed decisions about their own healthcareand providing clear information about the use of their health data. Moreover, patients should have the opportunity to consent to the use of AI tools in their care, thus reinforcing their agency. to ask questions about AI involvement in their treatment can enhance trust and engagement in the healthcare process.Justice in healthcare ethics emphasizes fairness and equity in the distribution of resources and access to care. The implementation of AI technologies must address potential disparities that could arise from biases embedded within AI systems. If these -representative disadvantage certain demographic groups, exacerbating existing inequalities in healthcare. To mitigate this risk, stakeholders must prioritize the development of Furthermore, ongoing assessment of AI algorithms for biased outcomes is critical to ensuring equitable treatment for all patients, regardless of their background.In addition to these principles, the concept of accountability, determining responsibility (Ahmad et al., 2019)in the event of an error or adverse outcome becomes complex. Clear guidelines and frameworks must be established to delineate the responsibilities of AI developers, healthcare providers, and institutions. This includes establishing protocols for accountability that outline who is liable when AI systems make mistakes, as well as mechanisms for patients to seek redress in such cases. Creating a culture of accountability can help foster trust in AI technologies, reassuring patients that their care is in capable hands.

The ethical considerations surrounding also encompass transparency. Patients and providers alike must understand how Transparent AI systems can demystify the technology, enabling patients to feel more confident in the recommendations they receive. This transparency can also extend to the development process, where stakeholders are encouraged to engage in open dialogue about the goals,. By fostering a collaborative approach that involves patients, clinicians, and technologists, can enhance the ethical deployment of AI.Furthermore, Medical education should incorporate training on the ethical dimensions of AI, equipping future healthcare providers with the skills to critically evaluate AI tools and their applications in clinical practice. This educational approach not only prepares healthcare professionals to navigate ethical dilemmas but also reinforces their role as advocates for patient welfare.The responsibility of stakeholders extends beyond the immediate deployment of AI systems; it includes a commitment to continuous evaluation and improvement of these technologies. As AI evolves, so its use in A proactive stance on ethics involves ongoing research into the societal implications of AI,(Ahmad et al., 2019) as well as the development of adaptive policies that can respond to new challenges as they arise., ethicists, and policymakers are essential for creating a dynamic framework that addresses ethical concerns in real time.Moreover, the global nature of healthcare necessitates consideration of cultural and ethical differences across various regions. The values and norms surrounding healthcare can vary significantly from one culture to another, influencing perceptions of AI and its ethical implications. As AI technologies are adopted globally, it is crucial to engage with local stakeholders to understand their unique ethical contexts and relevance and acceptability of AI technologies in diverse healthcare settings. Finally, of care. Technology should augment rather than replace the compassionate, patient-centered approach that is the hallmark of effective healthcare. By prioritizing the ethical foundations of AI, stakeholders can harness its potential to improve health outcomes while ensuring that the dignity and humanity of patients remain at the forefront of healthcare delivery.In conclusion, the ethical foundations rest on, non-maleficence, autonomy, justice, accountability, transparency, and continuous education. the healthcare sector can address the myriad challenges associated with this transformative innovation. A collaborative approach, grounded in ethical principles,(Aylak et al., 2021).

REGULATORY LANDSCAPE OF AI IN HEALTHCARE: OVERVIEW OF LAWS, GUIDELINES, AND STANDARDS

evolving as governments and organizations worldwide strive to establish frameworks. As AI systems increasingly play critical roles, (Bistron & Piotrowski, 2021)the need for comprehensive regulations is paramount. This landscape encompasses a variety of laws, guidelines, and standards that aim.applications. The FDA's approach focuses on the intended use of the software and its potential risks to patients. This includes a risk-based classification system that categorizes AI tools into different classes, premarket approval. In April 2021, the FDA released guidance outlining a "Software Precertification Program," designed to expedite the approval process for software developers who demonstrate a commitment to quality and safety in their AI technologies. This initiative highlights the agency's recognition In the European Union, the regulatory landscape is characterized by the comprehensive guidelines for the assessment and approval of medical devices, including AI-based tools. The EU's approach emphasizes the importance of safety and efficacy, requiring developers to provide clinical evidence demonstrating the performance of their AI systems. Additionally, while fostering innovation in the healthcare sector. Data privacy is sets stringent guidelines for the protection of patient information, mandating that any AI system handling protected health information (PHI) complies with its provisions. Similarly, Protection Regulation (GDPR) in the EU imposes strict requirements on data processing and privacy, including the need for informed consent when using personal data for AI training. These regulations necessitate that healthcare organizations and AI developers prioritize patient Guidelines from professional organizations also The World Health Organization (WHO) the ethical health, transparency, accountability, and inclusivity. These guidelines serve as a foundation for developing ethical AI applications that prioritize patient welfare and societal benefit. Similarly,(Brady & Neri, 2020) the American Medical Association (AMA) has published recommendations on AI in healthcare, advocating for transparency in used effectively and ethically.Standards organizations, such as for AI in healthcare. focuses on AI standards development, including guidelines for the ethical and societal implications of AI technologies.

These standards aim to establish best practices for the design, various sectors, including. By providing a common framework for AI development, these standards can facilitate interoperability and promote the safe use of AI technologies across different healthcare settings.The regulatory landscape must also address which often and improve. This presents challenges for traditional regulatory approaches, which address this issue, regulators are exploring adaptive regulatory frameworks that allow for ongoing evaluation and modification of AI systems post-deployment. Such frameworks would ensure that AI tools remain effective and safe throughout their lifecycle, incorporating real-world data and user feedback into their assessment.Collaboration among stakeholders is essential for shaping an effective regulatory landscape for AI in healthcare related to AI implementation. This collaborative approach can help ensure that regulations are not only protective of patient rights but also conducive to innovation. By fostering an environment of trust and collaboration(Amisha et al., 2020), stakeholders in healthcare.Moreover, international cooperation a cohesive regulatory framework for AI in healthcare. As AI technologies transcend national borders, harmonizing regulations can facilitate the global adoption of AI innovations while ensuring that safety and ethical standards are maintained. Initiatives such as the OECD's Principles on Artificial Intelligence and collaborations among regulatory agencies worldwide aim to create common guidelines and share best practices for AI governance. By fostering international dialogue, stakeholders can address the challenges posed by AI in healthcare more effectively and promote responsible innovation across the globe.

PATIENT AUTONOMY AND CONSENT IN AI-DRIVEN HEALTHCARE: NAVIGATING COMPLEXITIES

the principles of patient autonomy and informed consent take on new dimensions, reflecting both the promise and challenges posed by advanced. As AI systems become integral to diagnostics, treatment recommendations, and patient monitoring, ensuring that patients retain control over their healthcare decisions becomes increasingly complex. This complexity is compounded by the rapid evolution of AI technologies, which often "black boxes," for patients to The concept of informed consent is central to respecting patient autonomy, requiring interventions. In the context of AI, obtaining informed consent involves several unique challenges. For instance, patients must understand not only the treatment or diagnostic processes but also how AI systems contribute to those processes. This includes an awareness of how their personal health data will be used, the algorithms employed, and the potential implications of AI-driven decisions on their health outcomes. As AI tools can analyze vast amounts of data and provide recommendations that may not be easily interpretable, healthcare providers face the challenge of that is comprehensible and meaningful to patients.Moreover, systems, often, further. Traditional consent models may not suffice when the algorithms underlying AI applications are continually evolving. This raises questions about the necessity for ongoing consent: Should patients be re-informed periodically about changes in AI systems that might affect their care? The answer to this question is crucial, as it underscores the need for transparency and continuous communication between healthcare providers and patients.

A proactive approach to consent can help build trust and empower patients to engage meaningfully with their healthcare decisions.In addressing these complexities, healthcare providers must strive to create a patient-centered approach to informed consent that respects individual preferences and values. (Brady & Neri, 2020) This involves engaging patients in conversations about AI technologies in a manner that fosters understanding and encourages dialogue. Educational initiatives from the outset.Another layer of complexity arises from disproportionately affect certain populations. If patients are unaware of biases in AI algorithms, they may inadvertently consent to treatments or diagnostic procedures that do not adequately reflect their individual circumstances or health needs. This and equity into AI design and implementation. Healthcare organizations must prioritize diversity tools are inclusive and representative of all patient populations. Therefore, it is crucial for healthcare organizations to maintain a balance between leveraging AI for improved outcomes while ensuring that human judgment and empathy remain integral to patient care. Establishing clear guidelines that delineate the roles of AI and human providers can help mitigate concerns regarding the erosion of patient autonomy.Additionally,(Boucher, 2019) as AI continues to permeate healthcare, there is a pressing need for ongoing research and discourse on the ethical implications of these technologies. Stakeholders—including ethicists, technologists, healthcare providers, and patients—should engage in discussions that explore the evolving nature of autonomy and consent in the age of AI. Such discourse can inform best practices, regulatory developments, and educational initiatives that promote a culture of ethical AI usage in healthcare.In conclusion, patient autonomy and requires a multifaceted approach that prioritizes transparency, education, and shared decision-making. healthcare delivery, stakeholders must work collaboratively to ensure that informed consent processes are adapted innovations. By fostering a culture of understanding and respect for patient autonomy, the healthcare sector Ultimately, the goal is to create a healthcare environment where patients feel empowered to make informed choices about their care, supported by both advanced technologies and compassionate human interactions.

DATA PRIVACY AND SECURITY IN AI-DRIVEN HEALTHCARE: PROTECTING SENSITIVE INFORMATION

operational efficiencies. However, this rapid advancement brings significant challenges related to data privacy and security, particularly given the sensitive nature of healthcare information. As AI systems rely heavily on vast amounts of personal health data for training and operational effectiveness, ensuring the protection of this information is paramount. The complexities surrounding data privacy in necessitate a that addresses regulatory compliance, ethical considerations, and technological safeguards. At the core of data privacy in healthcare is the regulatory framework designed to protect patient information, as failure to adhere to these regulations can result in severe penalties and damage to reputations. Additionally,, emphasizing patient (Chan & Zary, 2019)consent, data minimization, and the right to be forgotten. As AI technologies often cross borders, understanding and complying with varying regulations becomes a critical challenge for healthcare organizations.One of the driven healthcare is the potential for unauthorized access and data breaches. Cybersecurity threats are increasingly sophisticated, targeting healthcare systems that may not have robust defenses in place. The consequences of data breaches can be devastating, not only compromising patient privacy but also undermining trust in healthcare systems. Therefore, implementing strong secure access controls, and regularly conducting vulnerability assessments and penetration testing. Moreover, healthcare organizations must cultivate AI systems themselves introduce unique privacy concerns, particularly regarding how data is processed and used. Machine learning algorithms typically require large datasets to function effectively, raising questions about data anonymization and de-identification. While techniques exist to anonymize data, there is always a risk that de-identified information power of AI while minimizing risks to patient privacy.In addition to technical safeguards, ethical considerations must guide their consent should be obtained before data collection and processing occur. This requires healthcare organizations to adopt transparent practices that clearly outline the purposes for which data is collected, how it will be used, and the measures taken to protect it. Engaging patients in discussions about data privacy not only fosters trust but also empowers them to make informed choices regarding their health information.

The role of data governance is critical in managing healthcare. Establishing robust data governance frameworks can help organizations create clear policies regarding data collection, usage, sharing, and retention. This includes defining potential vulnerabilities and ensuring adherence to data governance policies.(Carter et al., 2020)Furthermore, as AI systems continue to evolve, so too must the approaches to data privacy and security. security measures stay ahead of emerging threats. This involves leveraging advanced technologies,. Blockchain can provide a decentralized and tamper-proof way of managing healthcare data, ensuring that records are secure and accessible only to authorized parties. By integrating such innovative.Another key patient data for research and development purposes. AI technologies can drive significant advancements in medical research, but using patient data without proper safeguards raises ethical concerns. To address this, researchers must prioritize transparency and ethical considerations when utilizing data for AI training.

BIAS AND FAIRNESS IN AI DECISION-MAKING: ADDRESSING DISPARITIES AND INEQUITIES

As across law enforcement, concerns regarding bias and fairness have come to the forefront. These systems, while capable of processing vast amounts of data and generating insights, can inadvertently perpetuate or exacerbate existing disparities and inequities if not designed and implemented thoughtfully. to promote fairness are crucial steps toward ensuring that these Furthermore, can introduce bias. (Chan & Zary, 2021)The choices made during the development process, including feature selection and model tuning, can significantly impact how AI systems interpret data and make predictions. If the developers are not vigilant about potential biases in their models, they may inadvertently reinforce existing inequalities. This emphasizes the need for interdisciplinary collaboration during the AI development process, involving not only data scientists but also ethicistsThe implications of biased AI decision-making are profound and far-reaching. In healthcare, disparities, disproportionately affecting marginalized communities. In criminal justice, AI systems used for risk assessments may reinforce racial profiling, resulting in unfair sentencing and parole decisions. These examples illustrate that bias in AI can have life-altering consequences, perpetuating systemic injustices and eroding trust in institutions that deploy these technologies. Addressing these issues is not just a technical challenge; it is a moral imperative to promote social justice and equity.(European Commission, 2019)Another critical strategy involves ongoing auditing to make necessary adjustments. These evaluations should be transparent and involve diverse stakeholders, including community representatives and independent auditors, to ensure a comprehensive understanding of how AI systems impact various populations. Creating an open feedback loop where users can report concerns about bias can further enhance the accountability of AI systems. Education and ethical AI practices, including the recognition of biases and the importance of inclusive data collection. Building a culture of awareness within organizations can empower teams to prioritize fairness in their AI projects, fostering a commitment to social responsibility.

Moreover, engaging with affected communities can provide valuable insights into their experiences and needs, informing more equitable AI design.Additionally, establishing provide a structure for addressing bias Policymakers and industry leaders must collaborate to create, accountability, and fairness in AI systems. These regulations should require organizations to disclose their data sources, methodologies, and potential biases, enabling stakeholders to critically assess the fairness of AI applications. Such, ensuring perceived as tools for positive change rather than instruments of oppression.Promoting diversity within the tech industry is also essential for addressing bias in AI. workforce perspectives development process, reducing the likelihood of overlooking potential biases. Companies should prioritize hiring practices that, fostering an inclusive environment that encourages collaboration and innovation. By elevating underrepresented voices, attuned to the needs of all communities.Finally, fostering within organizations is Leaders must champion the importance expectations for their teams. This commitment should extend to the entire lifecycle of AI systems, from conception to deployment and beyond.

FDA REGULATION OF AI/MEDICAL DEVICES: CLEARANCE, APPROVAL, AND POST-MARKET SURVEILLANCE

The FDA employs II (moderate risk), and Class III (high risk). Most AI medical devices fall into Class II, requiring a premarket notification known as 510(k). This process involves presenting data that show the AI application's performance and safety profiles are comparable to existing devices. Given the complexities associated with AI algorithms necessitating robust validation studies and clinical data.For higher-risk devices classified as Class III, such as AI applications that provide significant diagnostic or therapeutic interventions, the FDA requires The PMA process is time-consuming and resource-intensive, reflecting the FDA's commitment to ensuring that high-risk AI medical devices meet stringent standards before reaching the market. As the landscape of AI technologies evolves, the FDA has recognized the need for adaptive regulatory strategies that can accommodate the continuous learning capabilities of AI algorithms. This has led to initiatives such as the "Digital Health Innovation Action Plan," which aims to create a more efficient and predictable regulatory pathway for digital health technologies, including AI applications.A pivotal aspect of the FDA's approach to regulating emphasis on transparency and validation. Given that AI algorithms can be opaque, or "black boxes," understanding their decision-making processes is vital for gaining clinician and patient trust. To address this, the FDA encourages the use of explainable AI (XAI) techniques that make AI predictions more interpretable. In addition, manufacturers are urged to conduct thorough validation studies that assess the performance of AI models across diverse populations, the FDA aims to enhance confidence in AI technologies among healthcare providers and patients alike.Post-market surveillance is another critical component medical devices. (European Commission, 2018) Once a device is cleared or approved, ongoing monitoring is essential to assess its real-world performance and identify potential safety concerns.

The FDA utilizes several mechanisms for post-market surveillance,, which collects reports of adverse events and device defects. This data is crucial for detecting trends that may indicate underlying issues with an AI application, such as algorithmic bias or decreased performance over time. Manufacturers are also required to conduct post-market studies as a condition of approval to gather additional data on device safety and effectiveness, ensuring that the AI system continues to operate as intended after it has been introduced to the market.Furthermore, the FDA is exploring innovative approaches to enhance post-market surveillance of AI-driven devices. The agency has recognized that traditional monitoring methods may not suffice for AI systems that continuously evolve. As such, the FDA is considering frameworks for adaptive learning and real-time monitoring that can facilitate ongoing evaluation of AI performance. For instance,, and other data sources could provide valuable insights into the long-term safety and efficacy of AI medical devices. These documents provide clarity on the regulatory pathway, emphasizing the need for robust data sets that reflect a wide range of demographics and clinical scenarios.(Floridi et al., 2020) This guidance is particularly important given the potential for AI algorithms to inherit biases from training data, which can lead to inequitable outcomes. By promoting inclusive data practices, the FDA the FDA is tasked with the challenge of adapting its regulatory framework to keep pace with innovation while safeguarding public health. The agency is committed to fostering an environment that encourages the responsible development of AI-driven medical devices while ensuring that safety and efficacy remain paramount. Initiatives such as the FDA's Digital Health Center of Excellence aim to support innovation In conclusion, the regulation of AI and medical devices by the FDA encompasses a multifaceted approach that includes clearance, approval, and post-market surveillance.

HIPAA AND DATA PROTECTION IN AI-DRIVEN HEALTHCARE: COMPLIANCE AND RISK MANAGEMENT

AI-driven healthcare applications often rely on vast datasets, which may include protected health information (PHI). The use of such data for training AI algorithms necessitates adherence to HIPAA regulations, which dictate how PHI can be collected, used, and disclosed. Healthcare providers, insurers, and technology vendors utilized for AI development is de-identified or appropriately anonymized, minimizing the risk of compromising patient privacy. Furthermore, when AI systems process PHI, organizations must establish and maintain adequate safeguards, confidentiality..Organizations must(Grote & Berens, 2020) conduct thorough evaluations to identify potential vulnerabilities associated with AI implementations. This includes assessing the security of AI algorithms, the systems that house them, and the data inputs and outputs. Risk management strategies should be developed to address identified threats, incorporating best practices in cybersecurity, data protection, and user training. By proactively identifying and mitigating risks, likelihood of costly breaches.Moreover, transparency is essential in AI-driven particularly when it involves algorithms that may influence their treatment or diagnosis. Healthcare providers must ensure that AI systems are explainable, meaning that their decision-making processes can be interpreted and understood by both healthcare professionals and patients. This transparency not only fosters trust but also aligns with HIPAA's emphasis on patient rights and informed consent.Collaboration among stakeholders is another vital component of effective compliance and risk management. addressing the unique challenges posed by the healthcare environment. By establishing clear protocols demonstrate their commitment to safeguarding patient data.In conclusion,(Hamet & Tremblay, 2017) the intersection of HIPAA compliance and AI-driven healthcare prioritizing data protection, conducting thorough risk assessments, ensuring transparency, fostering collaboration, and staying informed about regulatory developments, healthcare providers can effectively navigate the complexities of integrating AI technologies while upholding the principles of patient privacy and security. As the healthcare landscape continues to evolve, a steadfast commitment to compliance and risk management will be essential in harnessing the full potential of AI to improve patient care and outcomes.

LIABILITY AND ACCOUNTABILITY IN AI-DRIVEN HEALTHCARE: MALPRACTICE, NEGLIGENCE, AND ERROR

However, this innovation also raises critical questions regarding liability and accountability, particularly in the context of malpractice, negligence, and errors. As AI systems become increasingly involved in clinical decision-making, the delineation of responsibility for adverse patient outcomes becomes complex. Understanding the legal implications of AI-driven healthcare is essential for practitioners, organizations, and policymakers alike to navigate this evolving landscape effectively.At the core of liability in healthcare is the concept professionals who directly provide patient care. However, as AI systems take on roles that influence clinical decisions, it becomes challenging to determine whether the responsibility lies with the healthcare provider, the developers of the AI technology, or the healthcare organization that implements the system. This ambiguity complicates the legal framework surrounding malpractice, as existing laws may not adequately address the nuances introduced by AI.Negligence, similarly, poses a significant concern in AI-driven healthcare. To establish negligence, one must prove. With (Ho et al., 2020)AI systems assisting in diagnostics or treatment recommendations, questions arise about whether the technology itself can be deemed negligent if it provides inaccurate recommendations. Additionally, if a healthcare provider relies on AI-generated information, does that provider fulfill their duty of care by following the AI's recommendations, or do they bear responsibility for verifying the accuracy of those recommendations.

This gray area creates uncertainty regarding accountability and may result in legal challenges that could reshape the interpretation of negligence in medical practice.Error in AI systems—whether stemming from faulty algorithms, inadequate training data, or misinterpretation of results—can lead to significant patient harm. When errors occur, determining liability becomes crucial. If an AI system misdiagnoses a condition or recommends an inappropriate treatment, the question arises: who is liable? The developers of the AI technology, the healthcare organization that deployed it, or the medical personnel who acted upon its recommendations? Courts may need to evaluate whether the AI system met industry standards and whether healthcare providers exercised reasonable diligence in utilizing the technology. This multifaceted nature of accountability necessitates a collaborative approach among stakeholders to address potential legal ramifications.To effectively protocols and guidelines regarding the use of AI technologies. This includes implementing rigorous validation processes for AI systems engage in ongoing training to understand the limitations and capabilities of AI tools, ensuring they maintain an active role in patient care rather than becoming passive users of technology. Trust in AI technologies their care are reliable and safe. This trust can be fostered through transparency about how AI tools work, the data used for their development, and the safeguards in place to protect patient interests. Healthcare organizations should actively communicate the roles of AI and human providers in patient care, clarifying the accountability structures that exist to protect patients.intersection of liability and accountability in AI-driven healthcare presents complex challenges that require careful consideration from multiple stakeholders. As AI systems continue to reshape clinical decision-making, the legal frameworks surrounding malpractice, negligence, and errors must adapt to ensure clarity and protection for patients and providers alike. (Hee Lee & Yoon, 2021)By establishing robust protocols, fostering a culture of accountability, and developing comprehensive regulatory frameworks, the healthcare industry can effectively navigate the legal landscape of AI. Ultimately, the goal should be to enhance patient safety and care while responsibly leveraging the capabilities of AI technology. The journey toward integrating AI in healthcare demands collaboration, innovation,

AI-DRIVEN DIAGNOSIS AND TREATMENT: CLINICAL VALIDATION AND EVIDENCE-BASED MEDICINE

enhance patient care through improved accuracy, efficiency, and personalized medicine. However, the successful implementation of AI in clinical settings hinges on rigorous clinical validation and alignment with evidence-based medicine (EBM). These two pillars are crucial to ensuring that AI systems not only perform effectively but also uphold the standards of care that healthcare professionals and patients expect.Clinical validation effectiveness in real-world clinical environments. This involves extensive trials, including retrospective studies using existing patient data and prospective studies where the AI system is tested in live clinical settings. These evaluations are essential for determining the algorithm's accuracy, sensitivity, specificity, and overall clinical utility. For instance, an AI diagnostic tool designed to detect diseases, such as diabetic retinopathy or breast cancer, must demonstrate that it can consistently identify conditions with a level yield false positives or negatives, leading to misdiagnosis or inappropriate treatment plans.In parallel(Johnson, 2019), the principles of evidence-based medicine serve as a guiding framework for integrating AI into clinical practice. nterventions to individual patient needs. However, to align AI applications with EBM, the evidence supporting these algorithms must be robust and derived from high-quality clinical research. This necessitates a collaborative approach among clinicians, data scientists, and researchers to ensure that AI tools are grounded in scientifically validated evidence.The challenge of integrating AI with EBM also involves addressing biases inherent in training data. AI systems outside that group, potentially exacerbating health inequities. Therefore, it is imperative that the development of AI applications incorporates diverse and representative datasets to enhance their generalizability and fairness. Ongoing validation processes should also include assessments of how well AI systems perform across different populations and clinical scenarios.Furthermore, must understand how AI systems generate recommendations or diagnoses to incorporate them effectively into their decision-making processes. This requires explainable AI (XAI) models that not only provide results but also elucidate the rationale behind their conclusions. By ensuring that AI tools are interpretable, clinicians can better integrate them into their practice while remaining vigilant about their limitations. This transparency also fosters patient trust, as individuals are more likely to accept AI-driven recommendations when they understand the underlying reasoning and evidence supporting those recommendations. Regulatory frameworks also play a pivotal.

As AI technologies advance, regulatory bodies must adapt their oversight mechanisms, establishing standards for data privacy and security, and ensuring that AI tools are continuously monitored and updated based on emerging evidence. Such regulatory efforts are vital to maintaining the integrity of the healthcare system and protecting patient safety in the face of rapidly evolving technologies.Incorporating AI into clinical workflows also requires thoughtful consideration of how these tools interact with existing practices and healthcare teams. The implementation of AI systems should enhance, rather than replace, the clinician's role in patient care. AI can act as a powerful adjunct, providing insights that enable healthcare providers to make more informed decisions(Ho et al., 2020). For example, in radiology, AI algorithms can assist radiologists by identifying potential abnormalities in imaging studies, allowing for more accurate, while AI contributes to more efficient and precise diagnostics.Moreover, equipped with the knowledge and skills necessary to understand, interpret, and effectively utilize AI tools in their practice. This includes ongoing professional development and interdisciplinary enhance their capacity to integrate AI technologies while upholding the principles of evidence-based medicine.the intersection of AI-driven with clinical validation and evidence-based medicine represents a transformative opportunity for healthcare. By ensuring that AI systems undergo rigorous validation and align with the best available evidence, healthcare providers can enhance diagnostic accuracy, personalize treatment options, and ultimately improve patient outcomes. Addressing challenges related to bias, transparency, regulation, and education is essential to harnessing the of AI in improving healthcare delivery and ensuring patient safety. The journey toward AI-driven healthcare necessitates a commitment to excellence, accountability, and patient-centered care in an increasingly complex medical landscape.

AI-ASSISTED DECISION-MAKING: CLINICIAN-AI COLLABORATION AND HUMAN OVERSIGHT

has marked a significant clinical decisions are made, facilitating between clinicians and AI systems. AI-assisted decision-making harnesses the computational power of, thereby augmenting the capabilities of healthcare professionals. However, this innovative partnership necessitates a careful balance between leveraging AI's strengths and ensuring robust human oversight to maintain patient safety and ethical standards.At the heart.(Kelly et al., 2019) For example, in diagnostic imaging, AI algorithms can rapidly analyze radiological images, flagging potential abnormalities that may require further investigation. This capability allows radiologists to focus on more complex cases and enhances their efficiency. By combining the analytical prowess of AI with the contextual understanding of seasoned clinicians. This synergy is particularly beneficial in situations involving large volumes of data, where human capacity to process information may be limited.However, the effectiveness of this collaboration hinges on the quality the AI systems in use. AI models must undergo rigorous validation This involves comprehensive training on diverse datasets to mitigate biases and enhance the generalizability of the algorithms. When clinicians trust the AI systems they work with, they are more likely to integrate these tools into their practice effectively. Continuous validation and monitoring of AI performance are essential to adapting these systems to evolving clinical practices and ensuring they remain reliable over time.

Human oversight is a critical component of AI-assisted decision-making, as it serves as a safeguard against potential pitfalls of algorithm-driven recommendations. While AI can process data at remarkable speeds experiences, emotions, and ethical considerations to the table. Therefore, healthcare professionals must maintain an active role in interpreting AI outputs and making final decisions regarding patient care. For instance, an AI algorithm may suggest a particular treatment based on statistical outcomes, but it is the clinician's responsibility to consider factors such as patient preferences, comorbidities, and unique clinical contexts. This oversight ensures that patient care remains personalized and ethically sound.(Kelly et al., 2019)Moreover, effective communication between clinicians and AI systems is paramount. For AI-assisted decision-making to be successful, clinicians need clear, interpretable information from, they are better equipped to make informed decisions that align with evidence-based practices. This transparency not only enhances trust but also empowers clinicians to engage in collaborative discussions with patients about their care options.In addition to enhancing decision-making processes, pivotal supporting clinicians during high-pressure situations. For example, in emergency medicine, where timely decisions are critical, AI systems can rapidly analyze patient data and suggest potential interventions, allowing clinicians to focus on patient stabilization. However, the specific needs of the patient.the potential for over-reliance on technology, and the importance of informed consent must be carefully navigated. Engaging in ongoing ethical discussions within healthcare teams can help identify potential pitfalls and foster a culture of ethical practice in the use of AI.with patients, empowering them to understand and accept AI-driven recommendations. This patient-centered approach enhances the overall care experience and reinforces the partnership between clinicians, AI systems, and patients.In conclusion,(Luxton, 2014) AI-assisted decision-making represents a transformative opportunity for enhancing clinical care can leverage advanced analytics to improve diagnostic accuracy, personalize treatment options, and optimize patient outcomes. Ensuring the success of this partnership requires rigorous validation of AI systems, effective communication, ongoing education for clinicians, and a commitment to ethical practices.

for training and operation, including protected health information (PHI). This creates an attractive target for cybercriminals, who may seek to exploit weaknesses in data management and storage practices. Data breaches can lead to unauthorized access to sensitive information, resulting in identity theft, fraud, and other malicious activities. In addition to the immediate harm to patients, such breaches can have long-lasting repercussions for healthcare organizations, including legal liabilities, financial penalties, and reputational damage. Therefore, healthcare entities must prioritize Moreover, AI algorithms. For instance, in diagnostic imaging, an attacker could subtly alter an image to mislead an AI algorithm, potentially leading to incorrect diagnoses. This not only endangers patient safety but also raises questions about the reliability of AI-driven decision-making. To mitigate this risk, organizations need to implement robust validation processes for AI systems, continuously(Luxton, 2014) monitoring their performance and resilience against potential attacks. By establishing protocols for identifying and addressing vulnerabilities in AI algorithms, healthcare providers Another significant cybersecurity threat in AI-driven healthcare is the severely disrupt healthcare operations, delaying patient care and compromising treatment plans.

The urgency of healthcare services often pressures organizations to comply with ransom demands, exacerbating the cycle of cybercrime. To combat ransomware, healthcare entities should adopt a proactive approach that includes regular data backups, comprehensive incident response plans, and employee training on recognizing phishing attempts and other social engineering tactics. By fostering a culture of cybersecurity awareness, organizations can bolster their defenses against potential ransomware threats. (Lee et al., 2021)The increasing (IoT) in healthcare further compounds the cybersecurity challenges. These devices, while enhancing patient monitoring and data collection, can introduce vulnerabilities into healthcare systems. stringent security measures for all connected devices, including regular software updates, secure network configurations, and thorough risk assessments. Ensuring that IoT devices are securely integrated into the healthcare ecosystem is essential for maintaining overall system integrity.In addition to protecting patient data and AI systems, healthcare organizations must also focus on securing the underlying infrastructure that supports these technologies. This includes safeguarding networks, servers, and cloud, can help mitigate the risk of cyberattacks.Collaboration among stakeholders is critical in addressing cybersecurity threats in AI-driven healthcare. Healthcare organizations, regulatory bodies, and cybersecurity establish best practices for safeguarding patient data and systems. By sharing information about emerging threats and vulnerabilities, stakeholders can collectively enhance their defenses and promote a culture of cybersecurity across the industry. This collaborative approach can also facilitate the development of standardized protocols for incident reporting and response, Finally, as AI technologies continue in cybersecurity practices. Healthcare organizations should invest in emerging technologies, such as. These technologies can analyze patterns in cyber threats and detect anomalies in real time(Lecun et al., 2015), In conclusion, the cybersecurity landscape in AI-driven healthcare is fraught with challenges that require a multi-faceted approach to safeguard patient data and systems. By prioritizing data protection, implementing robust security measures for AI algorithms and connected devices, and fostering a culture of cybersecurity awareness, healthcare organizations in the healthcare system.

HEALTHCARE ORGANIZATIONAL READINESS FOR AI ADOPTION: CHANGE MANAGEMENT AND LEADERSHIP

However, for healthcare organizations to successfully integrate AI technologies, they must demonstrate a high level of organizational readiness, which encompasses change management strategies and effective leadership. This readiness is critical to navigating the complexities associated with AI implementation and ensuring that the technology is leveraged to its fullest potential.Organizational readiness for AI adoption involves assessing the current infrastructure, workforce capabilities, and cultural attitudes within healthcare settings(Murphy et al., 2021). Organizations must evaluate their technological landscape to determine whether existing systems can support AI tools comprehensive datasets to function effectively. Organizations should also ensure that their IT infrastructure is robust enough to handle the computational demands of AI algorithms while maintaining data security and compliance with regulations.A significant aspect of readiness, as they help mitigate resistance and foster a culture of adaptability. Effective change management requires a clear communication plan that outlines the benefits of AI, the expected changes to workflows, and the support available to staff throughout the transition. Engaging employees Leadership is a critical factor in driving organizational readiness for AI adoption. overall strategic goals. Effective leadership involves not only setting a vision but also modeling the behavior and attitudes necessary for embracing change. Leaders should foster an organizational culture that values innovation, collaboration, and continuous improvement. By championing AI initiatives and demonstrating commitment to the necessary changes, leaders can inspire confidence and motivate staff to engage with new technologies. Additionally, fostering interdisciplinary collaboration is essential for successful AI implementation. Healthcare organizations must create environments where data scientists, clinicians, IT professionals, and administrative staff work together to design, deploy, and refine AI systems. This collaborative approach ensures various stakeholders and enhances the likelihood of successful integration into clinical workflows.(Murphy et al., 2021). Regular interdisciplinary meetings and workshops can facilitate knowledge sharing and promote a unified with AI adoption.Furthermore, organizations should establish metrics and evaluation frameworks to assess the monitor the effectiveness of AI implementations and make data-driven decisions to refine and optimize their use of technology. Continuous evaluation also facilitates the identification of areas for improvement and allows organizations d emerging technologies. In addition, healthcare organizations the AI adoption process. Change is often met with challenges, and organizations must develop contingency plans to manage any unforeseen issues.

Leaders should encourage a mindset of resilience and adaptability among staff, reinforcing the idea that setbacks are a natural part of the innovation process. By cultivating a supportive environment that emphasizes problem-solving and continuous learning, organizations can navigate challenges more effectively.Another important consideration is the need for ongoing support and resources for staff following AI implementation. The transition to AI-driven workflows may necessitate adjustments in roles and responsibilities, and employees may require continued training and support to adapt to these changes. Organizations should establish mechanisms for ongoing education, mentorship, and access to technical assistance to help staff integrate AI tools into their daily practices. This commitment to supporting staff Ultimately, the successful adoption of. Organizations must assess their readiness, invest in workforce development, and foster interdisciplinary collaboration to realize the benefits of AI technologies. By prioritizing these elements, healthcare organizations can create an environment that is conducive to innovation and resilience, enabling them to harness the power of AI to improve patient outcomes and drive operational excellence. As the healthcare landscape continues to evolve, organizations that embrace AI with a proactive and thoughtful approach will be better positioned to thrive in an increasingly digital future. The journey toward AI adoption, and collaborative effort from all stakeholders involved.

WORKFORCE DEVELOPMENT AND TRAINING FOR AI-DRIVEN HEALTHCARE: EDUCATING CLINICIANS AND STAFF

First and foremost, understanding the foundational concepts of AI is crucial for healthcare professionals. Training programs must begin with an introduction to AI, machine learning, and data analytics, emphasizing how these technologies function and their applications in clinical settings. This foundational knowledge helps demystify AI and fosters a culture of acceptance and engagement among healthcare workers. By learning the basic principles, clinicians and staff can better appreciate the capabilities and limitations of AI tools, which is vital for making informed decisions in patient care.In addition to foundational training, continuous education is essential in a rapidly evolving field like AI. The healthcare landscape is characterized by constant technological advancements, necessitating ongoing professional development to keep staff updated on the latest tools, methodologies, and best practices. Organizations should implement regular training sessions, workshops, and seminars that focus on emerging AI applications,.(Sestino & De Mauro, 2022)One of the critical aspects of workforce training is ensuring that clinicians understand how to interpret AI outputs accurately. they are not infallible. Clinicians must be trained to critically evaluate AI-generated recommendations and understand the context in which these tools operate. This involves developing skills in data interpretation, understanding algorithmic biases, and recognizing when to question or override AI suggestions. By fostering critical thinking skills, Interdisciplinary collaboration is another key component of effective workforce development. AI implementation in healthcare often involves various stakeholders, including data scientists, IT professionals, and clinicians. Training programs should encourage collaboration across disciplines, allowing team members to understand each other's roles and perspectives. Interdisciplinary training initiatives can include joint workshops and simulation exercises that bring together diverse expertise to solve complex healthcare challenges fosters a sense of shared ownership over AI projects.Moreover, practical, hands-on training is essential for developing the technical skills required to operate AI tools effectively. Simulation-based learning environments can provide clinicians and staff with opportunities to engage with AI systems in a controlled setting, allowing them to gain experience without the risk of compromising patient safety.

These simulations can include scenarios where staff practice using AI-assisted diagnostic tools, engaging in decision-making processes, and responding to AI-generated alerts. Such experiential learning helps build confidence and competence in utilizing AI technologies in real-world situations.(Senthilraja, 2021)Ethical considerations surrounding AI use in healthcare must also be integrated into workforce training programs. By emphasizing ethical principles, organizations can ensure that staff are prepared to navigate the moral complexities associated with AI technologies, ultimately fostering a more equitable healthcare system.Leadership driving workforce development for AI integration. Healthcare leaders must advocate for training initiatives, allocate resources, and establish a clear vision for how AI will be utilized within the organization. By demonstrating a commitment to workforce education, leaders can inspire staff to embrace AI technologies and actively participate in their implementation. Additionally, leaders should encourage feedback from employees regarding training needs and experiences, facilitating continuous improvement in educational programs.Furthermore, organizations should leverage external partnerships to enhance workforce development. Collaborations with academic institutions, technology vendors, and industry experts can provide access to cutting-edge training resources, curriculum development, and best practices. These partnerships can also facilitate knowledge exchange and help organizations healthcare(Yoon et al., 2020). By integrating external expertise into workforce training initiatives, healthcare organizations can enhance the overall quality and effectiveness of their educational programs.Evaluation and assessment are vital components of any workforce training program. Organizations should establish training initiatives, including pre- and post-training assessments, participant feedback, and performance evaluations. By systematically assessing training outcomes, organizations can in the context of ongoing AI advancements in conclusion, workforce development and training are pivotal to the successful adoption of AI in healthcare. By equipping clinicians and staff with the and ethical considerations is essential. Leadership commitment, external partnerships, evaluation mechanisms, and a culture of innovation further strengthen workforce readiness for AI integration. As healthcare continues to evolve in the digital age, a well-prepared workforce will be instrumental in harnessing the full potential of AI to improve patient outcomes and drive operational excellence. Through strategic investments in workforce development, healthcare organizations can position themselves as leaders in the AI-driven future of healthcare.

AI-DRIVEN HEALTHCARE POLICY AND GOVERNANCE: INSTITUTIONAL, NATIONAL, AND GLOBAL PERSPECTIVES

The rapid, necessitating robust policy and governance frameworks at institutional, national, and global levels. As AI technologies become increasingly central to healthcare delivery, the need for comprehensive policies that ensure ethical use, data privacy, and equitable access becomes paramount. Effective governance structures are crucial for navigating the complexities associated with AI deployment, fostering innovation while safeguarding public health and safety.At the institutional level, healthcare organizations must develop tailored policies designed and implemented with consideration for bias and fairness. Institutional governance frameworks should incorporate interdisciplinary oversight, involving clinicians, data scientists, ethicists, and patient representatives decision-making processes. Such collaborative approaches not only enhance the credibility of AI initiatives but also build trust among stakeholders.On a national level changing landscape of AI technology. National policies should also prioritize equitable access to AI-driven healthcare solutions, ensuring that underserved populations benefit from technological advancements rather than being left behind.At the global level, the need for harmonized policies and governance structures is increasingly critical as AI technologies transcend national borders.

These organizations can help develop guidelines that promote best practices for AI deployment, emphasizing ethical considerations, data sharing, and global health equity. A coordinated global approach is essential to address the challenges posed by varying regulatory environments, ensuring that AI technologies are deployed responsibly and effectively across different contexts.(Senthilraja, 2021)Global governance of AI in healthcare must also take into using AI technologies in diverse cultural settings. Policymakers must relevance of policies but also fosters trust and acceptance of AI technologies in healthcare systems worldwide. Additionally, international collaborations successes in AI implementation.contribute to reducing, rather than exacerbating, health disparities.social implications at institutional, national, and global levels. Institutions must prioritize transparency, accountability, and workforce development to effectively implement AI technologies while fostering a culture of ethical responsibility. National governments must establish clear regulatory guidelines that promote innovation while safeguarding patient rights and equity in access to AI-driven healthcare solutions. On a global scale, harmonized policies and collaborative efforts are essential to address the challenges posed by AI in diverse healthcare contexts. By prioritizing ethical considerations, data sharing, and bias mitigation, stakeholders can work together to ensure that AI technologies enhance healthcare delivery and improve patient outcomes for all. As AI continues to evolve, proactive governance and responsive policy frameworks will be crucial in navigating the complexities of this transformative technology in the healthcare sector.

EMERGING TRENDS AND INNOVATIONS IN AI-DRIVEN HEALTHCARE: OPPORTUNITIES AND CHALLENGES

The landscape of healthcare is undergoing a seismic shift as artificial intelligence (AI) technologies emerge and evolve, presenting both remarkable opportunities and significant challenges. The potential of AI to enhance clinical decision-making, streamline operations, and personalize patient in healthcare. Personalized medicine, driven by AI algorithms, is poised to revolutionize treatment approaches by tailoring outcomes. However, the complexity of integrating genomic data with clinical practice presents challenges in terms of data management, ethical considerations, and the need for specialized training for healthcare providers another significant challenge systems.Moreover, the regulatory landscape surrounding AI in healthcare is still evolving. Policymakers face the daunting task of developing regulations that foster innovation while ensuring patient safety and ethical use of AI technologies. accountability of AI applications in healthcare. Collaboration among government agencies, industry stakeholders, and academic institutions.Interoperability remains a critical challenge as well. The successful integration of AI into healthcare systems depends on the seamless exchange of data across various platforms and applications. Fragmented health information systems can hinder the effective implementation of AI tools, limiting their ability to provide meaningful insights and recommendations. (Sestino & De Mauro, 2022) To overcome this barrier, stakeholders must prioritize the development of standardized data formats and protocols that facilitate interoperability among different healthcare technologies.

Finally, workforce readiness pressing need for healthcare professionals to develop the skills necessary to work alongside AI systems effectively. Educational programs must be adapted to include training on AI concepts, data analysis, present a wealth of opportunities for enhancing patient care, improving operational efficiencies, and personalizing treatment approaches. Predictive analytics, advanced diagnostic imaging, telemedicine, and personalized medicine are all poised to reshape the healthcare landscape significantly. However, these advancements also bring forth a series of challenges, including data privacy concerns, algorithmic bias, regulatory complexities, interoperability issues, and workforce readiness. (van der Aalst et al., 2017) To maximize the potential of AI in healthcare, stakeholders must collaboratively address these challenges through robust policy frameworks, ethical guidelines, and comprehensive training programs. By doing so, the healthcare industry can navigate the complexities effectively, safeguarding patient rights, enhancing public trust, and promoting equitable access to healthcare innovations. A well-structured roadmap for success in implementing these frameworks involves several critical components: stakeholder engagement, ethical guidelines, regulatory standards, continuous evaluation, and education.First and foremost, engaging stakeholders across the healthcare ecosystem is crucial for developing effective ethical and regulatory frameworks(van der Aalst, 2016). This engagement should include a diverse array of participants, including healthcare professionals, patients, technology developers, ethicists, and policymakers. By fostering dialogue among these groups, stakeholders can collaboratively identify potential ethical dilemmas, regulatory challenges, and best practices in AI implementation. This collaborative approach not only ensures that diverse perspectives are considered but also enhances buy-in from all parties involved, which is vital for the successful adoption of AI technologies.The next step informed consent, algorithmic transparency, and the mitigation of bias. For instance, organizations must prioritize the protection of patient data by implementing strict protocols for data handling, storage, and sharing. Informed consent processes should be transparent, allowing patients to understand how their data will be used in AI applications. Moreover, guidelines must emphasize the importance of developing AI algorithms that are free from bias, ensuring equitable treatment across diverse patient populations. By establishing these ethical principles, organizations can create a foundation of trust and accountability in AI applications.Continuous evaluation and improvement of AI systems are critical components of the roadmap for implementing ethical and regulatory frameworks. Organizations should establish metrics and benchmarks to assess the performance of AI technologies continually.

This evaluation process should include feedback mechanisms that allow healthcare providers and patients to report any concerns or adverse events associated with AI applications. regulatory implications of AI in healthcare. Organizations must invest in comprehensive educational programs that cover the fundamental concepts of AI, data ethics, and regulatory compliance. Training should be tailored to various roles within the healthcare ecosystem, from clinicians to administrators, to ensure that all stakeholders are equipped to engage with AI technologies responsibly. By fostering a knowledgeable workforce, organizations can mitigate risks and enhance the overall effectiveness of AI implementations.Furthermore, the rapid pace of AI innovation requires that ethical and regulatory frameworks be adaptable and responsive to emerging technologies. Policymakers and regulatory bodies must remain engaged with the latest developments in AI research and application, ensuring that regulations keep pace with advancements. This adaptability can be achieved through ongoing collaboration with industry experts, academic institutions, and patient advocacy groups to review and revise policies regularly. A flexible regulatory approach allows for the incorporation of new knowledge and best practices, promoting a dynamic and responsible integration of AI in healthcare.sharing agreements. Establishing clear protocols for data sharing that prioritize patient privacy and security is critical. Collaborative agreements should outline the ethical use of shared data, ensuring that all parties involved adhere to established guidelines. By fostering responsible data-sharing practices, organizations can enhance the effectiveness of AI technologies while maintaining public trust. In conclusion, implementing ethical and requires a strategic roadmap for success. Engaging diverse stakeholders, establishing clear ethical guidelines, developing comprehensive regulatory standards, and fostering continuous evaluation are all essential components of this process.(Stanfill & Marc, 2019) Education of AI technologies responsibly. Furthermore, organizations must prioritize transparency and public engagement, ensuring that patients and stakeholders are informed and involved in discussions surrounding AI in healthcare. By embracing these principles, healthcare organizations can successfully integrate good in improving health outcomes and patient care.

CONCLUSION

However, this potential comes with significant ethical dilemmas and regulatory complexities that must be navigated thoughtfully. To ensure that AI serves as a positive force in healthcare, stakeholders must commit to developing and implementing comprehensive frameworks that prioritize ethical considerations, regulatory compliance, and patient-centric approaches.AI technologies.Additionally, cannot be overstated. Governments and regulatory agencies must take an active role in defining standards for AI technologies, ensuring that these systems are safe, effective, and transparent. This involves not only Regulatory agility is crucial; as AI technologies evolve, so too must the frameworks that govern their use. Collaborative efforts between regulatory bodies, industry leaders, and healthcare professionals will be essential to create adaptive policies Furthermore, fostering interdisciplinary collaboration is vital in addressing the. This collaboration should extend to engaging patients and advocacy groups in discussions about the ethical dimensions of AI, ensuring that their voices are heard and their concerns are addressed. By prioritizing interdisciplinary dialogue, stakeholders can develop more comprehensive and effective solutions to the challenges posed by AI in healthcare.healthcare solutions.Moreover, transparency must be a guiding principle in the implementation of AI technologies. Healthcare organizations should prioritize open communication with patients and the public regarding how AI systems function, the data they utilize, and the potential risks and benefits involved. This transparency can help demystify AI In conclusion, the journey towards effectively addressing ethical and regulatory challenges in AI-driven healthcare is complex but essential. By prioritizing patient rights, safeguarding stakeholders can create an environment where AI technologies enhance patient care and operational efficiencies. Interdisciplinary collaboration, education, and transparency are critical components of this effort, enabling healthcare organizations to navigate the complexities of AI responsibly. As the healthcare landscape continues to evolve, in healthcare holds great promise, but it is the responsibility of all stakeholders to ensure that this promise is realized in a manner that is ethical, transparent, and beneficial to society as a whole. patient care.

REFERENCES

Aamir, M., Bazai, S., Bhatti, U. A., Dayo, Z. A., Liu, J., & Zhang, K. (2023, January). Applications of machine learning in medicine: Current trends and prospects. In *2023 Global Conference on Wireless and Optical Technologies (GCWOT)* (pp. 1-4). IEEE. DOI: 10.1109/GCWOT57803.2023.10064665

Aamir, M., Rahman, Z., Abro, W. A., Bhatti, U. A., Dayo, Z. A., & Ishfaq, M. (2023). Brain tumor classification utilizing deep features derived from high-quality regions in MRI images. *Biomedical Signal Processing and Control*, *85*, 104988. DOI: 10.1016/j.bspc.2023.104988

Aamir, M., Rahman, Z., Dayo, Z. A., Abro, W. A., Uddin, M. I., Khan, I., Imran, A. S., Ali, Z., Ishfaq, M., Guan, Y., & Hu, Z. (2022). A deep learning approach for brain tumor classification using MRI images. *Computers & Electrical Engineering*, *101*, 108105. DOI: 10.1016/j.compeleceng.2022.108105

Ahmad, O. F., Stoyanov, D., & Lovat, L. B. (2019). Barriers and pitfalls for artificial intelligence in gastroenterology: Ethical and regulatory issues. *Techniques and Innovations in Gastrointestinal Endoscopy*, *22*(2), 80–84. DOI: 10.1016/j.tgie.2019.150636

Ahmad, O. F., Stoyanov, D., & Lovat, L. B. (2019). Barriers and pitfalls for artificial intelligence in gastroenterology: Ethical and regulatory issues. *Techniques and Innovations in Gastrointestinal Endoscopy*, *22*(2), 80–84. DOI: 10.1016/j.tgie.2019.150636

Amisha, M., Malik, P., Pathania, M., & Rathaur, V. K. (2020). Overview of artificial intelligence in medicine. *Journal of Family Medicine and Primary Care*, *8*(7), 2328. DOI: 10.4103/jfmpc.jfmpc_440_19 PMID: 31463251

Aylak, B. L., Oral, O., & Yazici, K. (2021). Using artificial intelligence and machine learning applications in logistics. *El-Cezeri Journal of Science and Engineering*, *8*, 74–93.

Bistron, M., & Piotrowski, Z. (2021). Artificial intelligence applications in military systems and their influence on the sense of security of citizens. *Electronics (Basel)*, *10*(7), 871–890. DOI: 10.3390/electronics10070871

Boucher, P. (2019). How artificial intelligence works. STOA Panel for the Future of Science and Technology. Available at: https://www.europarl.europa.eu/stoa/en/document/EPRS_BRI(2019)634420

Brady, A. P., & Neri, E. (2020). Artificial intelligence in radiology: Ethical considerations. *Diagnostics (Basel)*, *10*(4), 231–240. DOI: 10.3390/diagnostics10040231 PMID: 32316503

Carter, S. M., Rogers, W., Win, K. T., Frazer, H., Richards, B., & Houssami, N. (2020). The ethical, legal, and social implications of using artificial intelligence systems in breast cancer care. *The Breast : Official Journal of the European Society of Mastology*, *49*, 25–32. DOI: 10.1016/j.breast.2019.10.001 PMID: 31677530

Chan, K. S., & Zary, N. (2019). Applications and challenges of implementing artificial intelligence in medical education: Integrative review. *JMIR Medical Education*, *5*(1), e13930. DOI: 10.2196/13930 PMID: 31199295

Council of the European Union. (2011). Directive 2011/24/EU of the European Parliament and of the Council of 9 March 2011 on the application of patients' rights in cross-border healthcare. Available at: https://eur-lex.europa.eu/LexUriServ/LexUriServ.do?uri=OJ:L:2011:088:0045:0065:en:PDF

European Commission, Directorate-General for Communications Networks, Content and Technology. (2019). Ethics guidelines for trustworthy AI. Publications Office. Available at: https://data.europa.eu/doi/10.2759/177365

European Commission, Directorate-General for Research and Innovation, European Group on Ethics in Science and New Technologies. (2018). Statement on artificial intelligence, robotics and 'autonomous' systems: Brussels, 9 March 2018. Publications Office. Available at: https://data.europa.eu/doi/10.2777/786515

Floridi, L., Cowls, J., King, T. C., & Taddeo, M. (2020). How to design AI for social good: Seven essential factors. *Science and Engineering Ethics*, *26*(3), 1771–1796. DOI: 10.1007/s11948-020-00213-5 PMID: 32246245

Grote, T., & Berens, P. (2020). On the ethics of algorithmic decision-making in healthcare. *Journal of Medical Ethics*, *46*(3), 205–211. DOI: 10.1136/medethics-2019-105586 PMID: 31748206

Guan, Y., Aamir, M., Rahman, Z., Ali, A., Abro, W. A., Dayo, Z. A., ... & Hu, Z. (2021). A framework for efficient brain tumor classification using MRI images.

Hamet, P., & Tremblay, J. (2017). Artificial intelligence in medicine. *Metabolism: Clinical and Experimental*, *69*, S36–S40. DOI: 10.1016/j.metabol.2017.01.011 PMID: 28126242

Hee Lee, D., & Yoon, S. N. (2021). Application of artificial intelligence-based technologies in the healthcare industry: Opportunities and challenges. *International Journal of Environmental Research and Public Health*, *18*, 1–18. PMID: 33401373

Ho, C. W. L., Ali, J., & Caals, K. (2020). Ensuring trustworthy use of artificial intelligence and big data analytics in health insurance. *Bulletin of the World Health Organization*, *98*(4), 263–269. DOI: 10.2471/BLT.19.234732 PMID: 32284650

Johnson, S. L. J. (2019). AI, machine learning, and ethics in health care. *Journal of Legal Medicine*, *39*(4), 427–441. DOI: 10.1080/01947648.2019.1690604 PMID: 31940250

Kelly, C. J., Karthikesalingam, A., Suleyman, M., Corrado, G., & King, D. (2019). Key challenges for delivering clinical impact with artificial intelligence. *BMC Medicine*, *17*(1), 195–204. DOI: 10.1186/s12916-019-1426-2 PMID: 31665002

Lecun, Y., Bengio, Y., & Hinton, G. (2015). Deep learning. *Nature*, *521*(7553), 436–444. DOI: 10.1038/nature14539 PMID: 26017442

Lee, M. S. A., Floridi, L., & Singh, J. (2021). Formalizing trade-offs beyond algorithmic fairness: Lessons from ethical philosophy and welfare economics. *AI and Ethics*, *1*(4), 529–544. DOI: 10.1007/s43681-021-00067-y

Luxton, D. D. (2014). Recommendations for the ethical use and design of artificial intelligent care providers. *Artificial Intelligence in Medicine*, *62*(1), 1–10. DOI: 10.1016/j.artmed.2014.06.004 PMID: 25059820

Murphy, K., Di Ruggiero, E., Upshur, R., Willison, D. J., Malhotra, N., Cai, J. C., Malhotra, N., Lui, V., & Gibson, J. (2021). Artificial intelligence for good health: A scoping review of the ethics literature. *BMC Medical Ethics*, *22*(1), 14. DOI: 10.1186/s12910-021-00577-8 PMID: 33588803

Senthilraja, M. (2021). Application of artificial intelligence to address issues related to the COVID-19 virus. *SLAS Technology*, *26*(2), 123–126. DOI: 10.1177/2472630320983813 PMID: 33390088

Sestino, A., & De Mauro, A. (2022). Leveraging artificial intelligence in business: Implications, applications, and methods. *Technology Analysis and Strategic Management*, *34*(1), 16–29. DOI: 10.1080/09537325.2021.1883583

Stanfill, M. H., & Marc, D. T. (2019). Health information management: Implications of artificial intelligence on healthcare data and information management. *Yearbook of Medical Informatics*, *28*(1), 56–64. DOI: 10.1055/s-0039-1677913 PMID: 31419816

Van Der Aalst, W. M. P. (2016). Green data science: Using big data in an "environmentally friendly" manner. In ICEIS 2016—Proceedings of the 18th International Conference on Enterprise Information Systems.

Van Der Aalst, W. M. P., Bichler, M., & Heinzl, A. (2017). Responsible data science. *Business & Information Systems Engineering*, *59*(5), 311–313. DOI: 10.1007/s12599-017-0487-z

Washington, D. C.U.S. Department of Labor, Employee Benefits Security Administration. (2004). *The Health Insurance Portability and Accountability Act*. HIPAA.

Yoon, J., Drumright, L. N., & Van Der Schaar, M. (2020). Anonymization through data synthesis using generative adversarial networks (ADS-GAN). *IEEE Journal of Biomedical and Health Informatics*, *24*(8), 1. DOI: 10.1109/JBHI.2020.2980262 PMID: 32167919

Chapter 3

Advanced Biomedical Signal Processing Techniques for Real-Time Health Monitoring Systems

Palak Mangal
VIT Bhopal University, India

D. Lakshmi
https://orcid.org/0000-0003-4018-1208
VIT Bhopal University, India

ABSTRACT

In recent years, the intersection of biomedical signal processing and communication technologies has significantly accelerated healthcare innovations, particularly in real-time health monitoring systems. This paper presents the core principles of biomedical signal processing, focusing on techniques for signal acquisition and preprocessing that are essential in improving data quality and reliability. Effective signal acquisition is a key challenge, as physiological signals—such as ECG, EEG, and EMG—are often affected by noise and artifacts from internal and external sources. Ultimately, this study demonstrates how advancements in electronics and communication engineering are driving significant progress in biomedical signal processing, leading to better health outcomes and more efficient patient care. Additionally, the paper examines the critical role of advanced filtering techniques in reducing noise and enhancing signal clarity, which is particularly important in wearable medical devices.

1.0 INTRODUCTION

The healthcare industry has undergone a profound transformation over the past few decades, largely driven by technological advancements that have reshaped patient care and outcomes. One of the most significant innovations in this revolution is the integration of biomedical signal processing and communication technologies, which has enabled the development of real-time health monitoring systems. These systems harness the power of electronics and communication engineering to continuously track, analyze,

DOI: 10.4018/979-8-3693-9816-6.ch003

and interpret physiological signals, providing a wealth of data that can improve diagnosis, treatment, and patient management. The motivation behind this integration lies in the desire to enhance the accuracy, timeliness, and accessibility of healthcare services, particularly through innovations such as wearable devices and remote patient monitoring. By leveraging advanced signal acquisition techniques, preprocessing methods, and machine learning (ML) algorithms, these technologies can address key challenges such as noise reduction, data quality enhancement, and personalized health insights. The role of communication technologies, including the integration of IoT (Internet of Things), is critical in ensuring seamless data transmission and enabling real-time monitoring, thereby facilitating better decision-making and early intervention. This paper explores how these cutting-edge advancements in biomedical signal processing and communication technologies contribute to improving the efficiency of health monitoring systems, while highlighting their potential to reduce the burden on healthcare systems globally. Ultimately, this integration offers a promising pathway toward next-generation healthcare solutions that can enhance the quality of care, empower patients, and reduce healthcare costs. (Rangayyan et al., 2024)

This chapter discusses different preprocessing techniques, including filtering, normalization, and artifact removal, are thus crucial to ensuring the accuracy of subsequent analyses. A major highlight of this study is the application of advanced ML algorithms to classify physiological signals. The use of ML in biomedical signal processing allows for the identification of subtle patterns in complex datasets, enabling early detection of diseases and more accurate diagnostic decisions. Central to this process is feature extraction, where essential characteristics of signals are identified and extracted to optimize the performance of ML models. Feature extraction methods such as wavelet transforms, time-frequency analysis and Principal Component Analysis (PCA) are instrumental in improving model accuracy and efficiency.

Filters like adaptive noise cancellation and wavelet denoising are employed to isolate meaningful physiological information from background noise, making these devices more reliable for continuous monitoring.

Emerging trends, such as the integration of Internet of Things (IoT) technologies, are transforming healthcare delivery by enabling real-time remote health monitoring and data transmission (JARIAL et al., 2024). IoT-based systems facilitate continuous tracking of vital signs and deliver personalized care by leveraging vast amounts of patient data. This convergence of biomedical signal processing, IoT, and personalized medicine promises to reshape the healthcare landscape by enhancing patient outcomes, improving care delivery, and reducing healthcare costs.

1.1 The Role of Biomedical Signal Processing in Healthcare

The healthcare industry has witnessed a profound transformation over the past few decades, driven largely by technological advancements. Among the most significant innovations is integrating biomedical signal processing and communication technologies, which have enabled real-time health monitoring systems. These systems leverage the power of electronics and communication engineering to continuously track, analyze, and interpret physiological signals, offering immense potential for improving patient care and outcomes. Biomedical signals, such as Electrocardiograms (ECG), Electroencephalograms (EEG), and electromyograms (EMG), provide critical information about the body's internal state. However, these signals are often contaminated by noise, artifacts, and other interferences that can compromise the accuracy and reliability of health monitoring systems (Khang et al,. 2024).

1.2 Challenges in Signal Acquisition and Preprocessing

Signal acquisition is one of the most crucial stages in the biomedical signal-processing pipeline, as the integrity of the collected data directly impacts the accuracy and reliability of the entire health monitoring system. The effectiveness of biomedical signal acquisition systems depends not only on the quality of sensors and hardware used but also on the system's ability to filter out unwanted noise and artifacts that can distort physiological signals. As the field advances towards miniaturized, wearable devices, maintaining high-quality signal acquisition becomes increasingly challenging due to constraints such as limited power, small form factors, and the presence of environmental noise. These challenges are further complicated by the non-stationary nature of many biomedical signals, where characteristics such as amplitude and frequency may change over time.(Anwer et al., 2024)

To address these obstacles, researchers have developed a range of advanced preprocessing techniques. Signal filtering, normalization, and artifact removal are essential for enhancing signal quality, but they must also be tailored to the specific characteristics of the signal and the noise sources. Adaptive noise cancellation (ANC) plays a vital role in this context, as it can dynamically adjust to varying noise patterns, particularly in non-stationary environments, allowing for effective removal of noise while preserving the integrity of the signal. Moreover, feature extraction methods help identify the most relevant components of the signal, enabling the extraction of meaningful information for subsequent analysis, even in the presence of noise or interference. Together, these preprocessing techniques ensure that the signals used for analysis are both accurate and reliable, forming a solid foundation for health monitoring systems. Failure to effectively address these preprocessing challenges—such as poor noise rejection or inadequate feature extraction—can undermine the entire diagnostic process, leading to inaccurate assessments or delayed interventions.

1.3 The Integration of ML and Communication Technologies

In recent years, machine learning (ML) has emerged as a powerful tool for enhancing biomedical signal processing, offering a significant leap forward in the analysis of complex physiological data. ML algorithms, such as support vector machines (SVM), random forests, and deep learning techniques like convolutional neural networks (CNNs) and recurrent neural networks (RNNs), have shown exceptional ability to identify subtle patterns within large datasets that would be difficult to detect manually. These algorithms have demonstrated remarkable success in automating the classification of physiological signals such as ECG, EEG, and EMG, making it possible to predict a range of diseases with higher accuracy and efficiency. For example, SVMs have been applied in detecting arrhythmias from ECG signals, while deep learning models like CNNs are increasingly used for early detection of brain disorders through EEG signals. These ML techniques not only enhance diagnostic decision-making but also enable personalized healthcare delivery by tailoring treatment plans based on an individual's unique physiological profile.

Additionally, techniques such as wavelet transform, time-frequency analysis, and Principal Component Analysis (PCA) have significantly improved feature extraction, enhancing the quality and relevance of the data used in machine learning models. These methods allow for better handling of non-stationary signals and improve the accuracy of disease predictions, as they extract more meaningful features from complex signals. In real-world applications, ML-powered systems are already being used to predict cardiovascular events, detect early signs of neurological diseases like epilepsy and Alzheimer's, and identify mental health conditions through continuous monitoring of physiological signals.(Adebayo et al,. 2024)

The integration of these ML-based systems with the rapid growth of the Internet of Things (IoT) and the evolution of 5G and upcoming 6G networks is transforming healthcare delivery. IoT-based systems now enable continuous, remote monitoring of patients, transmitting real-time physiological data to healthcare providers. This constant flow of data, paired with ML algorithms, allows for timely detection of potential health issues and real-time intervention. The advancements in wireless communication and data transfer, particularly through high-speed 5G and future 6G networks, have made it possible to track vital signs, monitor chronic conditions, and provide personalized care more efficiently. This not only reduces the need for in-hospital visits but also significantly improves patient outcomes by enabling proactive healthcare (Olaleye et al., 2024). For instance, patients with chronic heart conditions can now receive continuous ECG monitoring via wearable devices, with ML algorithms predicting potential complications and alerting healthcare providers before serious issues arise.

2.0 FUNDAMENTALS OF BIOMEDICAL SIGNALS

Biomedical signals are electrical signals that are generated by biological processes and can be measured to assess the physiological state of the human body. These signals are fundamental to healthcare monitoring and diagnostics, as they provide real-time insights into bodily functions and help in detecting abnormalities that might signal underlying medical conditions.

The measurement of these signals is a critical component of health monitoring systems, and their accurate acquisition, preprocessing, and analysis are essential for effective diagnosis and treatment (Bhatele et al., 2023). In this section, we will examine three key types of biomedical signals commonly used in health monitoring systems: Electrocardiogram (ECG), Electroencephalogram (EEG), and Electromyogram (EMG). Additionally, we will explore the characteristics of these signals and the challenges faced in their acquisition.

2.1 Types of Biomedical Signals

2.1.1. Electrocardiogram (ECG)

The ECG is one of the most widely used biomedical signals to monitor and evaluate the electrical activity of the heart. It records the heart's rhythm and electrical impulses as waveforms that provide information about heart rate, the timing of each heartbeat, and the presence of any abnormalities, such as arrhythmias or heart attacks (Ukil et al., 2022).

- Signal Characteristics: The ECG signal consists of P waves, QRS complexes, and T waves, each corresponding to different stages of the cardiac cycle (atrial depolarization, ventricular depolarization, and ventricular repolarization).
- Challenges in Acquisition: The ECG signal is susceptible to interference from various external sources such as power line noise and electromagnetic interference. Additionally, motion artifacts from the patient (such as body movement) can distort the signal, making it difficult to obtain accurate readings in ambulatory settings.

2.1.2 Electroencephalogram (EEG)

An EEG records the electrical activity of the brain by measuring voltage fluctuations resulting from ionic current flows within the neurons. It is primarily used to assess brain function, diagnose neurological conditions like epilepsy, sleep disorders, and brain injuries, and monitor brain activity during surgeries (Chaddad et al., 2023).

- Signal Characteristics: EEG signals are categorized into different frequency bands, including delta, theta, alpha, beta, and gamma waves, each associated with different states of brain activity, such as sleep, relaxation, or cognitive tasks.
- Challenges in Acquisition: EEG signals are extremely low in amplitude, which makes them susceptible to various sources of noise, including muscle activity (electromyographic noise) and electrical interference. Furthermore, the signals are often affected by the patient's movement or the placement of electrodes, making signal acquisition a delicate process.

2.1.3. Electromyogram (EMG)

The EMG records the electrical activity produced by skeletal muscles. It is used to assess muscle function, diagnose neuromuscular diseases, and evaluate muscle response during physical activities or rehabilitation exercises (Boyer et al., 2023).

- Signal Characteristics: The EMG signal consists of a combination of motor unit action potentials (MUAPs) and the electrical activity from muscle fibers. The signal's characteristics depend on muscle fiber type, muscle contraction force, and the location of the electrode.
- Challenges in Acquisition: The EMG signal is vulnerable to interference from nearby muscles, electrical noise, and skin impedance. The placement of electrodes is crucial for accurate signal detection, and proper skin preparation is necessary to minimize noise and improve the signal-to-noise ratio.

2.2 Characteristics and Challenges in Data Acquisition

The acquisition of biomedical signals is a critical step in health monitoring systems, as it directly influences the quality and accuracy of subsequent analyses. Biomedical signals, such as ECG, EEG, and EMG, are inherently complex and can be influenced by various internal and external factors, making their acquisition both challenging and essential. One of the key characteristics of these signals is their low amplitude, which often requires sensitive equipment to capture accurate data (Arooj et al., 2022). For instance, the ECG signal, which records the electrical activity of the heart, is typically measured in millivolts, and small variations in signal strength can represent significant health changes. Similarly, EEG signals from the brain are typically weak, requiring precise signal acquisition technologies to detect and differentiate between various brain states. Another characteristic is the non-stationarity of biomedical signals. These signals can vary over time due to physiological changes or external factors, making it difficult to maintain consistent data quality during acquisition. This non-stationarity requires advanced techniques in signal processing to handle variations and ensure that the acquired data is accurate for diagnostic purposes. For example, EEG signals can fluctuate due to changes in brain activity, while EMG signals may be influenced by muscle fatigue or movement artifacts. A major challenge in signal acquisition is the presence of noise and artifacts (Xiong et al., 2022). Physiological signals are often contaminated by various types of noise, including electromagnetic interference, motion artifacts, and powerline noise. These external interferences can distort the signal, leading to inaccurate readings. Electromyographic signals (EMG), for example, are particularly susceptible to movement artifacts, as the placement of sensors can be influenced by muscle contractions or environmental vibrations. Similarly, EEG signals may be contaminated by electrical noise from nearby equipment or by patient movement. Overcoming these challenges requires the use of advanced filtering and signal conditioning techniques to isolate the true physiological signal from the noise. Furthermore, sensor placement and sensor reliability also pose significant challenges in the acquisition process. The positioning of sensors, especially for wearable or portable devices, can affect the accuracy of the measurements (Ayerbe et al., 2022). Improper electrode placement can lead to poor signal quality or the introduction of additional noise. Additionally, sensor drift or malfunction over time can compromise long-term monitoring. To address these issues, researchers and engineers continuously innovate in the design of non-invasive, wearable sensors that are more robust and accurate in diverse real-world conditions

3.0 SIGNAL ACQUISITION AND PREPROCESSING

Signal acquisition and preprocessing are fundamental stages in the process of biomedical signal processing. These stages ensure that raw physiological signals, such as ECG, EEG, and EMG, are accurately captured and cleaned for further analysis. The quality of signal acquisition and the effectiveness of preprocessing directly impact the reliability of health monitoring systems (Lu et al., 2023). This section will explore sensor technologies, common noise sources and artifacts, and preprocessing techniques, including amplification and Analog-to-Digital Conversion (ADC), which play a critical role in ensuring high-quality data for real-time monitoring.

3.1 Sensor Technologies and Data Acquisition Circuits

The acquisition of biomedical signals begins with the use of various sensors and data acquisition circuits designed to detect and measure physiological activity from the human body. Electrodes are the most common sensor type for biomedical signal acquisition. For instance, ECG signals are typically captured using Ag/AgCl electrodes placed on the skin, as they offer high conductivity and low skin impedance, ensuring the accuracy of heart signal measurements. EEG signals, on the other hand, are detected using electrodes placed on the scalp. These electrodes can be either wet (with a conductive gel) or dry, with dry electrodes gaining popularity for their ease of use, particularly in wearable applications. EMG signals are captured through surface or intramuscular electrodes, depending on the specific requirements of muscle activity measurement (Lynch et al., 2022). In terms of data acquisition circuits, these sensors are connected to amplifiers and analog front-end (AFE) circuits, which are responsible for boosting weak biomedical signals to levels suitable for processing. Low-noise amplifiers (LNAs) are employed to amplify the signals without introducing additional noise, while the AFE ensures that the analog signal is filtered, amplified, and prepared for conversion into a digital format. Wearable sensors have become increasingly important in continuous health monitoring, and these devices are designed to be lightweight, non-intrusive, and capable of operating for extended periods. Flexible and stretchable sensors are being developed to improve the comfort and performance of these wearable systems, making them more suitable for long-term monitoring (Chidolue et al,. 2023).

3.2 Noise Sources and Artifacts

Biomedical signals are often contaminated by various noise sources and artifacts, which can significantly degrade the quality of the acquired data. One of the most common sources of noise is power line interference, which introduces 50/60 Hz oscillations that can corrupt ECG and EEG signals. Additionally, electromyographic noise can occur in ECG and EEG recordings due to the electrical activity of muscles, such as those caused by eye movement or facial muscle contractions. This is especially problematic in wearable devices, where the patient's motion can inadvertently generate noise in the signal (Iwamoto et al., 2022). Electromagnetic interference from nearby electronic devices, such as smartphones or medical equipment, can also distort the signal, making accurate signal processing more challenging.

Another major issue is motion artifacts, which occur when the patient moves during the signal acquisition process. For example, walking, shifting positions, or even normal breathing can create distortion in ECG, EEG, and EMG signals. The placement of electrodes is also crucial in reducing signal distortion, as skin impedance variations can introduce noise, especially in ECG and EMG signals (Ranjan et al., 2022). High skin impedance can cause weak or unstable signals, while low impedance can lead to excessive noise. Effective management of these noise sources is essential for ensuring reliable biomedical signal acquisition.

3.3 Preprocessing Techniques

Once the biomedical signals are acquired, preprocessing is essential for removing noise, amplifying weak signals, and preparing the data for further analysis. Signal amplification is one of the first steps in preprocessing. Since physiological signals are generally weak, amplifiers, particularly low-noise amplifiers (LNAs), are used to increase the signal strength without introducing additional noise. After amplification, the signals are typically passed through band-pass filters that allow only the frequency components of interest to pass through, removing unwanted high- and low-frequency noise.

Next, the analog signals are converted to digital form using analog-to-digital converters (ADCs). ADCs sample the analog signals at a specific rate, ensuring that the digital representation accurately reflects the original signal. The sampling rate is determined by the Nyquist criterion, which states that the sampling frequency must be at least twice the highest frequency component of the signal to prevent aliasing. The resolution of the ADC, typically measured in bit depth, determines how precisely the amplitude of the signal is represented, with higher bit-depth ADCs providing greater precision but requiring more power and resources (Werner de Vargas et al., 2023).

To further clean the signal, artifact removal techniques are applied. These can include methods such as wavelet transforms, which decompose the signal into different frequency components and allow for effective filtering of noise without affecting the underlying signal. Principal Component Analysis (PCA) is another technique used to reduce signal dimensionality while preserving the most significant features, which can help eliminate noise in multichannel recordings. Kalman filtering, an adaptive filtering technique, is also useful for estimating the signal in real-time, particularly when noise characteristics vary dynamically.

Finally, normalization is often applied to adjust the signal amplitude and ensure that all components are within a consistent range, making them easier to analyze and compare. By employing these preprocessing techniques, biomedical signals are significantly improved, making them suitable for more accurate analysis, classification, and interpretation.

4.0 ADVANCED SIGNAL PROCESSING TECHNIQUES

Advanced signal processing techniques play a pivotal role in improving the quality and accuracy of biomedical signal analysis. These techniques are particularly important in real-time health monitoring systems, where the need for precise and timely information is crucial for patient care. This section explores some of the most effective advanced signal processing methods currently employed in biomedical signal analysis, including time-frequency analysis, nonlinear filtering, adaptive algorithms, and compressed sensing. Each of these methods provides distinct advantages in terms of handling complex biomedical signals, minimizing noise, and ensuring efficient data transmission for real-time applications (Zhang et al,. 2022).

4.1 Time-frequency Analysis

Time-frequency analysis is a fundamental technique in biomedical signal processing, as it enables the analysis of non-stationary signals—signals whose frequency content changes over time. This is particularly useful for biomedical signals such as ECG, EEG, and EMG, which exhibit varying frequency components over time. One of the most widely used methods for time-frequency analysis is the Wavelet Transform. The wavelet transform allows for multi-resolution analysis, where the signal is decomposed into components at different frequency scales, providing both time and frequency information simultaneously. This capability is particularly beneficial for identifying transient features in the signal, such as abrupt changes in ECG waveforms or spikes in EEG that could indicate irregularities or health issues. Wavelet-based methods, including Continuous Wavelet Transform (CWT) and Discrete Wavelet Transform (DWT), are employed to detect events at multiple time scales with high accuracy, making them suitable for real-time applications in wearable health monitoring devices (Pachori et al., 2023).

Another key technique is the Short-Time Fourier Transform (STFT), which breaks down a signal into small overlapping segments and applies the Fourier transform to each segment. This method provides a frequency representation of the signal over time, but unlike wavelet transform, STFT uses fixed time and frequency resolutions. While it is less flexible than wavelet transform, STFT is still widely used due to its simplicity and efficiency in capturing the frequency content of stationary or quasi-stationary signals. Both wavelet transforms and STFT are commonly used in conjunction with filtering techniques to extract significant features for classification, anomaly detection, and disease prediction (Vuojamo et al., 2022).

4.2 Nonlinear Filtering and Adaptive Algorithms

Biomedical signals are often affected by complex, nonlinear noise and artifacts, which traditional linear filters may not effectively remove. As a result, nonlinear filtering techniques have gained increasing importance in biomedical signal processing. Nonlinear filters, such as the median filter and wavelet thresholding, are highly effective in removing impulsive noise and preserving sharp transitions in biomedical signals. For instance, median filtering is commonly used to eliminate spike noise in ECG signals without distorting the R-peaks or other important features of the heart's electrical activity (Satpathy et al., 2022).

Additionally, adaptive algorithms play a crucial role in real-time processing, where signal characteristics and noise conditions vary over time. These algorithms adjust filter parameters dynamically to minimize the error between the desired and actual signal. One of the most widely used adaptive algorithms is the LMS (Least Mean Square) algorithm, which adapts the filter coefficients based on the error signal, making it useful for applications where noise characteristics change unpredictably. Adaptive filtering is particularly effective in canceling out interference from power lines or other external sources, especially in environments where biomedical signals need to be recorded over long periods, such as during remote patient monitoring (Jin et al., 2023). Moreover, Kalman filters, which are based on statistical estimation, can be used for real-time prediction and correction of the signal, improving the accuracy of measurements by compensating for missing or corrupted data.

4.3 Compressed Sensing for Efficient Data Transmission

In the era of real-time health monitoring, especially in mobile and wearable devices, efficient data transmission and storage have become key concerns due to bandwidth limitations and power constraints. Compressed sensing (CS) has emerged as a revolutionary approach to address these challenges by enabling the acquisition of sparse signals at a lower sampling rate than traditionally required, without sacrificing signal quality. The core principle behind compressed sensing is that many biomedical signals, such as ECG or EEG, are inherently sparse in some transformed domain, meaning that they contain a limited number of significant components compared to the total number of samples (Sekar et al., 2022).

Through compressed sensing, these signals can be directly sampled in a compressed form, effectively reducing the amount of data that needs to be transmitted. This is achieved by leveraging the sparsity of the signal in a certain basis (e.g., wavelet or Fourier domains) and using optimization algorithms to recover the full signal from a small number of measurements. In practical terms, this reduces the need for high sampling rates and large storage capacities while maintaining signal fidelity. Compressed sensing is particularly useful in the context of wearable medical devices, where low power consumption and efficient data transmission are crucial for continuous, long-term monitoring (Ma et al., 2023). It also reduces the burden on wireless communication channels, enabling faster and more reliable transmission of health data, which is vital for real-time applications, such as remote monitoring and telemedicine.

Moreover, the integration of compressed sensing with other advanced techniques such as ML further enhances its potential by allowing for more efficient feature extraction and signal reconstruction. The combination of compressed sensing with ML algorithms enables real-time anomaly detection and disease prediction with minimal computational and bandwidth requirements.

5.0 APPLICATIONS AND CASE STUDIES

The rapid advancements in biomedical signal processing have paved the way for innovative applications in real-time health monitoring. These applications are revolutionizing healthcare delivery by enabling remote patient monitoring, enhancing wearable health devices, and improving the efficiency of smart hospital systems. This section explores three key applications of biomedical signal processing: remote patient monitoring, wearable health devices, and smart hospital systems. Each of these areas demonstrates how signal processing techniques are being leveraged to improve patient outcomes, optimize healthcare workflows, and ensure better management of chronic conditions (Paganelli et al., 2022).

5.1 Remote Patient Monitoring

Remote Patient Monitoring (RPM) is one of the most transformative applications of biomedical signal processing, especially in the context of telemedicine. RPM allows healthcare providers to monitor patients' vital signs and other physiological parameters from a distance, facilitating continuous care and reducing the need for in-person visits. Using wearable sensors and mobile technologies, patients can transmit real-time data such as ECG, heart rate, blood pressure, and oxygen saturation to healthcare professionals. Signal processing techniques are crucial in these systems for extracting meaningful information from the raw data, detecting anomalies, and providing timely alerts to both patients and healthcare providers (Shaik et al., 2023).

Advanced signal processing methods like adaptive filtering, wavelet transforms, and ML algorithms are integrated into RPM systems to enhance signal accuracy, reduce noise, and ensure the reliability of data transmission over wireless networks. For example, by processing ECG signals remotely, systems can detect arrhythmias or other heart conditions early, enabling healthcare providers to take prompt action. Similarly, EEG signals can be continuously monitored for signs of seizure activity, alerting caregivers before a potential seizure occurs. The combination of these technologies in RPM systems has been shown to significantly improve patient outcomes, especially for chronic disease management, elderly care, and post-surgical recovery (Tang et al., 2022).

Case studies like the Philips eICU program and AliveCor's KardiaMobile demonstrate the successful application of remote monitoring systems in real-world settings. These platforms leverage advanced signal processing and wireless communication to provide healthcare providers with real-time, actionable insights, enhancing patient care while reducing hospital readmissions.

5.2 Wearable Health Devices

Wearable health devices are rapidly becoming an integral part of personal health management, offering individuals the ability to monitor their health in real-time. These devices—ranging from fitness trackers to more sophisticated medical-grade wearables—use sensors to capture various physiological signals such as ECG, EMG, EEG, and accelerometer data. The data collected by these sensors is processed using advanced signal processing techniques to extract meaningful features, which can be used for both health monitoring and disease detection.

Wearables are particularly useful for continuous monitoring of heart health, detecting early signs of cardiovascular diseases, and tracking physical activity. For example, smartwatches with built-in ECG sensors can detect arrhythmias, such as atrial fibrillation, and provide users with the ability to share results with healthcare professionals remotely (Prieto-Avalos et al., 2022). AliveCor's KardiaMobile is a prominent case study in this field, offering a portable ECG device that allows users to perform an ECG test in just 30 seconds and send the results directly to their doctor. This real-time monitoring capability enhances early detection of heart conditions, enabling timely interventions before more serious complications arise. Similarly, wearable EEG headsets can monitor brain activity in patients with neurological disorders, such as epilepsy, and predict seizures through real-time signal processing of EEG data. This is particularly beneficial for patients who may not have easy access to frequent medical appointments.

EMG-based wearables, such as those used in muscle rehabilitation, monitor muscle activity and provide valuable feedback for patients undergoing physical therapy or those managing musculoskeletal disorders.

The importance of advanced signal processing in wearable health devices cannot be overstated. Techniques such as real-time filtering, motion artifact removal, and feature extraction are essential to ensure the accuracy of measurements, especially when the device is worn during daily, dynamic activities. For example, wearables like the Fitbit, Apple Watch, and Oura Ring have made significant strides in this area by incorporating algorithms that minimize motion-related noise and improve signal clarity. These devices not only enable users to track their vitals, such as heart rate and sleep patterns, but also promote health awareness and early intervention by alerting users to potential health concerns, such as abnormal heart rates or irregular sleep cycles. These advancements in wearable technology are empowering individuals to take charge of their health, offering a proactive approach to disease prevention and management (Dai et al,. 2022).

5.3 Smart Hospital Systems

Smart hospital systems integrate cutting-edge technologies such as biomedical signal processing, the Internet of Things (IoT), artificial intelligence (AI), and big data analytics to significantly enhance healthcare delivery within hospital settings. These systems are designed to continuously monitor patient health, optimize hospital workflows, and improve patient safety through real-time data collection and analysis. Biomedical signal processing plays a vital role in ensuring the accuracy and reliability of the data generated by a variety of hospital sensors, including vital signs monitors, infusion pumps, diagnostic equipment, and wearable devices. By applying advanced signal processing techniques, these systems can extract meaningful information from complex physiological signals, improving both clinical accuracy and response times.

In critical care settings like ICUs, smart hospital systems use advanced monitoring systems to continuously process signals such as ECG, blood pressure, oxygen saturation, and other vital signs. These systems are equipped with AI-driven algorithms that can detect early warning signs of patient deterioration, such as arrhythmias, septic shock, or respiratory distress. Upon identifying critical changes in patient conditions, the system automatically triggers alerts to clinical staff, enabling rapid interventions to prevent further complications. Machine learning (ML) algorithms also analyze historical and real-time patient data to uncover subtle patterns, predict adverse events, and assist in decision-making, reducing the likelihood of medical errors and improving clinical outcomes.

In addition to real-time patient monitoring, smart hospital systems leverage the IoT to interconnect various medical devices, enabling centralized monitoring and control. By creating a network of interconnected devices, the IoT allows for seamless communication between equipment and clinicians, ensuring that important data from multiple sources is synchronized and processed in real-time. For example, in a smart ICU, an array of devices continuously monitors patients' vital signs, analyzes trends over time, and shares the data with healthcare professionals via a centralized platform. This integration of IoT technology ensures that critical information is accessible at the point of care, enhancing clinicians' ability to make timely, informed decisions.

Furthermore, AI-driven analytics work synergistically with biomedical signal processing to enhance operational efficiency across the hospital. AI models can analyze large volumes of hospital data, from patient records to inventory management, to optimize resource allocation, streamline workflows, and reduce hospital bottlenecks. These systems can predict patient admission rates, manage staffing schedules, and monitor the supply chain, contributing to more efficient hospital operations. Ultimately, the integration of IoT with biomedical signal processing and AI is fundamental in creating a dynamic, responsive, and data-driven healthcare environment, where both patient monitoring and hospital operations are continuously improved to ensure better care and operational efficiency. (Kwon et al., 2022).

Case studies such as the Mount Sinai Health System in New York and the St. Gallen University Hospital in Switzerland have demonstrated the potential of smart hospital systems in improving patient outcomes. These hospitals have integrated biomedical signal processing techniques with IoT-enabled devices and AI to enhance monitoring, patient care, and operational efficiency.

6.0 EMERGING TRENDS AND FUTURE DIRECTIONS

The field of biomedical signal processing is evolving rapidly, driven by breakthroughs in Artificial Intelligence (AI), quantum computing, and advanced telecommunications technologies like 6G networks. These innovations promise to reshape how healthcare is delivered, improving both the quality and accessibility of care (Krishnamoorthy et al., 2023). This section delves into two of the most promising emerging trends in biomedical signal processing: the integration of AI and quantum computing in signal processing, and the role of 6G networks in transforming healthcare systems.

6.1 AI and Quantum Computing in Signal Processing

AI has already had a profound impact on biomedical signal processing, particularly through the use of ML algorithms that can analyze large, complex datasets in real time. AI-powered tools have enhanced signal classification, anomaly detection, and predictive modeling, enabling early disease detection and more accurate health monitoring. However, the integration of quantum computing into this space could revolutionize the way we process and analyze biomedical signals.(Mallow et al., 2022)

Quantum computing, with its ability to process vast amounts of data simultaneously, offers exponential improvements in computational power compared to classical computers. Quantum algorithms could enable the rapid processing of high-dimensional signal data, which would be particularly beneficial in areas such as genomic signal processing and multimodal sensor fusion. For instance, biomedical signal processing in EEG or ECG could benefit from quantum ML algorithms, enabling faster and more accurate classification of complex signals with lower computational overhead.

In particular, quantum-enhanced ML could be leveraged to improve signal feature extraction, anomaly detection, and predictive health analytics. Quantum computers can also handle large datasets with complex correlations, such as those encountered in multi-sensor and multi-modal health monitoring systems, where data from different sensors (ECG, EEG, EMG, etc.) must be fused to provide a holistic view of the patient's health status (Chauhan et al., 2022).

AI algorithms will likely evolve alongside quantum computing to enable quantum AI, which combines the strengths of quantum computing and machine learning. This hybrid approach will allow for real-time, highly accurate predictions of patient health conditions, improving the decision-making capabilities of healthcare providers and enhancing personalized medicine.

6.2 6G Networks for Healthcare

The advent of 6G networks is expected to revolutionize healthcare by offering ultra-fast, low-latency, and highly reliable communication capabilities. While 5G networks have already shown promise in supporting real-time health monitoring systems through faster data transmission and enhanced connectivity, 6G will take this to a new level, enabling an entirely new era of connected healthcare. One of the key features of 6G networks will be their ability to support massive device connectivity, which will be crucial for deploying large-scale Internet of Medical Things (IoMT) systems. These systems will enable continuous monitoring of patients through interconnected devices—such as wearables, smart implants, and remote sensors—all transmitting large volumes of biomedical data in real-time. 6G networks will facilitate this by providing extremely high bandwidth and Ultra-Reliable Low-Latency Communication (URLLC), ensuring that critical health data can be transmitted instantaneously with minimal delay. This is particularly important for remote surgeries or telemedicine applications, where real-time data streaming is essential for patient safety and surgical precision. (Srinivasu et al., 2022)

The improved data throughput and reduced latency of 6G networks will also make it feasible to transmit high-resolution, complex medical images and live biomedical signals, such as EEG or ECG data, from remote locations to healthcare providers or specialists. This enhanced communication capacity will enable remote diagnosis, allowing patients in rural or underserved areas to access medical expertise without the need for travel. Moreover, 6G networks will integrate AI and ML into the network itself, providing intelligent routing of data, predictive maintenance of medical devices, and even real-time decision support for healthcare providers (Ahmad et al., 2023) . The low power consumption associated with 6G will be crucial for the efficient operation of wearable health devices, which rely on long battery life for continuous monitoring.

One of the most promising applications of 6G in healthcare will be the development of smart hospitals, which leverage advanced network capabilities for seamless integration across all hospital systems. These systems will include smart medical devices, patient tracking, and automated healthcare workflows—all interconnected via the 6G network to ensure optimal resource utilization, patient safety, and real-time communication among healthcare providers. For example, in a smart hospital, real-time processing of patient signals will enable immediate action and remote monitoring, while AI and ML algorithms in the network can predict patient needs, optimize bed management, and even improve medical equipment management. (Amer et al., 2023)

In addition, 6G networks will play a transformative role in enabling immersive healthcare applications such as augmented reality (AR) and virtual reality (VR) for telemedicine. With the ultra-low latency and high throughput capabilities of 6G, AR and VR will be able to provide more effective and interactive telehealth experiences, from remote surgeries to rehabilitation and patient education. For example, in remote surgeries, surgeons can use AR to overlay critical patient information or 3D imaging onto their field of view, improving precision and reducing the risk of errors. VR will also enhance telemedicine by providing virtual consultations where patients and doctors can interact in a highly immersive, 3D environment, enhancing communication and ensuring better patient engagement. In the realm of rehabilitation, patients can use VR for guided physical therapy sessions, allowing them to perform exercises in a controlled, virtual space while receiving real-time feedback from healthcare providers. The combination of 6G's capabilities with AR and VR in telemedicine will enable more complex and specialized healthcare applications that were previously impractical, offering a more immersive, efficient, and precise approach to remote healthcare. (Bhardwaj et al., 2022.)

Ultimately, the innovations in biomedical signal processing not only promise to improve patient outcomes but also to reduce healthcare costs, enhance patient satisfaction, and ensure a more efficient and equitable healthcare system. As these technologies evolve, they will continue to play a critical role in bridging the gap between technology and healthcare, driving the future of next-generation health solutions.

REFERENCES

Adebayo, T. S., Özkan, O., & Eweade, B. S. (2024). Do energy efficiency R&D investments and information and communication technologies promote environmental sustainability in Sweden? A quantile-on-quantile KRLS investigation. *Journal of Cleaner Production*, *440*, 140832. DOI: 10.1016/j.jclepro.2024.140832

Ahmad, H. F., Rafique, W., Rasool, R. U., Alhumam, A., Anwar, Z., & Qadir, J. (2023). Leveraging 6G, extended reality, and IoT big data analytics for healthcare: A review. *Computer Science Review*, *48*, 100558. DOI: 10.1016/j.cosrev.2023.100558

Amer, N. S., & Belhaouari, S. B. (2023). Eeg signal processing for medical diagnosis, healthcare, and monitoring: A comprehensive review. *IEEE Access : Practical Innovations, Open Solutions*, *11*, 143116–143142. DOI: 10.1109/ACCESS.2023.3341419

Anwer, S., Li, H., Antwi-Afari, M. F., Mirza, A. M., Rahman, M. A., Mehmood, I., Guo, R., & Wong, A. Y. L. (2024). Evaluation of data processing and artifact removal approaches used for physiological signals captured using wearable sensing devices during construction tasks. *Journal of Construction Engineering and Management*, *150*(1), 03123008. DOI: 10.1061/JCEMD4.COENG-13263

Arooj, A., Farooq, M. S., Akram, A., Iqbal, R., Sharma, A., & Dhiman, G. (2022). Big data processing and analysis in internet of vehicles: Architecture, taxonomy, and open research challenges. *Archives of Computational Methods in Engineering*, *29*(2), 793–829. DOI: 10.1007/s11831-021-09590-x

Ayerbe, E., Berecibar, M., Clark, S., Franco, A. A., & Ruhland, J. (2022). Digitalization of battery manufacturing: Current status, challenges, and opportunities. *Advanced Energy Materials*, *12*(17), 2102696. DOI: 10.1002/aenm.202102696

Bhardwaj, V., Joshi, R., & Gaur, A. M. (2022). IoT-based smart health monitoring system for COVID-19. *SN Computer Science*, *3*(2), 137. DOI: 10.1007/s42979-022-01015-1 PMID: 35079705

Bhatele, K. R., Gupta, V., Gupta, K., & Shrivastava, P. (2023). The fundamentals of biomedical image processing. In *Research Anthology on Improving Medical Imaging Techniques for Analysis and Intervention* (pp. 23–42). IGI Global.

Boyer, M., Bouyer, L., Roy, J. S., & Campeau-Lecours, A. (2023). Reducing noise, artifacts and interference in single-channel emg signals: A review. *Sensors (Basel)*, *23*(6), 2927. DOI: 10.3390/s23062927 PMID: 36991639

Chaddad, A., Wu, Y., Kateb, R., & Bouridane, A. (2023). Electroencephalography signal processing: A comprehensive review and analysis of methods and techniques. *Sensors (Basel)*, *23*(14), 6434. DOI: 10.3390/s23146434 PMID: 37514728

Chauhan, V., Negi, S., Jain, D., Singh, P., Sagar, A. K., & Sharma, A. K. (2022, April). Quantum computers: A review on how quantum computing can boom AI. In *2022 2nd International Conference on Advance Computing and Innovative Technologies in Engineering (ICACITE)* (pp. 559-563). IEEE. DOI: 10.1109/ICACITE53722.2022.9823619

Chidolue, O., & Iqbal, T. (2023, March). System monitoring and data logging using PLX-DAQ for solar-powered oil well pumping. In *2023 IEEE 13th Annual Computing and Communication Workshop and Conference (CCWC)* (pp. 0690-0694). IEEE. DOI: 10.1109/CCWC57344.2023.10099099

Dai, B., Gao, C., & Xie, Y. (2022). Flexible wearable devices for intelligent health monitoring. *VIEW*, *3*(5), 20220027. DOI: 10.1002/VIW.20220027

Iwamoto, K., Ochiai, T., Delcroix, M., Ikeshita, R., Sato, H., Araki, S., & Katagiri, S. (2022). How bad are artifacts?: Analyzing the impact of speech enhancement errors on ASR. *arXiv preprint arXiv:2201.06685*. DOI: 10.21437/Interspeech.2022-318

Jarial, R. K., Dubey, A., & Dubey, A. (2024). Real-Time Health Monitoring Using IoT Sensors. In *Advanced Research in Electronic Devices for Biomedical and mHealth* (pp. 181–211). Apple Academic Press.

Jin, K., Chai, H., Su, C., Yin, X., & Xiang, M. (2023). A novel adaptive nonlinear Kalman filter scheme for DVL-aided SINS alignment in underwater vehicles. *Signal Processing*, *209*, 109045. DOI: 10.1016/j.sigpro.2023.109045

Khang, A., Hahanov, V., Litvinova, E., Chumachenko, S., Avromovic, Z., İsmibeyli, R., & Anh, P. T. N. (2024). Medical and Biomedical Signal Processing and Prediction Using the EEG Machine and Electroencephalography. In *Computer Vision and AI-Integrated IoT Technologies in the Medical Ecosystem* (pp. 109–124). CRC Press. DOI: 10.1201/9781003429609-7

Krishnamoorthy, S., Dua, A., & Gupta, S. (2023). Role of emerging technologies in future IoT-driven Healthcare 4.0 technologies: A survey, current challenges and future directions. *Journal of Ambient Intelligence and Humanized Computing*, *14*(1), 361–407. DOI: 10.1007/s12652-021-03302-w

Kwon, H., An, S., Lee, H. Y., Cha, W. C., Kim, S., Cho, M., & Kong, H. J. (2022). Review of smart hospital services in real healthcare environments. *Healthcare Informatics Research*, *28*(1), 3–15. DOI: 10.4258/hir.2022.28.1.3 PMID: 35172086

Lu, S., Lu, J., An, K., Wang, X., & He, Q. (2023). Edge computing on IoT for machine signal processing and fault diagnosis: A review. *IEEE Internet of Things Journal*, *10*(13), 11093–11116. DOI: 10.1109/JIOT.2023.3239944

Lynch, J. P., Sohn, H., & Wang, M. L. (Eds.). (2022). *Sensor technologies for civil infrastructures: Volume 1: Sensing hardware and data collection methods for performance assessment*. Woodhead Publishing.

Ma, W., Zhu, L., & Zhang, R. (2023). Compressed sensing based channel estimation for movable antenna communications. *IEEE Communications Letters*, *27*(10), 2747–2751. DOI: 10.1109/LCOMM.2023.3310535

Mallow, G. M., Hornung, A., Barajas, J. N., Rudisill, S. S., An, H. S., & Samartzis, D. (2022). Quantum computing: The future of big data and artificial intelligence in spine. *Spine Surgery and Related Research*, *6*(2), 93–98. DOI: 10.22603/ssrr.2021-0251 PMID: 35478980

Olaleye, D. S., Oloye, A. C., Akinloye, A. O., & Akinwande, O. T. (2024). Advancing green communications: The role of radio frequency engineering in sustainable infrastructure design. *International Journal of Latest Technology in Engineering* [IJLTEMAS]. *Management & Applied Science*, *13*(5), 113.

Pachori, R. B. (2023). *Time-frequency analysis techniques and their applications*. CRC Press. DOI: 10.1201/9781003367987

Paganelli, A. I., Mondéjar, A. G., da Silva, A. C., Silva-Calpa, G., Teixeira, M. F., Carvalho, F., Raposo, A., & Endler, M. (2022). Real-time data analysis in health monitoring systems: A comprehensive systematic literature review. *Journal of Biomedical Informatics*, *127*, 104009. DOI: 10.1016/j.jbi.2022.104009 PMID: 35196579

Prieto-Avalos, G., Cruz-Ramos, N. A., Alor-Hernandez, G., Sánchez-Cervantes, J. L., Rodriguez-Mazahua, L., & Guarneros-Nolasco, L. R. (2022). Wearable devices for physical monitoring of heart: A review. *Biosensors (Basel)*, *12*(5), 292. DOI: 10.3390/bios12050292 PMID: 35624593

Rangayyan, R. M., & Krishnan, S. (2024). *Biomedical signal analysis*. John Wiley & Sons. DOI: 10.1002/9781119825883

Ranjan, R., Sahana, B. C., & Bhandari, A. K. (2022). Motion artifacts suppression from EEG signals using an adaptive signal denoising method. *IEEE Transactions on Instrumentation and Measurement*, *71*, 1–10. DOI: 10.1109/TIM.2022.3142037

Satpathy, S. K., Panda, S., Nagwanshi, K. K., Nayak, S. K., & Ardil, C. (2022). Adaptive non-linear filtering technique for image restoration. *arXiv preprint arXiv:2204.09302*.

Sekar, K., Devi, K. S., & Srinivasan, P. (2022). Compressed tensor completion: A robust technique for fast and efficient data reconstruction in wireless sensor networks. *IEEE Sensors Journal*, *22*(11), 10794–10807. DOI: 10.1109/JSEN.2022.3169226

Shaik, T., Tao, X., Higgins, N., Li, L., Gururajan, R., Zhou, X., & Acharya, U. R. (2023). Remote patient monitoring using artificial intelligence: Current state, applications, and challenges. *Wiley Interdisciplinary Reviews. Data Mining and Knowledge Discovery*, *13*(2), e1485. DOI: 10.1002/widm.1485

Srinivasu, P. N., Ijaz, M. F., Shafi, J., Woźniak, M., & Sujatha, R. (2022). 6G driven fast computational networking framework for healthcare applications. *IEEE Access : Practical Innovations, Open Solutions*, *10*, 94235–94248. DOI: 10.1109/ACCESS.2022.3203061

Tang, M., Nakamoto, C. H., Stern, A. D., & Mehrotra, A. (2022). Trends in remote patient monitoring use in traditional medicare. *JAMA Internal Medicine*, *182*(9), 1005–1006. DOI: 10.1001/jamainternmed.2022.3043 PMID: 35913710

Ukil, A., Marin, L., Mukhopadhyay, S. C., & Jara, A. J. (2022). AFSense-ECG: Atrial fibrillation condition sensing from single lead electrocardiogram (ECG) signals. *IEEE Sensors Journal*, *22*(12), 12269–12277. DOI: 10.1109/JSEN.2022.3162691

Vuojamo, V., Turunen, V., & Orelma, H. (2022). Time–frequency analysis in R n. *The Journal of Fourier Analysis and Applications*, *28*(1), 6. DOI: 10.1007/s00041-021-09894-3

Werner de Vargas, V., Schneider Aranda, J. A., dos Santos Costa, R., da Silva Pereira, P. R., & Victória Barbosa, J. L. (2023). Imbalanced data preprocessing techniques for machine learning: A systematic mapping study. *Knowledge and Information Systems*, *65*(1), 31–57. DOI: 10.1007/s10115-022-01772-8 PMID: 36405957

Xiong, L., Li, S., Tang, G., & Strobl, J. (2022). Geomorphometry and terrain analysis: Data, methods, platforms and applications. *Earth-Science Reviews*, *233*, 104191. DOI: 10.1016/j.earscirev.2022.104191

Zhang, X. D. (2022). *Modern signal processing*. Walter de Gruyter GmbH & Co KG. DOI: 10.1515/9783110475562

Chapter 4

Advancements and Emerging Trends in Deep Learning–Based Transformers for Medical Image Processing

Uzair Aslam Bhatti
https://orcid.org/0000-0002-8743-2783
School of Information and Communication Engineering, Hainan University, China

Muhammad Aamir
College of Computer Science and Artificial Intelligence, Huanggang Normal University, China

Zia Ur Rehman
https://orcid.org/0000-0001-8233-567X
College of Computer Science and Artificial Intelligence, Huangguang Normal University, China

Jameel Ahmed Bhutto
https://orcid.org/0000-0003-4896-7205
College of Computer Science and Artificial Intelligence, Huangguang Normal University, China

Mughair Aslam Bhatti
Department of Robotics and Artificial Intelligence, SZABIST, Pakistan

Ahsan Ahmad Nizamani
Central South University, Changsha, China

Abdul Haseeb Nizamani
Central South University, Changsha, China

ABSTRACT

The U-net Architecture is a U-shaped neural network developed from Fully Convolutional Networks FCNs in medical image segmentation. However, the traditional Convolutional Neural Networks (CNNs), like the one in U-Net, poses challenges in addressing long-distance relationships relating to the subject matter hence making their applicability to several segmentation tasks somewhat restrained. To counteract this, extending Transformer modules into U-shaped designs has received considerable interest, as an approach to boosting feature extraction and segmentation effectiveness. This paper also presents an extensive analysis of U-Net and Transformer-related methods and sorts medical image segmentation models based on the position of the Transformer modules.

DOI: 10.4018/979-8-3693-9816-6.ch004

1. INTRODUCTION

It discusses that deep learning has brought significant changes in feature learning by allowing the neural network models to identify representations by its own. In this article, I consider this capability, which has been enhanced through the incorporation of gradient descent, as a catalyst for progress in a range of domains (Alhatami et al., 2024; Ali et al., 2023; Andrade-Miranda et al., 2023). In the field of computer vision, Convolutional Neural Networks (CNNs) have performed quite well, that they have become deeper in order to solve more challenging problems. The fully convolutional U-shaped network U-Net provided skip connections during down-sampling to recreate low feature detail while simultaneously acquiring global features, dramatically enhancing the segmentation efficiency. Since the success of U-Net, it became the base for medical image segmentation and it has finally inspired several derivatives tailored for specific medical applications(Asif et al., 2024a; Asif et al., 2024b;).

However, due to the intrinsic inductive bias of CNNs they are unable to model long range dependencies effectively thus hampering the performance of segmentation. This is a limitation that transformers, with their self-attention mechanism, do not have to overcome as they guard against long-range relationships. The Vision Transformer (ViT) continued the use of Transformer for computer vision by treating an image as a set of patches and processing patch tokens as sequences as in Natural Language Processing (NLP). In the following models like SETR and DETR, the role and possibility of using Transformers in vision tasks like segmentation and object detection were established(Azad et al., 2023; Bhatti et al., 2024; Bhatti et al., 2024;).

However, there are still some problems in employing Transformers for medical image segmentation, which are annotation challenges, highly imbalanced classes, low contrast, and less distinct boundaries in medical images. A small number of medical data also affects the quality of pre-training strategies for the Transformer models in this area. Therefore, it is crucial to find new solutions to apply Transformers in medical imaging(Bhatti et al., 2023; Bhatti et al., 2024).

Transformer has recently emerged as an innovative component for medical image segmentation within the U-shaped network topology; this paper systematically discusses the architectural features and design options for this model(Gao et al., 2024; Han et al., 2024;). We examine the strong and weak points of Transformer-based U-Net models, discuss how Transformer-based models can overcome the shortcomings of U-Net, and provide information about the use of Transformer-based U-Net for medical image processing tasks. Moreover, this paper present future direction towards the advancement of these hybrid model to revolutionize the medical image segmentation.

2. MEDICAL IMAGE SEGMENTATION

Medical image segmentation, a vital task in computer vision, focuses on pixel-level classification to precisely delineate target objects within medical images. These datasets are typically derived from advanced imaging modalities like MRI, CT, and ultrasound (Azad et al., 2023; Bhatti et al., 2024a). Traditional segmentation methods, such as thresholding, region-growing, and edge-detection techniques, offer simplicity and low hardware requirements but often depend heavily on manual tuning to achieve high-quality feature representation. In contrast, deep learning-based segmentation models automate feature learning with minimal manual input, delivering superior performance at the cost of significant computational resources for training(Bhatti et al., 2024b; Bhatti et al., 2023a; Bhatti et al., 2024c; Bhatti et al., 2024d; Bhatti et al., 2023b).

With advancements in GPU technology and memory capacity, training complex deep learning networks has become more accessible, driving their adoption in diverse applications, including medical image analysis. CNN-based segmentation models have been extensively used for tasks such as tumor detection, skin lesion analysis, and retinal vessel segmentation. Among these, U-Net has emerged as a cornerstone in medical image segmentation, particularly in computer-aided diagnosis and intelligent medical systems. U-Net's design, featuring skip connections to combine low-level and high-level features, has demonstrated significant success across various medical domains (Bhatti et al., 2023c; Bhatti et al., 2024e).

Despite their strengths, CNNs face inherent limitations, including difficulty capturing long-range dependencies and a reliance on fixed-size convolution kernels, which restrict their generalizability. Additionally, the unique challenges of medical images, such as fuzzy boundaries, low contrast, and varying target sizes, demand effective extraction of global contextual information (Bhatti et al., 2024f; Bhatti, Tang, & Wu, 2023). The introduction of Transformers, leveraging a self-attention mechanism originally developed for NLP, addresses these challenges by enabling models to capture long-range dependencies and global context. This capability has driven the adaptation of Transformer-based architectures to medical image segmentation, opening new avenues for improved accuracy and robustness. This paper explores the evolution of segmentation techniques, emphasizing the transition from traditional methods to CNN-based approaches and the recent integration of Transformer models. We highlight the strengths and limitations of each paradigm, focusing on the role of U-Net and its Transformer-enhanced variants in overcoming the challenges of medical image segmentation.

3. U-SHAPED NETWORK

Medical image segmentation is one of the essential and challenging tasks in the medical field, further comprehensive identification and definition of the anatomical structures and pathological change from different medical imaging modalities as MRI, CT, and ultrasound (Bristi et al., 2023; Cao et al., 2023; Chen et al., 2023a). The U-Net architecture have turned out to be the perfect solution due to its unique design which make it perfect in capturing details and the bigger picture in an image. Basic U-Net structure is shown in Figure. 1.

Figure 1. U-Net architecture

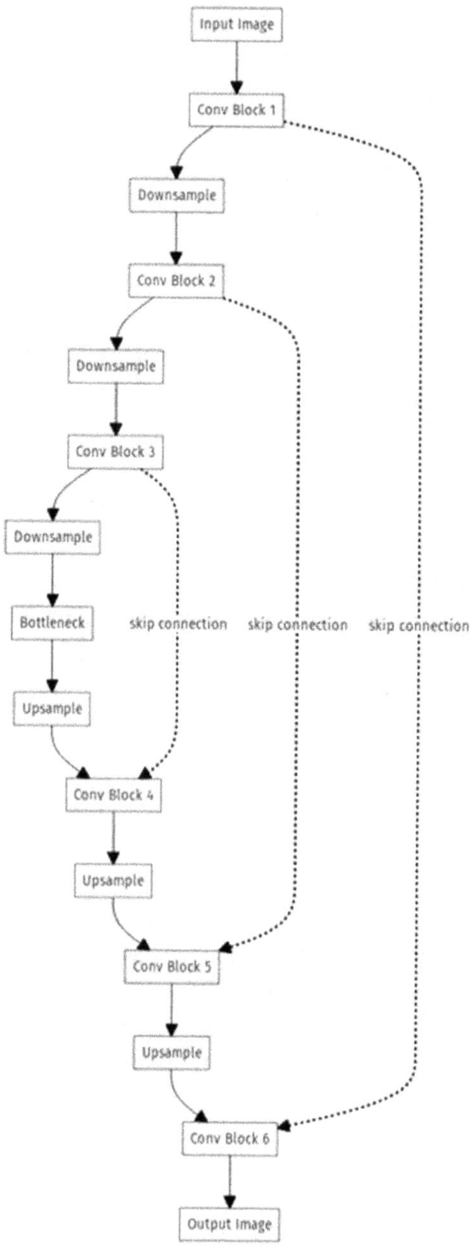

A U-shaped Network (U-Net) architecture is commonly visualized as follows:
Components:

1. Encoder (Contraction Path):
   - Series of convolutional layers followed by pooling layers.
   - Extracts features while reducing spatial dimensions (downsampling).

    - Captures the high-level context of the image.
2. Bottleneck:
    - The central part of the U-Net where features are processed at the lowest resolution.
    - Often consists of convolutional layers without pooling.
3. Decoder (Expansion Path):
    - Series of upsampling layers followed by convolutional layers.
    - Reconstructs the image resolution while refining segmentation details.
4. Skip Connections:
    - Directly connect corresponding layers in the encoder and decoder.
    - Preserve spatial information and fine details lost during downsampling.

a. Implementation of U-Net and Its Variants for 2D Applications

For multi-scale feature fusion, U-Net introduces encoder-decoder architecture, containing down-sampling for feature extraction, up-sampling to backing up for the missing information and skip connections. This integration enhances the ability of the model to include local and global features into consideration, making convergence to an optimum to be faster and an accuracy of medical image segmentation tasks to be higher(Chen et al., 2024; Chen, Lu, & Xie, 2023).

Since the introduction of U-Net, several modifications have been made based on the same. For example, U-Net++ introduced a concept of decreasing the difference in the feature maps of the encoder section and the decoder section. It achieves this by first introducing intermediate dense skip pathways through which the network can enhance the integration of the feature maps(Chen et al., 2023b; Cheng et al., 2023). This change makes the process of transition between different resolution levels more consistent, therefore provides better accuracy of the segmentation.

Another evolution to this is ResUNet which substitute the traditional convolutional layers of U-Net with residual blocks of ResNet. These residual connections resolve the vanishing gradient issue allowing the architecture to extend compatible with deeper networks without compromising a lot of performance(Cheng, Tang, Bhatti, & Li, 2024; Dong et al., 2023; Fahim, Fadil, & Bhatti, 2023; Fu et al., 2024). Building upon this, ResUNet++ includes Squeeze-and-Extraction (SE) Blocks after each residual block. These SE Blocks essentially use channel attention mechanisms which discard unwanted incoming features to the decoder. It improves the effectiveness of recombined multi-scale feature maps compared with the single-time concatenation procedure in the standard U-Net(Gao et al., 2024; Han et al., 2024a).

These improvements have ensured that U-Net and numerous derivatives are now vital resources in applications such as tumor detection, organ segmentation, and lesion delineation, where accuracy and speed are critical.

b. Application of U-net and its variants in 3D formulate

In 3D image segmentation, U-shaped networks have been extended to deal with volume data to overcome difficulties of 3D imaging modalities as MRI or CT scans. V-Net is one of the most well-known 3D adaptations as the authors remove 2D convolutional layers and apply the 3D convolutions to process the volume data. This is especially important for an accurate segmentation because this approach includes spatial dependencies in all three dimensions. Since there may be a considerable difference in the number of foreground and background classes typical for medical imaging, the authors of V-Net utilize Dice loss to improve the outcomes of segmentation(Han et al., 2024b; Hasnain et al., 2024a; Hasnain et al., 2024b).

Equally, 3D U-Net extends the original U-Net architecture by replacing the 2D operations with the 3D ones. This Flex offers high criterion and elastic characteristics fit well for semi-automatic and fully automatic feature a-segmentation as well. The application of 3D convolutions makes it possible for the network to get important representations from volumetric data and obtain a comprehensive understanding of the interior structures of the human body from the medical images (He & Bhatti, 2024; He et al., 2023a; He, Gou, & Wu, 2023; He et al., 2023b; He et al., 2023c; Huang et al., 2023a).

Its subsequent advancement, named nnU-Net, builds on that and states that data handling – preparation, normalization, denormalization, and specification of hyperparameters – is of equal significance to the deep learning algorithm. Due to a thorough optimization of each of these aspects related to particular datasets and tasks, nnU-Net has achieved a high level of segmentation accuracy with great efficiency, and these findings prove that a more general strategy goes beyond the architecture of the network(Huang et al., 2024a; Huang et al., 2024b; Joysoyal et al., 2024; Lei et al., 2023; Li & Bhatti, 2024; Li et al., 2023a). These 3D adaptations were originally developed and used for medical applications, but have since found their way into other industries including environment and geography. The ability to deal with 3D data has cemented the applications for U-shaped networks across a broad spectrum of use, guaranteeing its applications and value.

4. TRANSFORMER

Fusion of Transformer-based architectures on to U-shaped networks has been a paradigm shift for medical image segmentation, where Transformers excel at global dependency modeling, while U-Net excelled at hierarchical feature modeling(Li et al., 2024; Li et al., 2023b; Liang et al., 2023; Lin et al., 2023; Liu et al., 2023a; Liu, Feng, Huang, & Bhatti, 2024). These hybrid architectures making use of the Transformer's self-attention mechanism successfully incorporate both long-range dependencies and local context information, thus achieving superior segmentation accuracy in even hard tasks.

Figure 2. Transformers functioning according to need

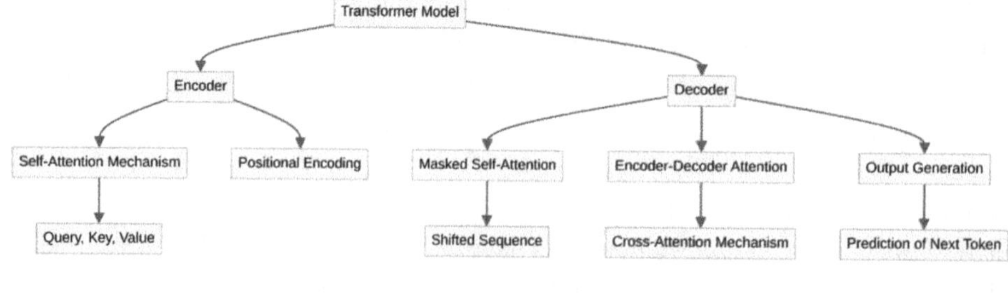

a. Transformer as Encoder:

In case of a U-shaped network architecture, encoder component can be deemed worthy to extract the required features. Putting the Transformer in the encoder takes advantage of this self-attention to attain dependencies from the low resolution input image, in addition to hierarchical feature extraction which is familiar to convolution operations in convolutional neural networks.

TransUNet

Proposed by Chen et al in 2021, TransUNet is the first work in the Transformer U-shaped network domain, which focuses on medical image segmentation. The technique involves downsampling of image patches within the encoder and serially feeding them through conventional transformer blocks(Liu, Kaul, & Wang, 2023; Liu et al., 2023b; Liu et al., 2024; Luo et al., 2023; Nawaz et al., 2024a). This architecture takes advantage of the Transformer in understanding long-range relationships and enhancing segmentation performance, particularly for the feature map rate at which the SeedNet fails due to low resolution(Nawaz et al., 2024b; Nawaz et al., 2024c; Nawaz et al., 2024d; Nawaz et al., 2023). However, in the case of TransUNet we are experiencing large fixed size block sizes and high attention computation which could be optimized in the following way.

MedT

To overcome the issues related to the size of the dataset, the positioning embeddings of MedT have a gate mechanism included. This mechanism helps generalization ability of the model and makes it a good solution for various medical imaging tasks.

X-Net

X-Net is a dual-encoder-decoder network and the primary segmentation encoder is designed using the Transformers. Further, an auxiliary encoder-decoder based on the convolution performs image reconstruction as the proxy task thus enhancing the feature representation in the Transformer-based encoder(Nizamani et al., 2023; Noor et al., 2024; Pang et al., 2023; Peng et al., 2024a). This dual structure improves the capacity of the network to learn features relevant to its meaningful utilization.

LeViT-UNet

LeViT Vision Transformer is lightweight and fast and when deployed in the encoder portion of the LeViT-UNet model, bent on delivering high segmentation precision with relative low computational cost. It has been exceptionally good on Synapse data set, where it has been placed among the best models based on speed and accuracy(Peng et al., 2024b; Pham et al., 2024; Pu et al., 2024).

TransFuse

BiFusion Block connects CNNs and Transformers in TransFuse and combines their beneficial feature extraction abilities. It further uses a pre-trained model, the DeiT (Data-Efficient Image Transformer), to achieve parameter efficiency without a compromise on feature extraction capability.

Swin UNETR

This model is based on Swin Transformer trained with contrastive learning and random augmentation tasks on large scale CT dataset. Swin UNETR demonstrate the superiority of the pre-training strategy before fine-tuning for 3D medical image segmentation tasks since pre-training on non-target datasets(Reja et al., 2023; Roy et al., 2023; Shao et al., 2024).

b. Transformer in the Decoder Only

Limited use of the Transformer only in the decoder is aimed at enhancing the utilization of the features extracted by encoder.

Segtran

The compressed and expanded attention modules of Segtran are derived from the Set Transformer ISAB (Induced Squeezed Attention Block). The first decreases the effort to compute attention, whereas the second, based on single-head Transformers, improves feature differentiation(Sun et al., 2023; Sun et al., 2024; Tang et al., 2024a). The semantic and the local continuity is also addressed in Segtran with the help of a learnable sine positional encoding.

This architecture brings performance gain in the second stage of segmentation which is decoding stage because high semantic and fine-grained details are important at this step.

c. Transformer in Both the Encoder and the Decoder

Training the Transformers both in the encoder and in the decoder can allow for the capturing of global context during the feature extraction phase and of further improving it during the reconstruction phase. But this endangers a huge number of retrievals to be made in many cases and often entails a vast amount of computational work.

nnFormer

nnFormer combines CNN and Transformer layers in its encoder and decoder systems in a theoretical way. Multi-scale supervision applied in it make sure that the features of the resolutions are precise. Since ImageNet pre-trained Transformer modules are utilized, the computation burden is reduced while segmentations are made more accurate in this manner(Tang et al., 2024b; Wang et al., 2023; Wu et al., 2023a).

D-Former

D-Former integrates dilated convolution with Transformer modules, which it incorporates local and global context in its architecture. On datasets similar to Synapse, this approach thus reached rather competitive performance while providing a correct segmentation of the input image(Wu et al., 2023b; Xu et al., 2024a; Xu et al., 2023a).

MISSFormer

The Medical Image Segmentation Transformer (MISSFormer) alleviates the problem of sequence length in the attention mechanism through matrix compaction of K and V. There is an emergence of a new skip connection known as the enhanced transformer context bridge that allows proper incorporation of low and high-frequency features. MISSFormer performs all the multi-organ segmentation tasks with relatively less amount of time compared to Swin UNet, though it yields a high level of accuracy(Xu et al., 2023b; Xu et al., 2023c; Yan et al., 2023).

MT Net

Reminder: MT Net effectively use external attention mechanisms for capturing inter-sample relationships and greatly enhancing the performance of segmentation.

PCAT-UNet

In PCAT-UNet, we incorporate convolutional self-attention within and between patches, to achieve a good compromise between global and local features.

d. Transitional Connections

In turn, connecting transformers to each other provides an opportunity to learn global relations from low-resolution feature maps at transitional connections between the encoder and decoder(Yang et al., 2024a; Yang et al., 2023a; Yang et al., 2024b; Yu et al., 2024; Yuan et al., 2023a; Zhang et al., 2024a).

UCATR

UCATR augments the classic Transformer architecture into the bottleneck stage of the U-Net for the extraction of global context from low-resolution images. skip connections, cross-attention mechanisms improve the segmentation quality by paying attention to important features.

TransBTS

The TransBTS family brings Transformers at the transition level. TransBTSv2 increases the dimensions of the feature space, and has a better parameterization of attention calculation and richer features than those in multiple stacking Transformers.

MS-TransUNet++

To cut the costs of the attention calculation, this model applies depth-wise convolutions, additionally, multiple skip connections help in feature recovery and accuracy of the segmentation.

e. Transformer in Skip Connections

Features related to skip connections can improve the integration of multi-modal features based on transformers situated in these connections. Transformers can better align two feature maps to improve fusion, and skip connections directly connect the encoder and decoder.

HTNet

HTNet incorporates Transformer modules into skip connections features deep and complex mechanisms known as RAPP (Residual Atrous Spatial Pyramid Pooling) as well as HCA (Hierarchical Context Attention). These modules improve the multi-scale contextual awareness for segmentation and global pixel interaction, further improving the segmentation result.

f. Transformer in the Output Block

The transformers in the output block further enhance the extremely local, highly detailed segmentation map.

RTNet

For DR segmentation, RTNet utilizes a Relation Transformer in the attention module to identify lesion-vascular relationships . Although being quite effective, addressing this issue resulted in the utilization of multiple attention modules that greatly increase the computational complexity of SWiMNet.

As has been noted in most Transformer-based U-shaped segmentation networks, the Transformer is commonly placed in the encoder section. This preference is justified by the Transformer's ability to target contextual relations which are essential for feature representation. Whereas incorporating Transformers in the decoder helps in feature reconstruction, this positioning cannot achieve optimal usage of the model's global dependencies(Zhang et al., 2024b). By applying Transformers at transitional stages or within the skip connections, there is the optimum of efficiency and performance. Transitional connections facilitate in capturing global relationships with low computational use because features maps are coarser. In the same manner, the addition of Transformers in skip connections provides better correspondence of encoder and decoder features for efficient feature integration. Depending on the task at hand then the appropriate position of the Transformer should be applied. Essentially, it is suggested to place the Transformer in the encoder for activities where fine-grained feature extraction is needed. Furthermore, feature integration is better achieved by using the Transformer in the decoder or skip connections for the tasks. There are future works that could be employed to employ the advantages of the transformer with lighter attention modules but the computational cost will be cheaper(Zhang et al., 2024c).

5. SEGMENTATION DATASETS

From the table 1, several datasets can be deduced to form a rich base upon which segmentation models can be enhanced especially in medical imaging and other areas. These datasets are designed to meet these requirements in a variety of applications such as organ segmentation, disease diagnosis and histology. For example, the BCV and The Segmentation Decathlon datasets include multi-organ segmentation tasks, which allow one to create models for a very wide range of problems. BraTS, TNBC, and LiTS datasets are Limited diseases such as brain tumor disease, new breast cancer, and liver tumor respectively, promote precision diagnostic accuracy and treatment methodologies(Zhang et al., 2024d). In histopathology applications such as GLAS and PanNuke, extracting Gland and nucleus is vital in cancer investigation. Also, retinal imaging datasets such as renew, drive, stare, chase_db1 are for the segmentation of the blood vessels and lesions that are essential for diabetic retinopathy analysis. Additional segmentation tasks including dermatological and gastrointestinal are also accomplished through

ISIC and Kvasir that concern themselves with melanoma and polyp classifying, respectively. Altogether, these datasets stress the significance of domain-dependent resources to establish and assess state-of-the-art segmentation models which has an extensive impact not only in the health care field but in a number of other domains too.

Table 1. Datasets of segmentation

Dataset	Focus Area	Modality	Applications	Notes
BCV (Beyond the Cranial Vault)	Multi-organ segmentation	CT	Abdominal organ segmentation.	Commonly used for evaluating segmentation in abdominal regions.
ACDC (Automated Cardiac Diagnosis Challenge)	Cardiac segmentation	MRI	Left and right ventricular segmentation, myocardium delineation.	Focuses on cardiac MRI analysis.
Brain US	Brain lesion and structure segmentation	Ultrasound	Detecting lesions and anatomical features in the brain.	Useful in analyzing brain conditions via ultrasound imaging.
GLAS (Gland Segmentation)	Colon histology segmentation	Histopathology	Gland segmentation in colon histology images.	A benchmark for histopathological gland analysis.
DSB18 (2018 Data Science Bowl)	Nucleus segmentation	Microscopy	Nucleus segmentation in diverse cellular images.	Benchmark for cellular and nuclei segmentation.
TNBC (Triple Negative Breast Cancer)	Breast cancer segmentation	Histopathology	Detection and segmentation of regions with triple-negative breast cancer.	Focused on aggressive cancer types.
BraTS (Brain Tumor Segmentation)	Brain tumor segmentation	MRI	Segmentation of low-grade and high-grade gliomas.	Widely used for glioma analysis and treatment planning.

6. MAMBA BASED SEGMENTATION

Mamba-based segmentation is a process that moves beyond the simple usage of the Mamba formula into today's method of deep learning(Aamir et al., 2018a). The Mamba algorithm, that originated from the morphological image processing, is effective for segmenting objects regarding geometric and structural features, and thus is most effective where the contact boundaries are most significant. This segmentation methodology is particularly outstanding in the analysis of those complex images that may have indefinite structures and unusual shapes; this is through the use of morphological operators including dilation, erosion, opening and closing to improve on the form and contours of objects. When incorporated into these deep learning platforms, operations developed with Mamba for segmentation will effectively link older image processing methods and more sophisticated neural network techniques(Aamir et al., 2019a; Aamir et al., 2018b).

Precisely, the use of Mamba-based segmentation has been well implemented in the application of medical imaging whereby precise boundary detection is crucial. For example, in tumor segmentation, the method improves the opportunity of precise detail on the edge of the tumor, which is important for diagnostic and therapeutic purposes. When combined with CNNs or Transformer structures, Mamba-based segmentation can also perform global and local contextual analysis while maintaining the structural coherence of segmented regions. Moreover, its capability to combine with many a prior/pre- and post-processing methods like denosing or edge detection makes it desirable in complex imaging conditions.(Aamir et al., 2017a; Aamir et al., 2019b; Guan et al., 2021a; Guan et al., 2021b; Guan et al., 2021c)

Borrowing aspects of Mamba into U-shaped architectures such as U-Net or its derivatives adds morphological constancy to the architecture and brings improvements in segmentation using more forgivable boundaries. This is especially beneficial in large or more varied data sets especially for histopathology or multi-organ CT scans. Further, derived Mamba-based segmentation is much faster, if not real-time, it makes it possible to be used in applications such as surgical navigation or even automated diagnostic platforms. These features, in combination with the perfect ability to work in the multi-scale feature extraction make this method a perspective tool in the image segmentation(Aamir et al., 2023c; Aamir et al., 2019c; Guan et al., 2021d; Aamir et al., 2019d; Aamir et al., 2018c).

7. CHALLENGES AND PROSPECTS

7.1 Challenges

Transformers have been found to give excellent results in those applications where there are long dependency models. However, using them in medical image segmentation introduces certain difficulties that are based on the nature of the medical datasets and the complexity of the Transformers(Aamir et al., 2019e; Aamir et al., 2018d; Aamir et al., 2019f). These problems are significant to solve for deployment in medical imaging tasks, as indicated below.

1. Small Medical Image Datasets

The first is the lack of big annotated medical image datasets which are available for whatever ai is going to be trained on. Putting labels in the medical image also demands a lot of effort, takes a lot of time and is very expensive. This limitation is quite limiting since it limits the number of large datasets which are required for training of deep learning models. Transformers, especially, benefit greatly from large sample sizes since self-attention is used to effectively capture global dependencies. So, when we do not have wide and extensive sets of data, we then risk developing models that over-fit, thus may not be portable and efficient in other contexts (Guan et al., 2021e; Aamir et al., 2023d; Guan et al., 2021f). This issue requires the use of approaches like transfer learning or semi-supervised learning, or unsupervised learning to leverage small sample size.

2. Many images during diagnosis or treatment need high quality and, therefore, high resolution.

These medical images usually have high resolutions to provide clear images of the internal human anatomy particularly when distal limb parts are involved since they are used in diagnosis and planning processes in treatment. Actually conceived for natural language processing tasks, images should be serialized into sequences before being processed for Transformers. Owing to approaches like Vision Transformer (ViT) where images are transformed into patches, high-resolution medical images are seen as long sequences. These long sequences greatly enhance computational and memory requirements, because the computational cost of self-attention is proportional to the square of the sequence length. This challenge hinders the scalability of Transformers for medical imaging, especially for real-time learning, and so the hypothesis inspires the need to research better attention mechanisms.

3. Another factor responsible for poor health among women is that most of the women lack position information.

Positional information is critical in medical image segmentation because structures depend on the surrounding space. Specifically, while convolution based architectures such as convolutional neural networks CNNs have inherent positional relationships given by the local receptive fields, the base Transformer architecture described here does not. To overcome this, positional embeddings are incorporated within the input sequences to ensure that the model understands spatial relation. However, these embeddings are specific to the given dataset, and can be sensitive to the imaging modality. This variability, when coupled with other factors, can result in suboptimal performance which underlines the requirement for the creation of far more structurally invariant and generally applicable approaches to encoding positional information.

4. Specially, the self-attention mechanism only performs within patch calculation.

Since it is computationally expensive, stand-alone pixel-wise attention is generally not used, and attention is usually calculated between patches of images. Though this patch-based approach help to reduce computational load the drawback is that it loses the ability to model the fine-grained intra-patch relationship in the image as demonstrated in the ViT architecture. This drawback is especially intriguing for medical image segmentation since often, microaneurysms or other subtle structures may need pixel distinctions, whereas tumor edges are typically thin. Failing to account for such relations results in imprecise definition of small structures, or even loss of the boundaries, which directly impacts segmentation success. To this end, there remains a need for better approximations to fully recover the original pixels by using fully fledged hybrid models/ attention mechanisms/ or some refined kernel that can provide both faster convergence rate and accurate pixel by pixel estimation.

7.2 Prospects

Building on the advancements in hybrid networks combining Transformers and U-shaped architectures, several promising research directions and future prospects are outlined:

- Semi-Supervised and Unsupervised Learning: To meeting the scarcity of labeled data in medical imaging, Transformers can be used to obtain global representations from large-scale data by solving auxiliary tasks. Besides, it is possible to improve classification performance and generalization in the case of semi-supervised or unsupervised training through obtaining high-confidence pseudo-labels.

- Integration of Prior Knowledge: It is possible to incorporate the knowledge about shapes and positional priors that would allow the model to concentrate on important features while avoiding multiple fittings of essentially the same thing. This might entail the use of anatomical priors for more accurate representation of structural relationships into designs for better performance for medical image segmentation.
- Multimodal Image Fusion: In this way, features from one imaging modality can be complemented with information of features from another imaging modality. For example, the integration of T1-weighted MRI for the structural information visualization, while T2-weighted MRI for the lesion location can produce a better and more accurate segmentation.
- Optimized Sampling Methods: Standard subsampling and up-sampling in U-shaped network tend to discard useful high frequency information and create duplicate information. Enhancing better advanced sample methods within the deliberation procedure can monetarily assist in maintaining a richness of noteworthy aspects while simultaneously subduing model intricacy, thereby greatly enhancing model accuracy as well as computational speed.

The outlined research directions emphasize potential future improvements in terms of the design and performance of additional networks with U-shaped structures constructed on the basis of hybrid Transformers to produce promising and clinically beneficial medical image segmentation outcomes.

8. CONCLUSION

The transformers have become a workhorse in deep learning proving their merit in capturing the global context through attention mechanism. This strength is particularly useful in medical image segmentation as dispersed target regions and variability in anatomical shapes are difficult to handle. In contrast to CNNs who make use of local receptive fields and have difficulties capturing long-term dependencies, transformers are designed to learn relation between each point in the image and any other and therefore produce highly accurate and consistent segmentation in cases for which it is challenging.

However, when applied to medical image segmentation, Transformers have main challenges that are as follows: A main limitation is the need to train on large data sets because the self-attention operates on high dimensional space that demands large data for generalization. The key problem with medical image datasets is that they are usually relatively small because of the time and expense associated with annotation. This lack of data hinders transformers from fully exploiting their potential and capacity hence resulting to suboptimalized solutions in the course of solving a problem.

To this end, combining Transformers with U-shaped networks can be seen as moderate solution. U-shaped architectures which we describe in the case of U-Net networks are good at capturing complicated dependencies on local spatial scales due to their encoder-decoder design and skip connections. By combining U-shaped networks with Transformer modules, the resulting hybrid models can harness the strengths of both approaches: the global context modeling of Transformers and the local feature extraction of U-shaped networks. This integration helps to improve the given model concerning the case of proper segmentation where both the big picture and intricate details are critical.

In this paper, we have proposed Transformer-based U-shaped networks and have divided them based on positions of Transformer modules in a network. For example, integration of the Transformer in the encoder captures global relations while integrating it in the decoder attentively reconstructs the segmentation maps with context information. Hybrid designs that incorporate Transformers within the encoder, such as TransUNet, and in the decoder, like MISSFormer, indicate the benefits of such approaches. These models indicate enhanced performance on tasks including the multi-organ segmentation and lesion detection on seldom huge datasets. This paper has presented and analyzed networks and synthesizes the change that may be expected when integrating U-shaped networks with Transformers. They also surpass the drawbacks that originate from each of the arbitrary structures and unveil aspects for further advancement of medical image segmentations. This capacity towards modelling both global and local details makes the Transformer based U-shaped network a path for future investigation and has potential to revolutionise medical imaging diagnostics by enhancing its efficiency.

REFERENCES

Aamir, M., Bazai, S., Bhatti, U. A., Dayo, Z. A., Liu, J., & Zhang, K. (2023). Applications of machine learning in medicine: Current trends and prospects. *2023 Global Conference on Wireless and Optical Technologies (GCWOT)*, 1-4. DOI: 10.1109/GCWOT57803.2023.10064665

Aamir, M., Pu, Y. F., Abro, W. A., Naeem, H., & Rahman, Z. (2017). A hybrid approach for object proposal generation. In *International Conference on Sensing and Imaging* (pp. 251-259). Springer. DOI: 10.1007/978-3-319-91659-0_18

Aamir, M., Pu, Y. F., Rahman, Z., Abro, W. A., Naeem, H., Ullah, F., & Badr, A. M. (2018). A hybrid proposed framework for object detection and classification. *Journal of Information Processing Systems, 14*(5), 1176–1194. DOI: 10.3745/JIPS.02.0095

Aamir, M., Pu, Y. F., Rahman, Z., Tahir, M., Naeem, H., & Dai, Q. (2018). A framework for automatic building detection from low-contrast satellite images. *Symmetry, 11*(1), 3. DOI: 10.3390/sym11010003

Aamir, M., Rahman, Z., Abro, W. A., Bhatti, U. A., Dayo, Z. A., & Ishfaq, M. (2023). Brain tumor classification utilizing deep features derived from high-quality regions in MRI images. *Biomedical Signal Processing and Control, 85*, 104988. DOI: 10.1016/j.bspc.2023.104988

Aamir, M., Rahman, Z., Abro, W. A., Bhatti, U. A., Dayo, Z. A., & Ishfaq, M. (2023). A progressive approach to generic object detection: A two-stage framework for image recognition. *Computers, Materials & Continua, 75*(3), 6351–6373. Advance online publication. DOI: 10.32604/cmc.2023.038173

Aamir, M., Rahman, Z., Abro, W. A., Tahir, M., & Ahmed, S. M. (2019). An optimized architecture of image classification using convolutional neural network. International Journal of Image. *Graphics and Signal Processing, 10*(10), 30–39. DOI: 10.5815/ijigsp.2019.10.05

Aamir, M., Rahman, Z., Dayo, Z. A., Abro, W. A., Uddin, M. I., Khan, I., Imran, A. S., Ali, Z., Ishfaq, M., Guan, Y., & Hu, Z. (2022). A deep learning approach for brain tumor classification using MRI images. *Computers & Electrical Engineering, 101*, 108105. DOI: 10.1016/j.compeleceng.2022.108105

Aamir, M., Rahman, Z., Pu, Y. F., Abro, W. A., & Gulzar, K. (2019). Satellite image enhancement using wavelet-domain based on singular value decomposition. *International Journal of Advanced Computer Science and Applications, 10*(6). Advance online publication. DOI: 10.14569/IJACSA.2019.0100667

Aamir, M., Rehman, Z., Pu, Y. F., Ahmed, A., & Abro, W. A. (2019). Image enhancement in varying light conditions based on wavelet transform. In 2019 16th International Computer Conference on Wavelet Active Media Technology and Information Processing (pp. 317-322). Chengdu, China. DOI: 10.1109/ICCWAMTIP47768.2019.9067714

Alhatami, E., & Bhatti, U. A. (2024). Advanced fuzzy denoising technique for agricultural remote sensing: Modified partition filter for suppressing impulsive. *IEEE Access : Practical Innovations, Open Solutions, 12*, 159025–159035. DOI: 10.1109/ACCESS.2024.3447704

Ali, A., Li, J., Chen, H., Bhatti, U. A., & Khan, A. (2023). Real-time spammers detection based on metadata features with machine learning. *Intelligent Automation & Soft Computing, 38*(3), 241–258. DOI: 10.32604/iasc.2023.041645

Andrade-Miranda, G., Jaouen, V., Tankyevych, O., Cheze Le Rest, C., Visvikis, D., & Conze, P.-H. (2023). Multi-modal medical transformers: A meta-analysis for medical image segmentation in oncology. *Computerized Medical Imaging and Graphics*, *104*, 101854. DOI: 10.1016/j.compmedimag.2023.102308 PMID: 37918328

Asif, M., Li, J. Q., Zia, M. A., Hashim, M., Bhatti, U. A., Bhatti, M. A., & Hasnain, A. (2024). Environmental sustainability in BRICS economies: The nexus of technology innovation, economic growth, financial development, and renewable energy consumption. *Sustainability (Basel)*, *16*(16), 6934. DOI: 10.3390/su16166934

Asif, M., Song, H., Zia, M. A., Ali, S., Awwad, E. M., Ghadi, Y. Y., & Al-Razgan, M. (2024). Shedding light on diagnostic precision: GANs for low light endoscopy image enhancements. *Journal of Cloud Computing (Heidelberg, Germany)*, *13*(1), 6. DOI: 10.1186/s13677-024-00133-9

Azad, R., Arimond, R., Aghdam, E. K., & Kazerouni, A.. (2023). Dae-former: Dual attention-guided efficient transformer for medical image segmentation. *Proceedings of the PRedictive Models in Medical Image Analysis Workshop*, 152-159. DOI: 10.1007/978-3-031-46005-0_8

Bhatti, M. A., Song, Z., & Bhatti, U. A., & M. S. (. (2024). AIoT-driven multi-source sensor emission monitoring and forecasting using multi-source sensor integration with reduced noise series decomposition. *Journal of Cloud Computing (Heidelberg, Germany)*, *13*(1), 65. DOI: 10.1186/s13677-024-00598-9

Bhatti, M. A., Zeeshan, Z., Syam, M. S., Bhatti, U. A., Khan, A., Ghadi, Y. Y., & Alsenan, S. (2024). Advanced plant disease segmentation in precision agriculture using optimal dimensionality reduction with fuzzy C-means clustering and deep learning. IEEE Journal of Selected Topics in Applied Earth Observations and Remote Sensing.

Bhatti, U. A., Bazai, S. U., Hussain, S., Fakhar, S., Ku, C. S., Marjan, S., Yee, P. L., & Jing, L. (2023). Deep learning-based trees disease recognition and classification using hyperspectral data. *Computers, Materials & Continua*, *77*(1), 681–697. DOI: 10.32604/cmc.2023.037958

Bhatti, U. A., Bhatti, M. A., Tang, H., Syam, M. S., Awwad, E. M., Sharaf, M., & Ghadi, Y. Y. (2024). Global production patterns: Understanding the relationship between greenhouse gas emissions, agriculture greening and climate variability. *Environmental Research*, *118049*, 118049. Advance online publication. DOI: 10.1016/j.envres.2023.118049 PMID: 38169167

Bhatti, U. A., Hao, T., Khan, A., Ghadi, Y. Y., Bhatti, M. A., & Khan, K. A. (2024). Investigating the nexus between energy, socio-economic factors and environmental pollution: A geo-spatial multi-regression approach. *Gondwana Research*, *130*, 308–325. Advance online publication. DOI: 10.1016/j.gr.2024.02.007

Bhatti, U. A., Marjan, S., Wahid, A., Syam, M. S., Huang, M., Tang, H., & Hasnain, A. (2023). The effects of socioeconomic factors on particulate matter concentration in China's: New evidence from spatial econometric model. *Journal of Cleaner Production*, *417*, 137969. DOI: 10.1016/j.jclepro.2023.137969

Bhatti, U. A., Masud, M., Bazai, S. U., & Tang, H. (2023). Investigating AI-based smart precision agriculture techniques. *Frontiers in Plant Science*, *14*, 1237783. DOI: 10.3389/fpls.2023.1237783 PMID: 37496855

Bhatti, U. A., Mengxing, H., Li, J., Bazai, S. U., & Aamir, M. (2024). *Deep learning for multimedia processing applications: Volume One: Image Security and Intelligent Systems for Multimedia Processing*. CRC Press.

Bhatti, U. A., Mengxing, H., Li, J., Bazai, S. U., & Aamir, M. (2024). *Deep learning for multimedia processing applications: Volume Two: Signal Processing and Pattern Recognition*. CRC Press.

Bhatti, U. A., Tang, H., & Wu, S. (2023). Mangrove decline puts Pakistan's coasts at risk. *Science*, *382*(6671), 654–655. DOI: 10.1126/science.adl3073 PMID: 37943921

Bristi, S. D., Tatha, M. J., Ali, M. F., Bhatti, U. A., Sarker, S. K., Masud, M., Ghadi, Y. Y., Algarni, A., & Saha, D. K. (2023). A meta-heuristic sustainable intelligent Internet of Things framework for bearing fault diagnosis of electric motor under variable load conditions. *Sustainability (Basel)*, *15*(24), 16722. DOI: 10.3390/su152416722

Cao, J., Bhatti, U. A., Feng, S., Huang, M., & Hasnain, A. (2023). Air quality index predictions with a hybrid forecasting model: Combining series decomposition and deep learning techniques. 2023 IEEE 6th International Conference on Pattern Recognition and Artificial Intelligence.

Chen, B., Liu, Y., Zhang, Z., & Lu, G. (2023). Transattunet: Multi-level attention-guided U-net with transformer for medical image segmentation. *IEEE Transactions on Medical Imaging*, *42*(6), 1809–1820. DOI: 10.1109/tmi.2023.3226702 PMID: 37022247

Chen, L., Zhang, Y., Xu, B., Shao, K., Yan, J., & Bhatti, U. A. (2024). A lot-based VMD-CNN-BIGRU indoor mariculture water quality prediction method including attention mechanism. *International Journal of High Speed Electronics and Systems*, •••, 2540010. DOI: 10.1142/S0129156425400105

Chen, Y., Lu, X., & Xie, Q. (2023). Advanced transformer for medical image segmentation. *Biomedical Signal Processing and Control*, *85*, 104777. DOI: 10.1016/j.bspc.2023.105079

Chen, Y., Wang, T., Tang, H., Zhao, L., Zhang, X., Tan, T., Gao, Q., Du, M., & Tong, T. (2023). CoTr-Fuse: A novel framework by fusing CNN and transformer for medical image segmentation. *Physics in Medicine and Biology*, *68*(13), 1346–1356. DOI: 10.1088/1361-6560/acede8 PMID: 37605997

Cheng, M., Li, D., Zhou, N., Tang, H., Wang, G., Li, S., Bhatti, U. A., & Khan, M. K. (2023). Vision-motion codesign for low-level trajectory generation in visual servoing systems. *IEEE Transactions on Instrumentation and Measurement*, *72*, 1–14. DOI: 10.1109/TIM.2023.3326234

Cheng, M., Tang, H., Bhatti, U. A., & Li, D. (2024). Optimized sustainable manufacturing through fuzzy control in image-based visual servoing with velocity and field-of-view constraints. *IEEE Transactions on Fuzzy Systems*, 1–12. DOI: 10.1109/TFUZZ.2024.3455408

Dong, F., Li, J., Bhatti, U. A., Liu, J., Chen, Y. W., & Li, D. (2023). Robust zero watermarking algorithm for medical images based on improved NasNet-mobile and DCT. *Electronics (Basel)*, *12*(16), 3444. DOI: 10.3390/electronics12163444

Fahim, A., Fadil, H., & Bhatti, U. A. (2023). Forecasting the carbon emissions in African countries using EMD-GCN. 2023 IEEE 6th International Conference on Pattern Recognition and Artificial Intelligence.

Fu, B., Peng, Y., He, J., Tian, C., Sun, X., & Wang, R. (2024). HmsU-Net: A hybrid multi-scale U-net based on a CNN and transformer for medical image segmentation. *Computers in Biology and Medicine, 163*, 107279. DOI: 10.1016/j.compbiomed.2024.108013 PMID: 38271837

Gao, J., Zhang, Y., Geng, X., Tang, H., & Bhatti, U. A. (2024). PE-Transformer: Path enhanced transformer for improving underwater object detection. *Expert Systems with Applications, 123253*, 123253. Advance online publication. DOI: 10.1016/j.eswa.2024.123253

Guan, Y., Aamir, M., Hu, Z., Abro, W. A., Rahman, Z., Dayo, Z. A., & Akram, S. (2021). A region-based efficient network for accurate object detection. *TS. Traitement du Signal, 38*(2), 228–237. DOI: 10.18280/ts.380228

Guan, Y., Aamir, M., Hu, Z., Dayo, Z. A., Rahman, Z., Abro, W. A., & Soothar, P. (2021). An object detection framework based on deep features and high-quality object locations. *TS. Traitement du Signal, 38*(3), 319–328. DOI: 10.18280/ts.380319

Guan, Y., Aamir, M., Rahman, Z., Ali, A., Abro, W. A., Dayo, Z. A., Bhutta, M. S., & Hu, Z. (2021). A framework for efficient brain tumor classification using MRI images. *Mathematical Biosciences and Engineering, 18*(6), 5399–5417. DOI: 10.3934/mbe.2021292 PMID: 34517512

Guan, Y., Aamir, M., Rahman, Z., Dayo, Z. A., Abro, W. A., Ishfaq, M., & Hu, Z. (2021). A dual-tree complex wavelet transform-based model for low-illumination image enhancement. *Wuhan University Journal of Natural Sciences, 26*(5), 405–414. DOI: 10.19823/j.cnki.1007-1202.2021.0051

Han, H., Hasnain, A., Bhatti, U. A., Yue, Y., He, Y., Wei, G., & Rahman, W. (2024). Assessing the spatio-temporal impact of the COVID-19 pandemic lockdown on air quality in Jiangsu province, China. *Environment, Development and Sustainability*, •••, 1–21. DOI: 10.1007/s10668-024-04914-w

Han, H., Zeeshan, Z., Talpur, B. A., Sadiq, T., Bhatti, U. A., Awwad, E. M., Al-Razgan, M., & Ghadi, Y. Y. (2024). Studying long term relationship between carbon emissions, soil, and climate change: Insights from a global Earth modeling framework. *International Journal of Applied Earth Observation and Geoinformation, 130*, 1–12. DOI: 10.1016/j.jag.2024.103902

Hasnain, A., Hashmi, M. Z., Bhatti, U. A., Wei, G., Jinru, L., & Asif, M. (2024). Prediction of particulate matter pollution using a long short-term memory model in Zhejiang Province, China. *Environmental Monitoring and Assessment, 196*(5), 487. DOI: 10.1007/s10661-024-12644-9 PMID: 38687422

Hasnain, A., Hashmi, M. Z., Khan, S., Bhatti, U. A., Min, X., Yue, Y., He, Y., & Wei, G. (2024). Predicting ambient PM2.5 concentrations via time series models in Anhui Province, China. *Environmental Monitoring and Assessment, 196*(5), 487. DOI: 10.1007/s10661-024-12644-9 PMID: 38687422

He, B., & Bhatti, U. A. (2024). Smart cities and smart networks: AI applications in urban geography and industrial communication. *International Journal of High Speed Electronics and Systems*, •••, 2440122. DOI: 10.1142/S0129156424401220

He, K., Gan, C., Li, Z., Rekik, I., Yin, Z., Ji, W., Gao, Y., & Wang, Q. (2023). Transformers in medical image analysis. *Intelligent Systems, 38*, 186–194. DOI: 10.1007/s10701-023-00488-0

He, K., Gou, F., & Wu, J. (2023). Image segmentation technology based on transformer in medical decision-making system. *IET Image Processing*, *17*(3), 391–399. DOI: 10.1049/ipr2.12854

He, S., Bao, R., Grant, P. E., & Ou, Y. (2023). U-Netmer: U-Net meets transformer for medical image segmentation. arXiv preprint. https://arxiv.org/abs/2304.01401

He, Y., Nath, V., Yang, D., Tang, Y., & Myronenko, A. (2023). Swinunetr-v2: Stronger swin transformers with stagewise convolutions for 3D medical image segmentation. *Proceedings of the Medical Imaging Conference*, 134-142. DOI: 10.1007/978-3-031-43901-8_40

Huang, H., Xie, S., Lin, L., Tong, R., & Chen, Y. W.. (2023). ClassFormer: Exploring class-aware dependency with transformer for medical image segmentation. *Proceedings of the AAAI Conference on Artificial Intelligence*, 88-96. DOI: 10.1609/aaai.v37i1.25171

Huang, M., Zhang, X. S., Bhatti, U. A., Wu, Y. Y., Zhang, Y., & Ghadi, Y. Y. (2024). An interpretable approach using hybrid graph networks and explainable AI for intelligent diagnosis recommendations in chronic disease care. *Biomedical Signal Processing and Control*, *91*, 105913. DOI: 10.1016/j.bspc.2023.105913

Huang, M., Zou, J., Zhang, Y., Bhatti, U. A., & Chen, J. (2024). Efficient click-based interactive segmentation for medical image with improved Plain-ViT. *IEEE Journal of Biomedical and Health Informatics*, *6*, 1–12. Advance online publication. DOI: 10.1109/JBHI.2024.3392893 PMID: 38656851

Joysoyal, R., Uddin, S. S., Islam, T., Sarker, S. K., Li, L., Ahsan, F., Bhatti, U. A., & Zafir, E. I. (2024). Blockchain for sustainable city transformation: A review on Bangladesh. *Engineering Reports*, *12948*(9), e12948. Advance online publication. DOI: 10.1002/eng2.12948

Lei, T., Sun, R., Wang, X., Wang, Y., & He, X. (2023). CiT-Net: Convolutional neural networks hand in hand with vision transformers for medical image segmentation. arXiv preprint. https://arxiv.org/abs/2305.04536 DOI: 10.24963/ijcai.2023/113

Li, D., & Bhatti, U. A. (2024). MSTFNet: A Mamba and dual Swin-transformer fusion network for remote sensing image classification for precision agriculture land processing. Available at *SSRN*, 5033170. DOI: 10.2139/ssrn.5033170

Li, G., Jin, D., Yu, Q., & Qi, M. (2023). IB-TransUNet: Combining information bottleneck and transformer for medical image segmentation. *Journal of King Saud University. Computer and Information Sciences*, *36*(12), 6606–6615. DOI: 10.1016/j.jksuci.2023.02.012

Li, J., Bhatti, U. A., Nawaz, S. A., Huang, M., Ahmad, R. M., & Ghadi, Y. Y. (2024). Remote-sensing image classification: A comprehensive review and applications. Deep Learning for Multimedia Processing Applications, 18-47.

Li, Z., Li, Y., Li, Q., Wang, P., Guo, D., & Lu, L. (2023). Lvit: Language meets vision transformer in medical image segmentation. *Proceedings of the Medical Imaging Conference*, 61-68. https://doi.org/DOI: 10.1109/medimaging.2023.00009

Liang, Z., Zhao, K., Liang, G., Li, S., Wu, Y., & Zhou, Y. (2023). MAXFormer: Enhanced transformer for medical image segmentation with multi-attention and multi-scale features fusion. *Knowledge-Based Systems*, *271*, 108530. DOI: 10.1016/j.knosys.2023.110987

Lin, X., Yu, L., Cheng, K. T., & Yan, Z. (2023). The lighter the better: Rethinking transformers in medical image segmentation through adaptive pruning. *IEEE Transactions on Medical Imaging*, *42*(10), 3124–3135. DOI: 10.1109/TMI.2023.3247814 PMID: 37027664

Liu, K., Li, P., Zhang, Y., Ren, J., Wang, X., & Bhatti, U. A. (2023). *Self-awakened particle swarm optimization BN structure learning algorithm based on search space constraint.* CMC-Computers Materials & Continua. DOI: 10.32604/cmc.2023.039430

Liu, Q., Feng, S., Huang, M., & Bhatti, U. A. (2024). Chronobridge: A novel framework for enhanced temporal and relational reasoning in temporal knowledge graphs. *Artificial Intelligence Review*, *57*(12), 1–33. DOI: 10.1007/s10462-024-10983-0

Liu, Q., Kaul, C., & Wang, J. (2023). Optimizing vision transformers for medical image segmentation. ICASSP 2023-2023 IEEE International Conference on Acoustics, Speech and Signal Processing, 5869-5873. DOI: 10.1109/ICASSP49357.2023.10096379

Liu, Y., Zhu, Y., Xin, Y., Zhang, Y., Yang, D., & Xu, T. (2023). MESTrans: Multi-scale embedding spatial transformer for medical image segmentation. *Computer Methods and Programs in Biomedicine*, *230*, 107367. DOI: 10.1016/j.cmpb.2023.107493 PMID: 36965298

Liu, Z., Li, J., Ashraf, M., Syam, M. S., Asif, M., Awwad, E. M., Al-Razgan, M., & Bhatti, U. A. (2024). Remote sensing-enhanced transfer learning approach for agricultural damage and change detection: A deep learning perspective. *Big Data Research*, *100449*, 100449. Advance online publication. DOI: 10.1016/j.bdr.2024.100449

Luo, Y., Li, J., Bhatti, U. A., Huang, M., Dong, F., & Li, Y. (2023). Robust zero-watermarking algorithm for medical images based on direction gradient histogram and DCT. 2023 IEEE 6th International Conference on Pattern Recognition and Artificial Intelligence.

Nawaz, S. A., Li, J., Bhatti, U. A., Shoukat, M. U., & Ahmad, R. M. (2024). Deep learning applications in digital image security: Latest methods and techniques. Deep Learning for Multimedia Processing Applications, 110-153.

Nawaz, S. A., Li, J., Bhatti, U. A., Shoukat, M. U., Li, D., & Raza, M. A. (2024). Hybrid watermarking algorithm for medical images based on digital transformation and MobileNetV2. *Information Sciences*, *653*, 119810. DOI: 10.1016/j.ins.2023.119810

Nawaz, S. A., Li, J., Li, D., Shoukat, M. U., Bhatti, U. A., & Raza, M. A. (2024). Medical image zero watermarking algorithm based on dual-tree complex wavelet transform, AlexNet, and discrete cosine transform. *Applied Soft Computing*, *112*, 112556. https://doi.org/10.xxxx/xxxxx

Nawaz, S. A., Li, J., Shoukat, M. U., Bhatti, U. A., & Raza, M. A. (2023). Hybrid medical image zero watermarking via discrete wavelet transform-ResNet101 and discrete cosine transform. *Computers & Electrical Engineering*, *112*, 108985. DOI: 10.1016/j.compeleceng.2023.108985

Nizamani, A. H., Chen, Z., Nizamani, A. A., & Bhatti, U. A. (2023). Advance brain tumor segmentation using feature fusion methods with deep U-Net model with CNN for MRI data. *Journal of King Saud University. Computer and Information Sciences*, *35*(9), 101793. DOI: 10.1016/j.jksuci.2023.101793

Noor, R., Wahid, A., Bazai, S. U., Khan, A., Fang, M., Syam, M. S., & Bhatti, U. A. (2024). DLGAN: Undersampled MRI reconstruction using deep learning-based generative adversarial network. *Biomedical Signal Processing and Control*, *93*, 106218. DOI: 10.1016/j.bspc.2024.106218

Pang, Y., Liang, J., Huang, T., Chen, H., Li, Y., & Zhang, Z. (2023). Slim UNETR: Scale hybrid transformers to efficient 3D medical image segmentation under limited computational resources. *Proceedings of the International Conference on Medical Imaging*, 333-342. https://doi.org/DOI: 10.1109/medimaging.2023.1005077

Peng, M., Liu, Y., Khan, A., Ahmed, B., Sarker, S. K., Ghadi, Y. Y., Bhatti, U. A., Al-Razgan, M., & Ali, Y. A. (2024). Crop monitoring using remote sensing land use and land change data: Comparative analysis of deep learning methods using pre-trained CNN models. *Big Data Research*, *36*, 100448. DOI: 10.1016/j.bdr.2024.100448

Peng, M., Liu, Y., Qadri, I. A., Bhatti, U. A., Ahmed, B., Sarhan, N. M., & Awwad, E. M. (2024). Advanced image segmentation for precision agriculture using CNN-GAT fusion and fuzzy C-means clustering. *Computers and Electronics in Agriculture*, *226*, 109431. DOI: 10.1016/j.compag.2024.109431

Pham, T. H., Li, X., & Nguyen, K. D. (2024). Seunet-trans: A simple yet effective unet-transformer model for medical image segmentation. *IEEE Access : Practical Innovations, Open Solutions*, *12*, 4567–4576. DOI: 10.1109/ACCESS.2024.3451304

Pu, Q., Xi, Z., Yin, S., Zhao, Z., & Zhao, L. (2024). Advantages of transformer and its application for medical image segmentation: A survey. *Biomedical Engineering Online*, *23*(1), 34. DOI: 10.1186/s12938-024-01212-4 PMID: 38310297

Reja, R. K., Amin, R., Tasneem, Z., Abhi, S. H., Bhatti, U. A., Sarker, S. K., Ain, Q., & Ghadi, Y. Y. (2023). A new ANN technique for short-term wind speed prediction based on SCADA system data in Turkey. *Atmosphere (Basel)*, *14*(10), 1516. DOI: 10.3390/atmos14101516

Roy, S., Koehler, G., Ulrich, C., & Baumgartner, M. (2023). Mednext: Transformer-driven scaling of convnets for medical image segmentation. *Proceedings of the Medical Imaging Conference*, 162-170. DOI: 10.1007/978-3-031-43901-8_39

Shao, K., Li, D., Tang, H., Zhang, Y., Xu, B., & Bhatti, U. A. (2024). Adaptive temporal convolutional network (ATCN) and internally-optimized transformer for dissolved oxygen prediction in aquaculture. Available at *SSRN*, 5039613. DOI: 10.2139/ssrn.5039613

Sun, G., Li, J., Bhatti, U. A., Ma, J., Dong, F., & Li, Y. (2023). Robust zero-watermarking algorithm for medical images based on AGAST-LATCH and DCT. 2023 26th ACIS International Winter Conference on Software Engineering.

Sun, X., Bhatti, U. A., Huang, M., & Zhang, Y. (2024). EF-UV: Feature enhanced fusion of U-Net and VIT transformer for brain tumor MRI image segmentation. *Journal of Medical Imaging and Health Informatics*, *12*(1), 1–12.

Tang, H., Chen, D., Zhang, Y., Xu, B., Bhatti, U. A., & Yu, M. (2024). Bidirectional interaction techniques based on device digital twin model. 2024 39th Youth Academic Annual Conference of Chinese Association of, 1-10. https://doi.org/DOI: 10.1109/YACCA.2024.03245

Tang, H., Zhang, Z., Zhang, Y., Xu, B., & Bhatti, U. A. (2024). Plug-and-work edge collaborator design for customised manufacturing. 2024 39th Youth Academic Annual Conference of Chinese Association of Automation.

Wang, M. S., Khan, A., Lin, Y., Jiang, Z., Tang, H., & Yousef, S. (2023). Deep reinforcement learning enables adaptive-image augmentation for automated optical inspection of plant rust. *Frontiers in Plant Science*, *14*, 1142957. DOI: 10.3389/fpls.2023.1142957 PMID: 37484461

Wang, X., Li, J., Bhatti, U. A., & Huang, M. (2023). Robust zero-watermarking algorithm for medical images based on maximally stable extremal regions and DCT. 2023 IEEE 6th International Conference on Pattern Recognition and Artificial Intelligence.

Wu, J., Ji, W., Fu, H., Xu, M., Jin, Y., & Xu, Y. (2024). Medsegdiff-v2: Diffusion-based medical image segmentation with transformer. *Proceedings of the AAAI Conference on Artificial Intelligence*, *38*(1), 4239–4246. DOI: 10.1609/aaai.v38i6.28418

Wu, Y., Zhang, L., Bhatti, U. A., & Huang, M. (2023). Interpretable machine learning for personalized medical recommendations: A LIME-based approach. *Diagnostics (Basel)*, *13*(16), 2681. DOI: 10.3390/diagnostics13162681 PMID: 37627940

Wu, Y., Zhang, L., Bhatti, U. A., Huang, M., & Zhang, Y. (2023). Interpretable medical recommendations based on SHAPs. 2023 IEEE 6th International Conference on Pattern Recognition and Artificial Intelligence.

Xu, B., Luo, C., Tang, H., Bhatti, U. A., Wang, X., & Jiang, W. (2024). Advancing transparency in AI-based automatic modulation classification. *2024 IEEE/CIC International Conference on Communications in China (ICCC)*. DOI: 10.1109/ICCC62479.2024.10682007

Xu, G., Zhang, X., He, X., & Wu, X. (2023). Levit-unet: Make faster encoders with transformer for medical image segmentation. *Proceedings of the International Conference on Pattern Recognition and Computer Vision*, 242-250. DOI: 10.1007/978-3-031-19812-0_27

Xu, S., Xiao, D., Yuan, B., Liu, Y., Wang, X., Li, N., Shi, L., Chen, J., Zhang, J.-X., Wang, Y., Cao, J., Shao, Y., & Jiang, M. (2023). FAFuse: A Four-Axis Fusion framework of CNN and Transformer for medical image segmentation. *Computers in Biology and Medicine*, *162*, 107280. DOI: 10.1016/j.compbiomed.2023.107567 PMID: 37852109

Yan, Q., Liu, S., Xu, S., Dong, C., Li, Z., Shi, J. Q., Zhang, Y., & Dai, D. (2023). 3D medical image segmentation using parallel transformers. *Pattern Recognition*, *137*, 108278. DOI: 10.1016/j.patcog.2023.109432

Yang, J., Sadiq, T., Xiong, J., Awais, M., Bhatti, U. A., & Alizadehsani, R. (2024). A novel myocarditis detection combining deep reinforcement learning and an improved differential evolution algorithm. *CAAI Transactions on Intelligence Technology*, *9*(6), 1347–1360. Advance online publication. DOI: 10.1049/cit2.12289

Yang, J., Tu, J., Zhang, X., Yu, S., & Zheng, X. (2023). TSE DeepLab: An efficient visual transformer for medical image segmentation. *Biomedical Signal Processing and Control*, *70*, 104698. DOI: 10.1016/j.bspc.2022.104376

Yang, M., Li, J., Bhatti, U. A., Yuan, Y., & Zhang, Q. (2024). A novel robust watermarking algorithm for encrypted medical images based on non-subsampled shearlet transform and Schur decomposition. Deep Learning for Multimedia Processing Applications: Volume One. *Image.*

Yu, Z., Li, D., Du, P., Luo, W., Kou, K. I., Bhatti, U. A., Benger, W., Lv, G., & Yuan, L. (2024). Hypercomplex signal processing in digital twin of the ocean: Theory and application [Hypercomplex Signal and Image Processing]. *IEEE Signal Processing Magazine*, *41*(3), 33–48. DOI: 10.1109/MSP.2024.3389496

Yuan, F., Zhang, Z., & Fang, Z. (2023). An effective CNN and transformer complementary network for medical image segmentation. *Pattern Recognition*, *139*, 109179. DOI: 10.1016/j.patcog.2022.109228

Zhang, C., Aamir, M., Guan, Y., Al-Razgan, M., Awwad, E. M., Ullah, R., Bhatti, U. A., & Ghadi, Y. Y. (2024). Enhancing lung cancer diagnosis with data fusion and mobile edge computing using DenseNet and CNN. *Journal of Cloud Computing (Heidelberg, Germany)*, *13*(1), 91. DOI: 10.1186/s13677-024-00597-w

Zhang, C., Iqbal, I., Bhatti, U. A., Liu, J., Awwad, E. M., & Sarhan, N. (2024). ResNet50 in remote sensing and agriculture: Evaluating image captioning performance for high spectral data. *Environmental Earth Sciences*, *83*(23), 1–16. DOI: 10.1007/s12665-024-11950-2

Zhang, J., Fu, R., Wu, Y., & Aslam, B. U. (2024). Practical consensus of time-varying fuzzy positive multi-agent systems. *AIMS Mathematics*, *9*(11), 31119–31141. DOI: 10.3934/math.20241500

Zhang, N., Yu, L., Zhang, D., Wu, W., Tian, S., Kang, X., & Li, M. (2024). Ct-net: Asymmetric compound branch transformer for medical image segmentation. *Neural Networks*, *144*, 18–30. DOI: 10.1016/j.neunet.2023.11.034 PMID: 38006733

Zhang, Y., Chen, J., Ma, X., Wang, G., Bhatti, U. A., & Huang, M. (2024). Interactive medical image annotation using improved Attention U-net with compound geodesic distance. *Expert Systems with Applications*, *237*, 121282. DOI: 10.1016/j.eswa.2023.121282

Zou, Y., Ge, Y., Zhao, L., & Li, W. (2023). MR-Trans: MultiResolution Transformer for medical image segmentation. *Computers in Biology and Medicine*, *163*, 107280. DOI: 10.1016/j.compbiomed.2023.107456 PMID: 37696179

Chapter 5
Alzheimer's Disease Detection Using CNN Model

Affaan Shaikh
https://orcid.org/0009-0004-7590-7456
Neuratia Labs, India

ABSTRACT

Alzheimer's disease (AD) is a disease of the brain that slowly destroys memory and thinking ability. It is one of the most common forms of dementia in people over the age of 65 worldwide. Early detection of Alzheimer's disease helps medical personnel diagnose this disease, which certainly reduces the risk of death. Therefore, early detection of Alzheimer's disease is an important healthcare issue. In order to achieve accurate and timely diagnosis, and for detection of AD in its early stages, many Artificial Intelligence (AI) and Machine learning approaches have been proposed using data from brain imaging. AI and ML are used for many medical and health purposes, such as disease detection. In this chapter, the main focus is on the diagnosis and detection of Alzheimer's disease using CNN model. A Convolutional Neural Network (CNN) is a deep learning model specialized in detecting and classifying patterns in visual data, commonly used for tasks like image recognition, object detection, and classification.

1. INTRODUCTION

Neurodegenerative Diseases are the group of disorders that affect the brain and the nervous system. They can lead to problems with important functions such as breathing, thinking, talking, memory, balance and heart functions. It is a disease in which the nerve cells in the brain or peripheral nervous system lose their function over time and eventually die (Checkoway, Lundin, & Kelada, 2011).

These diseases are now increasing in the older population in recent years and its detection has become a challenging task for doctors and scientists. The most consistent risk factor for developing a neurodegenerative disorder, especially AD or PD, is increasing age (Tanner, 1992). Alzheimer's disease (AD), Parkinson's disease (PD), and amyotrophic lateral sclerosis (ALS) are three of the major neurodegenerative diseases (Checkoway, Lundin, & Kelada, 2011).

The World Alzheimer Report (2015) estimated that globally there were 46.8 million people living with some form of dementia. Alzheimer's disease (AD) and Parkinson's disease (PD) are the two most prevalent progressive neurodegenerative diseases (NDs) (Bharathi & Arunachalam, 2021).

DOI: 10.4018/979-8-3693-9816-6.ch005

Aside from Alzheimer's disease (AD), Parkinson's disease (PD), and amyotrophic lateral sclerosis (ALS), other notable neurodegenerative diseases include Huntington's disease, frontotemporal dementia, and multiple system atrophy (Tysnes & Storstein, 2017). These diseases differ in their underlying pathophysiology and symptoms, but they all share the common feature of neuron degeneration (Swerdlow, 2007). AD and PD, for instance, are linked with the accumulation of abnormal protein aggregates (such as amyloid plaques and tau tangles in AD, and Lewy bodies in PD), which disrupt cellular function.

The causes of neurodegenerative diseases are multifactorial, involving genetic, environmental, and lifestyle factors (Hardy & Selkoe, 2002). In addition to aging, which remains the most significant risk factor, genetic mutations (such as in the case of familial Alzheimer's disease or Huntington's disease) and environmental exposures (such as toxins or infections) have been identified as contributing factors (McGeer & McGeer, 2013). Studies have also highlighted the role of inflammation, oxidative stress, and impaired protein clearance mechanisms in the development of these diseases (Heneka et al., 2015).

The impact of these diseases on individuals and society is profound. Neurodegenerative diseases not only cause physical and cognitive disabilities in patients but also impose significant emotional, social, and economic burdens on families and caregivers. With the global aging population, the prevalence of these diseases is expected to increase, making early detection, diagnosis, and intervention even more crucial Zhou et al., 2020).

Recent advancements in diagnostic technologies, such as neuroimaging, cerebrospinal fluid biomarkers, and genetic testing, are helping to identify neurodegenerative diseases at earlier stages, providing hope for more effective treatment strategies. Additionally, research into novel therapies, including gene therapy, stem cell treatments, and targeted drug therapies, is underway, offering potential avenues for managing or even reversing the effects of these diseases in the future.

The need for further research into neurodegenerative diseases is critical, particularly in identifying early biomarkers, understanding disease mechanisms, and developing innovative treatment options to alleviate the suffering of millions of people globally (Tetzlaff, 2018).

2. LITERATURE REVIEW

Martinez-Murcia et al. (2019) utilized deep convolutional autoencoders for data analysis in Alzheimer's disease (AD). Tatiq and Barber (2018) suggested in their research that targeting modifiable vascular risk factors could prevent Alzheimer's, as these factors often coexist in the brain and share some modifiable risk factors. Williams et al. (2013) predicted cognitive functioning based on neuropsychological and demographic data using four different models: SVM, Decision Tree, NN, and Naïve-Bayes.

Mehmood et al. (2021) emphasised the early identification of Alzheimer's on magnetic resonance images through mild cognitive impairment detection using structured deep learning with multiple layers for brain tissue segmentation. EI-Latif et al. (2023) highlighted Alzheimer's disease as a neurodegenerative condition characterised by cognitive impairment and abnormal protein buildup in the brain, affecting millions worldwide.

Kavitha et al. (2022) described Alzheimer's Disease (AD) as a progressive neurological condition causing short-term memory loss, paranoia, and delusional ideas, often mistaken for the effects of stress or aging, impacting approximately 5.1 million people in the United States. Ahmed et al. (2018) discussed the increasing prevalence of Neuroimaging for Dementia, a chronic and progressive cognitive decline caused by disease or impairment, presenting a significant challenge in achieving accurate and timely diagnosis.

Patil et al. (2022) highlighted the natural deterioration of physical and neurological functions in individuals as part of the aging process, which can significantly impact some due to specific risk factors. KV et al. (2023) underscored Alzheimer's disease as a global health emergency affecting at least 6 million people globally and being a major contributor to dementia.

Checkoway et al. (2011) focused on neurodegenerative diseases, including Alzheimer's, Parkinson's, and ALS, presenting growing health challenges. Molecular epidemiology was emphasized as a tool aiding understanding, diagnosis, and management of these conditions, guiding future prevention-focused research.

3. MACHINE LEARNING

Machine learning (ML) is a rapidly advancing subfield of artificial intelligence (AI) that focuses on enabling systems to learn and make decisions without explicit programming. By analyzing data and identifying patterns, ML algorithms can automatically improve their performance over time, making them highly versatile and effective in tackling complex problems across diverse domains. The performance of this system can improve the learning experience without any complicated programming (Bishop, 2006). These algorithms identify a unique feature or pattern in the given input data that contributes to better decision making. These algorithms are mainly used in applications related to medical images, computer vision, biometric recognition, object recognition, automation, etc (Bishop, 2006; Murphy, 2012).

There are three types of machine learning (Bishop, 2006; Murphy, 2012), such as supervised learning, unsupervised learning and reinforcement learning. ML algorithms learn through experience and improve automatically. It finds techniques, trains models, and uses the learned approach to determine the output automatically (Alzubi, Nayyar, & Kumar, 2018).

ML is particularly transformative in medical and healthcare applications, where it is used for disease detection, drug discovery, patient monitoring, and personalized treatment plans. For instance, in the diagnosis of neurodegenerative disorders like Alzheimer's and Parkinson's diseases, ML can process large datasets of medical images, genetic information, and clinical data to identify early biomarkers, predict disease progression, and suggest treatment strategies. These capabilities have the potential to revolutionize healthcare by enabling earlier and more accurate diagnoses, which are critical for managing progressive conditions.

In addition to supervised, unsupervised, and reinforcement learning, other advanced ML techniques, such as semi-supervised learning and self-supervised learning, are gaining traction. Semi-supervised learning leverages both labeled and unlabeled data, which is particularly valuable in scenarios where labeled data is scarce or expensive to obtain, such as rare diseases. Self-supervised learning, on the other hand, uses the data itself to generate labels, significantly reducing dependency on manual annotation while improving efficiency.

Key advancements in ML include deep learning, which employs artificial neural networks to analyze complex and high-dimensional data. Deep learning has shown remarkable success in areas like natural language processing (NLP), image recognition, and autonomous systems. For example, convolutional neural networks (CNNs) are widely used for analyzing medical images, while recurrent neural networks (RNNs) are effective for sequential data, such as patient monitoring or EEG signal analysis.

Choosing the right machine learning algorithm and tailoring it to the specific dataset and application is crucial to achieving optimal results. Techniques such as hyperparameter tuning, cross-validation, and ensemble learning can enhance model performance and ensure robust predictions. Additionally, integrating domain knowledge into the model design can improve its relevance and accuracy.

Challenges remain in applying ML to real-world scenarios, particularly in healthcare. Issues like data privacy, the need for large and diverse datasets, and interpretability of ML models require careful consideration. Transparent and interpretable models, such as decision trees or explainable AI frameworks, are essential for building trust with medical professionals and patients. Furthermore, ethical concerns, such as algorithmic bias and the potential for misuse, must be addressed to ensure fair and equitable use of ML technologies.

Looking ahead, the integration of ML with other emerging technologies, such as the Internet of Things (IoT) and edge computing, is poised to expand its applications further. For instance, wearable health devices powered by ML can provide real-time monitoring and alerts for chronic conditions, enabling timely interventions and improving patient outcomes. As research and innovation in ML continue to advance, its potential to drive breakthroughs in science, healthcare, and other fields becomes increasingly evident.

Choosing the correct existing machine learning algorithm and applying accordingly is crucial to obtain satisfying results.

Figure 1. Roadmap followed

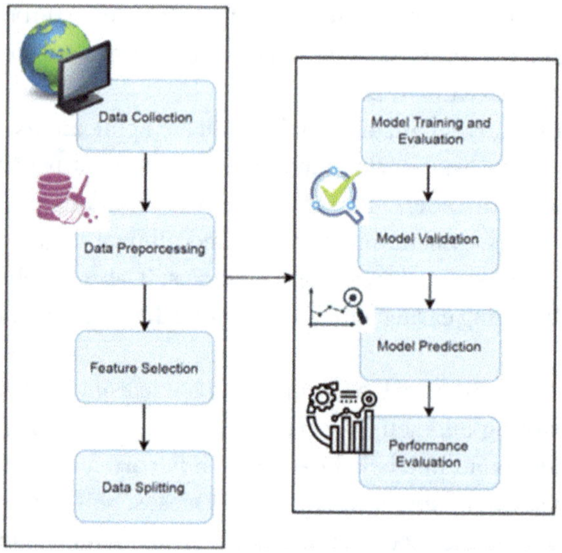

The Machine Learning techniques (Reddy et al., 2020; Abdulsahib & Khalaf, 2021) were applied to Alzheimer's disease datasets to bring a new dimension to predict Disease at an early stage. The raw Alzheimer's disease datasets are inconsistent and redundant, which affects the accuracy of algorithms (Gadekallu et al., 2023; Salman, Khalaf, & Abdulsahib, 2019). Before evaluating machine learning algorithms, the data must be effectively preprocessed for analysis by removing unwanted attributes, missing values and redundant data sets. Creating a machine learning model requires splitting the data into training and test sets. In the following data preparation step, the training data were used to create a model, which was then applied to test data to predict Alzheimer's Disease (Gadekallu et al., 2023; Srinivasu et al., 2021; Khalaf et al., 2020). The model was trained using the training data and the test data was used to test the unseen data. Cross-validation was performed by splitting the data set into three subsets. The model predictions are made using one subset of the data (test data), and the model performance is evaluated using the other subsets (training and validation data). The data had been preprocessed, and we randomly divided it into an 80:20 ratio, with 80% going to training and 20% gone to testing (Khalaf et al., 2020; Abdulsahib & Khalaf, 2018). Figure 1 describes the system workflow for predicting Alzheimer's Disease at an early stage (Khalaf et al., 2020; Abdulsahib & Khalaf, 2018). Figure 2 shows the representation of data splitting.

Figure 2. Dataset Splitting Workflow for Machine Learning Model Development

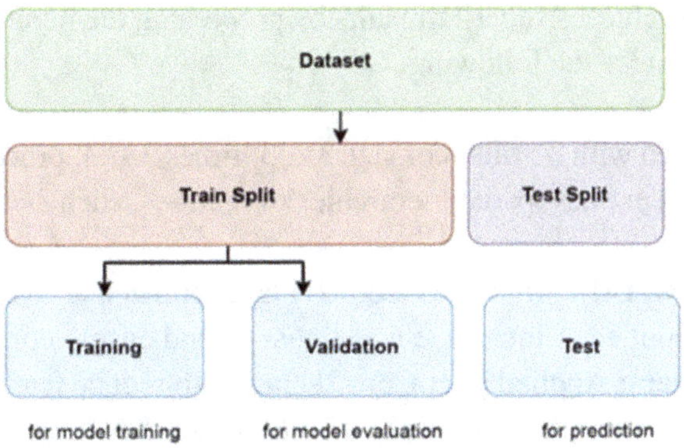

4. CONVOLUTIONAL NEURAL NETWORK MODEL

4.1 Model Building

The proposed Convolutional Neural Network (CNN) model is designed with a layered architecture to process and analyze MRI images efficiently. The architecture comprises multiple layers, each serving specific functions to extract and process features for Alzheimer’s disease detection.

1. **Base Model (6-layer CNN):**

The base model consists of six primary layers:

- o **Conv2D Layer:** Responsible for extracting features from the input images by applying convolutional filters.
- o **MaxPooling2D Layer:** Reduces the spatial dimensions of the feature maps, retaining the most significant information.
- o **Flatten Layer:** Converts the 3D feature maps into a 1D array for input to the fully connected layers.

- **Activation Layer (ReLU):** Introduces non-linearity to the model, enabling it to learn complex patterns.
- **Dropout Layer:** Helps prevent overfitting by randomly setting a fraction of the input units to zero during training.
- **Dense Layer:** Acts as a fully connected layer for decision-making and classification.

This model uses approximately 32 filters, each of size 3×33 \times 33×3, and the input to these layers consists of preprocessed MRI images.

2. **Extended Model (15-layer CNN):**

The extended CNN model is designed to enhance accuracy by incorporating more layers, allowing deeper feature extraction. It achieves superior results by processing the input data through all its bitwise filters. This architecture includes the following:

- **3 Conv2D Layers:** Each with 32 filters of size 3×33 \times 33×3, processing the input images sequentially. These layers extract spatial hierarchies of features, such as edges, textures, and higher-order features.
- **5 Activation Layers (ReLU):** After each Conv2D layer and dense layer, the Rectified Linear Unit (ReLU) activation is applied to introduce non-linearity and ensure computational efficiency.
- **3 MaxPooling2D Layers:** Applied after Conv2D layers to reduce feature map size while preserving important information, with a pool size of 2×22 \times 22×2.
- **1 Flatten Layer:** Converts the multi-dimensional feature maps into a 1D array suitable for fully connected layers.
- **2 Dense Layers:** The first dense layer has 64 neurons and applies ReLU activation, acting as a feature aggregator. The second dense layer has 2 neurons with a softmax activation, performing binary classification (e.g., Alzheimer's vs. Healthy).
- **1 Dropout Layer:** Includes a 50% dropout rate to minimize overfitting by randomly disabling neurons during training.

4.2 Model Workflow

1. **Input:**

The model accepts MRI images with a predefined input shape of (INPUT_SIZE,INPUT_SIZE,3)(\text{INPUT_SIZE},\text{INPUT_SIZE},3)(INPUT_SIZE,INPUT_SIZE,3). This shape accommodates RGB images, though grayscale images can also be preprocessed to fit this input structure.

2. **Initial Feature Extraction:**

The input is processed by the first Conv2D layer, where 32 filters of size 3×33 \times 33×3 are applied. This layer identifies low-level features like edges and corners. ReLU activation ensures that only positive feature values are propagated forward. A MaxPooling2D layer then downsamples the feature map, reducing its size to improve computational efficiency and mitigate overfitting.

3. **Deeper Feature Extraction:**

Two additional Conv2D layers follow, each extracting higher-level features from the images. These layers are also accompanied by ReLU activation and MaxPooling2D for downsampling.

4. **Flattening:**

After feature extraction, the output of the final MaxPooling2D layer is flattened into a 1D array by the Flatten layer, making it compatible with the fully connected layers.

5. **Fully Connected Layers:**
   - The first dense layer with 64 neurons aggregates the extracted features into a meaningful representation.
   - The Dropout layer, with a dropout rate of 0.5, reduces overfitting by deactivating 50% of neurons randomly during training.
   - The second dense layer, with 2 neurons and a softmax activation function, generates probability scores for the two output classes, enabling binary classification.

The deeper architecture allows the model to capture complicated patterns and relationships in the data, resulting in higher accuracy. The added Conv2D and activation layers improve feature extraction, while the dropout layer effectively addresses overfitting issues.

4.3 Training And Testing

The training of a Convolutional Neural Network (CNN) for Alzheimer's disease detection involves a systematic and comprehensive approach designed to optimize performance while ensuring robustness. This process leverages an organized Support Vector Machine (SSVM) framework and propagates its sub-gradient through the network. Although training CNN models is inherently complex, advancements in methods and frameworks have recently facilitated this task. Below is a detailed breakdown of the process, merging and refining the descriptions for clarity and quality.

4.3.1 Training Process

1. **Organized Framework and Sub-gradient Propagation:** The training process begins with the utilization of the SSVM framework, which organizes the training pipeline systematically. By employing an approximate sub-gradient method and a quick derivation strategy, the optimization of the CNN model becomes feasible. These strategies ensure efficient propagation of gradients through the network, even for challenging MRI data.
2. **Whole-image Training:** To enhance inference performance, the CNN model is trained on complete MRI images, mirroring the testing conditions where the model processes entire images. This alignment ensures that the model learns to handle complete data effectively, improving its real-world applicability.

3. **Iterative Refinement:** Training involves a multi-stage iterative refinement process. The initial model is trained on a dataset comprising MRI images ranging from mild dementia to severe dementia. This dataset provides a baseline for performance evaluation, highlighting areas for improvement. Hyperparameters are then adjusted, and certain layers are modified based on these findings to improve the model's accuracy. This refinement continues iteratively until the desired performance metrics are achieved.

4.3.2 Testing Process

1. **Evaluation on Hard Negative Samples:** Testing includes challenging the model with hard negative samples to evaluate its robustness and reduce false positives. This is crucial in building a resilient model capable of handling ambiguous or complex cases effectively.
2. **Five-stage Protocol:** The testing protocol is designed to comprehensively evaluate the model's performance and ability to generalize. This involves:
    - **Baseline Evaluation:** Initially, the model is trained and tested on the same dataset to establish a baseline for its performance. Metrics such as accuracy, precision, recall, and F1-score are assessed during this phase.
    - **Quality and Similarity Levels:** The model is tested at four levels using images of varying quality and similarity. This helps evaluate the model's adaptability and its capacity to handle diverse data characteristics.
    - **Calibration:** Based on the results, the model is recalibrated by fine-tuning hyperparameters or modifying layers. This iterative adjustment focuses on improving the model's weak areas identified during baseline evaluation.
    - **Cross-dataset Testing:** The refined model is tested on datasets with differing characteristics to measure its ability to generalize and learn from new data.
    - **Final Evaluation:** After successive iterations, the model is evaluated on datasets with decreasing similarity to the training data, ensuring its robustness across diverse scenarios.

4.3.3 End-to-End Training Benefits

End-to-end training of CNN models has proven advantageous in various applications, including Alzheimer's disease detection. By focusing on complete image datasets and iterative refinement, the model gains the following advantages:

- **Optimized Inference Performance:** Training on whole images ensures alignment with real-world testing scenarios, enhancing prediction accuracy.
- **Generalization Capability:** Cross-dataset testing fosters the model's ability to generalize across diverse MRI data, making it applicable in different clinical settings.
- **Adaptability:** Fine-tuning hyperparameters and modifying layers iteratively improve the model's learning capacity and adaptability to new datasets.

4.4 Validation

Validation of a CNN model is a crucial step in assessing its performance and generalisation capabilities. Approval of a CNN model includes assessing its exhibition on a different dataset (approval set) to guarantee that it sums up well to unseen data. This interaction recognizes potential overfitting and gives bits of knowledge into the model's general adequacy. validation of a CNN model ensures that it generalises well to unseen data and helps in making informed decisions regarding model architecture and hyperparameters. It plays a crucial role in the development and deployment of deep learning models.

Validation can be explained using following ways:

1. Data Splitting:
   - The dataset is usually split into three subsets: training set, validation set, and test set.
   - The training set is used to train the model, the validation set is used to tune hyperparameters and assess performance during training, and the test set is used for final evaluation after model training.
2. Training the Model:
   - During training, the CNN model learns to map input data to corresponding labels by minimising a chosen loss function.
   - The parameters of the model are iteratively updated using optimization algorithms (Koushik, n.d.).
3. Validation during Training:
   - At the end of each training epoch (a complete pass through the training dataset), the model's performance is evaluated on the validation set.
   - Metrics such as accuracy, pre precision, recall and F1-score can be calculated to evaluate the performance of the model (Deepchecks, n.d.).
   - If the model meets the desired performance criteria on the test set, it can be deployed for making predictions on real-world data.

5. WEBSITE DEVELOPMENT USING FLASK

5.1 PyCharm

PyCharm is a widely-used Python Integrated Development Environment (IDE) developed by JetBrains, designed to enhance productivity and streamline the coding process. Renowned for its robust features, PyCharm is particularly favored in web development projects for its powerful capabilities and user-friendly interface. It offers advanced code analysis tools, intelligent code completion, and seamless navigation, making it easier for developers to write, debug, and maintain their code efficiently.

PyCharm supports various web development frameworks, including Django and Flask, providing built-in tools to simplify tasks like template editing and database management. Its integrated development tools, such as version control systems (VCS), debugging utilities, and an interactive Python console, further optimize the development workflow. Additionally, PyCharm supports remote development, allowing developers to write and test their code on remote servers effortlessly.

The IDE also offers extensive customization options, plugins, and support for modern web technologies, including HTML, CSS, JavaScript, and TypeScript. PyCharm's ability to integrate with popular databases, testing frameworks, and deployment tools makes it a comprehensive solution for both novice and experienced developers.

Additionally, the PyCharm offers extensive support for the Flask framework, a popular choice for building web applications in Python (Aslam, Mohammed, & Lokhande, 2015).

5.2 Flask Framework

The background development of the server is done by the Flask micro framework.

- Advantages of using Flask for Web Development are

  (a) Flask's compatibility with Python makes it easy to integrate these components into web applications. Flask follows a minimalistic and lightweight design, making it easy to get started with building web applications. Its simplicity allows developers to focus on writing clean and efficient code (LMV Software, n.d.).
  (b) While Flask is lightweight, it's also highly scalable. Developers have the flexibility to start small and scale their applications as needed.
  (c) The Flask Framework can support multiple teams working in parallel, each focusing on a specific function. It has several open-source libraries, a built-in server, a testing unit, all of which are easy to learn and master.
  (d) There is a flexible Jinja 2 template engine in Flask to improve the front-end code, further enhancing the efficiency of development, and improving the maintenance.

- There is also a disadvantage of the flask framework and it is-

The Flask framework does not support database access, web form validation, and also user authentication.

- Overall, Flask's compatibility with Python, ease of development, simplicity, scalability, and strong community support makes it a great choice for building web applications (Aslam, Mohammed, & Lokhande, 2015).

5.3 Working

Within our Flask-based website designed for Alzheimer's disease detection, users are welcomed by a minimalistic interface featuring a prominent “Get Started” button on the homepage. This serves as the gateway for individuals seeking to utilise our Alzheimer's detection service.

Upon clicking the “Get Started” button, users are seamlessly transitioned to a dedicated page where they can actively engage with the Alzheimer's disease detection functionality. Here, they are prompted to select an MRI image, crucial for the subsequent detection process. The website facilitates this by providing a user-friendly file input option, allowing seamless uploading of the MRI image.

Subsequently, our Flask application takes charge of processing the uploaded MRI image through a pre-trained Convolutional Neural Network (CNN) model, specifically tailored for Alzheimer's disease detection. The CNN model meticulously analyses intricate patterns within the MRI data, aiming to discern potential indicators of Alzheimer's disease.

Following the completion of the image processing phase, the website promptly reveals the detection result. This outcome is communicated to the user through an intelligible format, such as a notification or a dedicated results section. The presentation is designed to clearly convey whether the MRI image exhibits signs indicative of Alzheimer's disease or not.

To further enhance user engagement and comprehension, the website incorporates thoughtful user feedback mechanisms. These may include informative messages or visual indicators, ensuring users grasp the significance of the Alzheimer's disease detection results. The objective is to provide a transparent and user-friendly experience, aiding individuals in understanding the implications of the analysis.

As users conclude their interaction with our website, they are presented with a conclusive message or a clear call-to-action. This may encourage further exploration of the platform or offer additional resources related to Alzheimer's disease, contributing to a comprehensive and informative user experience. Through this integration of a CNN model within a Flask framework, our website serves as a valuable tool for early Alzheimer's disease detection and education.

6. FLUTTER APPLICATION

Flutter is introduced as a compact User Interface (UI) tool intended to help cross-stage application improvement. By giving its own sources or options of interface parts, interface platforms instrument and quick advancement cycle, the structure intends to compare with local and cross-stage solutions. Flutter is a cross-platform framework aimed at developing high-performance mobile applications. In Flutter, every application is written using Dart. Google has developed and maintained a programming language called Dart (Tashildar et al., 2020).

Flutter adopts a highly efficient and versatile approach to cross-platform application development, enabling developers to create seamless, high-performing apps for multiple platforms with a single codebase. Developed by Google, Flutter provides its own set of application programming interfaces (APIs), a powerful rendering engine, and an array of foundational libraries to build visually appealing and functionally robust applications.

At the core of Flutter's architecture is its rendering engine, which eliminates the reliance on platform-specific UI components. Instead, Flutter directly renders its own user interface elements, such as buttons, text fields, and other widgets, ensuring consistency across Android, iOS, and other platforms. This approach enables Flutter to deliver a native-like look and feel, enhancing the user experience.

Flutter is built with a robust framework that includes its own graphics engine, Skia, which handles animations, graphics, and file management with precision. The rendering pipeline efficiently processes layout, painting, and compositing to deliver high-quality visuals and smooth animations. By avoiding overly complex layouts that require deep calculations for intricate widget trees, Flutter achieves a balance of simplicity, speed, and flexibility.

As an open-source software development kit (SDK), Flutter provides developers with the freedom to create apps that cater to the aesthetics and functionality expected by both Android and iOS users. Its pre-designed widgets follow Material Design and Cupertino standards, ensuring platform-specific familiarity while maintaining a unified development process.

In addition, Flutter's "hot reload" feature significantly speeds up the development cycle by allowing developers to see changes to the code in real time without having to restart the entire application. This boosts productivity and facilitates rapid iteration during the development process.

Flutter's versatility extends beyond mobile app development, supporting web, desktop, and embedded applications, making it a one-stop solution for building scalable and dynamic applications across various platforms. This makes Flutter a preferred choice for developers aiming to create intuitive, high-performance, and visually consistent applications for diverse user bases.

6.1 Figma Design

Figma has been an excellent tool to plan UI with superb features concerning Plan, Model, Coordinated effort, Plan Framework Module. Figma saves you time with incredible assets that cut down on manual undertakings and leave you additional time and mental ability for imagination.

As Figma is an open-source platform any e-developer or a beginner can use it and grow in terms of skills and professionally as well. One of the main benefits of Figma is that this platform is free to use for everyone just by signing up on Figma.com. The reason why we picked Figma for this projcct is because it allows users to work simultaneously in real time which makes collaboration easier and faster. Another reason why this User Interface is popular is because it gives an all-in-one solution to everything. Figma covers all that you want to make an application or any connection point like from conceptualising and wireframing to prototyping and sharing resources. Figma also generates CSS, Android and iOS code for developers to use (Figma, n.d.). The design for our Application is shown in Figure 4.

Figure 3. The Figma Design for the App

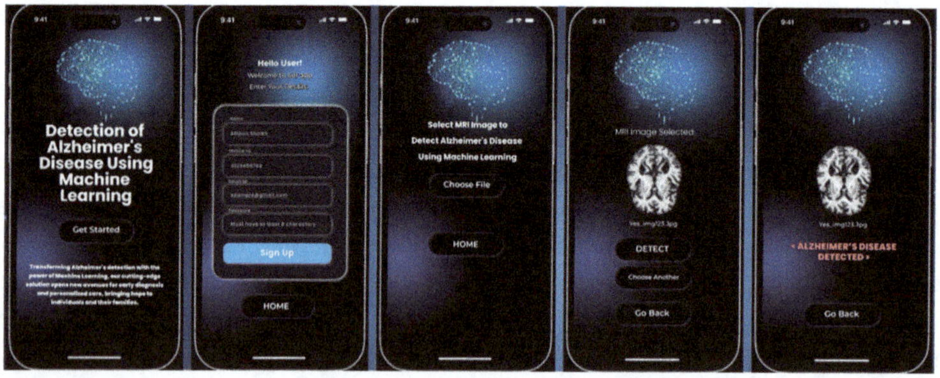

The Figma design is then exported to Flutter in VS code and then changes are made accordingly, to make the app responsive and workable. After the front end of the application is designs, the next task is to integrate our CNN model with the Flutter App.

6.2 Integration with the Model

The Flutter app provides a user-friendly interface for accessing the model's predictions, making it easy for farmers to use the system without any technical expertise (Shoaib et al., 2023).

Integrating the CNN model with the Flutter app involves several steps, including setting up a data server, creating APIs, and handling JSON data. Firstly, you need to deploy your ML model on a server that can handle inference requests from your Flutter app. This server can be hosted on cloud services like AWS, Google Cloud, or Azure. Once the model is deployed, you'll expose its functionality through APIs. APIs act as a bridge between the Flutter app and the ML model, allowing them to communicate seamlessly.

In terms of data flow, your Flutter app sends input data (such as user inputs or images) to the server through API requests. These requests typically include JSON-formatted data, as JSON is a lightweight data interchange format that is easy to parse and transmit. The server processes the input using the ML model, generates predictions, and sends the results back to the Flutter app in JSON format. The app can then parse the JSON response and display the predictions or take further actions based on the ML model's output.

This integration requires careful consideration of data formats, network communication, and error handling to ensure a smooth and efficient interaction between the Flutter app and the ML model deployed on the server. Additionally, proper security measures should be implemented to protect the data being transmitted between the app and the server.

Here's a more detailed breakdown of the process:

1. Deploying the ML Model on a Server

To make the CNN model accessible to the Flutter app, you need to deploy it on a server. This process involves several steps:

- **Model Preparation:** Ensure your trained CNN model (e.g., built using TensorFlow, PyTorch, or Keras) is converted into a format suitable for deployment, such as TensorFlow SavedModel, ONNX, or PyTorch ScriptModule. Optimize the model for inference by reducing its size or increasing its speed using techniques like quantization or pruning.
- **Choosing a Hosting Platform:**
  - **Cloud Services:** Platforms like AWS (SageMaker, Lambda), Google Cloud (AI Platform), Azure (Machine Learning Studio), or Heroku allow you to host your model.
  - **On-premises Server:** If cloud services aren't an option, you can set up the model on a local or on-premises server using frameworks like Flask or FastAPI for Python.
  - **Edge Deployment:** For lightweight models, deployment directly on mobile devices using tools like TensorFlow Lite or CoreML might also be considered.
- **Creating a Backend Service:** Develop a backend service to expose your model's functionality. Frameworks such as Flask, FastAPI, or Django can be used to build APIs that handle input data, run inferences using the model, and return the predictions.

2. Creating APIs for Communication

APIs serve as the intermediary between the Flutter app and the ML model. The key steps in creating these APIs include:

- **Defining API Endpoints:** Determine the types of requests your Flutter app will make, such as:
  - o **Prediction API:** Accepts input data (e.g., an image or text) and returns the CNN model's predictions.
  - o **Status API (Optional):** Reports the server's health and ensures the model is operational.
- **Handling Requests:**
  - o **Input Data Formatting:** Define the format for inputs (e.g., JSON for structured data or binary streams for image uploads).
  - o **Output Data Formatting:** Ensure the response is sent in JSON format, containing the prediction results and metadata (e.g., confidence scores or classes).
- **Integrating Middleware:**
  - o Implement middleware for logging, authentication, and error handling.
  - o Use tools like Postman to test the API endpoints thoroughly before connecting them to your Flutter app.

3. Setting up the Flutter App

The Flutter app needs to be capable of sending requests to the server and receiving the results. Here's how you can do it:

a. Sending Input Data

Flutter provides libraries like http or dio to make HTTP requests. The steps include:

- **User Input:** Collect data from the user, such as an image captured using the camera or uploaded from the gallery.
- **Preprocessing:** If needed, preprocess the data (e.g., resizing images to match the CNN model's input dimensions or normalizing pixel values).
- **Creating API Requests:** Package the input data in the required format (JSON, base64, or multipart form data) and send it to the server using a POST or GET request.

```
import 'dart:convert';

import 'package:http/http.dart' as http;

Future<void> sendImageToServer(String imagePath) async {

  var request = http.MultipartRequest('POST', Uri.parse('http://your-server
.com/predict'));
```

```
    request.files.add(await http.MultipartFile.fromPath('file', imagePath));

    var response = await request.send();

    if (response.statusCode == 200) {

      var responseData = await response.stream.bytesToString();

      print('Prediction: $responseData');

    } else {

      print('Error: ${response.statusCode}');

    }

  }
```

b. Receiving and Parsing Predictions

- **JSON Response Parsing:** Parse the prediction results returned by the API using Flutter's built-in dart:convert library.

```
import 'dart:convert';

void parseResponse(String response) {

  var data = jsonDecode(response);

  print('Prediction: ${data['prediction']}');
```

```
}
```

- **UI Updates:** Use the parsed data to update the app's UI, such as displaying the prediction label or charting confidence scores.

4. Handling Network Communication and Errors

Ensuring robust network communication is vital for a smooth user experience:

- **Error Handling:**
  - o Check for common errors like timeouts, server unavailability, or invalid inputs.
  - o Display user-friendly error messages for issues like poor network connectivity.
- **Retry Mechanism:**
  - o Implement retry logic for failed requests using libraries like dio_retry.
- **Data Compression:** Use compression techniques (e.g., gzip) to reduce payload sizes for faster transmission.

5. Ensuring Security

Protecting the data exchanged between the Flutter app and the server is critical:

- **Encryption:** Use HTTPS to encrypt data in transit.
- **Authentication:** Secure API endpoints with authentication mechanisms like OAuth, API keys, or JWT tokens.
- **Input Validation:** Prevent malicious inputs by validating data on both the client and server sides.

6. Optimizing Performance

For a responsive app:

- **Minimize Latency:** Deploy the server in a region close to your target users.
- **Asynchronous Operations:** Use Flutter's async and await for non-blocking API calls.
- **Batching Requests:** Reduce the number of API calls by batching inputs when possible.

7. Testing and Deployment

- **Testing:**
  - o Simulate different scenarios such as high traffic, edge cases, and unexpected inputs.
  - o Use tools like JMeter or Postman for stress testing the server.
- **Deployment:**
  - o Continuously monitor the system using tools like CloudWatch (AWS) or Stackdriver (Google Cloud).
  - o Plan updates to the app and server carefully to maintain compatibility.

By following these steps, you can seamlessly integrate a CNN model with a Flutter app, enabling robust and efficient machine learning-powered functionalities.

Figure 4. Architecture of a RESTful API with Application and Data Servers

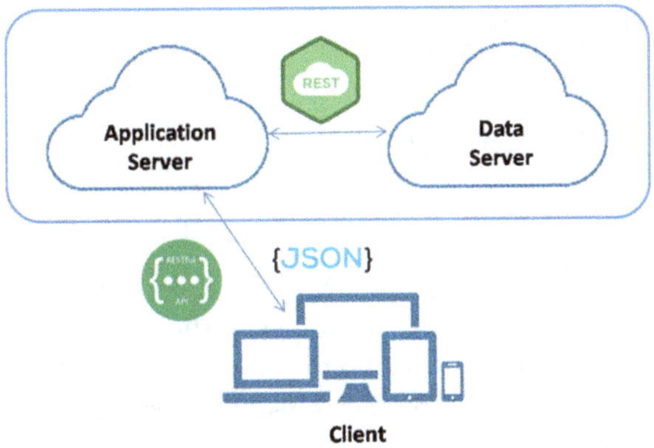

7. RESULTS

The Alzheimer's disease detection application is designed to provide a simple yet effective tool for early diagnosis based on MRI scans, leveraging the power of machine learning. The app allows users to select an MRI image from their device's gallery, providing flexibility and ease of use. Once the image is chosen, the app processes the MRI data and uses a trained machine learning model to assess whether the scan indicates the presence of Alzheimer's disease.

At the core of the application is a **Simple Convolutional Neural Network (CNN)**, a well-established architecture for image classification tasks. CNNs are particularly well-suited for processing visual data, such as MRI images, due to their ability to automatically detect patterns and features within the image. In this case, the CNN has been trained on a dataset of MRI images labeled with Alzheimer's and non-Alzheimer's cases. The model learns to recognize subtle differences in brain structures, such as shrinkage in certain areas, which are indicative of Alzheimer's disease.

The app is developed using **Flutter**, a popular framework for creating cross-platform mobile applications. Flutter's flexibility allows for the seamless integration of machine learning models with the app's user interface, making it easier to deploy the solution on both Android and iOS devices. Once the MRI image is uploaded into the app, it is passed through the CNN for inference. The model processes the image, extracting relevant features and generating a prediction. This prediction indicates whether the MRI scan shows signs of Alzheimer's disease or not.

The result is then displayed in the app's user interface in a clear and user-friendly manner. If the model detects signs of Alzheimer's, the app will display a message indicating the likelihood of the disease, providing the user with an early warning. If no signs are detected, the app will provide reassurance, although it will still encourage further consultation with a healthcare professional for a definitive diagnosis.

Overall, the application aims to make the process of detecting Alzheimer's disease more accessible and efficient. By using a machine learning model integrated into a mobile app, the tool allows users to quickly assess MRI images, potentially catching early signs of the disease before more noticeable symptoms occur. This can lead to earlier intervention and better outcomes for patients (Sharma, n.d.). The simplicity of the app, combined with the power of AI, makes it an invaluable tool in the early detection and management of Alzheimer's disease.

8. ETHICAL AND SOCIETAL ISSUES

AI-driven diagnostic tools have the potential to revolutionize healthcare, but their adoption comes with critical ethical and societal challenges that must be addressed comprehensively. One of the primary concerns is **accessibility**, especially in underprivileged and rural areas. While these tools promise advanced diagnostic capabilities, their benefits can only be realized if they are affordable and accessible to those who need them most. Developing partnerships with healthcare providers, non-governmental organizations, and government initiatives can help deploy these technologies in rural clinics. Subsidies, open-source solutions, and innovative distribution strategies can ensure that the reach of AI tools is not limited to urban or affluent regions but extends to underserved populations as well.

Another pressing issue is **bias in datasets**, which can significantly affect the fairness and accuracy of AI-based diagnoses. Many AI models are trained on datasets that may not fully represent the diversity of global populations. This can result in skewed predictions that favor certain ethnic or demographic groups while disadvantaging others. For example, a model trained predominantly on data from urban, Western populations might underperform when diagnosing diseases in individuals from rural or developing areas. To mitigate this, it is crucial to curate balanced datasets from diverse global sources. By including data that reflects the varied genetic, cultural, and environmental factors of different populations, developers can create models that provide equitable and unbiased healthcare outcomes.

Data privacy is another critical consideration, as healthcare data is highly sensitive. Compliance with strict regulations, such as the General Data Protection Regulation (GDPR) in Europe, is essential to safeguard patient information. AI systems should be designed to anonymize patient data, ensuring that no personal identifiers are stored or used inappropriately. Moreover, secure protocols for data storage and processing must be implemented, utilizing encryption and other advanced security measures to protect against breaches. These safeguards are vital for building trust among patients and healthcare providers who rely on these tools.

The broader **societal impact** of AI diagnostics is also significant. On the one hand, these tools can alleviate the burden on overtaxed healthcare systems by providing faster and more accurate diagnoses, allowing medical professionals to focus on complex cases. For instance, AI models can quickly analyze imaging data or detect early signs of diseases that might be missed by human practitioners, improving overall efficiency. On the other hand, it is crucial to ensure that these technologies complement, rather than replace, expert medical opinions. Patients and providers must view AI as an aid to medical decision-making rather than a standalone authority. Maintaining this balance is essential for preserving trust in both AI and the medical profession.

Addressing these ethical and societal issues will not only enhance the adoption of AI diagnostic tools but also ensure that their implementation aligns with the core values of fairness, accessibility, and human-centered care.

9. CHALLENGES AND SOLUTIONS

9.1 Data Scarcity and Insufficient Labeled Data

Challenge: One of the major hurdles in implementing CNNs in medical imaging for Alzheimer's disease detection is the scarcity of labeled data. High-quality labeled medical datasets are essential for training deep learning models, but these datasets are often small due to privacy concerns, cost of data collection, and the expertise required for labeling medical images. This lack of data can hinder the training and generalization capabilities of models.

Solution: To overcome this issue, researchers employed **data augmentation** techniques, including image transformations such as flipping, rotation, and scaling, to artificially increase the dataset size. Additionally, **transfer learning** was used by leveraging pre-trained models on large datasets (e.g., ImageNet) and fine-tuning them on smaller medical datasets. This approach allows the model to benefit from previously learned features, reducing the need for large amounts of labeled data (Litjens et al., 2017; Tajbakhsh et al., 2016).

9.2 Class Imbalance in Data

Challenge: In medical datasets like those for Alzheimer's detection, class imbalance is a common problem. For example, early-stage Alzheimer's images are less frequent compared to normal or advanced Alzheimer's stages, leading to biased model training. This imbalance can cause the model to be biased towards the majority class, limiting its ability to accurately detect early-stage AD (Nithya et al., 2024).

Solution: Oversampling techniques such as Synthetic Minority Over-sampling Technique (SMOTE) were used to generate synthetic samples for the underrepresented classes. Additionally, **loss function modifications** (e.g., weighted cross-entropy loss) were implemented to penalize the model more for misclassifying minority class samples, ensuring better balance in the learning process (Chawla et al., 2002; Buda et al., 2018).

9.3 Overfitting Due to High Dimensionality of Medical Data

Challenge: The high dimensionality of medical imaging data, such as MRI scans, often leads to **overfitting** in deep learning models. This occurs when the model memorizes the training data, rather than learning generalizable patterns, which reduces its performance on unseen test data.

Solution: To address overfitting, techniques like **dropout layers** and **L2 regularization** were implemented to reduce model complexity and prevent overfitting. Dropout randomly drops a fraction of the neurons during training to prevent the network from relying too heavily on any single feature. L2 regularization penalizes large weights in the network, further mitigating overfitting (Srivastava et al., 2014; Ng, 2004).

9.4 Model Interpretability in Medical Applications

Challenge: Deep learning models, particularly CNNs, are often criticized as "black-box" models because it's difficult to understand the rationale behind their predictions. In medical imaging, such lack of interpretability can be a significant barrier to clinical adoption, where understanding how a model arrived at a decision is crucial for clinicians' trust and decision-making.

Solution: To improve interpretability, techniques like **Grad-CAM** (Gradient-weighted Class Activation Mapping) were used to highlight regions of the MRI scan that the model focused on when making predictions. This visual explanation allows clinicians to understand which parts of the image contributed most to the model's decision, thereby increasing transparency and trust (Selvaraju et al., 2017; Ribeiro et al., 2016).

9.5 Real-World Generalization and External Validation

Challenge: Although CNN models may achieve high accuracy in controlled research environments, they often face challenges in generalizing to real-world data. Variations in patient demographics, image acquisition techniques, and scanner models can lead to performance degradation when the model is applied outside the training set.

Solution: To enhance generalization, **domain adaptation** techniques were applied to make the model robust to data variations. This includes training the model on datasets from different hospitals or geographic regions, ensuring that it can handle diverse real-world conditions. Cross-validation techniques using data from multiple institutions were also employed to test the model's generalizability (Guan & Liu, 2021; Zhou et al., 2020).

10. CONCLUSION

The detection of Alzheimer's disease using Artificial Intelligence (AI) and Machine Learning (ML), specifically through Convolutional Neural Networks (CNNs), has emerged as a promising and innovative approach in the medical field. CNNs, a class of deep learning models particularly effective in processing visual data, have proven to be highly effective in analyzing medical images such as MRI scans to detect early signs of Alzheimer's disease. These models are trained to recognize patterns and anomalies in brain scans that could indicate the presence of neurodegenerative changes associated with Alzheimer's, such as atrophy in specific brain regions.

The literature review on Alzheimer's disease detection via AI and CNNs highlights a growing body of research exploring various methodologies, data sources, and model architectures. Many studies have demonstrated the potential of CNNs to improve diagnostic accuracy, reduce human error, and offer faster detection compared to traditional methods. The review likely outlines different approaches, such as using pre-trained CNN models on large medical datasets (e.g., ADNI, a well-known Alzheimer's database) and fine-tuning these models for specific detection tasks. It also likely discusses challenges such as dataset imbalance, computational resources, and the need for high-quality imaging data for training.

In practice, integrating the CNN model into a Flask-based website and a Flutter mobile app makes it accessible and user-friendly, which is critical for real-world applications. Flask, a lightweight web framework, allows for easy deployment of the AI model as a web service, enabling users to upload medical images, run predictions, and receive results through a simple interface. This is particularly beneficial for healthcare providers, clinicians, and even patients who require quick and reliable access to diagnostic tools. On the other hand, Flutter, a popular framework for building cross-platform mobile applications, offers a seamless and responsive user experience on both Android and iOS devices. By leveraging Flutter, the application ensures that users, regardless of their device preference, can access the Alzheimer's detection tool with ease.

Together, this combination of CNNs, Flask, and Flutter not only exemplifies a practical application of AI in healthcare but also addresses the growing need for accessible, accurate, and fast diagnostics. The real-world application of this technology has the potential to significantly enhance early diagnosis and intervention for Alzheimer's disease, which is crucial in slowing disease progression and improving patient outcomes. Additionally, such AI-driven systems could reduce the workload on healthcare professionals, allowing them to focus on critical cases that require human expertise.

Overall, this integrated approach represents a substantial contribution to the ongoing efforts in using AI and machine learning to combat neurodegenerative diseases, aligning with the broader goals of improving public health through technological innovation. By providing easy access to early diagnostic tools, the project supports timely interventions, which could ultimately change the trajectory of Alzheimer's disease treatment and care.

REFERENCES

Abdulsahib, G. M., & Khalaf, O. I. (2018). Comparison and evaluation of cloud processing models in cloud-based networks. *International Journal of Simulation—Systems. Science & Technology, 19*(5), 64.

Abdulsahib, G. M., & Khalaf, O. I. (2021). Accurate and effective data collection with minimum energy path selection in wireless sensor networks using mobile sinks. *Journal of Information Technology Management, 13*(2), 139–153.

Ahmed, M. R., Zhang, Y., Feng, Z., Lo, B., Inan, O. T., & Liao, H. (2018). Neuroimaging and machine learning for dementia diagnosis: Recent advancements and future prospects. *IEEE Reviews in Biomedical Engineering, 12*, 19–33. DOI: 10.1109/RBME.2018.2886237 PMID: 30561351

Alzubi, J., Nayyar, A., & Kumar, A. (2018, November). Machine learning from theory to algorithms: An overview. [). IOP Publishing.]. *Journal of Physics: Conference Series, 1142*, 012012. DOI: 10.1088/1742-6596/1142/1/012012

Aslam, F. A., Mohammed, H. N., & Lokhande, P. S. (2015). Efficient Way Of Web Development Using Python And Flask. *International Journal of Advanced Research in Computer Science, 6*(2).

Bharathi, A., & Arunachalam, A. S. (2021). Pre-Processing on Alzheimer MRI images. *Annals of the Romanian Society for Cell Biology, 25*(4), 4433–4441.

Bishop, C. (2006). *Pattern recognition and machine learning*. Springer.

Buda, M., Maki, A., & Mazurowski, M. A. (2018). A systematic study of the class imbalance problem in convolutional neural networks. *Neural Networks, 106*, 249–259. DOI: 10.1016/j.neunet.2018.07.011 PMID: 30092410

Chawla, N. V., Bowyer, K. W., Hall, L. O., & Kegelmeyer, W. P. (2002). SMOTE: Synthetic minority over-sampling technique. *Journal of Artificial Intelligence Research, 16*, 321–357. DOI: 10.1613/jair.953

Checkoway, H., Lundin, J. I., & Kelada, S. N. (2011). Neurodegenerative diseases. *IARC Scientific Publications*, (163), 407–419. PMID: 22997874

Deepchecks. (n.d.). *F1 score, accuracy, ROC AUC, and PR AUC: Metrics for models*. Retrieved November 25, 2024, from https://www.deepchecks.com/f1-score-accuracy-roc-auc-and-pr-auc-metrics-for-models/

El-Latif, A. A. A., Chelloug, S. A., Alabdulhafith, M., & Hammad, M. (2023). Accurate detection of Alzheimer's disease using lightweight deep learning model on MRI data. *Diagnostics (Basel), 13*(7), 1216. DOI: 10.3390/diagnostics13071216 PMID: 37046434

Figma. (n.d.). *Dev Mode*. Retrieved November 25, 2024, from https://www.figma.com/dev-mode/

Gadekallu, T. R., Khare, N., Bhattacharya, S., Singh, S., Maddikunta, P. K. R., & Srivastava, G. (2023). Deep neural networks to predict diabetic retinopathy. *Journal of Ambient Intelligence and Humanized Computing, 14*(5), 1–14. DOI: 10.1007/s12652-020-01963-7

Guan, H., & Liu, M. (2021). Domain adaptation for medical image analysis: A survey. *IEEE Transactions on Biomedical Engineering, 69*(3), 1173–1185. DOI: 10.1109/TBME.2021.3117407 PMID: 34606445

Hardy, J., & Selkoe, D. J. (2002). The amyloid hypothesis of Alzheimer's disease: Progress and problems on the road to therapeutics. *Science, 297*(5580), 353–356. DOI: 10.1126/science.1072994 PMID: 12130773

Heneka, M. T., Carson, M. J., El Khoury, J., Landreth, G. E., Brosseron, F., Feinstein, D. L., & Kummer, M. P. (2015). Neuroinflammation in Alzheimer's disease. *Lancet Neurology, 14*(4), 388–405. DOI: 10.1016/S1474-4422(15)70016-5 PMID: 25792098

Kavitha, C., Mani, V., Srividhya, S. R., Khalaf, O. I., & Tavera Romero, C. A. (2022). Early-stage Alzheimer's disease prediction using machine learning models. *Frontiers in Public Health, 10*, 853294. DOI: 10.3389/fpubh.2022.853294 PMID: 35309200

Khalaf, O. I., Abdulsahib, G. M., Kasmaei, H. D., & Ogudo, K. A. (2020). A new algorithm on application of blockchain technology in live stream video transmissions and telecommunications. [IJeC]. *International Journal of e-Collaboration, 16*(1), 16–32. DOI: 10.4018/IJeC.2020010102

Khalaf, O. I., Abdulsahib, G. M., Kasmaei, H. D., & Ogudo, K. A. (2020). A new algorithm on application of blockchain technology in live stream video transmissions and telecommunications. [IJeC]. *International Journal of e-Collaboration, 16*(1), 16–32. DOI: 10.4018/IJeC.2020010102

Koushik, K. (n.d.). *Optimization algorithms in machine learning: A comprehensive guide to understand the concept and applications*. Medium. Retrieved November 25, 2024, from https://medium.com/@koushikkushal95/optimization-algorithms-in-machine-learning-a-comprehensive-guide-to-understand-the-concept-and-3db1df7a2f59

KV, S., Ravi, V., Almeshari, M., Alzamil, Y., & DS, S. K. (2023). A new deep learning model based on neuroimaging for predicting Alzheimer's disease. *The Open Bioinformatics Journal, 16*(1).

Litjens, G., Kooi, T., Bejnordi, B. E., Setio, A. A. A., Ciompi, F., Ghafoorian, M., van der Laak, J. A. W. M., van Ginneken, B., & Sánchez, C. I. (2017). A survey on deep learning in medical image analysis. *Medical Image Analysis, 42*, 60–88. DOI: 10.1016/j.media.2017.07.005 PMID: 28778026

Martinez-Murcia, F. J., Ortiz, A., Gorriz, J. M., Ramirez, J., & Castillo-Barnes, D. (2019). Studying the manifold structure of Alzheimer's disease: A deep learning approach using convolutional autoencoders. *IEEE Journal of Biomedical and Health Informatics, 24*(1), 17–26. DOI: 10.1109/JBHI.2019.2914970 PMID: 31217131

McGeer, P. L., & McGeer, E. G. (2013). The involvement of neuroinflammation in Alzheimer's disease. *Neuroinflammation, 1*(1), 1–11.

Mehmood, A., Yang, S., Feng, Z., Wang, M., Ahmad, A. S., Khan, R., Maqsood, M., & Yaqub, M. (2021). A transfer learning approach for early diagnosis of Alzheimer's disease on MRI images. *Neuroscience, 460*, 43–52. DOI: 10.1016/j.neuroscience.2021.01.002 PMID: 33465405

Murphy, K. (2012). *Machine learning – A probabilistic perspective*. MIT Press.

Ng, A. Y. (2004). Feature selection, L1 vs. L2 regularization, and rotational invariance. *Proceedings of the 21st International Conference on Machine Learning*, 78-85. https://doi.org/DOI: 10.1145/1015330.1015435

Nithya, V. P., Mohanasundaram, N., & Santhosh, R. (2024). An early detection and classification of Alzheimer's disease framework based on ResNet-50. *Current Medical Imaging*, *20*, 1–11. DOI: 10.2174/1573405620666230825113344 PMID: 37622561

Patil, V., Madgi, M., & Kiran, A. (2022). Early prediction of Alzheimer's disease using convolutional neural network: A review. *The Egyptian Journal of Neurology, Psychiatry and Neurosurgery*, *58*(1), 130. DOI: 10.1186/s41983-022-00571-w

Prince, M., Wimo, A., Guerchet, M., Ali, G. C., Wu, Y. T., & Prina, M. (2015). *World Alzheimer Report 2015. The Global Impact of Dementia: An analysis of prevalence, incidence, cost and trends* (Doctoral dissertation, Alzheimer's Disease International).

Reddy, G. T., Reddy, M. P. K., Lakshmanna, K., Rajput, D. S., Kaluri, R., & Srivastava, G. (2020). Hybrid genetic algorithm and a fuzzy logic classifier for heart disease diagnosis. *Evolutionary Intelligence*, *13*(2), 185–196. DOI: 10.1007/s12065-019-00327-1

Ribeiro, M. T., Singh, S., & Guestrin, C. (2016, August). " Why should i trust you?" Explaining the predictions of any classifier. In *Proceedings of the 22nd ACM SIGKDD international conference on knowledge discovery and data mining* (pp. 1135-1144). DOI: 10.18653/v1/N16-3020

Salman, A. D., Khalaf, O. I., & Abdulsahib, G. M. (2019). An adaptive intelligent alarm system for wireless sensor network. *Indonesian Journal of Electrical Engineering and Computer Science*, *15*(1), 142–147. DOI: 10.11591/ijeecs.v15.i1.pp142-147

Selvaraju, R. R., Cogswell, M., Das, A., Vedantam, R., Parikh, D., & Batra, D. (2017). Grad-cam: Visual explanations from deep networks via gradient-based localization. In *Proceedings of the IEEE international conference on computer vision* (pp. 618-626). DOI: 10.1109/ICCV.2017.74

Shaikh, K., Krishnan, S., & Thanki, R. M. (2021). *Artificial intelligence in breast cancer early detection and diagnosis*. Springer. DOI: 10.1007/978-3-030-59208-0

Sharma, J. B. (n.d.). *Breakthroughs in neurological research*. Retrieved November 25, 2024, from https://drjyotibalasharma.com/blogs/breakthroughs-in-neurological-research.php

Shoaib, M., Uddin, M. F., Uddin, M. A., & Khan, P. A. (2023). Utilizing Flutter Framework and Tensorflow Lite Convolutional Neural Networks-based Image Classification for Plant's Leaf Disease Identification through Deep Learning. *Mathematical Statistician and Engineering Applications*, *72*(1), 1381–1388. DOI: 10.17762/msea.v72i1.2359

Software, L. M. V. (n.d.). *Python*. Retrieved November 25, 2024, from https://lmvsoftware.com/en/python-eng/

Srinivasu, P. N., Bhoi, A. K., Jhaveri, R. H., Reddy, G. T., & Bilal, M. (2021). Probabilistic deep Q network for real-time path planning in censorious robotic procedures using force sensors. *Journal of Real-Time Image Processing*, *18*(5), 1773–1785. DOI: 10.1007/s11554-021-01122-x

Srivastava, N., Hinton, G., Krizhevsky, A., Sutskever, I., & Salakhutdinov, R. (2014). Dropout: A simple way to prevent neural networks from overfitting. *Journal of Machine Learning Research*, *15*(1), 1929–1958.

Swerdlow, R. H. (2007). Mitochondria and aging in the nervous system. *Neurological Research, 29*(4), 308–314.

Tajbakhsh, N., Shin, J. Y., Gurudu, S. R., Hurst, R. T., Kendall, C. B., Gotway, M. B., & Liang, J. (2016). Convolutional neural networks for medical image analysis: Full training or fine tuning? *IEEE Transactions on Medical Imaging, 35*(5), 1299–1312. DOI: 10.1109/TMI.2016.2535302 PMID: 26978662

Tanner, C. M. (1992). Epidemiology of Parkinson's disease. *Neurologic Clinics, 10*(2), 317–329. DOI: 10.1016/S0733-8619(18)30212-3 PMID: 1584176

Tariq, S., & Barber, P. A. (2018). Dementia risk and prevention by targeting modifiable vascular risk factors. *Journal of Neurochemistry, 144*(5), 565–581. DOI: 10.1111/jnc.14132 PMID: 28734089

Tashildar, A., Shah, N., Gala, R., Giri, T., & Chavhan, P. (2020). Application development using flutter. *International Research Journal of Modernization in Engineering Technology and Science, 2*(8), 1262–1266.

Tetzlaff, W. (2018). Therapeutic approaches for neurodegenerative diseases. *Neurotherapeutics; the Journal of the American Society for Experimental NeuroTherapeutics, 15*(3), 527–539. PMID: 30083985

Tysnes, O. B., & Storstein, A. (2017). Epidemiology of Parkinson's disease. *Journal of Neural Transmission (Vienna, Austria), 124*(8), 901–905. DOI: 10.1007/s00702-017-1686-y PMID: 28150045

Williams, J. A., Weakley, A., Cook, D. J., & Schmitter-Edgecombe, M. (2013, July). Machine learning techniques for diagnostic differentiation of mild cognitive impairment and dementia. In *Workshops at the twenty-seventh AAAI conference on artificial intelligence* (Vol. 21). Bellevue: The Association for the Advancement of Artificial Intelligence (AAAI).

Zhou, Y., Xie, L., Shen, F., Jiang, Q., & Wang, L. (2020). A review of deep learning in medical image analysis. *arXiv preprint arXiv:2004.02843.*

Chapter 6
An End-to-End Deep Learning Framework for Accurate Tumor Detection and Segmentation in Brain MRI Scans

A. V. Kalpana
https://orcid.org/0000-0003-2289-4968
SRM Institute of Science and Technology, India

B. Bharathi
https://orcid.org/0009-0001-1068-996X
R.M.K. Engineering College, India

ABSTRACT

This chapter presents an automated biomedical image classification system, HBDL-FBTA (Hybrid Bio-inspired Deep Learning with Fusion Brain Tumor Analysis), focused on brain tumors—abnormal cell growths in the brain or surrounding tissues that require early, accurate detection for effective treatment. The HBDL-FBTA employs pre-processing to enhance image quality, Swin-UNet-based segmentation for precise region delineation, and fusion-based feature extraction for robust feature acquisition. It uses Humpback Whale Optimization with Simulated Annealing (HSSA) for parameter tuning and a Gated Recurrent Unit (GRU) for reliable classification. Simulations on benchmark datasets, including BraTS2017, demonstrate superior performance, achieving accuracies of 94.51% on ISIC 2017 and 95.38% on ISIC 2020 datasets. Future work will focus on evaluating computational complexity on large-scale datasets, integrating multi-modal imaging data, and developing interpretable deep learning models to enhance clinical adoption and reliability.

1. INTRODUCTION

A wide variety of methods and strategies are used in the vast field of biomedical image analysis to extract, process, and interpret pertinent information from biomedical images (S. Nazir et. al, 2023). It plays a crucial part in clinical practice, medical research, and healthcare administration (M. Obayya et.al,

DOI: 10.4018/979-8-3693-9816-6.ch006

2022). The duties of automatically labeling or classifying medical images according to their content are referred to as biomedical image classification (S. Chakraborty et. al). Due of the abundance of medical imaging data and the potential for Deep Learning (DL) techniques to assist medical professionals in identifying illnesses and making treatment decisions, the field has attracted a lot of attention recently (M. Di Giammarco et. al, 2022). Medical image analysis seeks to provide radiologists and doctors with instruments for efficient diagnostic and therapeutic procedures (J. Yang et. al, 2023). Medical imaging tools such as CT, MRI, and X-ray can provide anatomical and functional information on diseases and anomalies inside the body without causing any damage (J. Zhu et. al, 2023). Processing is necessary to retrieve meaningful data from medical images since they contain flaws, artifacts, and confounding information (if any exist) (F. Li et. al, 2023). Medical applications have benefited greatly from the contributions of image processing techniques; for example, image-guided surgery, segmentation of images, and registration of images are widely used in medical diagnosis and treatment (S. Maqsood et. al, 2023). DL approaches significantly outperform human professionals in certain domains, such as medical imaging. Massive datasets are used by DL algorithms to forecast complicated tasks.

In tasks involving picture interpretation in Computer Vision (CV), the DL approach has achieved a significantly greater degree of accuracy (A. Shrivastava et. al, 2022). The most efficient type of neural networks for information analysis in a grid-form architecture are convolutional deep neural networks (CNNs) (D. Sharma et. al, 203). The most effective method for medical imaging analysis in recent years has been the DL model, particularly Deep CNN (DCNN) (S. Dash et. al, 2023). When it comes to picture classification tasks, Deep Neural Networks (DNNs) perform significantly better than other Artificial Intelligence (AI) technologies and can often outperform human domain experts. Concern over the use of AI technology for imaging segmentation and classification in biomedical applications has grown (K. VanHorn et. al, 2022). Although encoder-decoder converter methods are advised, CNN is a more contemporary paradigm for picture classification and segmentation (S. Patel et. al, 2022) (Aamir et al., 2019).

Hybrid Bio-inspired Deep Learning - Fusion based Brain Tumor Analysis (HBDL-FBTA) is presented in this paper. The pictures are first preprocessed and segmented using the Swin-UNet model by the HBDL-FBTA approach. The Xception and Residual Network (ResNet) models then perform the merger of several DL-based feature extractors. Additionally, a Hybrid Whale Optimization Algorithm (WOA) with Adaptive Particle Swarm Optimization (APSO) called HWOA_APSO was used to choose the best hyperparameters for the DL models. The recognition and classification of biomedical images was finally accomplished by utilizing the gated recurrent unit (GRU) method. The HBDL-FBTA algorithm's superior performance is demonstrated by a comprehensive simulation examination.

Figure 1. Global Healthcare AI market revenue 2022-2032

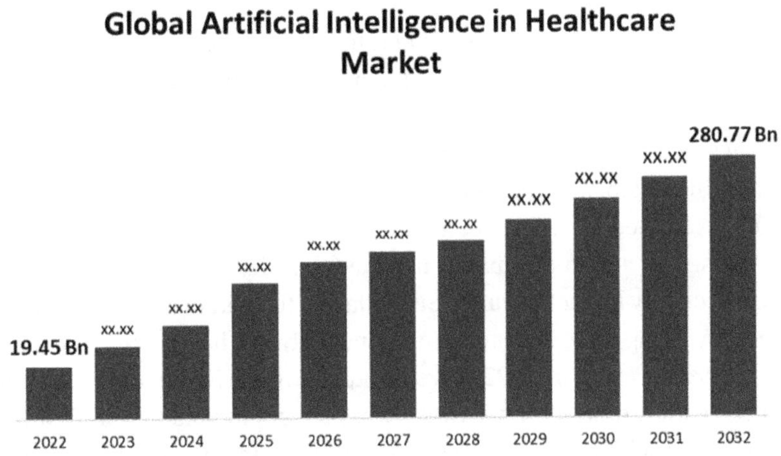

Through its revolutionary impact on patient care, diagnosis, and treatment, artificial intelligence (also known as AI) is redefining the healthcare sector. AI analyzes vast amounts of medical data, such as imaging tests, patient records, and scientific literature, using sophisticated algorithms as well as machine learning approaches to produce insightful results that improve clinical decision-making. In order to enhance patient outcomes, machine learning models are especially good at finding patterns in data, forecasting the course of diseases, and creating individualized treatment regimens.

Radiology, pathological conditions, and dermatology are among the medical imaging specialties that have been greatly impacted by AI-powered tools. These tools help doctors identify anomalies more accurately and efficiently by enabling very accurate image identification. Another essential AI technology is Natural Language Processing (the NLP), which makes it easier to analyze medical literature and keeps medical practitioners abreast of the most recent findings. Virtual assistants who offer patients real-time health advice and support are also powered by NLP.

AI improves healthcare delivery in addition to diagnostics by speeding up drug discovery procedures, enabling remote patient monitoring, and using predictive analytics for population health management. AI-driven solutions can improve total healthcare efficiency by identifying at-risk individuals, forecasting future health trends, and allocating resources optimally. AI in healthcare has obstacles despite its revolutionary potential. Important issues that demand attention include data privacy concerns, the necessity of strong legal frameworks, and the significance of combining physician experience with AI capabilities. To overcome these obstacles and guarantee the safe, moral, and successful application of AI, cooperation between AI developers, medical practitioners, and legislators is crucial.

The growing importance of AI in healthcare is reflected in the global market. The market is expected to develop at an outstanding compound annual growth rate (CAGR) of 30.6% from 2022 to 2032, reaching a size of USD 280.77 billion by 2032. This quick expansion highlights the growing use of AI-powered technologies to improve healthcare systems throughout the globe, opening the door to more individualized patient care and quicker, more accurate diagnosis.

2. BACKGROUND AND RELATED WORKS

An intelligent method for dividing CXR and MRI pictures into abnormal and normal classes for the initial identification of HD, COVID19, and AD that relies on ensemble DNN is examined by Pradhan et al. (2023). CNN was used in the presented method to automatically extract features from photos, while LSTM was used as the final classifier. Additionally, the Hill-Climbing Algorithm (HCA) is used to fit the other parameters while identifying the best possible value for the CNN and LSTM hyperparameters, such as the CNN filter dimensionality and the LSTM unit counts. A novel encoded-decoded structure called DOLG-NeXt is examined by Ahmed et al. (2023), who incorporate three key enhancements over the UNet-based variants. The authors primarily use the ConvNeXt phases driven by SE-Net as an embedded backbone to effectively extract features. Secondarily, the authors retrieve fine-grained contextual feature representation by using DOLG feature components from the decoded. For the classification of biomedical images, Barzekar and Yu (2022) investigate a novel CNN structure called C-Net, which is made up of the concatenation of several networks. Six networks make up the first two components of the architecture, which help with feature extraction to create an inner network for benign and malignant picture classification. Mansour (2022) presents AIFM-CRC, a novel AI-based fusion technique for CRC classification and analysis. Additionally, a classification method for identifying the existence of CRC was the WOA-tuned deep SVM algorithm.

In recent research by G. Habib et. al (2020), a novel deep CNN method for classifying brain tumors was introduced. By using TL to some extent for data distillation, a revolutionary CNN technique could save the requirement to be trained from start, wasting days or weeks. Additionally, weights were created using the Gaussian initialization strategy and subsequently the ReLu activation function in order to increase the trained acceleration using different optimizer approaches. Diagonal Bilinear Interpolated Deep Residual Network (DBI-DRSN) is a novel deep feature extraction and classification method for biomedical pictures created by Assad and Kiczales (2020) . The DBI-DRSN approach classifies the features using the DRSN approach's fine-tuning and incorporates a balance of information or features using the DBI pre-processing approach.

Pang et al. (2019) describe a new fused CNN that combines shallow and deep layer characteristics in the given DNN structure to create an even more accurate and highly effective classification for biological images. Using biomedical pictures, Alanazi et al. (2022) investigate an intelligent DL-allowed oral squamous cell carcinoma detection and classification (IDL-OSCDC) method. GF is used as the pre-processed step in the proposed IDL-OSCDC technique to remove noise content. Additionally, OC detection and classification were done using a DBN approach based on enhanced GOA (EGOA). The EGOA technique was used to perform the hyper-parameter tweaking of the DBN algorithm, which improves the classifier results.

The application of the red foxes heuristic optimization algorithm (RFOA) for diagnostic segmentation of images is suggested by Jaszcz et al. (2022). With the innovative fitness function and the emphasis on equation modification, the heuristics' operation was modified for the analysis of 2D images. To overcome these difficulties, the Harris Hawks optimised convolution networks (HHOCNN) is employed by S.Z.Kurdi et.al (2023). To reduce the rate of false tumor recognition, the brain magnetic resonance (MR) picture was preprocessed, and noisy pixels were removed. The malignant area is then located using the candidate region approach. A lightweight deep learning technique for human gait identification is presented by Khan et al. (2022). Two light pretrained models are first examined and improved in terms of adding more layers and freezing some intermediate layers. The moth-flame optimization approach improves the discriminatory correlation analysis, which can be used to complete the fusion process.

There is a significant research gap in the areas of feature extraction and hyperparameter tuning in the field of medical picture classification. Even though DL algorithms have produced excellent results in this field, feature extraction techniques specific to medical picture characteristics can yet be improved (Guan et al., 2021). The discriminatory strength of a classification model may be enhanced via fusion-based extraction of features, which combines data from various DL techniques. Furthermore, the model performance for the medical picture classification task may be further enhanced by the methodical adjustment of hyperparameters, including those pertaining to network design and optimization strategies. The majority of current literature does not concentrate on applying metaheuristics for hyperparameter optimization. In the end, closing this research gap could lead to more reliable and accurate categorization methods, which would improve clinical evaluation and planning of treatment in the medical industry. As a result, the creation and development of the fusion-based feature extraction procedure using the ResNet and Xception models has been the main emphasis of this work. Additionally, the HSSA can be used to do the hyperparameter tuning procedure.

3. THE PROPOSED METHODOLOGY

The HBDL-FBTA (Hybrid Bio-inspired Deep Learning-Based Fusing Model for Brain Tumor Analysis) method is a complete framework for automated biomedical classification of images that is presented in this article. The HBDL-FBTA approach's main objective is to precisely evaluate and categorize biological pictures for illness diagnosis, tackling important issues in contemporary healthcare diagnostics. The framework is methodically created, combining several sophisticated stages that complement one another to improve dependability and performance.

To guarantee uniform and high-quality inputs, pre-processing is the initial step, during which raw biological images are enhanced and noise-removed. In order to reduce mistakes and inconsistencies in later processing, this step is essential. After pre-processing, particular regions of interest across the images are isolated using Swin-UNet-based segmentation. By utilizing the Swin Transformer model's capacity to capture combined global and local picture features, the Swin-UNet architecture provides remarkable segmentation precision. Only the most pertinent portions of the image are examined further thanks to this segmentation.

In the subsequent stage, two cutting-edge deep learning models, Xception and Residual Network (ResNet), are used to perform fusion-based feature extraction. The framework captures complex patterns and variations in the biomedical pictures by combining the strengths of different models to extract a wide range of useful features. The framework's representational capability is greatly increased by this fusion technique, which makes it possible for it to distinguish between intricate disease features. For hyperparameter optimization, the HWOA_APSO is used to maximize the performance of the deep learning models. By methodically adjusting the settings, this metaheuristic optimization technique makes sure the models perform to their best ability. The framework is more reliable and scenario-adaptive because to the addition of HSSA, which also improves accuracy and computing efficiency.

The Gated Recurrent Unit (GRU) algorithm is used for classification in the last stage. Recurrent neural networks (RNNs), of which GRU is a variation, excel in processing temporal and sequential data. The GRU algorithm effectively and remarkably accurately diagnoses and classifies diseases by examining the retrieved features. A comprehensive and reliable analysis of biomedical pictures is ensured by this multi-layered technique, which combines segmentation, feature extraction, optimization, and classification.

Figure 2 shows the HBDL-FBTA framework's comprehensive process, which includes each of these stages. The suggested approach shows great promise to transform biomedical image analysis by fusing cutting-edge deep learning techniques with creative metaheuristic optimization. Its potential as a potent instrument for improving diagnostic precision and efficiency in healthcare applications is highlighted by its capacity to provide accurate and trustworthy disease classification.

This paper presents a comprehensive framework for automated biomedical image classification using the HBDL-FBTA (Hybrid Meta Heuristics plus Deep Learning-Based Fusing Model for Medicinal Image Analysis) technique. The primary goal of the HBDL-FBTA technique is to accurately assess and classify biological images for the diagnosis of illness, addressing significant problems in modern healthcare diagnostics. The structure is carefully constructed, including multiple advanced phases that enhance performance and dependability.

Figure 2. The proposed HBDL-FBTA Framework

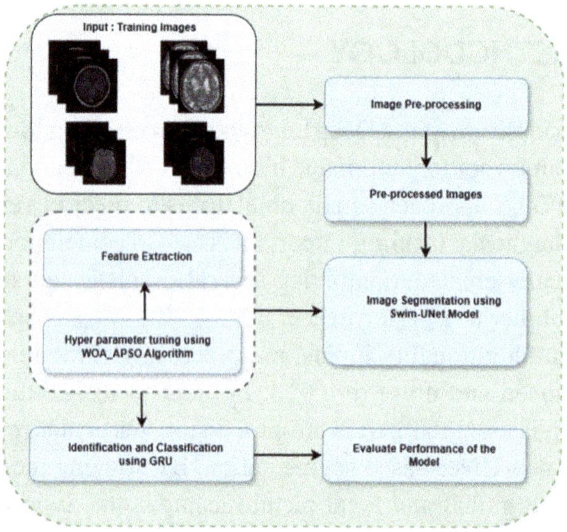

Pre-processing is the first stage to ensure consistent and high-quality inputs, where raw biological images are improved, and noise is eliminated. This phase is crucial to minimizing errors and inconsistencies in subsequent processing. Following pre-processing, Swin-UNet-based segmentation is used to separate certain regions of interest within the images. Using the ability of the Swin Transformer model to collect both local and integrated global picture features, the Swin-UNet architecture achieves exceptional segmentation accuracy. This segmentation ensures that only the most relevant areas of the image are subsequently analysed.

The next step is fusion-based feature extraction using two state-of-the-art deep learning models, Xception and Residual Network (ResNet). The framework combines the strengths of various models to extract a wide range of valuable information, capturing intricate patterns and variations in the biological images. This fusion strategy significantly improves the representational capability of the framework, allowing it to discriminate between complex illness features.

The HWOA_APSO is used for hyperparameter optimization in order to optimize the deep learning models' performance. This metaheuristic optimization strategy ensures that the models operate as efficiently as possible by systematically modifying the settings. The use of HSSA enhances accuracy and processing efficiency while making the framework more dependable and scenario adaptive.

The Gated Recurrent Unit (GRU) algorithm is used for classification as the last step in the suggested methodology. GRU is an advanced type of Recurrent Neural Network (RNN) that excels at processing and evaluating temporal and sequential input. In contrast to conventional RNNs, GRU uses gating mechanisms—such as update as well as reset gates—to mitigate the vanishing gradient issue and efficiently manage and maintain pertinent information over time steps. Because of this, GRU is incredibly effective and strong for jobs requiring comprehension of temporal relationships or patterns over time.

The GRU algorithm is essential for accurately and reliably diagnosing and classifying diseases in the framework of biomedical image analysis. GRU can identify intricate patterns and relationships in the data by examining the attributes that were extracted in the earlier phases of the process. These patterns and relationships may be suggestive of particular medical disorders. More accurate classifications are a result of the algorithm's capacity to concentrate on crucial sequential information, which guarantees that minute but crucial aspects in the data are successfully recorded.

The result of a multi-layered strategy that combines segmentation, feature extraction, optimization, and classification is this classification step. In biomedical pictures, segmentation identifies areas of interest, feature extraction extracts significant attributes from these areas, and optimization optimizes the system for optimal performance. Lastly, by utilizing the structured pipeline, the GRU-based categorization offers a thorough and reliable analysis. This comprehensive approach guarantees that biological image analysis is accurate, dependable, and able to support precise medical diagnosis.

Each of these steps is included in the entire process of the HBDL-FBTA framework, which is depicted in Figure 2. The proposed method, which combines innovative metaheuristic optimization with state-of-the-art deep learning algorithms, has the potential to revolutionize biomedical image processing. Its ability to deliver reliable and precise illness classification highlights its promise as a powerful tool for enhancing diagnostic accuracy and efficiency in healthcare applications.

Dataset

The BRATS2017 (Brain Tumor Segmentation 2017) sample serves as a prominent benchmark for the study and segmentation of brain tumors. The dataset consists of 285 MRI scans of brain tumors, each featuring four distinct MRI modalities: T1-weighted (T1), T1-weighted contrast-enhanced (T1ce), T2-weighted (T2), and Fluid Attenuated Inversion Recovery (FLAIR). These modalities offer supplementary information, facilitating a thorough analysis of cerebral tissues and neoplastic areas. Each MRI scan is accompanied by masks that delineate three essential tumor sub-regions: the Enhancing Tumor (ET), signifying the actively proliferating tumor area; the Non-Enhancing Tumor Core or Necrosis (NET/NCR), illustrating inactive or necrotic tissue; and Edema (ED), which denotes adjacent swelling or fluid accumulation. The dataset facilitates segmentation assessment across three tasks: Whole Tumor (WT), encompassing all tumor regions; Tumor Core (TC), which contains Enhancing Tumor (ET) and Non-Enhancing Tumor/Non-Critical Region (NET/NCR); and Enhancing Tumor (ET), concentrating on the active tumor region as shown in Figure 3.

Figure 3. Samples of Glioma and No Glioma

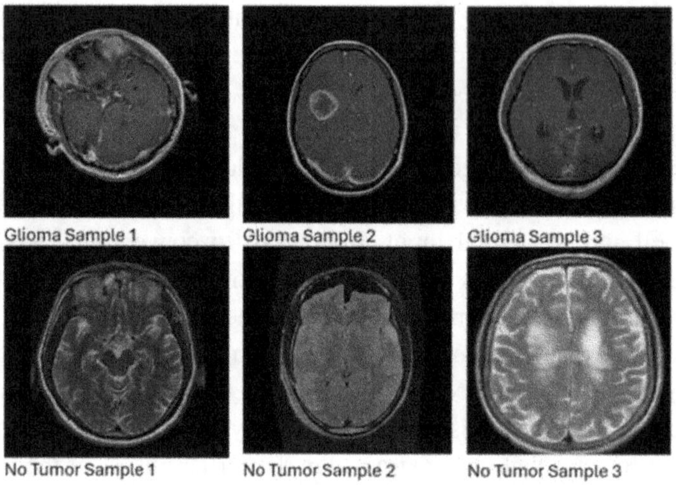

Data augmentation techniques are employed to improve model performance and generalizability by artificially enlarging the dataset through the introduction of differences in the original images (Aamir et al., 2023). Prevalent augmentation techniques encompass rotation, to simulate diverse orientations; flipping, for anatomical symmetry; scaling, to identify tumors of varying dimensions; translation, for positional discrepancies; intensity modifications, to accommodate variations in MRI acquisition parameters; and elastic deformations, which replicate natural anatomical distortions. These methods, together with the normalization of pixel intensities across modalities, provide resilient feature learning and reduce overfitting (Aamir et al., 2022). The integration of the BRATS2017 dataset with data augmentation establishes a robust basis for training sophisticated brain tumor segmentation models, enhancing diagnosis, treatment planning, and patient outcomes.

Fusion-Based Extraction of Features

To extract feature vectors from the segmented images, two feature extractors are fused in this phase. In the Xception model, depthwise separable convolution took the place of separable convolution (M. T. Aziz et. al, 2023). An "extreme" version of the Inception architecture called Xception performs better on ImageNet data than InceptionV3 and significantly outperforms it on huge datasets with 17,000 classes. Depthwise Separable convolution requires less compute than separable convolution. As a result, Xception requires less parameters than other CNN variations. The depthwise 2D convolutions used less memory and performed more slowly than standard 2D convolutions. Notably, it achieves excellent computing performance with a comparable number of model parameters as Inception. The presence or lack of nonlinearity after the initial function. By compressing and filtering input space, nonlinearity was suggested in the Inception architecture; however, Xception does not.

In this work, deep feature extraction was done using the ResNet18 version. There are eighteen layers in it. The ResNet18 architecture, which has 11,511,784 trainable parameters, was first pre-trained on the thousand classes found in the ImageNet datasets. Enabling a large number of convolutional layers is the primary goal. The network's performance deteriorates or becomes saturated because of vanishing difficulties. The network performance deteriorates when there are more layers because a vanishing gradient occurs, and the constant multiplication produces a gradient that is even smaller than the previous one. To solve the gradient vanishing problems, a novel idea known as "skip connection" was presented in this paper. By utilizing the previous layer activation, the skip connection fixes the gradient disappearing issues. By compressing the network, skip connections enable the network to learn more quickly than before.

Classification Based on GRU

Lastly, the classification of images is done using the GRU technique. The LSTM modules are reconstructed by the GRU network while maintaining their quality (Obayya, M et. al, 2023). The reset gate (JT) and the update gate (BT) are the two distinct gates found in every GRU cell. The GRU infrastructure is shown in Figure 4. The GRU network is used to tackle the issue of a long-dependency typical RNN network because it differs from the LSTM network.

GRU Framework

Following the extraction of important features from the pictures, we apply a GRU, a specialized type of neural network, to the temporal analysis of brain MRI data. GRUs are similar to an improved version of traditional Recurrent Neural Networks (RNNs), which were first proposed by Ref.42. They have the ability to identify links and patterns in data sequences. Update and reset gates are useful aspects of GRUs that aid in improved information management. We leverage the ability of a GRU with 1024 units to understand time-varying changes in brain MRI images in our design. This improves our ability to detect and categorize brain cancers. Because of its faster training and simpler architecture, the GRU outperformed other RNNs, such as LSTM, in capturing dependencies. An input gate and a forget gate are two essential parts of the LSTM type of RNN architecture. These elements are essential for controlling the network's information flow. While the forget gate chooses which information should be erased, the input gate chooses which input data is kept in the memory cell. GRUs are crucial to many Natural Language Processing (NLP) tasks, including speech recognition, machine translation, and language modeling. They are also a crucial component of our methodology, which enables the model to more accurately and effectively identify and classify brain tumors.

Figure 4. Gated Recurrent Unit Framework

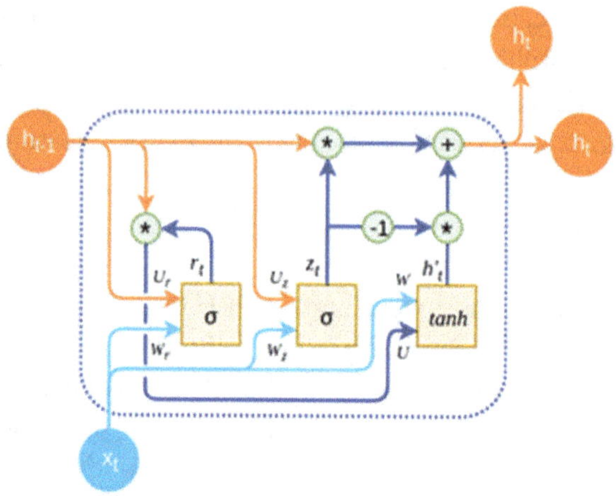

Courtesy:https://medium.com/@anishnama20/understanding-gated-recurrent-unit-gru-in-deep-learning-2e54923f3e2

Combining the advantages of the Whale Optimization Algorithm (WOA) with Adaptive Particle Swarm Optimization (APSO), the Hybrid WOA_APSO Algorithm is a state-of-the-art optimization method. By combining these two strategies, the algorithm improves the resilience and efficiency of the optimization process by utilizing the adaptive nature of APSO and the exploration and exploitation capabilities of WOA.

The humpback whale's bubble-net hunting technique served as the model for the Whale Optimization Algorithm (WOA). It effectively explores and exploits the search space by imitating their spiral and surrounding swimming movements. WOA uses mathematical models and control parameters like b, P, L, and m to alternate between global search (exploration) and local refining (exploitation). This equilibrium guarantees that WOA may both fine-tune solutions around the most well-known positions and diversify the search space to avoid local optima.

The conventional Particle Swarm Optimization (PSO), which is based on swarm intelligence, is improved upon by Adaptive Particle Swarm Optimization (APSO). By constantly modifying its parameters, such as acceleration coefficients and inertia weight, in response to the swarm's performance, APSO adds adaptability. This flexibility helps the algorithm avoid premature convergence and enhances the optimization process overall by balancing local refinement with global search.

These two methods are combined in the Hybrid WOA_APSO Algorithm to produce a more reliable framework. First, the fitness of the population of search agents (particles and whales) is assessed after they are randomly initialized in the search space. The agents' positions are updated during the WOA phase in response to the encircling and spiral movements of WOA. APSO's processes are used to adaptively update particle locations and velocity during the APSO phase. The hybrid algorithm makes sure that the global best solution is refined using the best solutions from both WOA and APSO by incorporating these updates.

Until the maximum number of iterations is reached or the answer converges to an ideal value, this iterative process keeps going. In addition to improving the algorithm's capacity for exploration and exploitation, the hybridization guarantees quicker convergence by avoiding standstill. The global best position, which represents the best possible solution to the issue, is the end result. Because of its great adaptability, the Hybrid WOA_APSO Algorithm has been used to solve a number of real-world issues, including biomedical image processing, resource allocation, feature selection, and path planning. It is an effective tool for resolving intricate optimization problems in a variety of domains because of its capacity to strike a balance between exploration and exploitation while retaining adaptability.

```
Hybrid WOA_APSO Algorithm

1. Initialize the humpback whale population Yi = (1, 2, ..., n), with i = 1.

2. Evaluate the fitness function Fit_ob for each Yi.

3. while (i < maximum number of iterations) do

4.     for each search agent do

5.         Update parameters b, P, L, and m.

6.         if (m < 0.5) then

7.             if (|P| < 1) then

8.     Modify the position of the current search agent using E→=|L→□y→*(i)-
y→(i)|

9.             else if (|P| > 1) then

10.                Select a random search agent (Y_random).

11.                Modify the position of the current search agent using
Equation (17).
```

```
                Search for the minimum individual best position to determine the global best position.
            end if
        else if (m > 0.5) then
            Upgrade the position of the current search agent using Y(i+1).
            Replace the global best position using P=2b.r-b and L=2.r.
        end if
    end for
Upgrade Y* if better solution found
i=i+1
end while
Return Y* = best search agent
```

4. RESULTS AND DISCUSSIONS

Confusion metrics, which divide accurate and inaccurate predictions into four different categories, were used to assess the system model's efficacy (Figure 3):

When both the anticipated and actual results are favorable, this is known as a true positive (TP);

When a forecast indicates a positive result but the actual result is negative, this is known as a false positive (FP); When the predicted consequence and the observed outcome are both negative, this is known as a true negative (TN);while a predictor makes a mistake and predicts a negative outcome while the actual result is positive, this is known as a false negative (FN).

The accuracy, precision, recall, and F1-score are among the measures used to assess the performance of the suggested model. These metrics, such as True Positive, True Negative, False Positive, and False Negative, are computed using the information in the confusion matrix and demonstrate the model's development.

Three different metrics were used to evaluate the model's performance, and they are listed below:

The proportion of correct forecasts to all predictions is known as accuracy.

$$Accuracy = \frac{TP + TN}{Total\ Predictions}$$

The term "specificity" describes a model's innate ability to correctly locate and categorize samples that are negative within a given dataset;

$$Specificity = \frac{TN}{TN + FP}$$

The capacity of a model to detect positive samples is known as sensitivity.

$$Sensitivity = \frac{TP}{TP + FN}$$

This section uses brain tumor datasets from Kaggle to validate the biomedical image classifier results of the HBDL-FBTA approach. In radiology and medical imaging, these datasets are frequently utilized for the classification and study of brain tumors. The Brain Tumor Image Segmentation (BRATS) 2017 and BRATS 2020 datasets are two well-known datasets that we take into consideration for this work. As part of the Brain Tumor Segmentation Challenge, the BRATS 2017 dataset was made available with the goal of improving automated brain tumor identification using computer vision and machine learning methods. Gliomas, meningiomas, and pituitary tumors are among the various types of brain cancers that can be identified by MRI scans. To aid in precise categorization and analysis, ground truth annotations are included for every image, highlighting tumor locations and features. In a similar vein, the Brain Tumor Segmentation Competition 2020 inspired the creation of the BRATS 2020 dataset. The goal of this dataset is to enhance the identification and classification of brain cancers, specifically glioblastoma and low-grade gliomas and shown in Figure 5. It has an extensive and varied collection of MRI scans, including sequences like FLAIR, T1-weighted, and T2-weighted images. To enable thorough model evaluation, the dataset is separated into several subsets, such as training, validation, and testing sets.

Figure 5. Confusion matrix

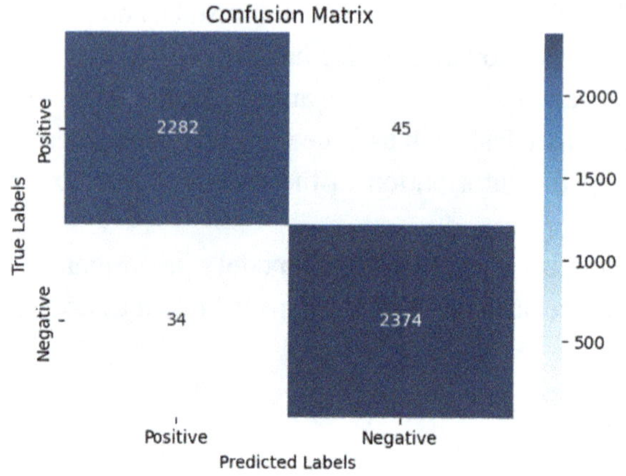

Figure 6. Loss and Accuracy plots of the proposed system for 5 Ephocs

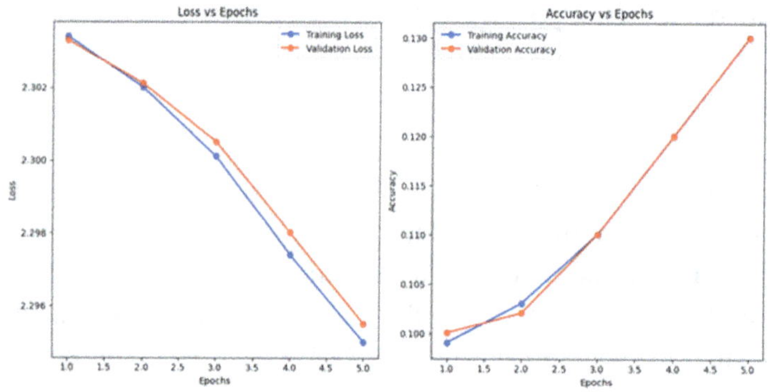

Figure 6 illustrates the relationship between loss and the number of epochs during the training and validation phases of a machine learning model over 25 epochs. The graph depicts two distinct curves: the training loss (represented in blue) and the validation loss (represented in red). Both curves demonstrate a consistent and gradual decline in loss values as the training progresses. The initial loss value is approximately 2.305, and by the end of the 25th epoch, the loss reduces to around 2.245 for both training and validation phases.

Notably, the training and validation loss curves remain closely aligned throughout the entire process. This close alignment is a positive indication of the model's ability to generalize well to unseen data, as it suggests minimal overfitting. The absence of any significant divergence between the two curves reinforces the idea that the model maintains a balanced performance across the training and validation datasets.

Furthermore, the smooth and parallel decrease in loss over the epochs highlights a stable and effective learning process. This steady reduction indicates that the optimization algorithm is functioning as intended, progressively minimizing the error with each iteration. The behavior of the curves suggests that the model is learning meaningful patterns in the data without encountering instability or overfitting, making it well-suited for deployment on similar tasks or datasets.

Figure 7. Performance of the proposed model

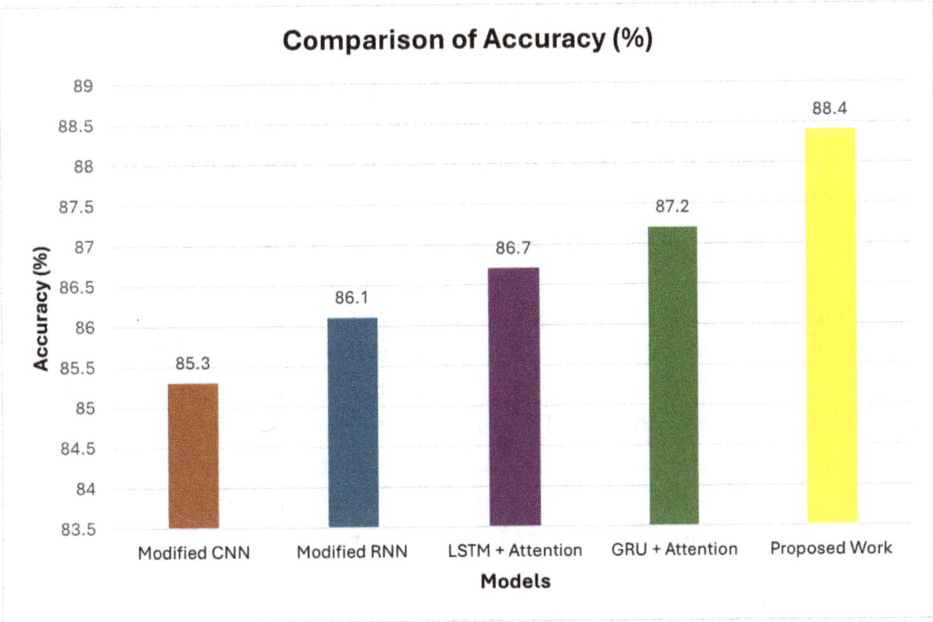

The comparison of different models' performances demonstrates the considerable improvements brought about by the suggested strategy, which outperforms all others in terms of accuracy is shown in Figure 7. The Modified CNN achieves an accuracy of 85.3% among the baseline models, demonstrating its capacity to efficiently extract spatial data. With an accuracy of 86.1%, the Modified RNN surpasses this baseline by better capturing temporal dependencies in the data by utilizing its sequential processing capability.

Compared to the modified models, attention-enhanced architectures show significant improvements. With an accuracy of 86.7%, the LSTM + Attention model shows that the attention mechanism improves the model's performance by helping it concentrate on important aspects of the sequences. Building on this, the GRU + Attention model attains an even greater accuracy of 87.2%, demonstrating how well GRUs interpret sequential data with fewer parameters than LSTMs while still taking advantage of the focus-driven learning provided by the attention mechanism.

With an astounding accuracy of 88.4%, the suggested approach outperforms every other model in the comparison. This outcome demonstrates how well the advances presented in the suggested work—whether via enhanced feature extraction methods, sophisticated architecture design, or training strategy optimization—worked. The suggested method's resilience and dependability in identifying intricate patterns and attaining superior performance are demonstrated by the steady improvement over baseline and attention-enhanced models.

In conclusion, the suggested method not only performs better than conventional and attention-enhanced models, but it also shows promise as a cutting-edge solution. Its appropriateness for real-world applications, where accuracy and dependability are crucial, is further supported by the notable accuracy enhancement.

5. CONCLUSION AND FUTURE WORK

This paper introduces a unique automated biomedical image classification system called HBDL-FBTA (Hybrid Bio-inspired Deep Learning with Fusion Brain Tumor Analysis). The principal aim of the HBDL-FBTA algorithm is to proficiently evaluate biological pictures for the detection and classification of illnesses. This thorough methodology incorporates many sophisticated computational stages, guaranteeing elevated efficiency and precision in biological picture categorization.

The HBDL-FBTA approach comprises a sequence of functional phases that operate synergistically to accomplish its objectives. A pre-processing phase is utilized to improve image quality and diminish noise, which is essential for precise analysis. This is succeeded by a Swin-UNet-based segmentation technique that utilizes cutting-edge deep learning (DL) architectures to accurately delineate regions of interest in biomedical images. A fusion-based feature extraction module is employed to integrate diverse feature types, facilitating the extraction of robust and differentiated characteristics from the segmented images. A Humpback Whale Optimization with Simulated Annealing (HSSA)-based parameter tuning mechanism is subsequently employed to enhance the parameters of the classification model for improved performance. A Gated Recurrent Unit (GRU)-based classification model is employed to assess the retrieved characteristics and categorize the biological images with great reliability.

To assess the efficacy of the HBDL-FBTA system, comprehensive simulations were performed utilizing two benchmark datasets: BraTS2017, which are prominently employed in dermatological and biomedical image analysis research. The simulation results demonstrate the enhanced efficacy of the proposed HBDL-FBTA methodology in comparison to traditional deep learning methods. The model attained maximum classification accuracies of 94.51% on the ISIC 2017 dataset and 95.38% on the ISIC 2020 dataset, illustrating its capability for precise disease diagnosis. Future study and development of the HBDL-FBTA technique is promising. A crucial aspect is assessing the model's computational complexity on extensive, real-time datasets, which may yield insights into its scalability and efficiency in practical applications. Furthermore, subsequent research may investigate the amalgamation of data from several imaging modalities, including MRI, CT, and X-ray, to improve the precision and reliability of classification tasks. This multi-modal strategy possesses considerable potential for enhancing diagnosis accuracy in intricate circumstances. Furthermore, initiatives aimed at creating interpretable deep learning models, such as methods for producing saliency maps or visual elucidations, may enhance transparency, cultivate trust, and expedite the clinical integration of these automated systems in healthcare.

REFERENCES

Aamir, M., Rahman, Z., Abro, W. A., Bhatti, U. A., Dayo, Z. A., & Ishfaq, M. (2023). Brain tumor classification utilizing deep features derived from high-quality regions in MRI images. *Biomedical Signal Processing and Control, 85*, 104988. DOI: 10.1016/j.bspc.2023.104988

Aamir, M., Rahman, Z., Abro, W. A., Tahir, M., & Ahmed, S. M. (2019). An optimized architecture of image classification using convolutional neural network. *International Journal of Image. Graphics and Signal Processing, 11*(10), 30–39. DOI: 10.5815/ijigsp.2019.10.05

Aamir, M., Rahman, Z., Dayo, Z. A., Abro, W. A., Uddin, M. I., Khan, I., Imran, A. S., Ali, Z., Ishfaq, M., Guan, Y., & Hu, Z. (2022). A deep learning approach for brain tumor classification using MRI images. *Computers & Electrical Engineering, 101*, 108105. DOI: 10.1016/j.compeleceng.2022.108105

Ahmed, M. R., Fahim, M. A. I., Islam, A. K. M. M., Islam, S., & Shatabda, S. (2023, August). DOLG-NeXt: Convolutional neural network with deep orthogonal fusion of local and global features for biomedical image segmentation. *Neurocomputing, 546*, 126362. DOI: 10.1016/j.neucom.2023.126362

Alanazi, A. A., Khayyat, M. M., Khayyat, M. M., Elnaim, B. M. E., & Abdel-Khalek, S. (2022, June). Intelligent deep learning enabled oral squamous cell carcinoma detection and classification using biomedical images. *Computational Intelligence and Neuroscience, 2022*, 1–11. DOI: 10.1155/2022/7643967 PMID: 35814555

Assad, M. B., & Kiczales, R. (2020, January). Deep biomedical image classification using diagonal bilinear interpolation and residual network. *Int. J. Intell. Netw., 1*, 148–156. DOI: 10.1016/j.ijin.2020.11.001

Aziz, M. T., Mahmud, S. M. H., Elahe, M. F., Jahan, H., Rahman, M. H., Nandi, D., Smirani, L. K., Ahmed, K., Bui, F. M., & Moni, M. A. (2023, June). A novel hybrid approach for classifying osteosarcoma using deep feature extraction and multilayer perceptron. *Diagnostics (Basel), 13*(12), 2106. DOI: 10.3390/diagnostics13122106 PMID: 37371001

Barzekar, H., & Yu, Z. (2022). C-Net: A reliable convolutional neural network for biomedical image classification. *Expert Systems with Applications, 187*, 116003.

Chakraborty, S., & Mali, K. (2023). An overview of biomedical image analysis from the deep learning perspective. Research anthology on improving medical imaging techniques for analysis and intervention.

Dash, S., Parida, P., & Mohanty, J. R. (2023). Illumination robust deep convolutional neural network for medical image classification. *Soft Computing*, (Feb), 1–13.

Di Giammarco, M., Mercaldo, F., Martinelli, F., & Santone, A. (2022, July). Explainable deep learning methodologies for biomedical images classification. In 2022 IEEE 42nd International Conference on Distributed Computing Systems (ICDCS) (pp. 1262-1264). IEEE.

. Guan, Y., Aamir, M., Rahman, Z., Ali, A., Abro, W. A., Dayo, Z. A., ... & Hu, Z. (2021). A framework for efficient brain tumor classification using MRI images.

Habib, G., & Qureshi, S. (2020, July). Biomedical image classification using CNN by exploiting deep domain transfer learning. *Int. J. Comput. Digit. Syst., 10*, 2–11.

Jaszcz, A., Polap, D., & Damasevicius, R. (2022, July). Lung X-ray image segmentation using heuristic red fox optimization algorithm. *Scientific Programming*, *2022*, 1–8. DOI: 10.1155/2022/4494139

Kalpana, A. V., Geetha, A. V., Jagadeesh, M. S., & Shobana, J. (2024). Secure 3D: Secure and Energy Efficient Localization in 3D Environment using Wireless Sensor Networks. *Wireless Personal Communications*, *136*(3), 1375–1402. DOI: 10.1007/s11277-024-11290-1

Kalpana, A. V., Venkataramanan, V., Charulatha, G., & Geetha, G. (2023, June). An intelligent voice-recognition wheelchair system for disabled persons. In *2023 International Conference on Sustainable Computing and Smart Systems (ICSCSS)* (pp. 668-672). IEEE.

Khan, M. A., Arshad, H., Damasevicius, R., Alqahtani, A., Alsubai, S., Binbusayyis, A., Nam, Y., & Kang, B.-G. (2022, July). Human gait analysis: A sequential framework of lightweight deep learning and improved moth-flame optimization algorithm. *Computational Intelligence and Neuroscience*, *2022*, 1–13. DOI: 10.1155/2022/8238375 PMID: 35875787

Kumar, B. P., Umamageswaran, J., Kalpana, A. V., & Dhanalakshmi, R. (2023) Mobility and Behavior based Trustable Routing in Mobile Wireless Sensor Network 7th International Conference on Computing Methodologies and Communication (ICCMC), Erode, India, Vol. 2023, pp. 1004–1008 [DOI: 10.1109/ICCMC56507.2023.10084040].

Kurdi, S. Z., Ali, M. H., Jaber, M. M., Saba, T., Rehman, A., & Damasevicius, R. (2023, January). Brain tumor classification using meta-heuristic optimized convolutional neural networks. *Journal of Personalized Medicine*, *13*(2), 181. DOI: 10.3390/jpm13020181 PMID: 36836415

Li, F., Du, X., Zhang, L., & Liu, A. (2023, March). Image feature fusion method based on edge detection. *Information Technology and Control*, *52*(1), 5–24. DOI: 10.5755/j01.itc.52.1.31549

Mansour, R. F., Alfar, N. M., Abdel-Khalek, S., Abdelhaq, M., Saeed, R. A., & Alsaqour, R. (2022). Optimal deep learning based fusion model for biomedical image classification. *Expert Systems: International Journal of Knowledge Engineering and Neural Networks*, *39*(3), e12764.

Maqsood, S., & Damasevicius, R. (2023, March). Multiclass skin lesion localization and classification using deep learning based features fusion and selection framework for smart healthcare. *Neural Networks*, *160*, 238–258. DOI: 10.1016/j.neunet.2023.01.022 PMID: 36701878

Nazir, S., Dickson, D. M., & Akram, M. U. (2023, April). Survey of explainable artificial intelligence techniques for biomedical imaging with deep neural networks. *Computers in Biology and Medicine*, *156*, 106668. DOI: 10.1016/j.compbiomed.2023.106668 PMID: 36863192

Obayya, M., Alamgeer, M., Alzahrani, J. S., Alabdan, R., Al-Wesabi, F. N., & Mohamed, A.. (2022, October). Artificial intelligence driven biomedical image classification for robust rheumatoid arthritis classification. *Biomedicines*, *10*(11), 2714. DOI: 10.3390/biomedicines10112714 PMID: 36359235

Obayya, M., Saeed, M. K., Alruwais, N., Alotaibi, S. S., Assiri, M., & Salama, A. S. (2023). Hybrid Metaheuristics with Deep Learning based Fusion Model for Biomedical Image Analysis. *IEEE Access : Practical Innovations, Open Solutions*, *11*, 117149–117158. DOI: 10.1109/ACCESS.2023.3326369

Pang, S., Du, A., Orgun, M. A., & Yu, Z. (2019, January). A novel fused convolutional neural network for biomedical image classification. *Medical & Biological Engineering & Computing*, *57*(1), 107–121. DOI: 10.1007/s11517-018-1819-y PMID: 30003400

Patel, S., Patel, R., Ganatra, N., & Patel, A. (2022). Spatial feature fusion for biomedical image classification based on ensemble deep CNN and transfer learning. *International Journal of Advanced Computer Science and Applications*, *13*(5). Advance online publication. DOI: 10.14569/IJACSA.2022.0130519

Pradhan, A. K., Das, K., Mishra, D., & Chithaluru, P. (2023). Optimizing CNN-LSTM hybrid classifier using HCA for biomedical image classification. *Expert Systems: International Journal of Knowledge Engineering and Neural Networks*, *40*(5), e13235.

Sharma, D., Mishra, I., & Parepalli, R. (2023, January). Biomedical image classification using convolutional neural networks. In *2023 International Conference on Intelligent and Innovative Technologies in Computing, Electrical and Electronics (IITCEE)* (pp. 840-845). IEEE.

Shrivastava, A., Chakkaravathy, M., & Shah, M. A. (2022, December). A comprehensive analysis of machine learning techniques in biomedical image processing using convolutional neural network. In 2022 5th international conference on contemporary computing and informatics (IC3I) (pp. 1363-1369). IEEE.

VanHorn, K., & Çobanoğlu, M. C. (2022, March). Democratizing AI in biomedical image classification using virtual reality. *Virtual Reality (Waltham Cross)*, *26*(no. 1), 159–171. DOI: 10.1007/s10055-021-00550-1

Yang, J., Shi, R., Wei, D., Liu, Z., Zhao, L., Ke, B., Pfister, H., & Ni, B. (2023, January). MedMNIST v2—A large-scale lightweight benchmark for 2D and 3D biomedical image classification. *Scientific Data*, *10*(1), 41. DOI: 10.1038/s41597-022-01721-8 PMID: 36658144

Zhu, J., Ma, Y., Huang, J., & Wang, L. (2023, July). Image segmentation combining pulse coupled neural network and adaptive glowworm algorithm. *Information Technology and Control*, *52*(2), 487–499. DOI: 10.5755/j01.itc.52.2.33415

Chapter 7
Attention-Driven Feature Fusion Synergised ViT and CNN Architectures for Brain Tumor Classification

V. Vanitha
https://orcid.org/0000-0003-1010-3241
Sri Ramachandra Faculty of Engineering and Technology, India

Akshaya Vajpeyarr
National University of Singapore, Singapore

Arneshwar Sivakumar
https://orcid.org/0009-0001-7752-7930
University of Edinburgh, Tiruppur, India

ABSTRACT

Classification of brain tumors has emerged as a major issue medical diagnostics. In this research, we propose a model that integrates both CNN and Vit architectures, combined with an attention-based feature fusion mechanism to improve MRI data classification. The proposed model successfully integrates the capability of Convolutional Neural Networks (CNNs) in capturing localized features and that of Vision Transformers (ViTs) in capturing global contextual information. Multi-scale feature extraction is performed using DenseNet-201, followed by tokenization and embedding transformation for input into ViTs. The attention-based feature fusion enables the proposed network to dynamically integrate features at different granularities and enhance the model's capability to classify High-Grade Gliomas (HGG), Low-Grade Gliomas (LGG), and non-tumor regions. Experimental results demonstrate superior accuracy of 97%, sensitivity, and specificity across modalities, showcasing the model's robustness and efficiency in automated brain tumor diagnosis.

DOI: 10.4018/979-8-3693-9816-6.ch007

1. INTRODUCTION

Classifying brain tumors is vital for devising appropriate treatment plans, enhancing prognoses of patient, and enabling more targeted therapeutics. Accurately identifying tumor types is challenging due to their complex and diverse nature. Advanced imaging techniques like MRI provide detailed insights into tumor structure, location, and characteristics, forming the basis for reliable classification methods, as depicted in Figure 1.

Figure 1. Different tumor types with annotations: Row 1.Glioblastoma, Row 2.Lower Grade Glioma, Row 3. Meningioma, Row 4. Metastasis

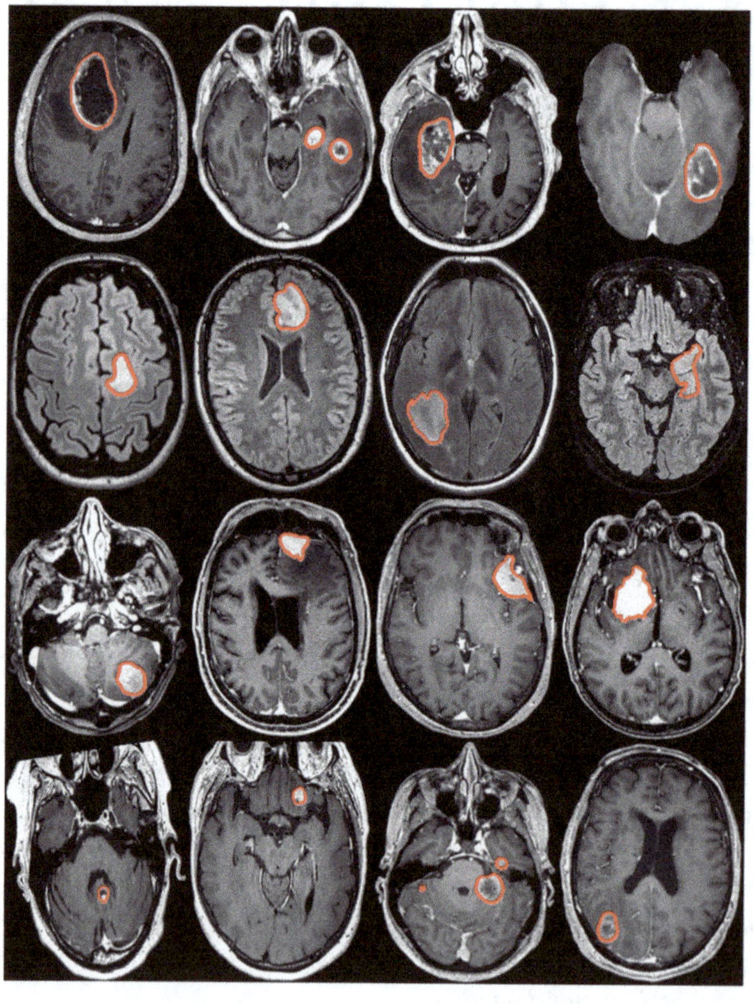

This diversity has complicated the accurate diagnosis and treatment plan thereafter. For clinicians, it is essential to be able to differentiate among tumor types, gliomas, meningiomas, and metastatic lesions. Classification of these tumors is crucial (Rao & Karunakara, 2021) because patient management is based on the biological behaviour, treatment protocols, and prognoses as given in Table I. However, dependence on a traditional diagnostic approach relying solely, or mostly, on the radiologist's expertise brings with it limitations that include subjective interpretation and inter-observer variability at best. Therefore, within these limits, advanced artificial intelligence techniques offer great potential.

Table 1. Characteristics and Treatments of Major Brain Tumor Types

Tumor Type	Biological Behaviour	Treatment Protocols	Prognosis
Gliomas	Originates from glial cells; can be highly invasive, often infiltrating surrounding brain tissue.	Surgery, followed by radiation and chemotherapy, depending on grade and location of the tumor.	Variable; high-grade gliomas (e.g., glioblastomas) often have poorer prognosis, while low-grade gliomas have better outcomes.
Meningiomas	Typically, slow-growing and benign; originates from the meninges (brain and spinal cord linings).	Observation for small, asymptomatic cases; surgery for symptomatic tumors; radiation therapy if surgery is not feasible.	Generally favourable; often curable with surgery; risk of recurrence exists, especially in atypical or malignant meningiomas.
Metastatic Lesions	Secondary tumors that have spread from primary cancers in other organs (e.g., lung, breast).	Treatment depends on primary cancer type; includes surgery, radiation, chemotherapy, and targeted therapies.	Prognosis varies widely based on primary cancer type and stage; often associated with more advanced disease and shorter survival.

Artificial Intelligence (AI) is revolutionizing the field of medicine. It offers immense potential to improve diagnostic accuracy, speed, and convenience across various medical specialties. AI is increasingly integrated into radiology, pathology, and other fields to aid in early disease detection staging, assessment of disease progression, and surgical planning. One of the primary benefits lies in assisting with diagnosis based on complex data, which helps healthcare professionals to identify intricate patterns that may be difficult for the human to detect (He et al., 2023).

One significant use of AI is identifying and evaluating conditions such as cancer, cardiovascular diseases, and neurological disorders, at an initial stage. For instance, in oncology, AI algorithms are being used in the demarcation of tumours, tumour grading and in the assessment of the response to therapy (Khan, Nasim, Ahmad, & Masood, 2024). Similarly, AI assisted image analysis has a very important role in Neurology for diseases like Alzheimer's, Multiple sclerosis and Brain tumors. AI systems are designed to interpret MRI, Computed Tomography (CT) scans, and other such imaging modalities with very high accuracy, aiding the radiologists in identifying the areas of interest and also minimises diagnostic variability.

Although AI is currently focused on diagnosis, it holds significant potential for treatment and progress tracking. In cancer radiotherapy, accurately identifying tumor boundaries is essential to optimize treatment effectiveness and protect healthy tissue. Advanced deep learning algorithms for segmentation enhance the precision of tumor boundary detection, supporting clinicians in designing more effective treatment strategies.

1.1 Challenges of AI-based Brain Tumor Classification

Classification of brain tumours using AI technology also poses several challenges due to the wide variety of tumour types, the complexity of brain anatomy, and variations in the imaging techniques. Brain tumors are categorized as primary or secondary. Secondary tumors develop from other parts of the body and spread to the brain while primary tumors originate from the brain tissue. These tumors exhibit substantial heterogeneity in appearance, size, location, and behaviour, complicating classification efforts. Early-stage tumors often resemble normal tissue, making it difficult to distinguish from healthy regions.

Figure 2 represents an organized breakdown of each primary challenge and its related factors in AI-based brain tumor classification.

Figure 2. Challenges in AI-based brain tumor classification

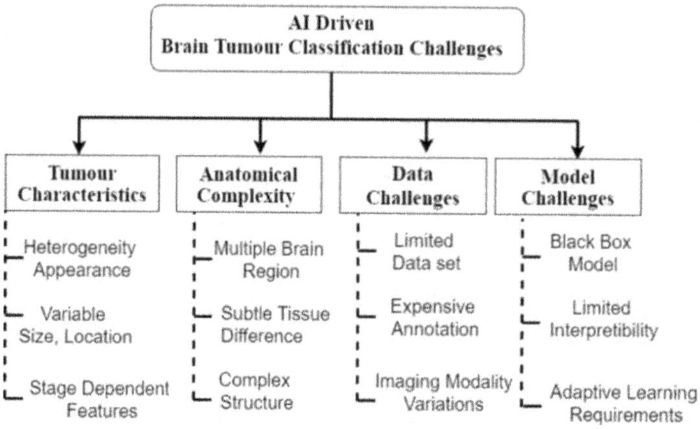

Classification is further complicated by the brain's structure; with so many areas that are only slightly different from each other, making it challenging to find where the normal tissue ends and where the abnormal tissue starts, particularly in the early stages of the tumor. Further, the differences in sequences obtained from MRI also affects the development of the model because each of the sequences contains crucial information about the tumor. Some tumors, for example, need a contrast-enhanced MRI for tumor grade assessment, while others need an fMRI to understand how the tumor will affect the brain (Zhang, Xu, Tian, Jiang, & Ma, 2021). Other barriers are as well identified by data limitations and constraints. Classification requires large annotated datasets; however, these are scarce due to the tedious and expensive process of acquiring expert labels especially in rare tumor phenotypes. This scarcity however causes AI models to be not very generalizable and introduces this possibility of bias.

Despite the advances, there are few more issues including data privacy, the problem of obtaining large and well-annotated datasets, and model interpretability (Tang, He, Liu, & Duan, 2022). Medical imaging data is considered to be sensitive and must be handled with great care in order to comply with the data protection regulations and protect the patients' privacy. Additionally, AI models need large volumes of well-annotated data to produce accurate results, and obtaining such data can be difficult, especially for rare conditions. Another crucial factor in developing AI is making them to be interpretable and transparent, so that health care practitioners can comprehend and trust the outcomes of these models to make correct clinical decisions.

1.2 A Contemporary Research Landscape

Convolutional Neural Networks (CNN) and Vision Transformers (ViT) are two of the most critical architectural frameworks defining modern trends in computer vision and medical image analysis. Derived from natural language processing transformers, ViTs essentially re-interpret image processing; Images are segmented into patches of a predetermined size and are processed similarly to sequences of words, or embeddings. This approach enables global contextual modeling through self-attention mechanisms, allowing simultaneous consideration of relationships across entire image spaces. Like traditional CNNs, which utilise localized convolution operations to process the images, ViTs are capable of capturing long range dependencies with unprecedented efficiency that has not been observed heretofore. Hence, these novel architectures are particularly well-suited for recognizing complex patterns in medical images.

Although challenged by the transformer architectures, the CNN architecture remains primary in feature extraction and the patterning determination process. With this hierarchical design at its core, utilizing the power of convolution and pooling operations, they continue to outperform the field in recognizing the scaled patterns of local spatial hierarchies and for detecting complex features in images. In recent research, the modifications of such general CNN structures, such as dilated convolution, SE blocks, and normalization layers, have become applicable to contemporary deep learning ecosystems.

The current research direction is gradually transferring to the combined architecture of ViT and CNNs that can complement each other. Researchers are exploring fusion techniques where local feature extraction and context perception are interactive. The goal of these hybrid models is to overcome the limitations of the individual architectures, establishing more robust, flexible neural networks. Their design allows for increasingly complex visual recognition challenges in diverse domains such as medical diagnostics and perception systems.

1.3 Feature Fusion: Concepts and Techniques

Feature fusion is a widely used technique that integrates data from multiple sources or representations to enhance model performance. In this context, the desired robustness and accuracy of predictions (Kittler, Hatef, Duin, & Matas, 1998) can be improved by exploiting complementary information to construct a more informative representation. Early, late, and hybrid fusion are several types of feature fusion.

Early fusion occurs at the feature level where several features are combined before being passed to the model. In this case, the model benefits by starting its learning process from the combined data. For instance, in the medical imaging application, early fusion might involve the fusion of MRI and CT health features' representation (Li, Jiang, Zhang, & Zhu, 2023). Late fusion, on the other hand, occurs after models have been developed and trained on different features whereas early fusion occurs prior to the models being built. Each model provides the probability over the classes, which are combined, for instance by averaging, voting, or stacking. Late fusion enables models to specialize in various features but lacks a way of optimally utilizing all the complementary information that can be derived from the raw data (Ahmed, Dada, & Samaila, 2023).

Early fusion and late fusion can be blended to integrate features at different stages of the modelling phase. This approach can be beneficial for complex tasks, such as classifying brain tumors, where both high- and low-level features are necessary (Xie et al., 2022; Batool & Byun, 2024). With a strategic fusion approach, models can extract a richer set of features in more challenging domains, thus improving their prediction accuracies.

1.4 Feature Fusion: Synergizing Architectural Capabilities in Medical Image Analysis

Combining both CNN and ViT using feature fusion presents a plausible solution to address the drawbacks of each in medical image analysis. CNNs are optimized for adopting the spatial organization of local details, hence useful in identifying minute details such as texture or lesion. On the other hand, ViTs are adept at modelling global dependencies by leveraging self-attention mechanisms, enabling them to understand broader contextual relationships across an image.

Patients' medical images including MRI, CT, histopathological images that are to be diagnosed, need local cues as well as global context cues. Feature fusion of CNN and ViT architectures combines these strengths, enabling enhanced feature extraction and interpretation. It is especially useful for tasks such as multi-class tumour classification, disease localisation, and detailed anomaly detection to which the global and local nature of the images seems crucial.

Benefits of integrating CNN and ViT include increased diagnostic accuracy, enhanced generalization across different datasets and a reduced risk of overfitting in complex models. Moreover, this synergy streamlines feature hierarchies, making the models more efficient.

Key advantages of feature fusion include:

- **Complementary Information:** Different model architectures excel at capturing different types of information. CNNs effectively extract local spatial features while ViTs model long-range dependencies well. These complementary features enable a more complete interpretation of input data.
- **Reduced Overfitting:** Feature fusion can reduce the likelihood of overfitting, which is an issue that often arises when using deep learning algorithms. By incorporating features learned from all these combined sources, the model becomes more robust to variability and noise.
- **Enhanced Performance:** Feature fusion improves the performance of deep learning algorithms consistently. Models can achieve higher accuracy, sensitivity and specificity results by using strengths of various architectures.
- **Improved Interpretability:** It can also enhance interpretability of deep learning models. Through visualization of the fused features, one can better understand how the model has arrived at the decision, and which aspects played a crucial role in leading the final prediction.

2. LITERATURE REVIEW

Brain tumor classification has gained significant attention in recent years, driven by advancements in deep learning techniques. Several approaches, including CNNs, transfer learning, Vision Transformers, and hybrid models, have been analysed in this section.

Aamir et al. (2022) proposed a multiscale CNN framework along with data augmentation and sliding window testing to reduce bias and prevent overfitting. Khan et al. (2020) developed an automated MM-Brain Tumor classifier utilizing deep learning, where VGG16 and VGG19 architectures were employed for precise feature selection. Contrast stretching was applied to enhance tumor visibility, and feature selection was conducted to reduce computational load. However, the study encountered several challenges, including the high similarity in tumor structures of certain types, the impact of low contrast in T1-weighted images on feature extraction, and the inherent complexities of multimodal classification.

Mohsen et al. (2017) utilized CNN, discrete wavelet transform (DWT) for feature extraction and principal component analysis (PCA) for dimensionality reduction, classifying MRIs into four broad categories. Their approach achieved classification accuracy comparable to traditional CNNs, with less equipment and faster computation. However, the study's limitations include the small dataset size and reliance on T2-weighted images, restricting its broader application.

Ari and Hanbay (2018) proposed an Extreme Learning Machine with Local Receptive Fields (ELM-LRF) for classifying MR images as benign or malignant. The main limitation is the small dataset, consisting of images from only 16 patients. In Srinivas et al. (2022), authors discussed the use of deep transfer learning techniques in classifying brain tumours based on MR images. VGG-16 yielded the best performance results after intensity normalization and re-sizing preprocessing the data. Badjie and Ülker (2022) developed a deep learning-based architecture that leverages pre-trained networks, fine-tuning them for tumor classification to effectively detect and differentiate various tumor types in MRI scans.

Mehrotra et al. (2020) evaluated various models including AlexNet, GoogLeNet, ResNet 50, ResNet 101, and SqueezeNet. However, they used only 696 MRI image samples which may not generalize well especially in large scale applications. Hao et al (18) introduced an innovative active learning framework leveraging transfer learning to minimize annotation costs. The performance yields an AUC of 82.89% on the test dataset and with augmentation all labelling costs are reduced by 40% mark.

Ali (2023) introduced ViT-BT, a Vision Transformer-based model designed for brain tumor classification. The ViT-BT framework enhances classification performance by first pre-training the Vision Transformer model and then fine-tuning it using specialized MRI brain tumor datasets with an accuracy of 98%. Reddy et al. (2024) implemented a variant of vision transformer for automatically classifying multiple classes of brain tumor from the MRI scan images. Several pre-trained models were compared in the study, with the FTVT-l16 model performing best with a test accuracy of 98.70%.

Tummala et al. (2022) proposed an ensemble of ViT models for tumor classification. Pretrained ViT models on ImageNet were fine-tuned and utilized for the classification task. The proposed model achieved an accuracy of 98.7%. Goceri (2023) leveraged advantages of CNN and ViT to develop a novel architecture for glioma classification through the effective integration of feature-combining modules. Experimental results demonstrated the approach's efficacy in classifying four glioma subtypes from histopathological images, achieving an accuracy of 96.75%.

Karagoz et al. (2024) introduced a self-supervised technique to address the issue of limited availability in datasets. The dual CNN & Vision Transformer approach is pre-trained and fine-tuned. Synthetic MRI imagery is used to balance datasets by augmenting them, thereby increasing classification efficiency and reducing overfitting. This model demonstrated excellent performance as well as generalization capability to other databases but the usage of fake images indicates that there may be some biases inherent to the generated synthetic images.

Asiri et al. (2023) introduced the FT-ViT model, a fine-tuned Vision Transformer leveraging image processing and deep learning techniques to classify tumors. The framework comprises multiple stages, including data preprocessing, patch extraction, feature concatenation, selection, learning, and fine-tuning. Trained on the CE-MRI dataset, which includes 5,712 brain tumor images, the FT-ViT achieved 98.13% accuracy. DeepTumorNet (Asiri et al., 2023) is a hybrid deep learning model designed for brain tumor classification. The architecture integrates a modified GoogLeNet with leaky ReLU activation. The results demonstrated that the model outperformed comparable methods, achieving an accuracy of 99.67% and a recall of 100%.

Vimala et al. (2023) utilized EfficientNets to classify brain tumors using the Figshare dataset. EfficientNetB2, fine-tuned with additional layers and Grad-CAM visualization for interpretability, outperformed other models. Dixon et al (2024) proposed a hybrid architecture combining ViT and CNNs for robust brain tumor classification. The framework integrates texture, structural, and deep features, leveraging Haralick features, local binary patterns, and ViT-derived features. Evaluations demonstrate superior performance on diverse brain MRI datasets. Aloraini et al. (2023) proposed a hybrid model for brain tumor classification, combining CNNs for local feature extraction and transformers for global feature attention. The model achieves average accuracies of 96.75% on the BraTS 2018 dataset and 99.10% on the Figshare dataset. Tabatabaei et al. (2023) proposed a two-branch parallel model combining a Transformer Module (TM), and CNN for brain tumor classification. Using a cross-fusion strategy, local and global features are integrated to enhance accuracy. The lightweight iResNet architecture outperformed other CNN variants, achieving 99.30% accuracy.

As indicated in the literature review, there are improvements for classification of brain tumours (Verma et al., 2023; Garg et al., 2024), however the studies present several issues that restricts the effectiveness for broader uses. One common issue identified is the limited or unbalanced datasets, as cited in Ari and Hanbay's (2018) and a similar case in Mehrotra et al (2020). These limitations impair transferability and reliability of the models, particularly within the clinical practice where numerous patient groups and imaging modalities are used. Further, the inclusion of synthetic data for augmentation as done in Karagoz, Nalbantoglu, & Fox (2024) pose some biases. Though synthetic data is beneficial since it can minimize the impact of small dataset; however, it will not always reflect real-world situations, thus the model's efficiency declines when tested on other datasets.

There are also major issues regarding the computational and training issues. Approaches by (Reddy et al., 2024; Tummala et al., 2022) need substantial computational resources for pretraining and fine-tuning, so they are not practically viable in resource constrained settings. In addition, many hybrid models such as DeepTumorNet (Asiri et al., 2023) are prone to overfitting due to the highly fine-tuned parameters and a limited amount of data. This may decrease the model's ability to generalize to the other datasets or other clinical applications.

The literature highlights some of the major difficulties in feature extraction, which have a direct relationship on the performance as well as the efficacy of the models used in brain tumor classification. One of the major challenges is that the structures of different types of tumors do not vary significantly, which poses a challenge to the models to discern in between them well. Additionally, low contrast in T1-weighted images poses a significant obstacle, as it hampers the extraction of meaningful features necessary for accurate classification. Multimodal classification is also inherently difficult because information derived from the various imaging modalities has to be combined and interpreted by the model. The aforementioned challenges imply that misclassifications are more likely to happen when the models are used in real clinical practice. This underscores the need to develop sophisticated feature extraction methods and reliable data fusion approaches.

The work shows the potential and limitations of Transfer Learning (TF), Vision Transformers (ViT), and ViT-CNN integrated models in brain tumour classification. TF models, often starting from VGG16 or ResNet, work well with feature extraction but fail at identifying tumor features when the size of the set of images is relatively small or unbalanced. It has been found that the use of ViTs is appropriate of large amounts of data and gets high accuracy but consumes a lot of computational power and does not capture local details. The ViT-CNN hybrids have better performance than the ViT and CNN approaches; however, they are complicated and may overfit on small datasets.

3. REVIEW OF APPROACHES IMPLEMENTED IN BRAIN TUMOR CLASSIFICATION

3.1 DenseNet-210

For the proposed hybrid model, DenseNet-201 serves as the primary CNN architecture. Figure 3 illustrates the detailed structure of DenseNet-20. The most distinctive feature of DenseNet-201 is connectivity, which implies the concatenation of the previous layer's features with all the subsequent layers. This connectivity structure enhances the flow of information which makes DenseNet-201 appropriate for extracting complex features in different applications. Let x_0 represent the input to the network, and $f_1,f_2,f_3,...f_{l-1},f_L$ denote the output from each of the L layers in the dense block. The input to layer l is the combined output from the earlier layers:

$$f_l=H([x_{0,}\ f_1,f_2,f_3,...f_{l-1}]) \qquad (1)$$

where H(·) represents the composite function applied in layer l, which typically includes operations like Batch Normalization, ReLU activation, and convolution.

Figure 3. Architecture of DenseNet-201

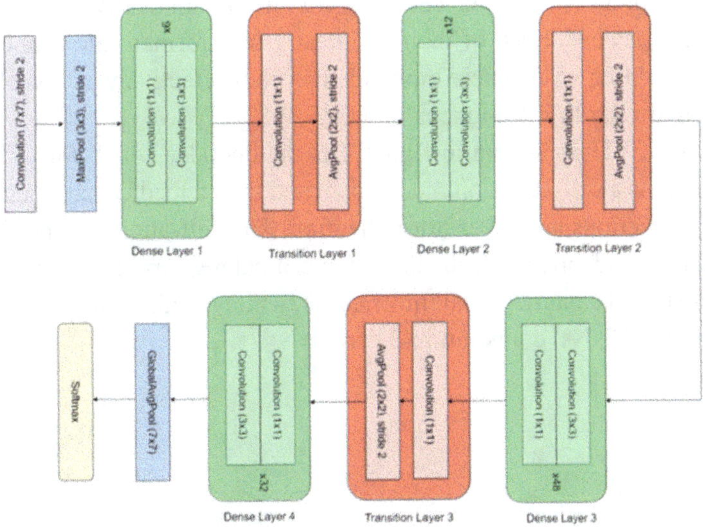

The structure of DenseNet is made of dense block and transition layers. A dense block has many convolutional layers, and each layer is connected with all other layers through dense connectivity. In this case there are transition layers between the dense blocks which assist in down sampling the feature maps using average pooling. Additionally, the growth rate, which determines the number of new features added by each layer, is kept relatively low to ensure computational efficiency while preserving model performance.

The output of DenseNet-201 features is passed through a Multilayer Perceptron with two fully connected layers, each containing 512 neurons each. These layers are interspersed with BN (Batch Normalization) to increase the stability of the learning process. Leaky ReLU is used as the activation function, defined as:

$$f(z) = \begin{cases} z\, z > 0 \\ \alpha z\, z \leq 0 \end{cases} \tag{2}$$

where α prevents dead neurons and is constant, allowing neurons to handle negative inputs.

3.2 Vision Transformer

The Vision Transformer represents a shift from conventional paradigms in computer vision to the currently popular Transformer models in natural language processing. In 2020, researchers at Google Brain developed ViT, applying the self-attention mechanism of Transformers to image data, in contrast to the standard sequence data used in NLP. This approach addresses the limitations of CNN such as restricted global context awareness. Thus, ViT became a notable architecture, particularly in large-scale image classification, achieving significant results and marking a new era in research.

ViT differs fundamentally from CNNs in the way it processes images. Traditional CNNs work hierarchically by extracting more and more abstract features from the localized receptive field to understand the image content. In contrast, ViT treats images as a sequence of fixed-sized grids. This is similar to how NLP models treat sentences as sequences of words. In this innovative approach, the input image is segmented into image patches. Each of them is linearly transformed into a one-dimensional vector through a learnable embedding layer. These embedded patches effectively act as tokens to be processed by Transformer models similar to word tokens in NLP.

The key component of ViT as shown in figure 4 is the encoder which forms the backbone of the model. Each block contains a self-attention mechanism and then a feedforward neural network with the addition of residual connections and layer normalization. The self-attention mechanism evaluates the dependencies of the patches adaptively, focusing on the critical regions of the image. This enable ViT to learn long-range contexts and capture global information, while avoiding the need for many parameters, as is the case of traditional CNNs' convolutional kernels.

Figure 4. Architecture of Vision Transformer

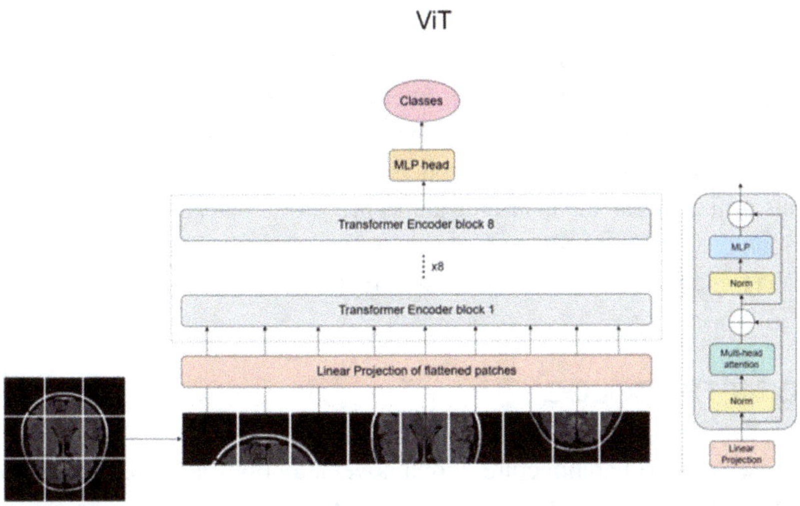

To preserve the spatial structure of the image, ViT adds learnable positional embeddings on the patch embeddings. This is because the Transformer models are naturally order-agnostic by default and do not inherently understand token layout. The model keeps the spatial structure by using positional embeddings to know the position of every patch in the image. When combined with the self-attention mechanism, these embeddings make ViT learn to capture the local and the global spatial structures, and thus perform even better in learning spatial patterns.

This concept, originally introduced in the BERT model for NLP tasks, serves as a global representation of the entire image in ViT. As the image is processed, the CLS token interacts with all other patches via the self-attention mechanism, collecting features that represent the overall content of the image. Once the image passes through the final Transformer encoder layer, the CLS token is passed through a linear classification layer, where it is used to generate the model's final prediction. By incorporating both local and global features, this approach enables ViT to effectively analyse and classify images.

The computational power and the large datasets deemed necessary for training ViT models effectively are substantial. Unlike CNNs that have certain built-in biases such as spatial hierarchies and local patterns (e.g., edges and textures), ViT is not affected by these inherent biases. For this reason, ViT models require pretraining on large datasets such as ImageNet-21k or JFT-300M to learn high quality representations. Then they can be fine-tuned using task specific datasets to perform well. This pretraining-finetuning approach of ViT enables it to generalize better and often outperforms CNN models in large-scale classification tasks.

Despite these advantages, the computational complexity of ViT is a big issue. However, the self-attention mechanism is highly resource intensive, scaling quadratically with the number of patches, which is especially significant given that ViTs work well with high-resolution images. The model needs to compute all patch interactions, resulting in quadratic memory and processing power scaling. However, while these high demands are required for ViT in resource limited settings they can be impractical. In order to address these challenges, researchers have developed solutions including sparse self-attention as well as these hierarchical Transformer architectures, which come at a reduced computational cost but maintain strong performance.

The rise in popularity of Vision Transformers has led to the development of various hybrid architectures that merge advantages from both fields of CNNs and transformers. Models like the Swin transformer and DeiT (Data-efficient Image Transformers) combine the power of local feature extraction achieved through the CNN structure with the global context-awareness of transformers. Conventional models provide a regional fit, making hybrid models appropriate for small datasets. For instance, Swin transformer models utilize hierarchical structuring to process images at varying resolutions to make it far less computationally expensive without compromising accuracy. These improvements help address the limitations of ViT and make these models more practical for real-world use.

4. PROPOSED METHODOLOGY

This work proposes a hybrid architecture with a novel attention-based feature fusion mechanism to classify the MRI of the BRaTS dataset into three categories.

The contributions of this work are:

1. **Novel Hybrid Architecture:** A hybrid framework that integrates the advantages of CNN and ViT is proposed. It aims to capture and integrate both global and local information from images.
2. **Attention driven Feature Fusion Module:** A novel feature fusion mechanism is proposed that combines features at various granularities using a cross-attention mechanism. This allows the module to seamlessly integrate global contextual patterns with localized details through the cross-attention mechanism. This dynamic fusion process also adjusts the importance of features while simultaneously increasing the variety of captured information, without merely including other features.

The proposed method consists of three interconnected components as shown in figure 5.

Figure 5. Hybrid CNN-ViT architecture with attention-based feature fusion mechanism

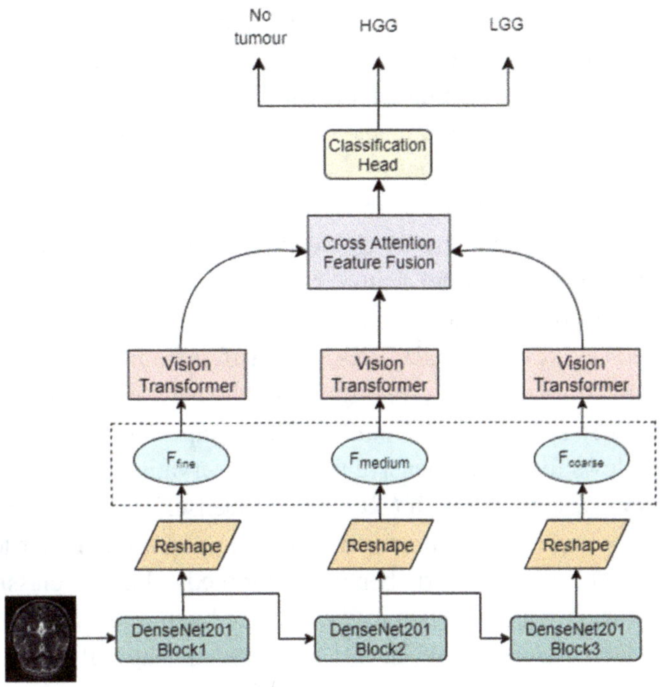

1. **CNN-Based Multi-Scale Feature Extraction**:

This component employs DenseNet-201 to generate feature maps at three distinct spatial scales: features at the coarse level (global structural patterns), medium level (intermediate anatomical details), and fine level (localized and textural information). The module produces detailed and diverse representations by extracting features across multiple scales.

2. **ViT Feature Refinement**:

The attention mechanism in these transformers enhances CNN-derived features with contextual information, resulting in structured and high-quality feature map representations.

3. **Cross-Attention Feature Fusion Model**:

This mechanism enables interaction between feature maps of different scales from the three ViTs, optimizing the feature maps with refinements and consolidating the integrated results into a single feature map. The cross-attention mechanism uses the information from the coarse, medium, and fine feature levels to yield a unified multi scale representation tailored to be used in classification.

The following section will detail each component of the architecture, elucidating its architecture and function in the overall system.

4.1 CNN-Based Multi-Scale Feature Extraction

DenseNet-201 is designed to have dense connectivity across its layers. This structure enhances the flow of gradients during backpropagation and improves feature reuse. The model is organized into several dense blocks, with each block extracting features at different levels of abstraction. For brain tumor classification, we aim to extract fine, medium, and coarse features from these blocks to capture various spatial patterns and structures in brain images.

The reasons for choosing DenseNet-201 as the CNN Component are as follows:

Dense Connectivity: Within each dense block, every layer utilizes feature maps from all preceding layers, enabling an efficient mechanism for feature reuse. This approach captures subtle and nuanced features, which are crucial for precise diagnosis.

Feature Preservation: Unlike traditional CNNs which suffer from feature loss, DenseNet-201 maintains and combines features from earlier layers throughout the network. This characteristic is crucial in medical imaging, where early-stage feature details can be as important as high-level semantic features. The dense connectivity allows for comprehensive feature preservation and aggregation.

Parameter Efficiency: Despite its depth (201 layers), DenseNet-201 achieves remarkable parameter efficiency. The dense connectivity pattern reduces the need for redundant feature maps, resulting in a more compact model. This is particularly beneficial for medical image classification, where model complexity and computational requirements must be balanced with precision.

Multi-Scale Feature Extraction: DenseNet-201's architecture naturally supports multi-scale feature extraction. The dense blocks capture features at different levels of abstraction, ranging from low-level texture details to high-level semantic representations. This multi-scale approach is ideal for medical image analysis, where tumors and pathological conditions can manifest in various subtle ways.

DenseNet-201, with its dense connections, parameter efficiency, and multi-scale feature extraction capabilities, provides high-quality hierarchical feature maps that are ideal for a hybrid CNN-ViT architecture. When combined with the Vision Transformer's long-range dependency modeling, this setup leverages the strengths of both paradigms, making it highly effective for challenging tasks like brain tumor classification.

Extraction of Fine Features (Dense Block 1)

Dense block 1 is responsible for extracting fine features, which includes low-level details and small anatomical structures. The input image, denoted as X_0, passes through the initial convolution layer before being processed by the dense block layers. Each convolution operation within this block takes the output from all previous layers, enabling the model to capture increasingly complex patterns. Mathematically, the output of the ith convolutional layer within Dense Block 1 is represented as:

$$Y_i=\sigma(W_i * X_i-1+b_i) \tag{3}$$

where W_i is the convolution kernel, b_i is the bias term, $*$ denotes the convolution operation, and σ is the non-linear activation function (ReLU). After processing through all layers in Dense Block 1, the output feature map, denoted as F_{fine}, represents the fine-grained details.

Extraction of Medium Features (Dense Block 2)

After extracting fine features from Dense Block 1, the next step is to capture medium features. These features are abstracted from the fine-level details and represent intermediate anatomical patterns, such as larger structures or patterns within the brain. The output from Dense Block 1, denoted as F_{fine} , is passed to Dense Block 2, where additional layers further process the features. The mathematical representation of this transition from Dense Block 1 to Dense Block 2 is as follows:

$$F_{medium}=f_{block}(F_{fine}) \tag{4}$$

where f_{block} refers to the operations performed within Dense Block 2, including additional convolutional layers and batch normalization. The resulting output F_{medium} contains medium-level features, which abstract away finer details and begin to capture larger anatomical structures. These medium features are essential for identifying intermediate tumor characteristics and structures that span across smaller regions in the image. Additionally, these features can also help detect relationships between different brain regions which are essential for accurate tumor diagnosis.

Extraction of Coarse Features (Dense Block 3)

Dense Block 3 captures the coarse features, which represent the highest level of abstraction in the feature extraction process. These coarse features are global, large-scale patterns that encompass significant structures, such as the entire tumor or other broader brain regions. The output from Dense Block 2, denoted as F_{medium} is passed to Dense Block **3** for further processing. The mathematical transition from Dense Block 2 to Dense Block 3 is represented as:

$$F_{coarse}=f_{block}(F_{medium}) \tag{5}$$

where f_{block} represents the operations within Dense Block 3, including further convolutions and batch normalization. The resulting output F_{coarse} contains coarse features, which are abstracted and provide a global understanding of the brain's structures. These coarse features are essential for recognizing the overall tumor region, its size, and its relationship with other parts of the brain. The coarse features provide the model with context about the tumor's location within the brain, which is critical for making final classification decisions.

Table II summarizes the dimensions of output at different stages of the DenseNet-201 architecture for an input size of 240×240×4. After the first convolution layer and pooling layer, the spatial dimensions are halved. Output size after initial convolution and pooling is 120×120×64 where 64 is the number of filters/channels. This serves as input to the first dense block.

Table 2. Dimensions of feature maps at various stages of DenseNet-201

Stage	Spatial Size	Channels
Initial Input	120×120	64
After Dense Block 1	120×120	92
After Transition 1	60×60	128
After Dense Block 2	60×60	384
After Transition 2	30×30	256
After Dense Block 3	30×30	1792

4.2 ViT Feature Refinement

The integration of Convolutional Neural Network with Vision Transformer represents a critical computational challenge in modern computer vision architectures. This transformation requires a sophisticated approach to convert hierarchical feature maps into a tokenized format compatible with transformer-based models. This section proposes a systematic approach for such transformation, with a focus on handling features at multiple granularities to enable hierarchical representation learning.

4.2.1 Mathematical Formulation of Feature Map Transformation

Let the CNN-extracted feature map at granularity level g {fine, medium, coarse} be denoted as be F_g, represented mathematically as:

$$F_g \in R^{W_{g \times H_g \times c_g}} \tag{6}$$

where H represents the height, W the width, and C the number of channels of the feature map. ViTs require tokenized inputs, where each token corresponds to a fixed-length vector. This necessitates:

1. Flattening of spatial dimensions height (H_g) and width (W_g) into a single dimension.
2. Projection of the resulting tokens into an embedding space of dimension d, which aligns with the ViT input specifications.

4.2.2 Tokenization and Embedding Transformation

Tokenization and embedding transformation are critical steps that adapt image data into a format suitable for processing by transformer architectures. The steps involved in this process is detailed below.

4.2.2.1 Flattening CNN Feature Maps.

The spatial dimensions $H_g \times W_g$ are flattened, converting the feature map F_g into a matrix F_g^{flat} as:

$$F_g \in R^{W_{g \times H_g \times c_g}} \tag{7}$$

For a feature map $F_g \in R^{64 \times 16 \times 16F}$, flattening produces $F_g^{flat} \in R^{256 \times 64}$ (i.e., 256 tokens, each of dimension 64).

4.2.2.2 Linear Projection to Embedding Space.

Flattened feature map F_g^{flat} is projected into a lower-dimensional space using a learnable linear projection matrix W_g^{proj} and the bias term b_g^{proj} as given in (8)

$$E_g = F_g^{flat} \cdot W_g^{proj} + b_g^{proj} \tag{8}$$

Where $W_g^{proj} \in R^{C_g \times d}$: Linear projection matrix that reduces C_g-dimensional tokens to d- dimensional embeddings. $b_g^{proj} \in R^d$: Bias term added to each token embedding.

The resulting token embeddings E_g are given by:

$$E_g \in R^{(H_g, W_g) X d} \tag{9}$$

4.2.2.3 Processing Tokenized Features with Vision Transformers.

The tokenized embeddings E_g are processed through a dedicated ViT block for each granularity level g:

$$F'_g = ViTBlock(E_g) \tag{10}$$

where $F'_g{}'$ represents the refined features. Each ViT block consists of:

- Multi-head self-attention (MHSA) layers for capturing long-range dependencies.
- Feedforward layers for non-linear transformations.

The independent processing of E_g at different granularities enables the model to extract multi-scale representations critical for downstream tasks.

4.3 Cross-Attention Feature Fusion Model

The proposed fusion technique addresses the challenge of effectively integrating multi-granularity feature representations. The model begins with three distinct feature maps extracted from different levels of granularity as shown in figure 6.

Figure 6. Multi Scale Feature Extraction using DenseNet-201

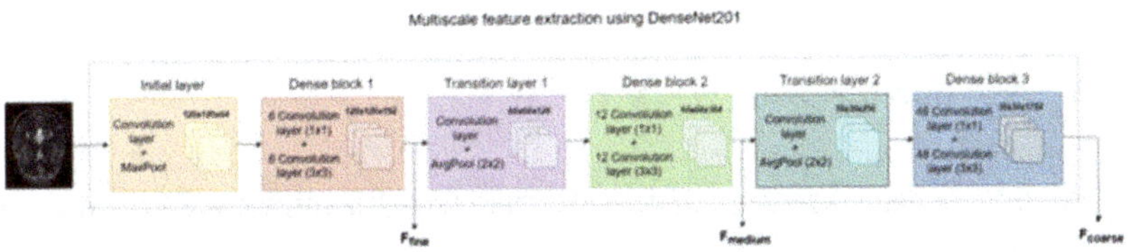

Let F'_1, F'_2, F'_3 represent feature maps extracted from coarse-, mid-, and fine-level ViTs, respectively. These feature maps, obtained after tokenization and embedding transformation, are of varying spatial resolutions and semantic granularity. To enable effective fusion, all feature maps are projected into a common feature dimension d:

$$F'_i = W_i F_i + b_i \tag{11}$$

$W_i \in R^{dXd'}$ where W_i *and* b_i are learnable projection parameters, and d′ is the original feature dimension.

4.3.1 Cross-Attention Blocks

To fuse information, three cross-attention blocks are defined, where each feature map alternates as the query while the remaining two serve as keys and values. The Cross-attention Feature fusion is depicted in figure 7.

Figure 7. Cross-Attention Feature Fusion

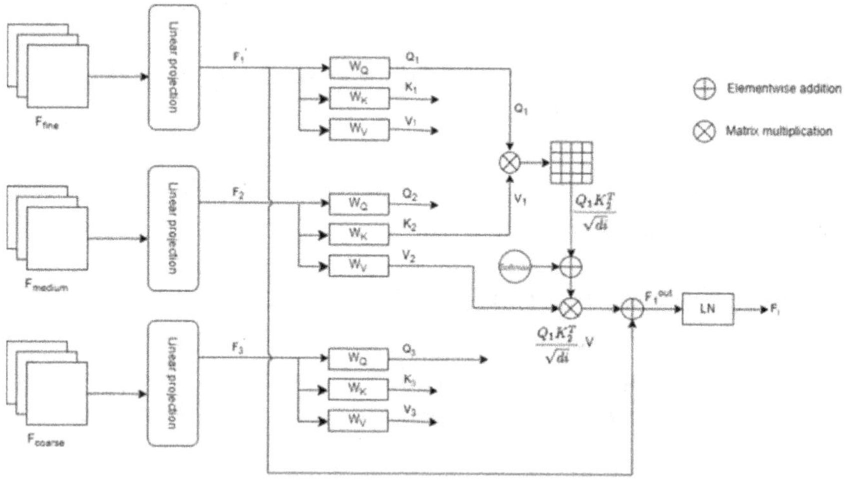

Block 1: Coarse-level features F'_1 as query.

$Q_1=F'_1W_Q$, $K_2=F'_2W_K$, $V_2=F'_2W_V$, K3= F'_3W_K, $V_3=F'_3W_V$

where W_Q W_k, W_v $\in R^{d\times d'}$ are learnable projection matrices for queries, keys, and values. The cross-attention output is computed as:

$$F_1^{out}= Softmax\left(\frac{Q_1K_2^T}{\sqrt{d'}}\right) V_2+ Softmax\left(\frac{Q_1K_3^T}{\sqrt{d'}}\right) V_3 \tag{12}$$

Block 2: Mid-level features F'_2 as query.

$Q_2=F'_2W_Q$, $K_1=F'_1W_K$, $V_1=F'_1W_V$, $K_3= F'_3W_K$, $V_3=F'_3W_V$

$$F_2^{out}= Softmax\left(\frac{Q_2K_1^T}{\sqrt{d'}}\right) V_1+ Softmax\left(\frac{Q_2K_3^T}{\sqrt{d'}}\right) V_3 \tag{13}$$

Block 3: Fine-level features F'_3 as query.

$Q_3=F'_3W_Q$, $K_1=F'_1W_K$, $V_1=F'_1W_V$, $K_2= F'_2W_K$, $V_3=F'_2W_V$

$$F_3^{out}= Softmax\left(\frac{Q_3K_1^T}{\sqrt{d'}}\right) V_1+ Softmax\left(\frac{Q_3K_2^T}{\sqrt{d'}}\right) V_2 \tag{14}$$

4.3.2 Residual Connections and Normalization

Residual connections and layer normalization are applied to each cross-attention output to stabilize training and enhance feature representation,

$$F_i^{res} = \text{LayerNorm}\left(F_i' + F_i^{out}\right) \tag{15}$$

4.3.3 Concatenation and Fully Connected Fusion

The residual outputs from all three blocks are concatenated:

$$F_{concat} = Concat\left[F_1^{res}, F_2^{res}, F_3^{res}\right] \tag{16}$$

The concatenated features are then passed through a multi-layer perceptron to generate the final fused feature representation:

$$F_{fused} = MLP\left(F_{concat}\right) \tag{17}$$

Algorithm: Attention Based Feature Fusion
Inputs:

- F_1', F_2', F_3' : Feature maps from ViTs at coarse, mid, and fine granular levels, with sizes $B\times N \times d_1$, $B\times N_2\times d_2$, $B\times N_3\times d_3$.
- d′: Common feature dimension for fusion.

Output:F_{fused}: Fused feature map.
1. Initialization:
1.1. Define projection matrices $W_1, W_2, W_3 \in R^{d\times d'}$.
1.2. Define bias vectors $b_1, b_2, b_3 \in Rd'$.
1.3. Define query, key, and value projection matrices $W_Q, W_K, W_V \in R^{d\times d'}$.
2. Linear Projection:
2.1. For each feature map Fi do:
2.2. Compute: $F_i' = W_i F_i + b_i$
3. Cross-Attention Blocks:
3.1. For i=1 to 3 (denoting granularities) do:
3.2. Set F_i' as the query: $Q_1 = F_1' W_Q$
3.3. For all other feature maps F_j' j≠i:
3.4. Compute keys and values: $K_j, V_j = F_i' W_K, F_i' W_V$
3.5. Compute cross-attention output: $F_i^{out} = \Sigma j Softmax\left(\frac{Q_i K_j^T}{\sqrt{d'}}\right) V_j$
3.6. Add residual connection and normalize: $F_i^{res} = \text{LayerNorm}\left(F_i' + F_i^{out}\right)$
End for
4. Concatenation:
4.1.Concatenate all residual outputs: $F_{concat} = Concat\left[F_1^{res}, F_2^{res}, F_3^{res}\right]$

5. Final Fusion:

5.1. Pass Fconcat through an MLP to integrate multi-granular features;

$F_{fused} = MLP(F_{concat})$

5. EXPERIMENTAL SETUP AND RESULT

5.1 Experimental Setup

Models were implemented using Python-based libraries and executed on a desktop equipped with a CPU-Intel Core i9-13900K CPU alongside a GPU - NVIDIA GeForce RTX 3090. A deep learning-based classification framework was developed for analyzing MRI using convolutional neural networks (CNNs). The framework performed multiclass classification to categorize tumors into four distinct types. The implementation utilized Python-based deep learning libraries, specifically Keras with TensorFlow backend, within the Anaconda environment.

5.2 Dataset

The BraTS 2015 (Brain Tumor Segmentation) dataset represents a significant milestone in medical imaging resources, comprising multimodal MRI scans from 220 high-grade glioma (HGG) cases and 54 low-grade glioma (LGG) cases. Each case in the dataset contains four distinct MRI sequences: T1-weighted (T1), T1-weighted with contrast enhancement (T1ce), T2-weighted (T2), and Fluid Attenuated Inversion Recovery (FLAIR).

Rigorous preprocessing was undertaken on the dataset to ensure standardization across all cases of the dataset. All images were manually annotated by expert neuroradiologists. A key feature of the BraTS 2015 dataset is the inclusion of detailed segmentation masks and classification labels. Tumor regions were annotated using a hierarchical segmentation approach: label 1 for necrosis, non-enhancing tumor, and cyst; label 2 for edema; label 4 for enhancing tumor; and label 0 for all other areas. These annotations serve as a benchmark for developing and testing of automated segmentation algorithms. The unique advantage of the BraTS 2015 dataset lies in the inclusion of both HGG and LGG cases, making it invaluable for creating classification and segmentation algorithms that are both effective and robust.

Samples of the four MRI modalities are illustrated in Figure 8. Each modality includes 155 slices, resulting in 620 images per case. For the 274 cases, this results in a total of 169,880 MRI images, as detailed in Table III. The dataset is divided into 80% for training and 20% for testing. For this study, we categorized the dataset into three classes:

- Class 1 represents High-Grade Gliomas (HGG) and includes Necrosis (1), Enhancing Tumor (4), and extensive Edema (2), as these features indicate aggressive tumor behaviour.
- Class 2 represents Low-Grade Gliomas (LGG) and includes images labelled as Non-enhancing Tumor (3).
- Finally, Class 0, labelled as non-tumor.

Figure 8. HGG and LGG Cases with Four MRI Modalities in the BraTS 2015 Dataset

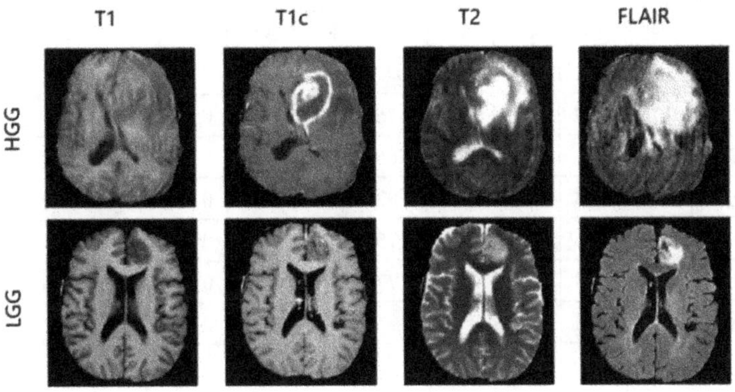

Table 3. BraTS 2015 Dataset Description and Train-Test Split statistics

Total Number of Patient Cases	**274**
Overall MR Images Count	169,880
Number of Modalities/Case	4
Resolution of Each Image	240 x 240
MR Images/Modality	155
Total MR Images per Patient	620
Training Datasets	
LGG images	43
HGG images	177
Total MR Images in Training Dataset	135,904
Testing Datasets	54
Total HGG & LGG Images	33,976

5.3 Results

5.3.1 Comparison with Transfer Learning Models and VIT

The proposed model's performance is evaluated against several alternative models, including MobileNetV3, EfficientNet, VGG16, ResNet50, DenseNet121, InceptionV4, Xception, and the baseline ViT. Table IV presents the comparative results. The proposed Hybrid CNN-ViT demonstrates superior performance in multi-modal feature fusion and classification tasks.

Table 4. Performance comparison across MRI modalities and models

MODEL	T1				FLAIR				T2				T1C			
	Acc	P	R	F1	Acc	P	R	F1	Acc	P	R	F1	Acc	P	R	F1
MobileNetV3	0.85	0.82	0.81	0.82	0.83	0.81	0.8	0.8	0.82	0.8	0.79	0.79	0.84	0.82	0.81	0.82
EfficientNet	0.81	0.78	0.76	0.77	0.79	0.77	0.76	0.76	0.78	0.76	0.75	0.75	0.81	0.77	0.76	0.77
VGG16	0.71	0.7	0.69	0.7	0.68	0.67	0.66	0.66	0.67	0.66	0.65	0.65	0.71	0.7	0.68	0.7
DenseNet121	0.86	0.83	0.83	0.83	0.84	0.83	0.82	0.82	0.83	0.82	0.81	0.81	0.86	0.83	0.83	0.84
InceptionV4	0.81	0.77	0.76	0.76	0.79	0.76	0.75	0.75	0.78	0.75	0.74	0.74	0.81	0.77	0.75	0.76
Xception	0.8	0.79	0.78	0.78	0.78	0.77	0.77	0.77	0.77	0.76	0.76	0.76	0.8	0.79	0.78	0.78
ViT	0.93	0.93	0.87	0.93	0.92	0.94	0.92	0.93	0.93	0.92	0.93	0.92	0.93	0.93	0.89	0.93
Proposed Model	**0.97**	**0.97**	**0.96**	**0.96**	**0.98**	**0.97**	**0.97**	**0.97**	**0.98**	**0.97**	**0.98**	**0.97**	**0.97**	**0.97**	**0.96**	**0.96**

Figure 9 compares the overall performance of various models.

Figure 9. Model Comparison: Overall Accuracy, Precision, Recall, F1-Score

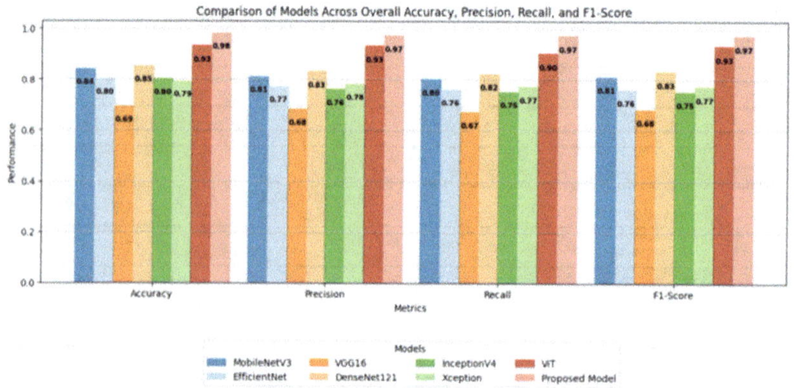

5.3.2 Performance across Imaging Modalities

Table V displays the effectiveness of the proposed model across different imaging modalities (FLAIR, T1, T1C, T2) for tumor classification, including HGG (Necrosis, Edema, Enhancing, Non-Enhancing), LGG, and No Tumor.

Table 5. Performance of hybrid model for classifying HGG, LGG, and No Tumor

Modality	HGG			LGG	No Tumour	Avg Performance Measure			
	Necrosis	Edema	Enhancing	Non-Enhancing	No Tumour	Acc.	P	R	F
	Individual Accuracy					Average Measure			
Flair	0.97	0.98	0.975	0.97	0.98	0.975	0.968	0.977	0.942
T1	0.97	0.97	0.96	0.96	0.97	0.966	0.955	0.956	0.954
T1c	0.97	0.97	0.96	0.96	0.97	0.966	0.945	0.957	0.956
T2	0.98	0.98	0.97	0.97	0.98	0.976	0.968	0.977	0.962

Among the four modalities, FLAIR and T2 exhibit superior performance, achieving high average accuracy values of 0.975 and 0.976, respectively, with excellent precision (0.968 and 0.968) and recall (0.977 and 0.977). T1C and T1 also perform well, with average accuracies of 0.966 each, though their precision and recall are slightly lower compared to Flair and T2. This analysis underscores the robustness of the model, particularly for FLAIR and T2 modalities, which consistently deliver strong results across all metrics and tumor categories. The results highlight the model's ability to effectively process diverse imaging inputs for accurate tumor classification.

5.3.3 Visualisation of Attention and Feature Maps

The feature maps of DenseNet 201 at multiple scales, as proposed in the architecture are depicted in figure 10 below. This figure shows feature maps of DenseNet201 at three different levels of abstraction after Dense Blocks 1, 2, and 3. Dense Block 1's feature maps represent low level and simple structures and basic patterns of the image. The feature maps of Dense Block 2 show intermediate level features, where the shapes and localized structures are more evident. The feature maps of Dense Block 3 extract highly abstract yet meaningful features by emphasizing the importance of small regions to the classification of brain tumors.

Figure 10. Feature Maps at Three Granularity Levels from DenseNet201 (a) After Dense Block 1 (b) After Dense Block 2 (c) After Dense Block 3

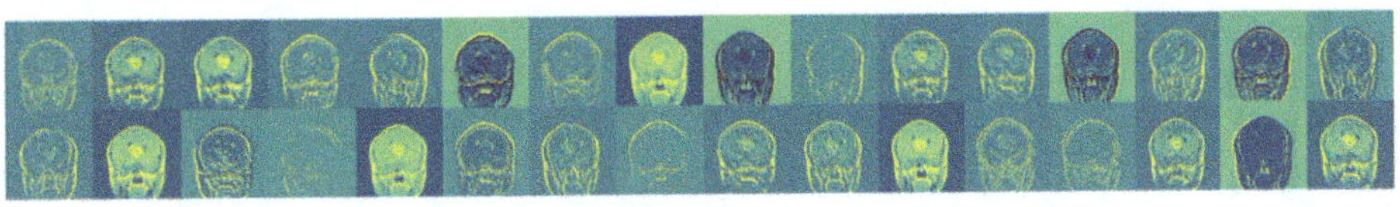

Figure 11 presents MRI scans along with their corresponding attention maps generated by the hybrid Vision Transformer model. These maps highlight the model's focus on specific tumor-related regions. In the MRI images, distinct tumor areas are visible, characterized by altered enhancement patterns and edema surrounding the lesion. The attention maps reflect the model's ability to pinpoint these regions indicating areas identified as containing tumor tissue. For example, in the first MRI, the attention map predominantly highlights a lower portion of the tumor, suggesting that the model is focusing on the necrotic or non-enhancing core. In the second MRI, the attention map shifts to areas surrounding the tumor, possibly capturing the peritumoral edema, which is also highlighted in the enhanced scan. The third and fourth MRIs show attention maps that focus on the enhancing regions, suggesting that the model accurately identifies contrast-enhanced tumor areas as key features. This targeted focus on different tumor characteristics such as necrosis, edema, and enhancing regions demonstrates the proposed model's capacity to differentiate between these pathological features, reflecting the model's sophisticated understanding of tumor morphology.

Figure 11. Visualization of MRI images (top) and their corresponding attention maps (bottom)

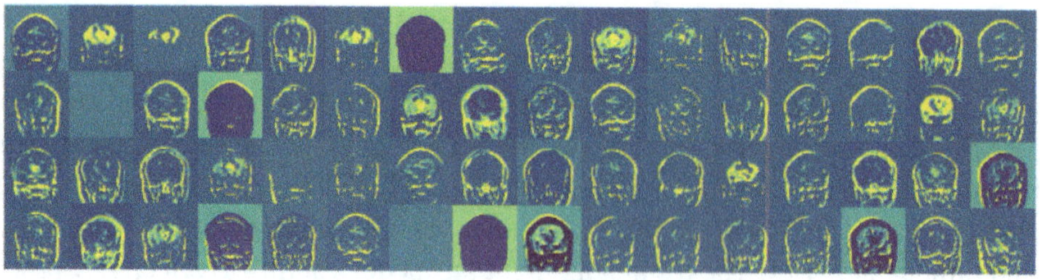

5.3.4 Loss-Accuracy Curve and Confusion Matrix Analysis

Figure 12 illustrates the accuracy and loss curves for DenseNet201, Vision Transformer (ViT), and the proposed model. For DenseNet201 the accuracy steadily increases but at a slow rate, stagnating around 0.85. The pattern observed in training accuracy and the validation accuracy graph suggests overfitting. While the training loss sharply decreases and converges to a very low value, the validation loss reduces more slowly, indicating minor generalization issues. The training and validation accuracy of ViT shows a gradual progress through epochs and stabilises at approximately 0.9. However, there is still a small gap between the training and validation accuracy, indicating potential overfitting. On the other hand, the proposed hybrid model achieves high accuracy (0.97) early in training, with both training and validation losses converging quickly to nearly zero. This suggests better efficiency and reduced overfitting in comparison to the baseline models, highlighting the proposed model's superiority over existing alternatives.

Figure 12. Training and Validation Accuracy - Loss plots for three models.10

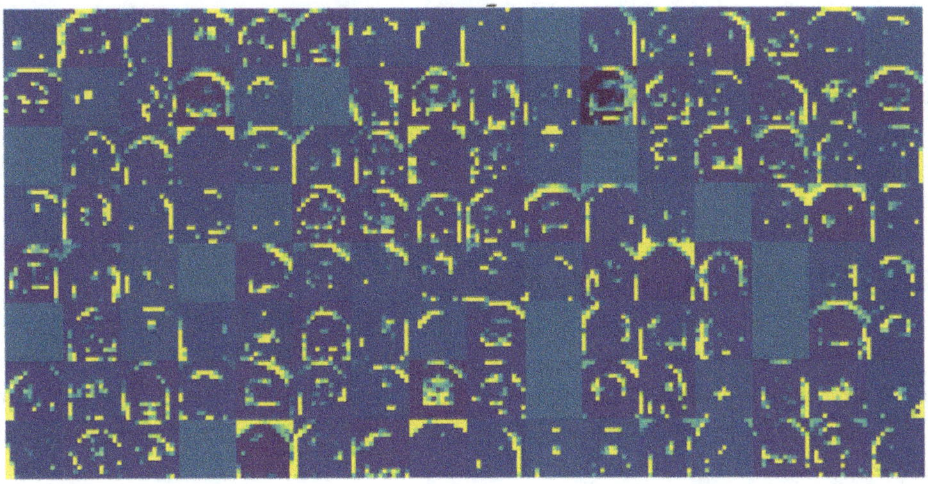

The normalized confusion matrix is shown in figure 13.

Figure 13. Normalised Confusion matrix for the proposed model

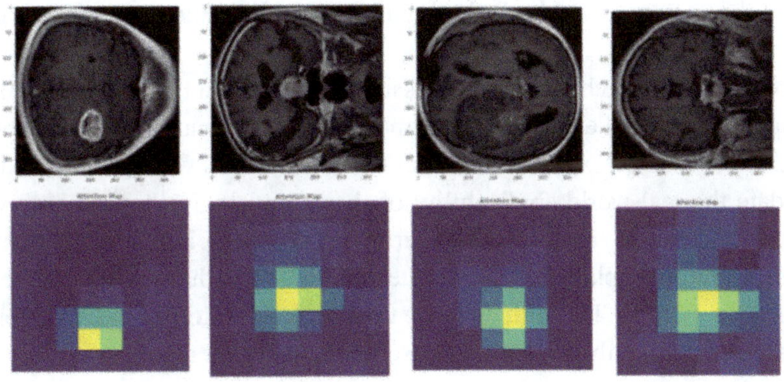

The proposed model provides a great classification of HGG with true positive rate of 0.98. However, a very small proportion of the HGG samples is misclassified to LGG (0.01) and Nontumor (0.01) also. This suggests that although the model is efficient in detecting aggressive results for tumor morphology, there might be some overlap of distinct features with LGG and Nontumor, which may be tuned or refined further in the future. As with LGG, the true positive rate of the model is 0.97 and reflects the ability of the model to effectively segment low-grade glioma areas. However, 0.02% of LGG samples are misclassified as HGG probably because the tumor characteristics of the two grades may be quite similar. Furthermore, it is detected that 0.01 of LGG samples are misclassified as Nontumor, which might stem from feature similarity or noise of input data. For Nontumor, the model achieves a true positive rate of 0.98, showcasing its ability to accurately detect non-tumor regions. A minimal proportion of these samples is misclassified as HGG (0.01) or LGG (0.01), which could result from background features or artifacts being incorrectly interpreted as tumor regions.

Overall, the high classification rates across all categories highlight the model's effectiveness. However, the minor misclassification rates suggest opportunities for improvement, particularly in refining the separation of overlapping features between HGG and LGG. Addressing these issues may involve enhancing the CNN feature extraction stages, fine-tuning the ViT layers, or incorporating additional data preprocessing techniques to minimize noise and improve accuracy.

6. CONCLUSION AND FUTURE WORK

The proposed model demonstrates robust performance by effectively leveraging hierarchical granularity, attention-based feature fusion, and multi-scale information. Features from Brain MRI tumor images are extracted at three granularity levels using DenseNet-201 and then processed through three Vision Transformers, capturing both local and global spatial patterns. The feature fusion technique based on attention incorporates the extracted features that are improved in distinguishing among classes of tumors by focusing on areas that may be relevant for tumor. The fused feature will be classified into HGG, LGG, and No Tumor categories. In that sense, the overall strength of the model developed surpasses the individual performances; whereas DenseNet201 stands with an accuracy of 86% and ViTs stood at 93% respectively. This hybrid approach gives high accuracy and generalization across different tumor types, demonstrating the model's potential as an efficient solution for automated brain tumor diagnosis. Future work will enhance the current model by including interpretability and involve clinician engagement to adopt in clinical settings.

The future work on hybrid architecture for classification of brain tumor will be directed towards the fine-tuning and optimization of the model. Furthermore, combining multiple image modalities, including MRI, PET, and CT, will also be explored for better classification as well as increased performance and stability. To validate the real-world applicability of these models, further research will be conducted to test them in clinical settings, ensuring they perform effectively in diverse patient populations and environments. Furthermore, explainability and interpretability modules will be added to ensure transparency in the decision making. This will enhance trust and facilitate clinical adoption by ensuring that the model's decisions are not only accurate but also understandable and justifiable.

REFERENCES

Aamir, M., Rahman, Z., Abro, W. A., Bhatti, U. A., Dayo, Z. A., & Ishfaq, M. (2023). Brain tumor classification utilizing deep features derived from high-quality regions in MRI images. *Biomedical Signal Processing and Control*, *85*, 104988. DOI: 10.1016/j.bspc.2023.104988

Aamir, M., Rahman, Z., Dayo, Z. A., Abro, W. A., Uddin, M. I., Khan, I., Imran, A. S., Ali, Z., Ishfaq, M., Guan, Y., & Hu, Z. (2022). A deep learning approach for brain tumor classification using MRI images. *Computers & Electrical Engineering*, *101*, 108105. DOI: 10.1016/j.compeleceng.2022.108105

Ahmed, H., Dada, M. O., & Samaila, B. (2023). Current challenges of the state-of-the-art of AI techniques for diagnosing brain tumor. *Materials Science and Engineering*, *7*(4), 196–208.

Ali, K. H. (2023). ViT-BT: Enhancing Brain Tumor Classification Using Vision Transformers. *SSRN*. https://ssrn.com/abstract=4959261

Aloraini, M., Khan, A., Aladhadh, S., Habib, S., Alsharekh, M. F., & Islam, M. (2023). Combining the Transformer and Convolution for Effective Brain Tumor Classification Using MRI Images. *Applied Sciences (Basel, Switzerland)*, *13*(3680), 3680. Advance online publication. DOI: 10.3390/app13063680

Ari, A., & Hanbay, D. (2018). Deep learning-based brain tumor classification and detection system. *Turkish Journal of Electrical Engineering and Computer Sciences*, *26*(5), 1–8. DOI: 10.3906/elk-1801-8

Asiri, A. A., Shaf, A., Ali, T., Shakeel, U., Halawani, H. T., Alghamdi, A. H., Irfan, M., Alshamrani, A. F. A., Mehdar, K. M., & Alqhtani, S. M. (2023). Exploring the power of deep learning: Fine-tuned Vision Transformer for accurate and efficient brain tumor detection in MRI scans. *Diagnostics (Basel)*, *13*(2094), 2094. Advance online publication. DOI: 10.3390/diagnostics13122094 PMID: 37370989

Badjie, B., & Ülker, E. D. (2022). A deep transfer learning-based architecture for brain tumor classification using MR images. *Information Technology and Control*, *51*(2), 332–344. DOI: 10.5755/j01.itc.51.2.30835

Batool, A., & Byun, Y. C. (2024). Brain tumor detection with integrating traditional and computational intelligence approaches across diverse imaging modalities-Challenges and future directions. *Computers in Biology and Medicine*, *175*, 108412. DOI: 10.1016/j.compbiomed.2024.108412 PMID: 38691914

Dixon, J., Akinniyi, O., Abdelhamid, A., Saleh, G. A., Rahman, M. M., & Khalifa, F. (2024). A Hybrid Learning-Architecture for Improved Brain Tumor Recognition. *Algorithms*, *17*(6), 221. DOI: 10.3390/a17060221

Goceri, E. (2023). Vision transformer based classification of gliomas from histopathological images. *Expert Systems with Applications*, *205*, 122672. DOI: 10.1016/j.eswa.2023.1226go72

. Guan, Y., Aamir, M., Rahman, Z., Ali, A., Abro, W. A., Dayo, Z. A., ... & Hu, Z. (2021). A framework for efficient brain tumor classification using MRI images.

Hao, R., Namdar, K., Liu, L., & Khalvati, F. (2021). A transfer learning–based active learning framework for brain tumor classification. *Frontiers in Artificial Intelligence*, *4*, 635766. DOI: 10.3389/frai.2021.635766 PMID: 34079932

He, K., Gan, C., Li, Z., Rekik, I., Yin, Z., Ji, W., Gao, Y., Wang, Q., Zhang, J., & Shen, D. (2023). Transformers in medical image analysis. *Intelligent Medicine, 3*(1), 59–78. DOI: 10.1016/j.imed.2022.07.002

Karagoz, M. A., Nalbantoglu, O. U., & Fox, G. C. (2024). Residual Vision Transformer (ResViT) Based Self-Supervised Learning Model for Brain Tumor Classification. *arXiv*. https://arxiv.org/abs/2411.12874

Khan, M. A., Ashraf, I., Alhaisoni, M., Damaševičius, R., Scherer, R., Rehman, A., & Bukhari, S. A. C. (2020). Multimodal Brain Tumor Classification Using Deep Learning and Robust Feature Selection: A Machine Learning Application for Radiologists. *Diagnostics (Basel), 10*(8), 565. DOI: 10.3390/diagnostics10080565 PMID: 32781795

Khan, S. M., Nasim, F., Ahmad, J., & Masood, S. (2024). Deep Learning-Based Brain Tumor Detection. *Journal of Computing & Biomedical Informatics, 7*(02).

Kittler, J., Hatef, M., Duin, R. P., & Matas, J. (1998). On combining classifiers. *IEEE Transactions on Pattern Analysis and Machine Intelligence, 20*(3), 226–239. DOI: 10.1109/34.667881

Li, M., Jiang, Y., Zhang, Y., & Zhu, H. (2023). Medical image analysis using deep learning algorithms. *Frontiers in Public Health, 11*, 1273253. DOI: 10.3389/fpubh.2023.1273253 PMID: 38026291

Mehrotra, R., Ansari, M. A., Agrawal, R., & Anand, R. S. (2020). A transfer learning approach for AI-based classification of brain tumors. *Machine Learning with Applications, 1*, 100003. DOI: 10.1016/j.mlwa.2020.100003

Mohsen, H., El-Dahshan, E. A., El-Horbaty, E. M., & Salem, A. M. (2017). Classification using deep learning neural networks for brain tumors. *Future Computing and Informatics Journal, 3*(1), 68–71. DOI: 10.1016/j.fcij.2017.12.001

Rao, C. S., & Karunakara, K. (2021). A comprehensive review on brain tumor segmentation and classification of MRI images. *Multimedia Tools and Applications, 80*(12), 17611–17643. DOI: 10.1007/s11042-020-10443-1

Reddy, C. K. K., Reddy, P. A., Janapati, H., Assiri, B., Shuaib, M., Alam, S., & Sheneamer, A. (2024). A fine-tuned vision transformer based enhanced multi-class brain tumor classification using MRI scan imagery. *Frontiers in Oncology, 14*, 1400341. DOI: 10.3389/fonc.2024.1400341 PMID: 39091923

Srinivas, C., Prasad, K. S. N., Zakariah, M., Alothaibi, Y. A., Shaukat, K., Partibane, B., & Awal, H. (2022). Deep Transfer Learning Approaches in Performance Analysis of Brain Tumor Classification Using MRI Images. *Computational Intelligence and Neuroscience, 2022*, 3264367. Advance online publication. DOI: 10.1155/2022/3264367 PMID: 35299683

Tabatabaei, S., Rezaee, K., & Zhu, M. (2023). Attention transformer mechanism and fusion-based deep learning architecture for MRI brain tumor classification system. *Biomedical Signal Processing and Control, 86*, 105119. DOI: 10.1016/j.bspc.2023.105119

Tang, W., He, F., Liu, Y., & Duan, Y. (2022). MATR: Multimodal medical image fusion via multi-scale adaptive transformer. *IEEE Transactions on Image Processing, 31*, 5134–5149. DOI: 10.1109/TIP.2022.3193288 PMID: 35901003

Tummala, S., Kadry, S., Bukhari, S. A. C., & Rauf, H. T. (2022). Classification of brain tumor from magnetic resonance imaging using vision transformers ensembling. *Current Oncology (Toronto, Ont.)*, *29*(10), 7498–7511. DOI: 10.3390/curroncol29100590 PMID: 36290867

Vimala, B. B., Srinivasan, S., Mathivanan, S. K., Mahalakshmi, P. J., & Dalu, G. T. (2023). Detection and classification of brain tumor using hybrid deep learning models. *Scientific Reports*, *13*(1), 23029. DOI: 10.1038/s41598-023-50505-6 PMID: 38155247

Xie, Y., Zaccagna, F., Rundo, L., Testa, C., Agati, R., Lodi, R., Manners, D. N., & Tonon, C. (2022). Convolutional neural network techniques for brain tumor classification (from 2015 to 2022): Review, challenges, and future perspectives. *Diagnostics (Basel)*, *12*(8), 1850. DOI: 10.3390/diagnostics12081850 PMID: 36010200

Zhang, H., Xu, H., Tian, X., Jiang, J., & Ma, J. (2021). Image fusion meets deep learning: A survey and perspective. *Information Fusion*, *76*, 323–336. DOI: 10.1016/j.inffus.2021.06.008

Chapter 8
Convolutional Neural Networks (CNNs) for Enhanced Decision-Making in Medical Imaging

Kehinde Iyioluwa Adeyinka
https://orcid.org/0009-0009-7685-6693
University of Science and Technology, Beijing, China

Taye Iyinoluwa Adeyinka
https://orcid.org/0009-0006-4357-6319
University of Science and Technology, Beijing, China

Joseph Wadefai Passing
https://orcid.org/0009-0006-7615-6900
University of Science and Technology, Beijing, China

ABSTRACT

The rapid development in medical imaging technologies has greatly enlarged the capacity to diagnose and treat a wide range of medical diseases. On the other hand, because of the increased complexity and number of medical pictures, it is challenging to provide timely and proper decision-making. Among deep learning methods, CNN has been an auspicious approach in automatically and effectively carrying out medical image analysis, thus enabling faster, more effective, and more reliable diagnostic procedures. This chapter examines the use of CNNs in medical imaging: multi-modal imaging data integration, image segmentation, and the identification of an illness are given special attention. We cover how CNNs can be applied to early diagnosis, augmenting clinical decision-making by capturing delicate patterns that human clinicians may lose. Also, we examine how CNN-based systems support real-time decision-making for emergency diagnosis and robotic surgery.

DOI: 10.4018/979-8-3693-9816-6.ch008

1. INTRODUCTION

Medical imaging has incredibly changed the healthcare industry with its non-invasive ways of identifying and monitoring various ailments and diseases. Traditional imaging methods, such as CT, MRI, ultrasound, and X-rays, have been crucial in clinical diagnosis for decades. but, the increasing data generation and heightened complexity of medical images has various challenges to healthcare workers. In return, AI systems that can support medical image interpretation have been developed in response to increasing demands for more effective decision-making tools. Convolutional Neural Networks are among the most efficient AI methods, among many other effective methods for automating image analysis.

Figure 1. Medical Image Techniques

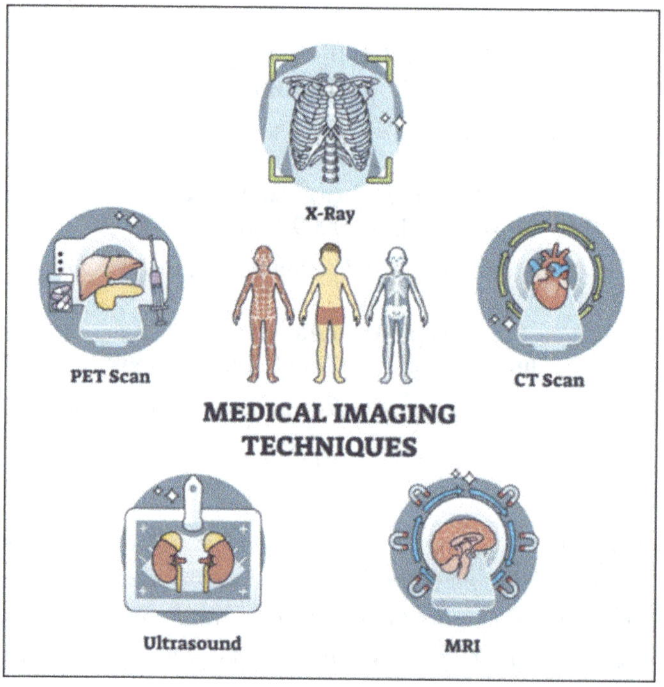

CNNs are a subset of deep learning architectures that are especially well-suited to medical image analysis because of their excellent processing accuracy in visual data. This is because CNNs play a critical role in modern medical imaging, automatically extracting relevant features from images and learning from extensive data to generate predictions with minimal human inpuy (LeCun, Bengio, & Hinton, 1998). Yann LeCun and colleagues first developed CNNs to automate image recognition tasks in the early 1990s (LeCun, Bengio, & Hinton, 2015). However, CNNs were not widely used in the big data explosion and computer power improvements, especially in the medical imaging industry. Identifying abnormalities in chest X-rays and categorizing brain cancers in MRI scans were among the early uses of CNNs in medical diagnostics (Shin et al., 2016). These days, CNNs are used in many different imaging modalities and applications, such as radiology, pathology, dermatology, and ophthalmology.

CNNs' architecture is one of the factors contributing to their success in medical imaging. Convolutional, pooling, and fully connected layers are among the several layers that make up CNNs. These levels enable the network to learn hierarchical feature representations of images automatically. CNNs are very good at diagnosing illnesses from complicated medical images because they can extract features without human assistance (Aamir et al., 2023). The increasing flexibility of CNNs has facilitated the application of these models to 3D imaging data, such as the MRI and the CT scans, further increased their applicability within the medical domain. Disease detection is one of the more popular applications of CNNs in medical imaging. Various CNN-based systems have been developed to detect diseases based on medical images, including neurological disorders, cardiovascular conditions, and cancers. For instance, CNNs have been applied in oncology for diagnosing skin cancer from dermatological images (Aamir et al., 2022), locating lung cancer from CT scans (Esteva et al., 2017), and detecting and classifying tumors from mammography images in breast cancer (Mridha et al., 2021). CNNs help improve diagnostic efficiency and reduce work pressure on radiologists by automating detection tasks, therefore making life-threatening conditions recognized more accurately and earlier. Besides, there is enormous potential for CNNs in neurological diagnosis. In neurology, CNN has been used to diagnose the early detection of Alzheimer's disease using MRI images (Kriegeskorte, 2015). CNNs have also identified strokes and brain hemorrhages from CT and MRI images, respectively, thus supporting doctors with valuable information in urgent situations where an immediate diagnosis is required (Rajpurkar et al., 2018).

In addition to standard radiology, CNNs are being investigated in dermatology, where they assist doctors in identifying skin cancers like melanoma from pictures of skin lesions (Esteva et al., 2017). CNNs' capacity to identify patterns in pictures that are hard for the human eye to pick up on can result in quicker and more accurate diagnoses, which could enhance patient outcomes. Image Segmentation and Its Influence on Decision-Making CNNs have significantly impacted even medical image segmentation. Image segmentation, which includes dividing an image into meaningful parts such as organs, tumors, or blood arteries, provides substantial assistance in the diagnosis, treatment planning, and observation of disease courses. Precise segmentation helps clinicians locate, size, and shape a tumor, which is essential in choosing the best course of therapy. CNNs automatically learn and extract features pertinent to the segmentation process, which makes them very useful for medical picture segmentation applications. Conventional picture segmentation methods frequently call for human contributions, which can be laborious and prone to have mistaken. On the other hand, CNN-based segmentation algorithms can effectively process enormous amounts of medical pictures, significantly reducing the time required for diagnosis. Moreover, it has been shown that CNNs outperform the performance of the traditional methods in such applications as detecting liver tumors from CT scans (Di et al., 2022), brain tumor segmentation from MRI scans (Guan et al., n.d.), and retinal vascular segmentation in ophthalmology (Wang et al., 2022).

The segmentation process done with CNNs makes much of a difference in clinical decision-making. Clinicians can make much better treatment decisions, surgical techniques, and tactics for monitoring, provided the segmentations are more accurate and detailed. For example, proper delineation of tumors for oncological cases helps to plan radiation treatment more precisely, sparing normal tissues and optimizing the dose to the tumor (Gul & Khan, 2023). In general, clinical practice, different imaging modalities are combined to provide a more complete picture of a patient's condition. Multi-modality imaging integrates information from various sources- CT, MRI, PET scans, and ultrasound- to give a more enhanced view of the anatomy and pathology. However, combining such imaging modalities has many challenges, especially in co-coordinating the data from several sources and ensuring that the pertinent information is captured. CNNs demonstrate promise in treating such problems by making it possible to fuse multi-modal medical pictures. Multi-modality imaging will enable physicians to exploit the strengths of each imaging modality: PET for metabolic activity, MRI for soft tissue contrast, and CT for comprehensive anatomical information. CNNs can help detect diseases that may not be as apparent if only one imaging modality is used and make more accurate predictions by combining various data. CNNs, for example, have been applied in oncology by combining CT and PET scans to segment and monitor tumor growth (Liang, Zadeh, & Morency, 2024). Multi-modal image data integration enhances decision-making by giving physicians a richer understanding of patient conditions. This, in some cases, could lead to improved treatment response monitoring, more accurate tumor staging, and earlier disease detection (Pei et al., 2023). Real-time decision-making plays a vital role in medicine, especially in critical care, where immediate diagnosis and treatment are necessary. The CNNs are finding their way into real-time decision-making systems where their accuracy and speed are critical, such as telemedicine platforms, robotic operations, and emergency diagnostics. CNN, can help guide the surgeon during robotic surgery by interpreting real-time visual feeds from surgical cameras and offering information about the surgical site. In order to direct the surgeon's actions appropriately, this can assist in identifying areas of concern, such as tumors or anomalies. Similarly, CNN-based systems can quickly analyze emergency medical pictures for clinicians, who must make quick decisions. Despite the above achievements, several obstacles must be overcome to unleash CNNs completely in medical imaging. One of the significant challenges is the need for extensive datasets with annotations for CNN training. Medical imaging datasets are often limited due to issues with high-quality labelled data, patient consent, and privacy concerns (Willemink et al., 2020), according to. Without question, solving this problem and ensuring the safety and ethics in data exchange will require collaboration among medical facilities, researchers, and regulatory agencies. Another challenge is the interpretability of CNN. While CNNs can provide accurate predictions, it is often hard to know from what the model has derived a specific decision (Alzubaidi et al., 2021). Accountability and transparency are most important in life-critical healthcare applications; thus, the "black-box" nature of deep learning models raises questions about their application. These challenges notwithstanding, CNNs have a promising future in medical imaging (Altaf, Shah, et al., 2019)]. The current limitations cited are expected to be removed by developments in explainable AI, generative models, and transfer learning. Moreover, using CNNs with other innovative technologies, such as robotics, augmented reality (Jayasundar & Kumar, n.d.), and personalized medicine, may transform healthcare delivery in ways never seen before. Indeed, convolutional neural networks have greatly improved decision-making in medical imaging. CNNs are helpful in diverse uses for physicians, such as multi-modal integration, image segmentation, and disease identification and diagnosis (Xu et al., 2024). Full integration of CNNs into real-time clinical decision-making and treatment planning is expected to proliferate further. At the same time, AI evolves, leading to better patient outcomes and lower healthcare expenses. In particular, before the CNN-based systems can be safely and effectively used in clinical practice, data accessibility, model interpretability, and regulatory considerations have to be addressed.

1.1 Literature review

Medical imaging has been considered a principal pillar of modern healthcare for several decades, providing doctors of various specialties with diagnostic aids. The demand for image analysis that is more automated, effective, and accurate has increased in the last few decades. Convolutional neural networks (CNNs) are one of the most promising technologies for automated medical image analysis, and their development has been accelerated by this spike in demand (Aamir et al., 2019). In image classification, detection, and segmentation tasks all critical for making decisions in medical practice—CNNs, a subset of deep learning algorithms, have shown remarkable performance.

This literature review aims to assess the use of CNNs in medical imaging, underlining advances, challenges, and possible applications of this technology to improve diagnosis and treatment decision-making in illness. The history of CNNs in medical imaging started when LeCun and associates initially created the convolutional architecture for pattern recognition tasks in the 1990s (LeCun, Bengio, & Hinton, 1998). Initially, CNNs were applied for non-medical applications such as natural language processing and handwritten digit recognition. Only after significant advances in computational powers and the availability of large datasets could CNNs significantly impact medical imaging (LeCun, Bengio, & Hinton, 2015). Currently, CNNs have been used for various tasks spanning disease classification, detection, segmentation, and even prognosis prediction. Since then, their use in the medical profession has proliferated (Tufail et al., 2021). Because of their automatic hierarchical extraction from images, CNNs are particularly adept at medical imaging. CNNs can learn spatial hierarchies of features straight from the raw data, unlike standard machine learning models, which have to be hand-engineered by features, as per (Du et al., 2020). In medical imaging, where the relevant entities, like cancers, lesions, and organs, may vary in size, shape, and texture between patients, this auto-feature extraction becomes essential. Particular benefits of CNNs show up in radiology, where they have transformed the practice of medicine with their ability to process and interpret images. Applications in radiology focused on the early detection and classification of malignancies present within chest X-rays (Moses et al., 2021). The field has since expanded to include a variety of imaging methods, such as MRI, CT, and ultrasound. Indeed, various studies have involved CNNs that outperform human radiologists, particularly in detecting a variety of minor abnormalities that would remain unnoticed otherwise. CNNs' main applications in medical imaging involve the identification and detection of diseases. Deep learning models can leverage the rich information contained in medical images, particularly those generated from radiological methods, for exact disease identification. CNNs are applied to the detection of illnesses in a number of medical conditions, including cancer, neurological disorders, and cardiovascular disorders.

In oncology, CNNs have been applied successfully to detect tumors within MRI, CT, and mammography images. The use of CNNs to identify breast cancer from mammograms is a good example. In the study by (Oyelade et al., 2022), CNN-based models could classify mammogram pictures with accuracy that matched that of skilled radiologists. Because of this capacity to identify microcalcifications, masses, and other minute characteristics suggestive of breast cancer, CNNs are very useful in early diagnosis (Al-Yasriy, et al., 2020). CNNs have also been used to detect lung cancer from chest CT scans. (Atmakuru, et al., 2024) investigated the efficiency of a deep CNN model in detecting lung cancer that could reach the accuracy level of human radiologists. This capacity is beneficial given the complexity and volume of chest CT images that can take much time and experience to examine. Automating the detection process can help reduce the burden on radiologists so that they can have more time for complicated patients or treatments. The CNNs have shown great promise in dermatology for detecting skin cancer from dermatological pictures, particularly melanoma. Winkler et al. (2023) showed that CNNs may outperform general practitioners in melanoma detection and classify skin lesions at a dermatologist-level performance. This article points out the potential of CNNs in those specialties where early identification is crucial to successful treatment. CNNs have also been used in neurology to diagnose neurological conditions such as stroke, brain tumors, and Alzheimer's disease (Gautam & Sharma, 2020). For instance, CNNs, when applied to MRI images, have shown great promise in detecting early signs of Alzheimer's disease (Yao, et al., 2023). One of CNNs' main capabilities is their ability to detect very slight changes in brain morphology, such as atrophy of the hippocampus. Such a possibility will significantly enhance early diagnosis and treatment planning. Another important domain in which CNNs' performance has significantly enhanced medical imaging is image segmentation. Segmentation refers to dividing an image into helpful regions, where one might identify specific organs, tumors, or lesions within medical images. Accurate segmentation is important for clinical decision-making in oncology, neurology, and cardiology, where precise demarcation of abnormal tissues plays a key role in diagnosis, treatment planning, and follow-up.

Conventional image segmentation techniques, that depends on physicians' manual demarcation, can be laborious and has no error. Conversely, CNN-based segmentation algorithms automate this procedure, yielding precise and repeatable outcomes that can save significant time in clinical settings (Xu et al., 2024). For example, CNNs have been successfully applied to the segmentation of liver lesions in CT images, brain tumors in MRI scans (Almotairi, et al., 2020), and retinal vessels in ophthalmology (Guthoff, et al., 1991). In all these cases, CNNs outperformed traditional segmentation methods, providing more accurate and reproducible results. CNN-based segmentation bears great impact on clinical decisions. Accurate tumor segmentation in oncology is important to determine tumors' location, size, and shape, all of which are critical factors for treatment planning. For example, during radiotherapy, correct tumor delineation ensures that radiation hits the right place while reducing maximum injury to healthy tissues (Burnet, et al., 2004). In neurology, accurate brain tumor segmentation can be used to guide surgical planning and to improve the monitoring of disease progression. Retinal vascular segmentation is essential in ophthalmology for diagnosing glaucoma and diabetic retinopathy, which can cause blindness if neglected. Another exciting recent development in the field of medical imaging is the integration of multimodal imaging techniques. These techniques can combine data from different multiples imaging modalities to produce a more rounded view of a patient's state. Multimodal imaging provides complementary information, like anatomical, functional, and metabolic data, that forms the basis for accurate diagnosis and treatment planning. Because CNNs can learn characteristics from different sources, they are particularly well-suited to multimodal medical imaging. For example, CNNs have been applied to combine the functional information of PET with the complete anatomical information of CT scans for cancer diagnosis (Sibille, et al., 2020). This integration will lead to more personalized treatment regimens due to its improved diagnosis and staging of tumors. CNNs have been applied to neurology for integrating images from PET and MRI to diagnose Alzheimer's disease. Combining structural MRI, which provides accurate anatomical information, with functional PET, which assesses metabolic activity, allows for the detection of early degenerative changes in the brain that may not be visible on any one scan (Teune, et al., 2010). Multi-modal imaging data can be integrated by CNNs, by offering a comprehensive view of the patient's state and this enhances clinical decision-making.

Real-time decision-making is integral to several therapeutic situations, mainly telemedicine, emergency care, and surgery. CNNs are increasingly being integrated into real-time decision-making systems like robotic surgery, emergency diagnostics, and telemedicine applications. In robotic surgery, CNNs can be applied to live video feeds from surgical cameras and supply doctors with real-time suggestions about the same. For example, CNNs help highlight critical structures like organs, blood arteries, and tumors that will help the surgeon make good decisions intraoperatively. According to Samuel (n.d.), CNN-based systems may also consider CT scans in emergency care for fast evaluation, thus assisting in diagnosing life-threatening conditions such as strokes and brain hemorrhages. CNNs are also enabling telemedicine applications, especially where the access to medical specialists is not available. Clinicians that are in deprived locations can get diagnostic support by using CNNs to assess medical images remotely. This ability to make accurate decisions on medical images, especially in remote and real-time situations, can significantly improve access to healthcare services. CNNs have many potential uses, yet there are drawbacks to using them in medical imaging. The requirement for sizable, annotated datasets in order to train CNN models is one of the main challenges. Concerns about patient privacy, legal limitations, and the challenge of acquiring high-quality labeled data frequently hinder medical imaging datasets (Willemink, et al., 2020). Another problem is class imbalance, which occurs when some diseases or illnesses are underrepresented in datasets. The consequence might be biased models which could generalize poorly to new data.

The interpretability of CNNs is another challenge. CNNs are frequently referred to as "black-box" models, which means it can be challenging to comprehend how the model makes its decisions, even though they have demonstrated exceptional performance in various medical imaging tasks (Razzak, Naz, & Zaib, 2018). The lack of interpretability is a major obstacle to the widespread use of CNNs in medical applications, where transparency and trust are crucial. Saliency maps and attention mechanisms that highlight areas in an image which influence a model's decision are two active research strategies to increase the Explainability of CNNs. With the continuous improvement in technology and its clinical applications, the future of CNNs in medical imaging also seems promising. CNNs have great potential for enhancing medical imaging decision-making when integrated with other AI approaches, including expert systems, reinforcement learning, and natural language processing. Additionally, further innovation within this domain will likely be fueled by the expanding availability of multi-modal datasets and growing processing capacity of modern systems. More importantly, more dependable, interpretable, and generalizable models need to be developed if CNNs are to see wide clinical practice (Salahuddin, et al., 2022). Ethical aspects related to data privacy and fairness are also under investigation concerning the design of medical imaging systems. CNNs play an important role and must be considered if technologies are to be used responsibly and equitably. Medical imaging has revolutionized due to convolutional neural networks, which improve disease detection, diagnosis, and decision-making. Particularly in radiology, oncology, neurology, and dermatology, the features they can extract automatically from medical images have led to remarkable improvements in accuracy and efficiency. Yet there are challenges regarding interpretability, generalizability, and limited datasets. While these may act as setbacks for CNNs, a bright future lies ahead with continued research toward advancing the technology and integration into clinical workflows. As these issues are ironed out, the importance of CNNs in the future is expected to be much more influential on healthcare and medical decision-making.

2. CNN ARCHITECTURES AND THEIR ROLE IN MEDICAL IMAGING

Because of their remarkable capacity to evaluate and comprehend intricate visual input, Convolutional Neural Networks (CNNs) are leading the way in deep learning applications in medical imaging. This section examines the most well-known CNN designs, how well they work for particular medical imaging applications, and how they can be tailored to handle high-dimensional data, like 3D medical scans.

Figure 2. CNNs architectures commonly used in medical imaging. (a) One CNN with 2 convolutional layers, 2 pooling layers, and a fully connected layer; (b) Node graph of 1D representation of a classical CNN structure; (c) Node graph of 1D representation of a multi-stream CNN structure; (d) Node graph of 1D representation of structure of a CNN for segmentation (U-NET with only one down-sampling stage)

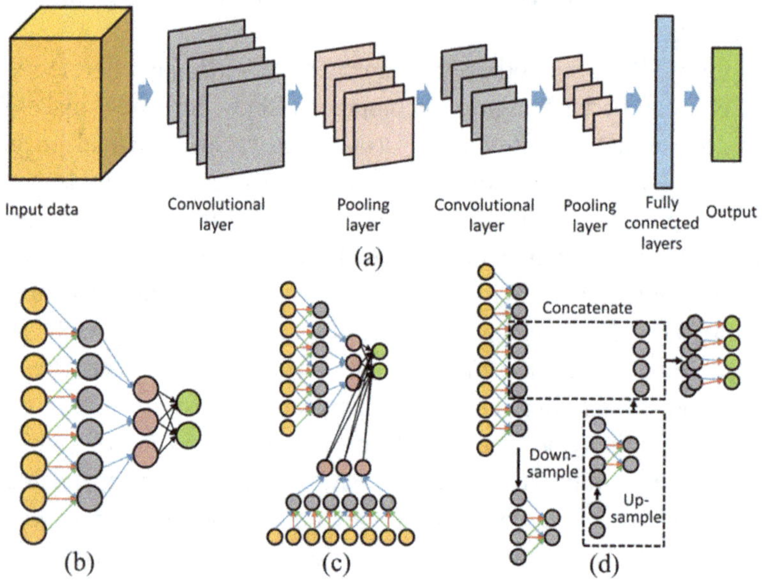

- **Examining Well-Known Medical Imaging Architectures**

Several CNN designs have become essential instruments for medical image analysis, with each being particularly good at specific tasks like anomaly detection, segmentation, and picture classification.

AlexNet (2012): One of the first CNNs to show off deep learning's capabilities in image recognition applications was AlexNet. AlexNet's eight-layer design uses dropout for regularization, ReLU activation, convolutional, and fully connected layers. Function in Medical Imaging: AlexNet has been applied to simple classification tasks, like identifying cancer in histopathological pictures or distinguishing normal from aberrant tissues in X-rays. Its comparatively straightforward architecture provides a framework for creating increasingly intricate networks.
VGGNet (2014): To capture fine features, VGGNet introduced deeper architectures with up to 19 layers using smaller 3x3 convolutional filters. Function in Medical Imaging: VGGNet is appropriate for jobs like spotting tiny changes in brain MRI imaging, such as gliomas or Alzheimer's disease, because of its capacity to represent complex patterns. However, because of its size and processing requirements, VGGNet frequently needs to be modified for use with medical data.
ResNet (2015): ResNet established the idea of residual learning, enabling efficient training of intense networks by utilizing shortcut connections to avoid superfluous layers. Function in Medical Imaging: Complex classification problems, including identifying several diseases from chest X-

rays (e.g., pneumonia, COVID-19, or tuberculosis), are especially well-suited for ResNet's deep architecture. It is also resilient in situations with little training data, which is a frequent medical imaging problem.

DenseNet (2017): ResNet is further enhanced by DenseNet, which reduces the parameters and allows feature reuse by connecting each layer to every subsequent layer. Function in Medical Imaging: Because of its effectiveness, DenseNet is perfect for applications needing high-resolution image analysis, such as identifying liver lesions in CT scans or diagnosing mammogram tumors.

U-Net (2015): A specific CNN architecture called U-Net was created for picture segmentation. It employs an encoder-decoder structure to forecast pixel-level outputs, in which the encoder gathers features, and the decoder reconstructs the image. Function in Medical Imaging: For segmentation tasks, such as identifying tumors, organs, and blood arteries in CT and MRI scans, U-Net has emerged as the industry standard. Planning radiation therapy and guiding surgeries benefit significantly from its capacity to record minute details.

2.1 Architecture Suitability Comparisons for Particular Tasks

Because of their distinct design elements, several architectures perform better on particular medical imaging tasks. Their appropriateness for three crucial medical imaging tasks is contrasted below:

Classification of Images:

AlexNet, VGGNet, ResNet, and DenseNet are the best-suited architectures.

These structures are quite effective for tasks like recognizing diseases (e.g., distinguishing whether skin lesions are benign or malignant) or detecting anomalies in X-rays and mammograms. Because of their deeper structures, ResNet and DenseNet excel at solving challenging categorization issues. When paired with object identification frameworks like Faster R-CNN, the best-suited architectures are ResNet and DenseNet.

Object detection is essential in medical pictures for locating certain regions of interest, like tumors or nodules. The feature-dense layers in DenseNet and the residual connections in ResNet improve the process of finding and classifying objects in photos. U-Net and its variations are the best-suited architectures.

U-Net's encoder-decoder architecture is perfect for pixel-wise segmentation tasks like recognizing tumor boundaries or separating blood vessels in retinal pictures. However, for precise segmentation in medical imaging, the spatial resolution must be maintained, aided by its skip connections.

2.1.1 Personalized CNN Adjustments for High-Dimensional Health Information

Complex, high-dimensional data, such as 3D volumes produced by MRI or CT scans, are frequently used in medical imaging. Conventional 2D CNNs need to be modified to handle volumetric data properly, even though they perform well for planar pictures like X-rays. To process volumetric input directly, 3D CNNs expand the conventional 2D convolution to a third spatial dimension. To extract characteristics from the depth dimension which is essential for comprehending spatial relationships inside medical scans 3D CNNs employ 3D kernels rather than 2D filters. Combining 2D and 3D CNNs is a new trend that aims to balance the spatial awareness of 3D CNNs with the computational efficiency of 2D CNNs. For instance, a hybrid model may employ 3D CNNs for context-aware classification and 2D CNNs for feature extraction. CNN architectures can incorporate attention modules to highlight important sections of an image while disregarding unimportant ones. This is especially helpful in medical imaging, where anomalies frequently take up a small portion of the image. Applications include the identification of microcalcifications in mammograms, which are a sign of breast cancer in its early stages. It highlights areas of the brain that are ischemia in order to diagnose stroke.

- **Learning Transfer:**

Transfer learning is fine-tuning a CNN for particular medical imaging applications after pretraining it on sizable, general-purpose datasets (like ImageNet). This method addresses the typical problem of little labelled data in medical fields. Uses include modifying pre-trained ResNet models to identify COVID-19 from chest X-rays. To address the lack of labeled data, GANs can produce artificial medical images to supplement training datasets. CNN architectures are frequently trained or optimized using these artificial pictures. Applications include creating a variety of tumor forms for segmentation model training.

2.2 CNNs for Medical Image Segmentation

In the healthcare industry, medical picture segmentation is a crucial task. Exact identification and analysis of features like tumors, organs, and blood vessels are essential for precise diagnosis, treatment planning, and disease monitoring. Conventional segmentation techniques mostly rely on human interaction, which is difficult in high-dimensional imaging data, time-consuming, and subject to unpredictability. This discipline has seen a revolution with the introduction of Convolutional Neural Networks (CNNs), which automate segmentation jobs with increased efficiency and accuracy. This part covers the significance of segmentation, the developments made possible by CNN-based designs such as U-Net, SegNet, and Mask R-CNN, and their practical uses in tasks like liver lesion identification, brain tumor analysis, and retinal vascular segmentation.

2.2.1 The Value of Medical Imaging Segmentation

Medical image segmentation entails dividing an image into meaningful areas to identify particular anatomical features or clinical characteristics. Segmentation is essential for applications that demand great precision because it offers pixel-level or voxel-level granularity, in contrast to classification jobs that assign a single label to an entire image. Determining tumor size, shape, and growth patterns requires knowing their borders. Thanks to accurate tumor segmentation, oncologists can arrange radiation therapy and surgical resection with precision, guaranteeing that the tumor is targeted while preserving healthy tissue. For instance, segmenting brain tumors in MRI scans is essential for directing neurosurgical treatments for glioblastoma. Assessing the size of organs, including the liver, kidneys, and heart, identifying structural anomalies, and tracking disease course depend on their segmentation. For example, liver segmentation in CT scans helps detect cirrhosis or track how well liver cancer treatment is working. The diagnosis of vascular disorders like atherosclerosis, diabetic retinopathy, and glaucoma depends heavily on the segmentation of blood vessels, such as coronary arteries or retinal vessels. Planning minimally invasive procedures like stent installation also requires vessel segmentation. Conventional segmentation techniques sometimes depend on expert manual delineation, which is time-consuming and prone to inter-observer variability. By automating the segmentation process, CNNs overcome these difficulties and produce reliable, repeatable findings on big datasets.

2.2.2 Segmentation Models Based on CNN

A number of CNN designs have been created and refined for segmenting medical images. These models are designed to handle medical data's particular difficulties, including limited annotated datasets, complicated anatomical variances, and high dimensionality.

U-Net which is One of the most often used architectures for segmenting biological images is U-Net. Its symmetric encoder-decoder topology with skip links, first presented by Ronneberger et al. (2015), enables the network to capture local and global context. The encoder compresses the input image into a low-dimensional representation, and the decoder reconstructs the segmentation map. The skip connections preserve fine-grained spatial information by bridging corresponding layers in the encoder and decoder, it is used in ;

- MRI image segmentation of brain tumors.
- CT imaging identification of lung nodules.
- Segmentation of retinal vessels in fundus pictures.

SegNet With an emphasis on computational efficiency, SegNet uses an encoder-decoder design. The decoder uses the encoder pooling indices to up-sample the feature maps produced by the encoder to maintain spatial information.

Applications:

- CT scans for the identification of liver lesions.
- Segmentation of skin lesions in dermatological pictures.

Mask R-CNN expands and Improves R-CNN speed by including a parallel branch for segmentation mask prediction and bounding box prediction. Because of its instance segmentation capability, it is perfect for identifying and separating specific items in a picture. Attention is a U-Net add-on that uses attention mechanisms to concentrate on the most pertinent areas of the image. This is especially helpful in medical imaging, where anomalies frequently take up a small portion of the image. 3D CNNs are made to handle volumetric data, like CT and MRI scans, whereas most CNNs work with 2D slices. To capture spatial context across several slices, they employ 3D convolutional kernels.

2.2.3 Applications in the Real World

Numerous medical imaging tasks have seen the successful application of CNN-based segmentation models. These apps show off their adaptability and revolutionary influence on therapeutic procedures. Accurate brain tumor segmentation is essential for radiation and surgical planning. In MRI scans, U-Net has been widely utilized to identify gliomas, giving neurosurgeons accurate tumor boundaries with which to work.

In a study by Kamnitsas et al. (2017), a multi-scale 3D CNN demonstrated state-of-the-art performance in brain tumor segmentation, greatly enhancing treatment planning. Liver segmentation in CT images is crucial for identifying lesions and tracking the course of the disease. SegNet and its variations have been used to segment the liver and detect anomalies such as metastases and hepatocellular cancer. For instance, CNN-powered automatic segmentation methods have been included in clinical systems to help radiologists detect liver cancers more quickly. Segmenting the retinal vessels is essential in diagnosing glaucoma and diabetic retinopathy in ophthalmology. Early diagnosis of these vision-threatening diseases is made possible by the incredible precision with which CNN-based models such as U-Net and Mask R-CNN have segmented retinal vessels from fundus images. The detection of nodules in chest CT imaging requires lung segmentation. CNN-based techniques have been used to segment the lungs and locate suspicious areas suggestive of lung cancer. These models increase diagnostic confidence and decrease false positives. CNNs are used in gastroenterology to identify polyps in colonoscopy pictures, which helps identify colorectal cancer early. Mask R-CNN has proven wildly successful at segmenting polyps at the instance level.

2.2.3 Medical Image Segmentation Challenges

Even while CNNs have shown incredible success, there are still several obstacles to overcome:

1. Restricted Annotated Information

Medical datasets are frequently tiny because of privacy issues and the expense of professional annotation. Data augmentation, transfer learning, and synthetic data production are employed to overcome this constraint.

2. Unbalanced Class:

Class imbalance results from anomalies taking up a minor portion of the image in many medical datasets. Loss functions like Dice loss and focused loss are intended to lessen this problem.

3. Interpretability:

CNNs are sometimes criticized for being opaque. Saliency maps and attention mechanisms are being used to improve interpretability. CNNs trained on a single dataset could not generalize well to data from other imaging modalities or institutions. Multi-center datasets and domain adaptation strategies are being investigated to increase resilience.

2.3 Integration of CNNs with Multi-modal Medical Imaging

Convolutional Neural Networks (CNNs) have become a potent tool for increasing diagnostic precision and offering a more thorough comprehension of a patient's condition when combined with multimodal medical imaging. In order to obtain complementary data regarding anatomical structures, functional activity, and tissue composition, multimodal imaging combines several imaging modalities, including ultrasound, Positron Emission Tomography (PET), Magnetic Resonance Imaging (MRI), and Computed Tomography (CT). Clinical professionals can improve diagnosis, treatment planning, and patient monitoring by integrating the advantages of these many imaging modalities. This section covers in detail the advantages of integrating several imaging modalities, the function of CNNs in merging data from these modalities, and actual case studies in neurology, cardiology, and oncology research.

1. Multimodal Imaging's Advantages for Medical Diagnostics

Every imaging modality offers distinct data that may be useful in diagnosing. However, because of its inherent limitations, depending only on one imaging approach can be restrictive. CT imaging Offers fine-grained pictures of the body's anatomy but does not reveal details on metabolic or tissue function. Using methods like functional MRI (fMRI), MRI imaging can offer both anatomical and functional information, as well as high-resolution pictures of soft tissues. By capturing metabolic activity, PET imaging can identify areas with aberrant cell activity and malignant tissues. Ultrasound allows for real-time imaging, which is especially helpful for imaging soft tissues like the liver and heart.

By combining various modalities, healthcare professionals can get a more complete picture of the patient's state. For example, physicians can locate metabolic activity within anatomical structures by combining PET and CT (PET/CT). Similarly, fMRI and structural MRI can be combined to analyze morphological changes in neural tissue and reveal information about brain function.

2. CNN-Based Methods for Combining Multimodal Data

CNNs are very good at combining and evaluating data from different sources. CNNs can be used for feature, decision, and pixel-level fusion, among other phases of fusing multimodal medical imaging data. Here, we go over some of the most essential methods for combining CNNs with multimodal data:

Early fusion entails integrating the raw pictures into a single data set from many modalities before putting them through the CNN. The network can quickly learn joint representations from several modalities with this method. For instance, the CNN model may concurrently learn anatomical structure and physiological activity by fusing MRI and PET data at the pixel level.

Example of Application: The combination of MRI and PET scans aids in the identification of brain tumors by revealing the tumor's location and metabolic features. CNNs initially use distinct routes to extract features from each modality in feature-level fusion, and then they combine the information afterward. This enables the network to acquire features unique to each modality before merging them for additional processing. Using distinct CNN branches for CT and MRI images and combining the data from both branches at a higher layer to predict the presence of cancer could be a popular method for detecting lung cancer. In late fusion, sometimes called decision-level fusion, each modality is processed separately using a different CNN model, and the predictions are subsequently combined. This method is easier to use because it does not use the interactions across modalities at intermediate levels. However, it might only sometimes be as successful as previous fusion strategies.

Application Example: CT and MRI scans can be analyzed separately to produce distinct predictions for heart problems. These are merged to produce a final diagnostic judgment in identifying cardiac disorders. CNNs can better manage complicated, multimodal data by focusing on the most pertinent information from each modality according to attention processes. Attention-based CNNs can improve the fusion process by dynamically balancing the significance of various modalities during training. To improve prediction accuracy in cancer diagnosis, an attention mechanism could assist the network in concentrating on areas of interest in the MRI and PET images, such as tumor hotspots, and assessing their relative relevance.

3. Multimodal CNN Applications Case Studies

The combination of CNNs and multi-modal imaging has significantly improved the diagnosis and prognosis of several multimodal. Here are a few noteworthy case examples that highlight the exceptional performance of multimodal.

a. Oncology (Diagnosis and Identification of Cancer)

Since tumors can be identified by metabolic activity (PET) and structural alterations (CT, MRI), cancer detection frequently necessitates a mix of modalities. Multi-modal CNN models have significantly enhanced the sensitivity and accuracy of cancer multi modulation of PET/CT for Lung Cancer:

The model combined the metabolic activity from PET scans with the anatomical data from CT scans using an early fusion technique. Compared to single-modality models, the resultant model greatly increased detection sensitivity and decreased false positives.

Findings: The multi-modal tumor location and the ability to distinguish between benign and malignant lesions. When MRI and PET images are combined, CNNs have demonstrated exceptional effectiveness in detecting gliomas in brain tumor diagnosis. While PET scans provide metabolic information that aids in identifying tumor activity, MRI scans provide precise physical features of the brain. CNNs trained on fused MRI and PET images are more accurate in differentiating between tumor and non-tumor regions. Researchers have reported improved tumor segmentation using the fusion model, which gives a more precise map of the tumor's extent—an essential tool for treatment planning.

b. Neurology (Alzheimer's and stroke brain imaging)

Multi-modal are very beneficial for neurological illnesses, including stroke and Alzheimer's. A more thorough examination of brain activity, anatomical integrity, and metabolic alterations is possible by combining structural MRI, functional MRI (fMRI), and PET. CNNs have been used to diagnose Alzheimer's disease by analyzing functional fMRI data as well as anatomical MRI scans. By combining structural and functional data, CNN models can evaluate alterations in brain morphology (such as hippocampus atrophy) and brain activity patterns suggestive of early AD.

Findings: Researchers have found that multi-modal CNNs are better than single-modality models in detecting biomarkers for early-stage AD and forecasting the start of Alzheimer's disease.

2.3.1 Combining CT and PET to Diagnose Strokes

PET scans measure metabolic activity in damaged brain regions, while CT scans detect ischemia areas to diagnose stroke. By integrating these modalities with CNNs, clinicians can anticipate patient outcomes, guide rehabilitation techniques, and provide more precise assessments of stroke severity.

Findings: The fusion model has demonstrated enhanced precision in identifying infarcted tissue and more accurate forecasting of functional recovery.

c. Cardiovascular Research (Heart Imaging and Heart Disease)

Multi-modal imaging is beneficial when diagnosing cardiovascular disease, where structural abnormalities (CT or MRI) and functional information (e.g., blood flow from PET or MRI) are joined.

Coronary artery disease can be evaluated by analyzing the myocardium's structural blockages and functional condition by combining CT angiography and MRI. CNNs trained on fused CT and MRI data can be utilized to predict the severity of CAD and detect stenosis. Compared to single-modality CNN models, multi-modal CNN models demonstrated higher accuracy in identifying coronary artery blockages and forecasting the likelihood of a heart attack. Whereas MRI scans provide anatomical features, PET scans provide functional information on metabolic activity for evaluating cardiac viability. By combining these modalities with CNNs, clinicians can anticipate which parts of the heart muscle are at danger of necrosis and which are still viable following a myocardial infarction. Following cardiac events, the fused PET/MRI models offer more accurate and dependable forecasts for patient outcomes.

4. Difficulties in CNN-Based Multimodal Medic Multimodal

Although there are many benefits to integrating CNNs with multi-modal also several drawbacks:

- **Data Alignment and Registration:**

One of the primary challenges in multimodal imaging is ensuring proper spatial alignment of data from several multimodal that result in inaccurate fusion, which may diminish the model's efficacy. To align modalities prior to CNN processing, sophisticated picture registration techniques are required.

- **Unbalanced Data:**

Data imbalance may result from different modalities' differing degrees of quality and availability. For instance, PET scans may be more costly or unavailable than CT scans. This imbalance must be addressed to train reliable multi-multimodal models' multimodal models.

- **Complexity of Computation:**

Since processing high-resolution images from various modalities enhances the model's complexity, training multi-modal CNNs demands significant multimodal. Hardware acceleration and effective algorithms are crucial to overcome these obstacles.

Interpretability:

Comprehending how the model integrates data from several modalities can be challenging because of the growing complexity of multi-modal CNNs. It is essential to develop methods multimodal model interpretability, particularly for clinical adoption. CNNs and multi-modal medical imaging have the potential to perform diagnostic procedures in several specialties, such as cardiology, neurology, and oncology. Clinicians can get a more thorough picture of a patient's condition by combining the advantages of various imaging modalities, which improves diagnosis and therapy planning. Even if there are obstacles related to interpretability, computational complexity, and data alignment, continuous research and development in multi-modal deep learning approaches assists in minimizing these difficulties and opens the door to more sophisticated and dependable healthcare solutions.

2.4 Role of Transfer Learning in Medical Imaging with CNNs

In medical imaging, transfer learning has become a crucial method that tackles one of the biggest problems in the field: the need for large, annotated datasets. Despite being detailed and crucial for diagnosis, medical imaging data is frequently challenging to gather and annotate because of patient privacy issues, legal constraints, and the labor-intensive nature of expert labeling. Transfer learning provides an answer by enabling models that have already been trained on extensive, general-purpose datasets, like ImageNet, to be optimized for particular medical imaging tasks. This method benefits healthcare applications since it lessens the computing load, speeds up the training process, and improves model performance.

Fundamentally, transfer learning adapts broad features discovered in non-medical datasets to the unique needs of medical imaging. For instance, convolutional neural networks (CNNs) that have been pre-trained on ImageNet a dataset containing millions of tagged natural images—have already mastered recognizing basic patterns like edges, textures, and forms. Since anatomical structures and disorders also display these patterns, these low-level traits are frequently transferred to medical pictures. When researchers refine these pre-trained models for organ segmentation, disease categorization, or tumor detection, they can achieve high accuracy even with a few datasets. There are numerous benefits of using transfer learning in medical imaging. First, it drastically reduces the time and computing power required for training. Using transfer learning, researchers can avoid pre-training on big datasets like ImageNet, which usually takes much computing power and training time, and instead concentrate on improving the model. Second, transfer learning enhances performance on specialized tasks by allowing the model to learn task-specific features from the medical dataset while maintaining the generalized knowledge learned during pre-training. This is particularly helpful in fields like medical imaging, where obtaining enough labeled data is complex.

Transfer learning has several significant applications in medical imaging. For example, pre-trained models such as ResNet and DenseNet have been refined in oncology to identify breast cancer in mammograms or identify lung cancer in CT scans. These models have demonstrated exceptional accuracy, frequently matching or outperforming human radiologists in detecting minute anomalies. CNNs already trained on ImageNet have also been modified for neurology tasks like MRI scan-based Alzheimer's disease identification. These models can forecast the early development of the disease and allow for prompt management by concentrating on characteristics such as cortical thinning and hippocampus atrophy. Significant benefits have also been seen in ophthalmology, where transfer learning is used to categorize retinal conditions from fundus pictures, such as glaucoma or diabetic retinopathy, improving early identification and treatment approaches. Transfer learning in medical imaging has drawbacks despite its benefits. The domain shift between the source dataset (such as ImageNet) and the target medical dataset is a significant drawback. Certain elements may be less transferable between natural and medical photos due to the significant differences in texture, scale, and context. To solve this, researchers frequently fine-tune the target dataset in great detail to ensure the model fits the new domain. However, this procedure can be computationally costly, especially with larger datasets and models.

Another difficulty is the requirement for domain-specific changes to pre-trained models' architecture. Medical imaging tasks frequently call for finer, more specialized features to properly categorize diseases or segment anatomical components, even though general-purpose models are excellent at learning broad features. For example, models built for object recognition must be modified for tasks like tumor delineation or vascular segmentation to carry out pixel-level segmentation.

Future developments in unsupervised and self-supervised learning are anticipated to expand transfer learning use in medical imaging significantly. These methods avoid the requirement for intensive manual annotation by enabling models to pre-train on big, unlabeled datasets. Because it allows models to learn from the intrinsic structure of the data—for example, by seeing patterns in unlabeled MRI scans or CT images self-supervised learning, in particular, shows promise for medical imaging. Furthermore, combining transfer learning with multi-modal imaging which combines data from many modalities, including CT, MRI, and PET could improve diagnostic precision and offer a more profound understanding of intricate medical disorders. In summary, transfer learning has emerged as a critical instrument in medical imaging, bridging the gap between the practical limitations of small annotated datasets and the enormous potential of CNNs. Researchers and medical professionals may diagnose and treat illnesses with surprising precision and speed by using pre-trained models and tailoring them to specific tasks. Transfer learning's influence on medical imaging is set to grow as methods like self-supervised learning and multi-modal integration advance, significantly altering the healthcare environment.

2.5 Ethical Considerations in the Use of CNNs for Medical Imaging

Unquestionably, introducing Convolutional Neural Networks (CNNs) into medical imaging has revolutionized healthcare by providing notable improvements in personalized medicine, treatment planning, and diagnostic precision. However, to guarantee that these technologies are applied responsibly and fairly, a number of ethical issues are raised by the use of CNNs in medical settings. These difficulties include algorithmic bias, data privacy, accountability, and balancing human control and AI autonomy.

- **Security and Privacy of Data**

As part of a patient's protected health information, medical imaging inevitably incorporates sensitive patient data, such as CT scans, MRI pictures, and X-rays. One of the most important ethical issues when using CNNs is protecting the security and privacy of this data. Medical data breaches may result in identity theft, unauthorized access, or improper use of medical records, which could have serious repercussions for patients. Strong data protection measures are necessary to combat this. Trust in AI-powered systems depends on adherence to laws like the General Data Protection Regulation (GDPR) in Europe and the US Health Insurance Portability and Accountability Act (HIPAA). Encryption, data anonymization, and secure data-sharing protocols are essential for protecting patient data. Furthermore, federated learning, which trains CNNs on decentralized data without sharing sensitive information, is a promising method for improving privacy and facilitating the creation of more efficient models.

- **Algorithmic Fairness and Bias**

In medical imaging, where diagnostic choices can have life-altering repercussions, bias in CNNs is a serious ethical concern. When CNNs are trained on data that is not representative of the heterogeneous patient population, biases may exist in the produced models. When used on patients from different demographics, for example, a CNN trained primarily on imaging data from a particular ethnic or demographic group may perform poorly. Disparities in healthcare outcomes and diagnostic accuracy may result from this. During model training, carefully considering dataset composition is necessary to address algorithmic bias. Building fair and equitable CNN models requires diverse, inclusive datasets representing the entire patient population range. The development process should also incorporate fairness measures and bias detection tools to find and eliminate biases prior to deployment. Models must also be continuously monitored and validated in clinical settings to guarantee consistent performance across various patient groups.

- **Responsibility and Liability**

Critical concerns regarding responsibility and liability are brought up by using CNNs in medical imaging, especially when the AI system makes a mistaken diagnosis or recommendation. Because CNNs are incapable of reasoning or justifying, it is difficult to assign blame for mistakes, in contrast to human therapists. Who is responsible if a CNN misidentifies a tumor or overlooks a severe abnormality—the algorithm's creators, the medical facility, or the physician using the system? Explicit criteria for using CNNs in medical decision-making must be established to allay these worries. AI systems ought to be seen as supplementary resources that enhance human knowledge rather than taking its place. Clinicians must still make the final decisions about diagnosis and treatment, with AI as a tool to help them do so. Before being used in clinical settings, CNN-based systems must also pass stringent validation and certification procedures to guarantee that they fulfill strict accuracy and dependability requirements.

- **Explainability and Transparency**

The "black-box" nature of CNNs raises yet another crucial ethical concern. Although these models excel at seeing trends and forecasting outcomes, their decision-making procedures could be more precise, making it easier for physicians to comprehend how particular results are produced. In therapeutic settings where responsibility and justification are crucial, this lack of transparency can cause problems and erode confidence in AI systems. Explainable AI (XAI) approaches for CNNs are being developed to solve the transparency problem. Techniques like attention mechanisms, Grad-CAM (Gradient-weighted Class Activation Mapping), and saliency maps offer visualizations that draw attention to the areas of an image that significantly influence the model's decision-making. These methods help doctors better comprehend and accept the AI's recommendations by providing interpretable outputs, which promotes improved decision-making.

- **Data Use in AI Development That Is Ethical**

Concerns about consent and ownership are just as significant as privacy regarding the ethical use of medical data in AI development. Patients frequently donate their data for particular medical uses, but ethical concerns surface when these datasets are used to train CNN models. Did patients receive enough information about how their data might be used? Does their data usage in AI research and development fall within their control? Transparency and informed consent are essential for ensuring ethical data use. Patients should have the option to opt out if they so desire and be fully informed about how their data will be utilized. Institutions should also consider ways to promote trust and cooperation by sharing the advantages of AI developments with the patients and communities that provide data.

- **AI Autonomy and Human Oversight in Balance**

As CNN-based systems become more autonomous, the balance between AI decision-making and human control is an issue. Although CNNs are incredibly fast and accurate in analyzing large volumes of imaging data, close supervision is necessary due to their incapacity to apply clinical judgment and lack of contextual knowledge. Without sufficient human intervention, reliance on AI systems might breed overconfidence in technology and raise the possibility of mistakes. A "human-in-the-loop" paradigm, in which medical professionals actively evaluate and validate AI-generated outcomes, is a moral way to include CNNs in medical imaging. This method guarantees that AI technologies improve patient care rather than degrade it by fusing the advantages of CNNs with human practitioners' experience and contextual awareness.

- **Frameworks for Ethics and Regulations**

Robust legal and moral frameworks are necessary to ethically and successfully use CNNs in medical imaging. These frameworks should cover essential topics like accountability, model validation, and data governance to guarantee that AI systems are as safe and effective as possible. Cooperation between legislators, medical organizations, and AI researchers is essential to creating uniform standards that encourage ethical AI deployment internationally.

3. RESEARCH OBJECTIVE

This chapter's primary goal is to examine how Convolutional Neural Networks (CNNs) are revolutionizing medical imaging, emphasizing how they improve patient outcomes, treatment planning, and diagnostic accuracy. The chapter's investigation of CNN integration in a range of medical imaging tasks, including segmentation, disease detection, and multi-modal data analysis, attempts to:

- Give a thorough explanation of CNN architectures designed for medical imaging tasks, covering their development, features, and applicability to specific medical applications.
- Stress the usefulness of CNNs in diagnosing ailments like cancer, neurological disorders, cardiovascular diseases, and retinal diseases, highlighting how they affect early identification and individualized treatment plans.
- Examine CNNs' function in segmentation, paying particular attention to how well they can distinguish anatomical features like tumors, organs, and vessels—all essential for making wise therapeutic decisions.
- Examine how CNNs are integrated with multi-modal medical imaging to demonstrate how integrating information from several imaging modalities (such as CT, MRI, and PET) improves diagnostic accuracy and offers a more profound understanding of intricate medical diseases.
- Discuss the practical and ethical issues surrounding using CNNs in clinical settings, such as interpretability, algorithmic bias, data privacy, and regulatory compliance, and offer strategies to overcome these obstacles.
- To offer a path for utilizing these technologies to transform healthcare, talk about the possible advancements and future directions in CNN-powered medical imaging, including federated learning, explainable AI, and real-time diagnostics.

In the end, the chapter aims to close the gap between CNN technology breakthroughs and their practical use in healthcare by fairly assessing their advantages, drawbacks, and moral implications. This goal aligns with the overarching mission of encouraging a more effective, fair, and patient-centered medical diagnosis and care method.

3.1 Research Methodology

This chapter's methodology takes an interdisciplinary approach to investigate how Convolutional Neural Networks (CNNs) are revolutionizing medical imaging. The chapter offers a thorough framework for comprehending CNN applications in medical diagnostics and treatment by integrating a systematic review of the literature, a comparative assessment of CNN architectures, an examination of real-world case studies, and an investigation of ethical and technical issues.

- **Methodical Literature Review**

This chapter synthesizes developments and difficulties in using CNNs for medical imaging by comprehensively evaluating previous research. Finding, assessing, and synthesizing research from reliable sources such as peer-reviewed journals, conference proceedings, and clinical reports are all part of the review process. We conducted a thorough search of scholarly databases like PubMed, IEEE Xplore, and SpringerLink using specific keywords like “deep learning for disease detection,” “CNN in medical imaging,” and “segmentation with CNNs.” The comprehensive study highlights the transformational promise and limitations of CNN technologies in healthcare by examining the state-of-the-art architectures and their applications in various medical contexts, from picture segmentation to illness diagnosis. The groundbreaking work of (Ronneberger, Fischer, & Brox, 2015) on U-Net, which transformed biomedical picture segmentation, and the thorough review of (Aamir et al., 2023), which described the wide range of uses of deep learning in medical imaging, are essential sources influencing this understanding. This pioneering research offers a framework for investigating later developments and uses.

- **CNN Architectures a Comparative Study**

An investigation of popular architectures was done to determine how successful CNNs are in medical imaging. The suitability of various architectures, including AlexNet, VGGNet, ResNet, DenseNet, and U-Net, for tasks including object detection, segmentation, and picture classification was assessed. Metrics, including computing complexity, accuracy, and efficiency, guided the comparison analysis.

For example, ResNet has become a mainstay for challenging classification tasks in medical imaging due to its capacity to minimize the vanishing gradient problem through residual connections (Gao et al., 2019). DenseNet is perfect for jobs requiring high-resolution analysis, including tumor segmentation in mammograms, because its densely connected layers further improve feature reuse and model efficiency (Alshehri, 2023). Meanwhile, U-Net remains the industry standard for medical picture segmentation because of its encoder-decoder design and skip links, which allow for exact localization (Yin et al., 2022).

This investigation demonstrates how CNN architectures have been modified to address the particular difficulties associated with medical imaging, including limited annotated datasets and high-dimensional data. Studies conducted by (Gupta et al., 2021) further support the usefulness of these structures in particular applications, such as the identification of Alzheimer's disease and the screening for diabetic retinopathy.

- **Investigation of Actual Case Studies**

The chapter looks at real-world case studies where CNNs have significantly influenced closing the gap between theoretical developments and clinical practice. These case studies offer valuable perspectives on how CNNs improve patient outcomes, expedite workflows, and increase diagnostic accuracy. Verma & Mishra (2024) showed how CNNs can use thermoscopic images to classify skin lesions as benign or malignant with dermatologist-level accuracy. This study demonstrated how CNNs can provide access to diagnostic tools and support clinical competence in areas with limited resources CNNs have been utilized in neurology to discover patterns of hippocampus atrophy linked to early-stage disease progression to detect Alzheimer's disease through MRI images. These models have demonstrated potential for enhancing patient care techniques and facilitating early intervention. Gulshan et al. (2020) showed how CNNs can identify diabetic retinopathy in ophthalmology by analyzing retinal fundus pictures. This allows for extensive screening programs that help avoid vision loss. These case studies highlight CNNs' adaptability to various medical specialties and demonstrate how they might revolutionize conventional diagnostic procedures.

- **Practical and Ethical Aspects to Consider**

This chapter also covers the ethical and practical aspects of using CNNs in medical imaging. Because medical imaging data is sensitive, data security and privacy are critical. Methods to improve privacy while fostering creativity are investigated, including federated learning and data anonymization, which enable models to be trained on decentralized data without sending sensitive information. Another serious issue is algorithmic prejudice. Disparities in healthcare delivery could result from CNNs performing differently if they were trained on datasets not representative of various populations (Norori et al., 2021). Fairness criteria to assess model performance across various demographic groups are necessary to tackle this issue, together with diverse and inclusive datasets. Clinical adoption requires interpretability and transparency. The chapter covers techniques that make CNN decisions more interpretable and help doctors comprehend the logic behind AI-driven recommendations, such as saliency maps and Grad-CAM.

3.2 Applications of CNNs in Medical Imaging

Medical imaging has revolutionized thanks to Convolutional Neural Networks (CNNs), which offer instruments that improve diagnostic precision, expedite processes, and permit individualized patient care. Their extensive use in various medical fields can be attributed to their capacity to process intricate visual data, spot trends, and generate predictions. The main uses of CNNs in medical imaging are examined below, demonstrating their revolutionary influence on healthcare.

1. Identification and Categorization of Diseases

Disease identification and categorization are among the most well-known uses of CNNs in medical imaging. CNNs frequently match or even exceed human proficiency in detecting anomalies in medical images and categorizing them into diagnostic groups.

- **Finding Cancer:** In oncology, CNNs are frequently used to identify malignancies in imaging modalities such as MRIs, CT scans, and mammograms. For instance, CNNs can spot microcalcifications or lumps in mammograms to diagnose early-stage breast cancer, allowing for prompt treatment. CNNs examine CT pictures to find pulmonary nodules in lung cancer that human radiologists would overlook. CNNs can classify skin cancer from dermoscopic images with dermatologist-level accuracy. This reduces physicians' workload and speeds up diagnostics.
- **Identification of Neurological Diseases:** In neurology, CNNs are used to identify and track conditions like multiple sclerosis, Alzheimer's disease, and brain tumours. CNNs can detect cortical thinning or hippocampus atrophy linked to early Alzheimer's disease by evaluating MRI data, which makes early diagnosis and treatment easier.
- **Evaluation of Cardiovascular Disease:** CNNs are used in cardiology to evaluate MRIs, CT scans, and echocardiograms to identify anomalies in heart valves, arrhythmias, and coronary artery disease. Cardiologists can prioritize high-risk patients with these algorithms' automated insights.
- **Applications in Ophthalmology:** CNNs have demonstrated efficacy in identifying eye conditions such as age-related macular degeneration, glaucoma, and diabetic retinopathy from retinal fundus pictures. CNN-powered systems, for example, can screen huge populations for diabetic retinopathy, lowering the prevalence of avoidable blindness.

2. Segmenting Images for Accurate Localization

One crucial use of CNNs in medical imaging is segmentation, the act of dividing an image into distinct parts. Segmentation makes it possible to pinpoint the exact location of diseased characteristics and anatomical structures, which is crucial for monitoring, diagnosis, and therapy planning.

- **Segmenting tumors:** In imaging modalities like MRI and CT, CNNs like U-Net and Mask R-CNN are often employed to define tumor boundaries. Precise tumor segmentation aids in radiation therapy, surgical planning, and treatment response monitoring.
- **Segmenting Organs:** Segmenting the liver, heart, and lungs can help assess organ size, detect abnormalities, and plan surgical or interventional procedures. For instance, liver segmentation in CT images is essential for tumor or lesion detection and tracking.
- **Segmenting Vessels:** CNN-based retinal vascular segmentation aids in the diagnosis of conditions like glaucoma and diabetic retinopathy. Vessel segmentation in cardiovascular imaging helps identify coronary artery blockages or stenoses, directing procedures like stent implantation.

3. Analysis of Multi-modal Images

Integrating data from several imaging modalities, including CT, MRI, PET, and ultrasound, is known as multi-modal imaging. CNNs are good at integrating these modalities to give a complete picture of a patient's health.

- **Cancer:** To enhance tumor detection and staging, CNNs can combine PET, which measures metabolic activity, with CT or MRI, which offers anatomical detail. This combination improves the precision of diagnosis and guides treatment plans.
- **The study of neurology:** Analysis using many modalities Combining structural MRI with functional imaging modalities such as PET or fMRI can help us gain a deeper understanding of brain abnormalities. CNN, for example, can examine the metabolic activity and structural alterations linked to brain malignancies or Alzheimer's disease.
- **Heart health:** CNNs in cardiac imaging can combine information from MRI and CT angiography to evaluate structural and functional heart problems, offering thorough diagnostic insights.

4. Prognosis and Predictive Analytics

In order to help clinicians, make data-driven decisions, CNNs are essential for forecasting disease outcomes and therapy responses.

- **The prognosis for Cancer:** CNNs trained on imaging data can forecast patient survival rates, metastasis probability, and tumor aggressiveness. These insights can inform patients about their prognosis and tailor treatments.
- **Cardiac Risk Evaluation:** CNNs use clinical and imaging data to forecast the likelihood of cardiac events like arrhythmias or heart attacks. These forecasts aid in setting priorities for high-risk patients' preventive care.
- **Results for the nervous system:** CNNs can help with rehabilitation planning in stroke care by predicting the degree of brain injury and the likelihood of recovery based on CT or MRI images.

5 Real-Time Decision-Making

By giving doctors prompt feedback and direction, real-time CNN applications revolutionize critical care and surgical operations.

- **Robotic Surgery:** CNNs, built into robotic surgical systems, analyze real-time video feeds to help surgeons navigate intricate anatomical structures. CNN, for instance, might draw attention to important regions, such as tumors or blood arteries, lowering the possibility of consequences.
- **Diagnostics for emergencies:** CNNs evaluate imaging data in real-time in emergency rooms to identify potentially fatal illnesses like internal injuries, brain hemorrhages, and strokes. These technologies guarantee prompt intervention by offering quick diagnostic support.
- **Telehealth:** CNN-powered telemedicine platforms make remote analysis of imaging data possible, making high-quality diagnoses available in environments with limited resources.

3.3 Challenges and Solutions in Applying CNNs to Medical Imaging

1 Scarcity of Data and Annotation: Access to sizable, high-quality annotated medical datasets is restricted due to privacy issues and the expense of expert labelling.

- To increase datasets, use data augmentation.
- Use Generative Adversarial Networks (GANs) to create artificial medical images.

- Use federated learning to enable cooperative training across institutions without exchanging raw data.

2 Unbalanced Class: Biased models result from datasets that must be more balanced between typical and atypical cases.

- Use either an under sampled majority class or an oversampled minority class.
- To deal with imbalances, use weighted loss functions such as focused loss.
- Create more instances of minority classes by employing artificial methods.

3 Interpretability: Because CNNs function as "black boxes," practitioners find it challenging to have faith in their judgment.

- Use explainable AI technologies like Grad-CAM and saliency maps to draw attention to key areas in the image.
- Create interpretable structures that support their predictions with textual or visual explanations.
- Generalization and Algorithmic Bias:

4 CNNs may perform poorly on diverse populations or unexplored datasets due to biases based on the composition of the training data.

- The solution is to use a variety of representative datasets to train models.
- Models can be adjusted for new populations by using domain adaptation approaches.
- To find and lessen biases during training, use fairness measures.

5 Including Clinical Workflows in Integration: Ensuring clinicians adopt and integrate CNN-based systems into current healthcare operations can be challenging.

- The solution is to provide user-friendly CNN system interfaces.
- Clinicians should receive instruction and training to comprehend and believe AI advice.
- Make sure AI tools enhance clinical knowledge rather than take its place.

6 Ethical and Regulatory Consideration: Addressing moral issues around data privacy and accountability while ensuring laws like HIPAA are followed.

- Make use of anonymous and secure data management procedures.
- Before deploying CNN models in clinical settings, thorough testing and validation must be conducted.
- Provide precise accountability structures for healthcare AI decision-making.

3.4 Result and Discussion

Results

Investigating Convolutional Neural Networks (CNNs) in medical imaging shows how revolutionary they may be in improving diagnostic precision, automating complex processes, and enabling individualized therapy. CNNs have demonstrated outstanding performance in tackling critical issues in medical diagnostics, ranging from illness detection to real-time clinical decision support. The main conclusions drawn from the analysis of CNN applications in medical imaging are listed below:

- **Enhanced Precision in Diagnosis:**

When it comes to identifying diseases like cancer, neurological disorders, and cardiovascular ailments, CNNs routinely outperform conventional image-processing approaches and frequently equal or even exceed human knowledge. For example, research shows that CNNs have a higher sensitivity and specificity than conventional techniques in detecting lung cancer in CT images and breast cancer in mammograms.

- **Effectiveness in Segmenting Images:**

Cutting-edge CNN designs like U-Net and Mask R-CNN have shown remarkable aptitude in segmenting anatomical features, including organs, arteries, and tumours. These models' increased accuracy in activities like tumor delineation makes better surgical results and treatment planning possible.

- **Combining Multi-Modal Imaging:**

CNNs combine information from several imaging modalities (CT et al.) to improve diagnostic insights. Multi-modal techniques have demonstrated notable gains in complicated diagnostic tasks like neurological illness assessment and cancer staging. Despite their efficacy, CNNs have drawbacks, such as limited data, algorithmic bias, and problems with interpretability. Although approaches like federated learning, explainable AI, and data augmentation show promise, further study and advancement are needed to overcome these constraints fully CNN-powered real-time clinical decision support systems are advancing surgical aid and emergency treatment, leading to better results in time-sensitive situations. CNNs are also advancing personalized medicine by using imaging and other data to customize therapies and diagnoses for specific patients.

Discussion

The results highlight CNNs' revolutionary influence on medical imaging and point to important areas for development. Below, we examine the consequences of these findings, along with their advantages, disadvantages, and prospects for the future.

- **CNNs' advantages in medical imaging**

CNNs' capacity to automatically learn and extract features from intricate medical images substantially improves over conventional techniques, which frequently depend on manually annotated images and hand-crafted features. CNNs have made significant strides in diagnostic efficiency and accuracy by utilizing sophisticated architectures and big datasets. U-Net has emerged as the industry standard for segmentation jobs, supporting activities like organ delineation and tumor localization. Because of these characteristics, imaging has a more significant role in precision medicine, enabling doctors to make better decisions.

- **Implementation Difficulties**

Despite their many advantages, CNNs can require more work to integrate into clinical workflows. Lack of data is still a significant obstacle, especially for rare diseases with few annotated datasets. Federated learning and data-sharing frameworks can help reduce this problem by facilitating cooperative model training across institutions without jeopardizing patient privacy. However, established protocols and a robust infrastructure are necessary to adopt these strategies broadly. Another important concern is algorithmic bias since CNNs frequently exhibit the biases found in their training data. This may result in disparities in diagnostic performance between various demographic groups. To solve this issue, efforts must be made to create representative, diverse datasets and apply training methods that consider fairness.

Another urgent issue with CNNs is their interpretability. More effort is required to guarantee that CNNs are transparent and reliable, particularly in high-stakes situations like cancer diagnosis or stroke detection, even though techniques like Grad-CAM and saliency maps provide some insights into model decision-making. CNNs in medical imaging have a bright future by tackling these issues and seizing new opportunities. The development of explainable AI will be essential for building clinician trust and making incorporating CNNs into clinical procedures easier. Furthermore, real-time diagnostics in resource-constrained environments will be made possible by developing lightweight CNN architectures and edge computing solutions, increasing access to high-quality healthcare.

Another intriguing approach is to integrate CNNs with other AI methods like reinforcement learning and natural language processing. For example, CNNs' prediction ability can be improved by integrating imaging data with genomic and electronic health record data, allowing for more individualized and comprehensive patient care. Lastly, the creation and application of CNN-based medical imaging systems must continue to be centred on ethical issues. Building systems that function effectively and support the principles of responsible and equitable healthcare will need to ensure patient privacy, responsibility, and fairness.

CONCLUSION

The diagnosis, tracking, and treatment of diseases have all changed dramatically due to the incorporation of Convolutional Neural Networks (CNNs) into medical imaging. CNNs have shown great promise in improving diagnostic precision, automating complex operations like segmentation, and facilitating real-time clinical decision-making by utilizing their extraordinary accuracy in analyzing complex imaging data. These developments signal a dramatic change in the healthcare industry, as AI-powered solutions are increasingly essential for enhancing patient outcomes and expediting processes. The results presented in this chapter demonstrate the revolutionary influence of CNNs in several fields, such as neurology, cardiology, ophthalmology, and oncology. CNNs have continuously outperformed conventional techniques in various fields, including early cancer detection, neurological problems, cardiovascular conditions, and more. With solutions ranging from tumor segmentation to multi-modal data integration, architectures like U-Net, ResNet, and DenseNet have proven essential to medical imaging jobs. In addition to increasing efficiency, these technologies make high-quality diagnostics more accessible, especially in impoverished areas.

CNN use in medical imaging has its challenges, however. These models' "black-box" nature, algorithmic bias, and lack of data pose severe obstacles to their wider use. Initiatives to overcome these constraints, such as explainable AI, federated learning, and data augmentation, are making more transparent and fair AI systems possible. Fostering confidence and acceptance among physicians and patients alike requires that CNNs be created and implemented responsibly, emphasizing patient privacy and fairness. In the future, customized medicine could greatly benefit from combining CNNs with other cutting-edge AI methods and data sources, including genomic data and electronic medical records. CNN-powered systems will become more widely available in resource-constrained environments as real-time applications and lightweight architectures proliferate, democratizing access to state-of-the-art diagnostics. Furthermore, ethical issues and legal frameworks must continue to play a crucial role in technological advancement to guarantee that the advantages of new technologies are shared equitably and responsibly.

To sum up, CNNs are a paradigm shift in medical imaging that is changing conventional methods and paving the way for the seamless integration of AI-driven technologies into healthcare in the future. CNNs have the potential to revolutionize medical diagnostics by tackling present issues and expanding on current developments, allowing for more accurate, effective, and individualized treatment for patients everywhere.

FUTURE WORK

Convolutional neural networks (CNNs) have a bright future in medical imaging thanks to continuous developments in artificial intelligence, computer technology, and medical research. Even though CNNs have already significantly increased diagnostic efficiency and accuracy, several unresolved issues and problems remain that can be resolved in future studies to increase their influence in healthcare Creating more reliable and broadly applicable CNN models is crucial for further research. Because imaging equipment, techniques, and patient demographics vary, current CNNs frequently need help performing consistently across datasets or populations. The main goal of future research should be the development of models that can successfully generalize across many clinical contexts. Strategies like domain adaptation, transfer learning, and the utilization of sizable, varied, multi-center datasets can be extremely important to increase model resilience and guarantee that CNNs operate dependably across a variety of applications.

Another exciting avenue is the integration of CNNs with data modalities other than imaging. More thorough and individualized diagnosis may be made possible by combining CNNs with information from genomics, laboratory testing, and electronic health records (EHRs). Indeed, customized medicine is possible if imaging data is combined with genetic profiles and patient histories to enable more accurate risk assessment and treatment planning. Future research will focus on creating multi-modal AI systems that can quickly process and easily understand data from multiple sources. Another important topic for further research is explainable AI (XAI). Because clinicians must comprehend and have faith in AI-generated conclusions, CNNs' black-box character remains a hurdle to their clinical use. Future research should focus on creating more interpretable CNN models, utilizing strategies like saliency maps, attention mechanisms, and post hoc explanation tools. In addition to increasing physician trust, improving interpretability will offer insights into illness mechanisms and decision-making procedures.

The future of CNNs in medical imaging will heavily rely on decentralized AI models and federated learning. These methods address data sharing and security concerns while facilitating cooperative model training across institutions and protecting patient privacy. To ensure that privacy-preserving AI systems can be deployed globally, future research should concentrate on refining federated learning algorithms to handle massive, high-dimensional medical imaging data effectively. Another exciting avenue is the creation of lightweight CNN systems, particularly for real-time applications and deployment in environments with constrained resources. These models should maximize their efficiency without sacrificing accuracy for use in portable diagnostic instruments, edge computing systems, and mobile devices. These developments have the potential to democratize access to AI-powered healthcare by providing high-quality diagnostics to underserved and rural areas. Future research should also cover the moral and legal issues surrounding the use of CNNs in clinical settings. This entails developing uniform assessment procedures for AI systems, guaranteeing justice and fairness in model performance, and putting in place explicit accountability structures. To overcome these obstacles and create standards for the ethical application of AI in healthcare, cooperation between ethicists, researchers, physicians, and legislators will be crucial.

Lastly, a significant area for further research is the incorporation of CNNs into real-time clinical operations. Real-time CNN applications can significantly improve clinical decision-making, from supporting surgeons during procedures to offering immediate diagnostic input in emergencies. Realizing this promise will require improvements in hardware acceleration, such as the usage of GPUs and TPUs, as well as the development of algorithms for low-latency performance. In conclusion, CNNs in medical imaging can potentially revolutionize healthcare in the future. Future research can fully realize CNNs' potential and enable more precise, effective, and egalitarian medical diagnostics and therapies by tackling issues with generalization, interpretability, data integration, and ethical considerations. The development of the upcoming generation of CNN-powered healthcare solutions will depend heavily on the continued cooperation of AI researchers, healthcare experts, and legislators.

REFERENCES

Aamir, M., Bazai, S., Bhatti, U. A., Dayo, Z. A., Liu, J., & Zhang, K. (2023, January). Applications of machine learning in medicine: Current trends and prospects. In *2023 Global Conference on Wireless and Optical Technologies (GCWOT)* (pp. 1–4). IEEE. DOI: 10.1109/GCWOT57803.2023.10064665

Aamir, M., Rahman, Z., Abro, W. A., Bhatti, U. A., Dayo, Z. A., & Ishfaq, M. (2023). Brain tumor classification utilizing deep features derived from high-quality regions in MRI images. *Biomedical Signal Processing and Control*, *85*, 104988. DOI: 10.1016/j.bspc.2023.104988

Aamir, M., Rahman, Z., Abro, W. A., Tahir, M., & Ahmed, S. M. (2019). An optimized architecture of image classification using convolutional neural network. *International Journal of Image. Graphics and Signal Processing*, *11*(10), 30–39. DOI: 10.5815/ijigsp.2019.10.05

Aamir, M., Rahman, Z., Dayo, Z. A., Abro, W. A., Uddin, M. I., Khan, I., Imran, A. S., Ali, Z., Ishfaq, M., Guan, Y., & Hu, Z. (2022). A deep learning approach for brain tumor classification using MRI images. *Computers & Electrical Engineering*, *101*, 108105. DOI: 10.1016/j.compeleceng.2022.108105

Al-Yasriy, H. F.. (2020). Diagnosis of lung cancer based on CT scans using CNN. In *IOP Conference Series: Materials Science and Engineering*. IOP Publishing. DOI: 10.1088/1757-899X/928/2/022035

Almotairi, S., Kareem, G., Aouf, M., Almutairi, B., & Salem, M. A.-M. (2020). Liver tumor segmentation in CT scans using modified SegNet. *Sensors (Basel)*, *20*(5), 1516. DOI: 10.3390/s20051516 PMID: 32164153

Alshehri, M. (2023). Breast cancer detection and classification using hybrid feature selection and DenseXtNet approach. *Mathematics*, *11*(23), 4725. DOI: 10.3390/math11234725

Altaf, F., & Shah, S. M.. (2019). Going deep in medical image analysis: Concepts, methods, challenges, and future directions. *IEEE Access : Practical Innovations, Open Solutions*, *7*, 99540–99572. DOI: 10.1109/ACCESS.2019.2929365

Alzubaidi, L., & Fadhel, M. A.. (2021). Review of deep learning: Concepts, CNN architectures, challenges, applications, future directions. *Journal of Big Data*, *8*(1), 1–74. DOI: 10.1186/s40537-021-00444-8 PMID: 33816053

Atmakuru, A., Chakraborty, S., Faust, O., Salvi, M., Datta Barua, P., Molinari, F., Acharya, U. R., & Homaira, N. (2024). Deep learning in radiology for lung cancer diagnostics: A systematic review of classification, segmentation, and predictive modeling techniques. *Expert Systems with Applications*, *255*, 124665. DOI: 10.1016/j.eswa.2024.124665

Burnet, N. G.. (2004). Defining the tumour and target volumes for radiotherapy. *Cancer Imaging; the Official Publication of the International Cancer Imaging Society*, *4*(2), 153–161. DOI: 10.1102/1470-7330.2004.0054 PMID: 18250025

Di, S., Zhang, Z., & Zhang, Z.. (2022). TD-Net: A hybrid end-to-end network for automatic liver tumor segmentation from CT images. *IEEE Journal of Biomedical and Health Informatics*, *27*(3), 1163–1172. DOI: 10.1109/JBHI.2022.3181974 PMID: 35696476

Du, P., & Liu, L.. (2020). Advances of four machine learning methods for spatial data handling: A review. *Journal of Geovisualization and Spatial Analysis*, *4*(1), 1–25. DOI: 10.1007/s41651-020-00048-5

Esteva, A., Kuprel, B., Novoa, R. A., Ko, J., Swetter, S. M., Blau, H. M., & Thrun, S. (2017). Dermatologist-level classification of skin cancer with deep neural networks. *Nature*, *542*(7639), 115–118. DOI: 10.1038/nature21056 PMID: 28117445

Gao, F., & Zhao, X.. (2019). Deep residual inception encoder–decoder network for medical imaging synthesis. *IEEE Journal of Biomedical and Health Informatics*, *24*(1), 39–49. DOI: 10.1109/JBHI.2019.2912659 PMID: 31021777

Gautam, R., & Sharma, M. (2020). Prevalence and diagnosis of neurological disorders using different deep learning techniques: A meta-analysis. *Journal of Medical Systems*, *44*(2), 49. DOI: 10.1007/s10916-019-1519-7 PMID: 31902041

Guan, Y., Aamir, M., Rahman, Z., Ali, A., Abro, W. A., Dayo, Z. A., Bhutta, M. S., & Hu, Z. A framework for efficient brain tumor classification using MRI images.

Gul, S., & Khan, M. S. (2023). A survey of audio enhancement algorithms for music, speech, bioacoustics, biomedical, industrial and environmental sounds by image U-Net. *IEEE Access : Practical Innovations, Open Solutions*, *11*, 144456–144483. DOI: 10.1109/ACCESS.2023.3344813

Gupta, V. B., & Kumar, R.. (2021). Retinal changes in Alzheimer's disease—Integrated prospects of imaging, functional and molecular advances. *Progress in Retinal and Eye Research*, *82*, 100899. DOI: 10.1016/j.preteyeres.2020.100899 PMID: 32890742

Guthoff, R. F.. (1991). Doppler ultrasonography of the ophthalmic and central retinal vessels. *Archives of Ophthalmology*, *109*(4), 532–536. DOI: 10.1001/archopht.1991.01080040100037 PMID: 2012556

Jayasundar, S., & Kumar, N. Augmented Reality and Deep Learning Integration for Enhanced Design and Maintenance in Mechanical Engineering.

Kriegeskorte, N. (2015). Deep neural networks: A new framework for modeling biological vision and brain information processing. *Annual Review of Vision Science*, *1*(1), 417–446. DOI: 10.1146/annurev-vision-082114-035447 PMID: 28532370

LeCun, Y., Bengio, Y., & Hinton, G. (1998). Gradient-based learning applied to document recognition. *Proceedings of the IEEE*, *86*(11), 2278–2324. DOI: 10.1109/5.726791

LeCun, Y., Bengio, Y., & Hinton, G. (2015). Deep learning. *Nature*, *521*(7553), 436–444. DOI: 10.1038/nature14539 PMID: 26017442

Liang, P. P., Zadeh, A., & Morency, L.-P. (2024). Foundations & trends in multimodal machine learning: Principles, challenges, and open questions. *ACM Computing Surveys*, *56*(10), 1–42. DOI: 10.1145/3663364

Moses, D. A., & Beasley, C.. (2021). Deep learning applied to automatic disease detection using chest x-rays. *Journal of Medical Imaging and Radiation Oncology*, *65*(5), 498–517. DOI: 10.1111/1754-9485.13273 PMID: 34231311

Mridha, M. F., & Biswas, S. R.. (2021). A comprehensive survey on deep-learning-based breast cancer diagnosis. *Cancers (Basel), 13*(23), 6116. DOI: 10.3390/cancers13236116 PMID: 34885225

Norori, N., Hu, Q., Aellen, F. M., Faraci, F. D., & Tzovara, A. (2021). Addressing bias in big data and AI for healthcare: A call for open science. *Patterns (New York, N.Y.), 2*(10), 100347. DOI: 10.1016/j.patter.2021.100347 PMID: 34693373

Oyelade, O. N., Ezugwu, A. E., Venter, H. S., Mirjalili, S., & Gandomi, A. H. (2022). Abnormality classification and localization using dual-branch whole-region-based CNN model with histopathological images. *Computers in Biology and Medicine, 149*, 105943. DOI: 10.1016/j.compbiomed.2022.105943 PMID: 35986967

Pei, X., & Liu, W.. (2023). A review of the application of multi-modal deep learning in medicine: Bibliometrics and future directions. *International Journal of Computational Intelligence Systems, 16*(1), 44. DOI: 10.1007/s44196-023-00225-6

Rajpurkar, P., Irvin, J., Ball, R. L., Zhu, K., Yang, B., Mehta, H., Duan, T., Ding, D., Bagul, A., Langlotz, C. P., Patel, B. N., Yeom, K. W., Shpanskaya, K., Blankenberg, F. G., Seekins, J., Amrhein, T. J., Mong, D. A., Halabi, S. S., Zucker, E. J., & Lungren, M. P. (2018). Deep learning for chest radiograph diagnosis: A retrospective comparison of the CheXNeXt algorithm to practicing radiologists. *PLoS Medicine, 15*(11), e1002686. DOI: 10.1371/journal.pmed.1002686 PMID: 30457988

Razzak, M. I., Naz, S., & Zaib, A. (2018). Deep learning for medical image processing: Overview, challenges, and the future. In *Classification in BioApps: Automation of Decision Making* (pp. 323–350).

Ronneberger, O., Fischer, P., & Brox, T. (2015). U-net: Convolutional networks for biomedical image segmentation. In *Medical Image Computing and Computer-Assisted Intervention–MICCAI 2015:18th International Conference,Munich, Germany,October 5-9, 2015, Proceedings, Part III* (pp. 234–241). Springer.

Salahuddin, Z., Woodruff, H. C., Chatterjee, A., & Lambin, P. (2022). Transparency of deep neural networks for medical image analysis: A review of interpretability methods. *Computers in Biology and Medicine, 140*, 105111. DOI: 10.1016/j.compbiomed.2021.105111 PMID: 34891095

Samuel, F. The Role of Convolutional Neural Networks in Analyzing CT Scans for Hemorrhages.

Shin, H.-C., Hwang, E.-J., & Zhao, L.. (2016). Deep convolutional neural networks for computer-aided detection: CNN architectures, dataset characteristics, and transfer learning. *IEEE Transactions on Medical Imaging, 35*(5), 1285–1298. DOI: 10.1109/TMI.2016.2528162 PMID: 26886976

Sibille, L., Seifert, R., Avramovic, N., Vehren, T., Spottiswoode, B., Zuehlsdorff, S., & Schäfers, M. (2020). 18F-FDG PET/CT uptake classification in lymphoma and lung cancer by using deep convolutional neural networks. *Radiology, 294*(2), 445–452. DOI: 10.1148/radiol.2019191114 PMID: 31821122

Teune, L. K., Bartels, A. L., de Jong, B. M., Willemsen, A. T. M., Eshuis, S. A., de Vries, J. J., van Oostrom, J. C. H., & Leenders, K. L. (2010). Typical cerebral metabolic patterns in neurodegenerative brain diseases. *Movement Disorders, 25*(14), 2395–2404. DOI: 10.1002/mds.23291 PMID: 20669302

Tufail, A. B., & Ali, M.. (2021). Deep learning in cancer diagnosis and prognosis prediction: A minireview on challenges, recent trends, and future directions. *Computational and Mathematical Methods in Medicine, 2021*, 9025470. DOI: 10.1155/2021/9025470 PMID: 34754327

Verma, N., & Mishra, P. K. (2024). A statistical review of skin disease detection models for different skin-tones. *Frontiers in Health Informatics*, •••, 6987–7005.

Wang, Z., Zheng, Y., & Hu, Z.. (2022). Artificial intelligence and deep learning in ophthalmology. In *Artificial Intelligence in Medicine* (pp. 1519–1552). Springer. DOI: 10.1007/978-3-030-64573-1_200

Willemink, M. J., Koszek, W. A., Hardell, C., Wu, J., Fleischmann, D., Harvey, H., Folio, L. R., Summers, R. M., Rubin, D. L., & Lungren, M. P. (2020). Preparing medical imaging data for machine learning. *Radiology, 295*(1), 4–15. DOI: 10.1148/radiol.2020192224 PMID: 32068507

Winkler, J. K., & Evers, S.. (2023). Assessment of diagnostic performance of dermatologists cooperating with a convolutional neural network in a prospective clinical study: Human with machine. *JAMA Dermatology, 159*(6), 621–627. DOI: 10.1001/jamadermatol.2023.0905 PMID: 37133847

Xu, X., & Wang, Z.. (2024). A comprehensive review on synergy of multi-modal data and AI technologies in medical diagnosis. *Bioengineering (Basel, Switzerland), 11*(3), 219. DOI: 10.3390/bioengineering11030219 PMID: 38534493

Xu, Y., & Zhang, L.. (2024). Advances in medical image segmentation: A comprehensive review of traditional, deep learning, and hybrid approaches. *Bioengineering (Basel, Switzerland), 11*(10), 1034. DOI: 10.3390/bioengineering11101034 PMID: 39451409

Yao, Z., Wang, H., Yan, W., Wang, Z., Zhang, W., Wang, Z., & Zhang, G. (2023). Artificial intelligence-based diagnosis of Alzheimer's disease with brain MRI images. *European Journal of Radiology, 165*, 110934. DOI: 10.1016/j.ejrad.2023.110934 PMID: 37354773

Yin, X.-X., & Li, Y.. (2022). [Retracted] U-Net-Based Medical Image Segmentation. *Journal of Healthcare Engineering, 2022*(1), 4189781. PMID: 35463660

Chapter 9
Transforming Medical Imaging With Convolutional Neural Networks (CNNs): Advances in Diagnosis and Treatment

Punam Kumari
https://orcid.org/0000-0001-8144-7573
Amity University, Bengaluru, India

ABSTRACT

Convolutional Neural Network (CNN) is a deep learning model for image recognition tasks. They automatically extract features from images for tasks like classification, segmentation, and object detection to enhance image processing accuracy. This chapter explores the pivotal role of CNNs in transforming medical imaging, driving significant advancements in diagnosis and treatment planning. Along with that, the chapter also delves into key CNN architectures such as ResNet, and U-Net, examining their applications in medical fields like radiology, pathology, and ophthalmology. Additionally, it discusses the integration of CNNs in real-time imaging systems and the impact of deep learning in reducing human error in diagnosis. Ethical considerations, including privacy, data security, and the need for explainable AI in medical settings, are also addressed. By examining cutting-edge CNN applications, this chapter highlights how deep learning is revolutionizing the future of healthcare through more accurate, efficient, and personalized medical services.

1. INTRODUCTION TO CNNS AND MEDICAL IMAGING

1.1 Contextualizing CNNs in Deep Learning

Convolutional Neural Networks (CNNs) are a specialized type of deep learning model, particularly designed for processing grid-like data, such as images (Aamir et al., 2019). Originally inspired by the structure and function of the visual cortex in animals, CNNs have revolutionized image recognition and

DOI: 10.4018/979-8-3693-9816-6.ch009

other visual tasks, making them essential in fields like medical imaging (Salehi et a., 2023), autonomous driving (Muhammad et al., 2020), and facial recognition (Wang, M., & Deng, W. 2021).

CNN Architecture

The architecture of CNNs consists of multiple layers designed to automatically and hierarchically learn features from input images. The key components of a CNN are:

a. **Convolutional Layers**: A convolutional layer in CNN applies filters to input data, extracting features like edges, textures, and patterns for analysis.
b. **Pooling Layers**: A pooling layer in CNN reduces the spatial dimensions of feature maps, retaining important information while minimizing computational complexity and overfitting.
c. **Fully Connected Layers**: A fully connected layer in CNN connects all neurons, integrating extracted features to make final predictions in classification or regression tasks
d. **Activation Functions**: An activation function introduces non-linearity in a neural network, enabling it to learn complex patterns and relationships in the data.

1.2 Medical Imaging in Healthcare

Medical imaging is a vital tool in modern healthcare, enabling physicians to visualize the internal structures of the body, diagnose diseases, guide treatments, and monitor the progress of medical conditions (Aamir et al., 2023). Various medical imaging techniques use different physical principles to create images of the body's internal anatomy. Here's an overview of the most used types of medical imaging:

1.2.1 Magnetic Resonance Imaging (MRI)

Overview: MRI uses powerful magnetic fields and radio waves to generate detailed images of soft tissues, such as the brain, muscles, and internal organs. It does not use ionizing radiation, making it safer for long-term use.

How it works: MRI machines create strong magnetic fields that cause protons in the body's water molecules to align. Radio waves are then sent through the body, which disrupt this alignment. When the radio waves are turned off, the protons re-align, and this realignment is detected by the MRI machine to form detailed images (Talagala, S. L., & Lowe, I. J. 1991).

Applications: MRI is used to diagnose and monitor conditions affecting the brain (stroke, tumors, multiple sclerosis), spine, joints, soft tissues, and organs such as the liver and heart.

Advantages: Excellent for imaging soft tissues, high-resolution images, non-invasive.

Disadvantages: Expensive, takes longer than other imaging methods, not suitable for patients with certain metal implants.

1.2.2 Computed Tomography (CT) Scans

Overview: CT scans use a series of X-ray images taken from different angles to create cross-sectional images (slices) of bones, blood vessels, and soft tissues. It is more detailed than standard X-rays and can visualize both bone and soft tissues in the body.

How it works: A CT scanner emits a series of X-rays as it rotates around the body. These X-rays pass through the body, and the data is processed by a computer to create cross-sectional images, which can be combined to form a 3D image of the scanned area (Cantatore, A., & Müller, P., 2011).

Applications: CT scans are used for diagnosing bone fractures, tumors, internal bleeding, and for planning surgeries. They are widely used in emergency medicine, oncology, and cardiovascular imaging.

Advantages: Fast, detailed imaging of bones and soft tissues, useful in emergencies.

Disadvantages: Involves exposure to ionizing radiation, may not be ideal for children or pregnant women.

1.2.3 X-rays

Overview: X-rays are a common imaging technique that uses ionizing radiation to create images of the inside of the body, primarily for examining bones and detecting fractures.

How it works: X-ray machines emit radiation that passes through the body and is absorbed in different amounts depending on the density of the tissues. Bones, being denser, absorb more X-rays and appear white on the X-ray film, while softer tissues allow more X-rays to pass through and appear darker (Pasveer, B., 1989).

Applications: X-rays are primarily used for imaging bones (fractures, dislocations, bone tumors), teeth, and the chest (pneumonia, lung infections). They are also used in mammography to screen for breast cancer.

Advantages: Quick, inexpensive, widely available, and non-invasive.

Disadvantages: Exposure to ionizing radiation, though minimal in diagnostic amounts, may still pose a risk with repeated exposure.

1.2.4 Ultrasound

Overview: Ultrasound uses high-frequency sound waves to create images of the inside of the body, primarily soft tissues. It is commonly used in obstetrics and gynecology, cardiology, and abdominal imaging.

How it works: An ultrasound machine sends sound waves into the body using a transducer. These waves bounce off tissues and organs, and the echoes are converted into images by the ultrasound machine (Powers, J., & Kremkau, F., 2011).

Applications: Ultrasound is commonly used for monitoring pregnancy, imaging the heart (echocardiography), and assessing the abdomen (gallbladder, kidneys, liver, and blood vessels). It is also used to guide needle biopsies and other minimally invasive procedures.

Advantages: Non-invasive, no ionizing radiation, real-time imaging, relatively inexpensive.

Disadvantages: Limited ability to image areas that contain gas (lungs, intestines) and bones, lower resolution compared to MRI and CT.

1.3 Why CNNs for Medical Imaging?

Convolutional Neural Networks (CNNs) have become a transformative tool in image analysis, especially for tasks involving complex pattern recognition, such as medical imaging. Below is a discussion of the suitability of CNNs for image analysis and why they excel at recognizing complex patterns in medical images.

1.3.1. Architecture and Hierarchical Feature Learning

- **Local Receptive Fields and Filters**: CNNs are built on layers of convolutions that use filters to detect patterns in small, localized areas of an image. These filters are learned during training and automatically adapt to detect simple features like edges, lines, or colors in the initial layers, and more complex patterns such as shapes, textures, and objects in deeper layers. This hierarchical learning enables CNNs to capture both low-level and high-level features, which is crucial for analyzing medical images that often require the identification of subtle, intricate patterns.
- **Pooling and Dimensionality Reduction**: CNNs use pooling layers (e.g., max pooling) to reduce the spatial dimensions of the image while retaining important information. This dimensionality reduction makes the network more efficient by reducing the number of parameters, while also making the model less sensitive to small translations or distortions in the image. For medical images, where slight variations may occur due to different imaging conditions or patient anatomy, this feature is highly valuable.
- **Multiple Layers and Deep Learning**: CNNs can stack multiple layers, each detecting increasingly abstract and complex features. In medical imaging, where diseases may manifest in subtle or multi-scale features (e.g., tiny lesions or complex organ shapes), the deep architecture of CNNs can capture these intricate details that traditional methods often miss.

1.3.2. Ability to Handle Complex Patterns in Medical Images

- **Recognition of Fine-Grained Patterns**: Medical images, such as MRI scans, CT scans, and X-rays, often contain highly complex and fine-grained patterns. These patterns are difficult to recognize using traditional image analysis techniques like manual feature extraction, which depends heavily on human expertise and handcrafted algorithms. CNNs, on the other hand, automatically learn the most relevant features directly from the data, making them far more adaptable to different types of images and diseases (Aamir et al., 2023).
- **Generalization Across Modalities**: CNNs are highly effective at recognizing patterns across various types of medical images, including X-rays, CT scans, MRIs, and ultrasound. For example, a CNN trained to detect tumors in a CT scan can be adapted to learn new patterns in mammograms with relatively minor adjustments. Traditional methods often require entirely new sets of features and manual tweaking for each imaging modality (Guan et al. 2021).

1.3.3. Superior Performance Over Traditional Methods

- **Automatic Feature Extraction**: Traditional image analysis methods rely on predefined features engineered by experts, such as edge detection, texture analysis, or pixel intensity thresholds. These handcrafted features often fall short when it comes to complex images like medical scans, which may require the identification of highly nuanced patterns (e.g., identifying early-stage cancer in dense tissue) (Aamir et al., 2022). CNNs remove the need for manual feature extraction, learning features automatically based on the dataset, leading to superior performance in complex pattern recognition.

- **End-to-End Learning**: CNNs work in an end-to-end manner, meaning they take raw image data as input and produce classification or detection results directly. In contrast, traditional methods often involve multiple stages of processing and manual intervention, which can introduce errors and reduce efficiency. The end-to-end learning process of CNNs makes them more accurate and streamlined for medical image analysis.
- **Robustness to Variability**: Traditional methods can struggle with variations in lighting, orientation, or image quality, which are common in medical imaging due to differences in equipment and patient conditions. CNNs are more robust to these variations because they learn patterns that are invariant to small changes in the input image. This adaptability ensures that CNNs perform well across a wide range of medical imaging conditions, making them more reliable than traditional techniques.

1.3.4. Handling Large and Diverse Datasets

- **Scalability**: Medical imaging datasets are often large and diverse, covering a wide range of diseases, anatomical variations, and imaging conditions. Traditional methods may become overwhelmed or require significant manual intervention when applied to large datasets. CNNs, on the other hand, excel at handling big data and can learn from millions of images, continuously improving their accuracy as more data becomes available.
- **Transfer Learning**: CNNs also allow for transfer learning, where a model trained on one large dataset (e.g., ImageNet) can be fine-tuned for medical imaging tasks with smaller datasets. This ability to leverage pre-trained networks significantly reduces training time and computational resources, making CNNs highly suitable for medical applications where labeled data may be scarce.

1.3.5. Examples of CNNs in Medical Image Analysis

- **Tumor Detection**: CNNs have been highly successful in detecting tumors in MRI and CT scans, where traditional methods may struggle to identify subtle changes in tissue structure. CNNs can pinpoint abnormal growths with high accuracy and speed, providing invaluable assistance to radiologists in diagnosing cancer (Chattopadhyay, A., & Maitra, M., 2022).
- **Retinal Disease Screening**: In ophthalmology, CNNs have been used to analyze retinal images for signs of diabetic retinopathy and age-related macular degeneration. The ability of CNNs to automatically detect tiny lesions in retinal images has made them a valuable tool for early disease detection (Muchuchuti, S., & Viriri, S., 2023).
- **Chest X-ray Classification**: CNNs have been used to analyze chest X-rays for conditions such as pneumonia, tuberculosis, and COVID-19. Their ability to quickly and accurately classify medical images can assist physicians in diagnosing respiratory conditions, especially in resource-constrained settings (Ibrahim et al., 2024).

2. UNDERSTANDING CONVOLUTIONAL NEURAL NETWORKS

2.1 Basic Architecture of CNNs

Convolutional Neural Networks (CNNs) have become the foundation of many applications in medical imaging and healthcare due to their powerful ability to process and analyze visual data. The layered structure of CNNs allows them to automatically learn and extract relevant features from medical images, making them highly effective for tasks such as disease diagnosis, tumor detection, and image segmentation. Here is a detailed explanation of how CNNs are structured.

2.1.1 Convolutional Layers

Structure: Convolutional layers are the fundamental building blocks of CNNs. These layers apply filters (or kernels) to the input image to detect patterns. Each filter slides over the input image (or feature map) and performs element-wise multiplication, followed by summation, to produce an output called a **feature map**.

- **Filters**: Filters are small matrices (e.g., 3x3 or 5x5) that detect specific features such as edges, corners, or textures.
- **Stride**: Stride refers to how far the filter moves during convolution. A stride of 1 means the filter moves one pixel at a time, while a larger stride skips pixels, reducing the feature map size.
- **Padding**: Padding is applied to preserve the size of the input when filters reduce the output size. For example, zero-padding adds extra pixels around the border of the image.

A pictorial representation of convolutional layer is depicted in Fig 1.

Figure 1. Process to calculate feature maps in convolutional layer

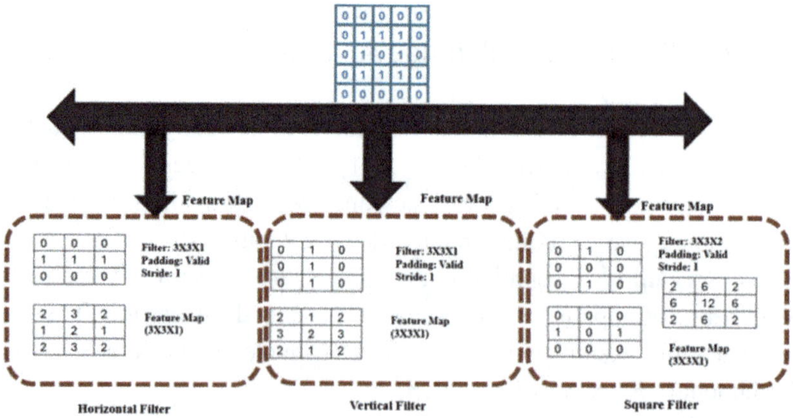

After applying series of filters to the input image, convolutional layer creates a stacks of feature map and use it as an input for next layer.

It is necessary to remember that the depth of the filter used for convolution should match that of input size. For example, for gray scale images depth of image (number of channel) is 1 so filter depth will be 1 whereas for RGB images filter depth will be 3.

Role in Medical Imaging:

In medical imaging, convolutional layers are responsible for extracting key features from images such as MRI scans, X-rays, CT scans, and ultrasound images. The early layers capture basic features (edges, contrasts), while deeper layers capture more complex patterns (e.g., organ shapes, abnormalities, tumors).

- **Example**: In cancer detection, convolutional layers can identify irregular tissue patterns or tumor boundaries that may be difficult for radiologists to spot with the naked eye.

Benefits:

- **Automatic Feature Learning**: CNNs automatically learn which features are most important for a specific medical task (e.g., detecting lesions or tumors).
- **Spatial Hierarchy**: Convolutional layers retain spatial information about where features are located, which is crucial in medical imaging where the position of anomalies is important for diagnosis.

2.1.2. Pooling Layers

Structure: Pooling layers are used to reduce the spatial dimensions (width and height) of the feature maps, while preserving important information. The most common type of pooling is max, min and average pooling.

- **Max Pooling**: A window (e.g., 2x2) slides over the feature map, and the maximum value in that window is retained while the rest are discarded.
- **Min Pooling**: A window (e.g., 2x2) slides over the feature map, and the minimum value in that window is retained while the rest are discarded.
- **Average Pooling**: Less common in practice, this takes the average value of each window rather than the maximum.

Stride in Pooling: Similar to the convolutional layer, pooling also uses stride to control how much the window moves over the image.

The pictorial representation of various pooling processes is illustrated in Figure 2.

Figure 2. Process to reduce spatial dimension of feature maps using various pooling layer

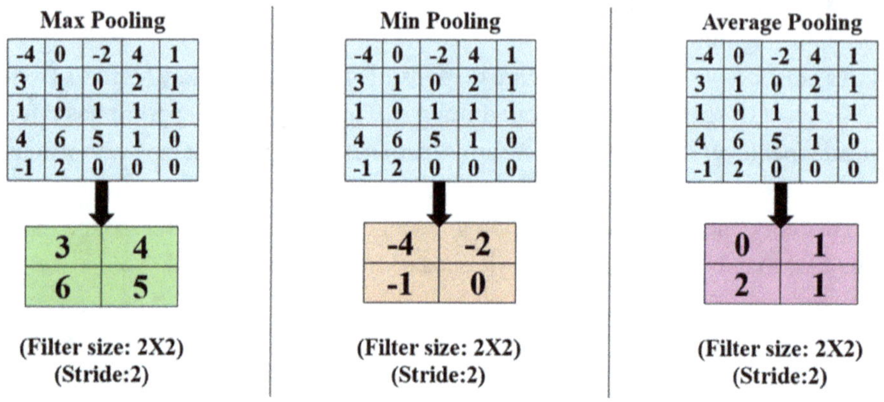

Role in Medical Imaging:

By keeping the most prominent features while downsampling, pooling helps focus on the most critical parts of the medical images.

- **Example**: In a CNN designed for lung disease detection from CT scans, pooling layers reduce the amount of data the model has to process, helping it focus on areas of the scan that show disease, like nodules.

Benefits:

- **Dimensionality Reduction**: Pooling layers reduce the computational cost of training without losing important features.
- **Invariance to Small Translations**: Pooling layers make the model less sensitive to small shifts or distortions in the image, which is important in medical imaging since patient positioning or imaging conditions can vary.

2.1.3 Fully Connected Layers

Structure: Fully connected layers are standard neural network layers where each neuron is connected to every neuron in the previous layer. After convolutional and pooling layers extract features from an image, these fully connected layers use these features for classification or regression tasks.

- **Neurons**: Each neuron receives input from every neuron in the previous layer, performs a weighted sum of these inputs, applies an activation function, and passes the result to the next layer.

Role in Medical Imaging:

Fully connected layers are used to make the final predictions in medical imaging tasks. After feature extraction through convolutional and pooling layers, these layers decide what the image represents (e.g., whether a scan shows the presence of a tumor or not).

- **Example**: In a CNN trained to classify MRI scans as either normal or cancerous, the fully connected layers aggregate the features extracted by the previous layers and output the probability that the scan shows cancer.

Benefits:

- **Feature Aggregation**: Fully connected layers combine features from across the image to make high-level decisions.
- **Final Classification**: These layers make the final decision in a classification task (e.g., healthy vs. diseased), essential for diagnostic applications in healthcare.

2.1.4. Activation Functions

Structure: Activation functions introduce non-linearity into CNN, allowing the network to learn complex relationships between inputs and outputs. Common activation functions include:

- **ReLU (Rectified Linear Unit)**: The most used activation function in CNNs, it outputs zero for negative inputs and the input itself for positive values.
- **Sigmoid**: Outputs values between 0 and 1, often used in binary classification tasks.
- **Softmax**: Used in the output layer for multi-class classification, producing a probability distribution over classes.

Role in Medical Imaging:
Activation functions allow CNNs to make complex, non-linear decisions about medical images, which is crucial for recognizing patterns in varying tissue densities, shapes, and textures.

- **Example**: In a CNN designed to detect multiple conditions from chest X-rays, a softmax activation function at the output layer could assign probabilities to conditions like pneumonia, tuberculosis, or a normal scan.

Benefits:

- **Non-Linearity**: Activation functions allow CNNs to model complex, non-linear relationships, which are often needed in medical tasks where simple linear models would fail.
- **Decision Making**: Functions like softmax provide probability distributions, which are useful in medical applications where multiple conditions need to be considered simultaneously.

The pictorial representation of the complete architecture of a convolutional neural network is shown in Fig 3.

Figure 3. Complete CNN architecture

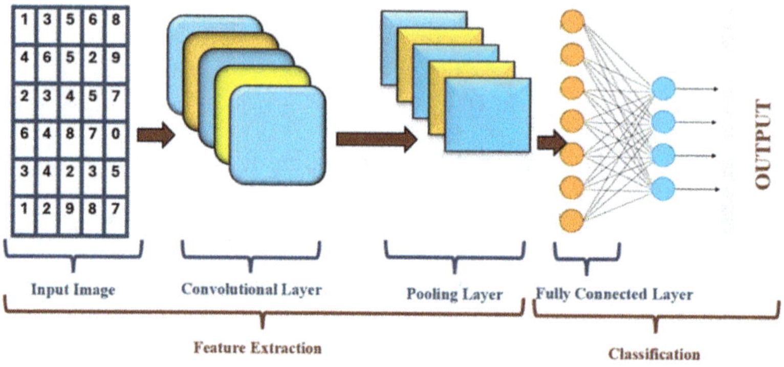

2.2 How CNNs Learn from Images: Training Process Overview

Convolutional Neural Networks (CNNs) learn from images through a structured training process that involves supervised learning, backpropagation, and gradient descent. These mechanisms allow the CNN to automatically detect and learn features from the images, enabling it to perform tasks like classification, object detection, or segmentation. Below is an explanation of each component of the training process for CNNs.

2.2.1. Supervised Learning in CNNs

Supervised learning is the foundation of CNN training (Aljuaid, A., & Anwar, M., 2022). In this paradigm, the network is trained using a labeled dataset where each image is associated with a specific label (or ground truth). CNN's objective is to learn the relationship between the input images and their corresponding labels so it can predict labels for new, unseen images.

- **Training Dataset**: The dataset consists of pairs of input images (e.g., MRI scans, X-rays) and their corresponding labels (e.g., "cancerous," "non-cancerous").
- **Prediction**: During training, the CNN processes each input image and outputs a prediction, which could be a class label (in classification tasks) or continuous values (in regression tasks).
- **Loss Function**: The predicted output is compared to the true label using a loss function. The loss function quantifies the difference between the predicted value and the true value, providing a measure of how well CNN is performing.

2.2.2 Backpropagation

Once the CNN makes predictions, backpropagation is used to adjust the network's internal parameters (i.e., weights and biases) to minimize the loss. Backpropagation is an algorithm that computes the gradient of the loss function with respect to each parameter in the network, allowing the network to learn from its mistakes and improve over time (Mizutani, H., 1994).

Steps of Backpropagation:

1. **Forward Pass**: During the forward pass, the input image is fed through the CNN, moving through the convolutional layers, pooling layers, fully connected layers, and activation functions. The network generates a prediction based on the input.
2. **Calculate Loss**: The loss function compares the predicted label to the true label. A common loss function for classification tasks is cross-entropy loss, while mean squared error is used for regression tasks.
3. **Backpropagation of Errors**: The backpropagation algorithm calculates how much each weight in the network contributed to the loss. This is done using the chain rule from calculus, allowing the CNN to trace the error backward from the output layer to each previous layer, calculating the gradient of the loss function with respect to each weight.
4. **Weight Update**: Once the gradients are calculated, the weights are updated to reduce the loss. This process is iteratively repeated, allowing the CNN to gradually learn and improve its accuracy.

2.2.3. Gradient Descent

Gradient descent is the optimization algorithm used to update the weights of CNN during training. The goal of gradient descent is to minimize the loss function by moving the network's parameters in the direction of the steepest descent (i.e., the negative gradient of the loss) (Cui, N., 2018).

Types of Gradient Descent:

- **Batch Gradient Descent**: In batch gradient descent, the entire dataset is used to compute the gradients before updating the weights. While this can lead to more accurate gradient calculations, it is computationally expensive and slow for large datasets.
- **Stochastic Gradient Descent (SGD)**: In SGD, the network updates the weights after each training example (or a small batch of examples), making it faster and more scalable for large datasets. However, the updates can be noisy, which may lead to oscillations in the loss function during training.
- **Mini-Batch Gradient Descent**: A compromise between the two, mini-batch gradient descent divides the dataset into small batches and updates the weights after each batch. It is commonly used in CNN training, as it balances speed and accuracy.

Learning Rate: The learning rate is a hyperparameter that controls the size of the steps taken during gradient descent. A high learning rate may cause the model to converge too quickly and overshoot the optimal solution, while a low learning rate may cause slow convergence or getting stuck in local minima.

Steps of Gradient Descent:

Step 1. Initialize Parameters

- Start by initializing the parameters (weights) randomly or using some heuristic.
- The initial values can affect how quickly the algorithm converges.

Step 2. Calculate the Loss

- Compute the loss (or cost) function, which measures the difference between the predicted values and the actual values. A common loss function is Mean Squared Error (MSE) for regression or Cross-Entropy for classification.

Step 3. Computing the Gradient

- Calculate the gradient of the loss function with respect to each parameter. The gradient indicates the direction and rate of the fastest increase of the loss function.

Step 4. Update Parameters

- Update the parameters in the direction opposite to the gradient to minimize the loss. The update is done using the formula:

$\theta=\theta-\alpha\cdot\nabla J(\theta)$ where: (1)

- Θ represents the parameters (weights)
- α is the learning rate (a small positive number that controls how big the update is)
- $\nabla J(\theta)$ is the gradient of the loss function.

Step 5. Repeat

- Repeat the process of calculating the loss, computing the gradient, and updating the parameters until convergence is reached (i.e., when the change in the loss function becomes negligible or a predetermined number of iterations is completed).

Step 6. Convergence

- The algorithm converges when the parameters no longer change significantly, meaning the loss function has reached a minimum (ideally global minimum, but sometimes local minimum).

Example: CNN Training in Medical Imaging
Consider a CNN trained to detect pneumonia from chest X-rays:

1. **Supervised Learning**: The CNN is trained on a labeled dataset of chest X-rays, where each X-ray has a label indicating whether the patient has pneumonia or not.
2. **Forward Pass**: During each iteration, an X-ray image is passed through the CNN. The network's filters and pooling layers extract features from the image, such as lung patterns and abnormalities, and the fully connected layers output a prediction (e.g., "pneumonia" or "no pneumonia").

3. **Loss Calculation**: The prediction is compared to the true label, and the cross-entropy loss is calculated.
4. **Backpropagation**: The backpropagation algorithm calculates how much each filter and weight contributed to the incorrect prediction and adjusts them accordingly.
5. **Gradient Descent**: Gradient descent is used to update the network's weights, moving them closer to the values that minimize the loss.

This iterative process continues over multiple epochs, and CNN gradually improves its ability to detect pneumonia in unseen chest X-rays.

2.3 Key Advantages of CNNs for Image Recognition Tasks

Convolutional Neural Networks (CNNs) have proven to be highly effective for image recognition tasks due to several key advantages that make them superior to traditional machine learning methods. Some of the most significant advantages include translation invariance, spatial hierarchy, and reduced preprocessing requirements.

2.3.1. Translation Invariance

Translation invariance refers to the ability of CNNs to recognize objects or patterns in images regardless of their position or orientation within the image. This property is crucial for tasks like object detection, facial recognition, and medical imaging, where an object can appear anywhere within the image, or may be slightly rotated or shifted.

Example: In facial recognition, CNNs can identify a person's face even if the face is slightly rotated or shifted within the image frame (Sohail et al., 2024).

2.3.2. Spatial Hierarchy

CNNs exploit the concept of spatial hierarchy through their deep layered architecture, which progressively builds higher-level representations of the input image. This hierarchy allows CNNs to automatically learn different levels of features, from low-level features like edges and corners to high-level features like shapes and complex objects.

- **Hierarchical Learning**: Early layers in a CNN learn basic features like edges and textures, while deeper layers combine these features to learn more complex structures like shapes, objects, or even specific entities like faces or organs.
- **Receptive Fields**: As you move deeper into the network, each neuron's receptive field (the part of the image it "sees") increases. This enables the network to capture both fine details and the broader context of the image.

Example: In medical imaging, early layers of a CNN might detect small details like tissue textures, while deeper layers recognize larger structures like organs or tumors, providing comprehensive analysis for diagnostic purposes.

2.3.3. Reduced Preprocessing Requirements

One of the major advantages of CNNs over traditional methods is their ability to learn features directly from raw data, minimizing the need for manual feature extraction or preprocessing. In traditional machine learning, significant effort is required to handcraft features from images, which is both time-consuming and error-prone. CNNs, however, automate this process.

Example: In traditional medical imaging analysis, radiologists or engineers might need to manually extract features like shape, texture, or intensity. CNNs bypass this step, learning all relevant features from the raw images, significantly streamlining the workflow (Kumar et al.,2024).

Other Key Advantages

2.3.4. Parameter Sharing and Local Connectivity

- CNNs utilize **parameter sharing**, where the same filter (or kernel) is applied across different regions of the image. This reduces the number of parameters compared to fully connected networks and allows CNNs to generalize better with less data.
- **Local connectivity** refers to how CNNs focus only on a small part of the image at a time, making them efficient for high-dimensional data like images.

2.3.5. Effective for Large-Scale Data

- CNNs are highly scalable and effective for handling large datasets, as seen in applications like ImageNet, which contain millions of images. CNNs can process high-resolution images with complex patterns and provide accurate results.

2.3.6. Robust to Noisy Data

- Due to their deep architecture and hierarchical feature learning, CNNs are often robust to noisy or imperfect data. They can still identify patterns even in the presence of distortions, blurs, or occlusions.

3. APPLICATION OF CNNS IN MEDICAL IMAGING

3.1 Disease Detection and Diagnosis

Convolutional Neural Networks (CNNs) have revolutionized early disease detection by significantly improving the accuracy and efficiency of medical image analysis. CNNs are widely used in diagnosing various conditions such as cancer (breast, lung, skin), Alzheimer's disease, diabetic retinopathy, and heart conditions. Below is an overview of how CNNs are applied in detecting these diseases.

3.1.1. Breast Cancer Detection

In the early detection of breast cancer, CNNs are trained on mammograms, MRI scans, or ultrasound images to identify abnormalities such as tumors or calcifications that may indicate the presence of cancer.

Example: Google's DeepMind has developed a CNN-based model that can outperform radiologists in breast cancer detection from mammograms by reducing both false positives and false negatives (McKinney SM, 2020).

3.1.2 Lung Cancer Detection

Lung cancer detection typically involves analyzing CT scans to identify suspicious nodules or lesions that could be early indicators of cancer.

CT Scans: CNNs are trained to recognize nodules of varying shapes and sizes in lung CT scans. They can assess features like the nodule's size, texture, and growth over time to determine whether it is cancerous (Javed et al., 2024).

Low-Dose CT Scans: CNNs have been employed in screening programs that use low-dose CT scans, particularly in high-risk populations, to detect lung cancer in its early stages.

3.1.3. Skin Cancer Detection

CNNs have demonstrated remarkable success in identifying skin cancers, including melanoma, by analyzing dermoscopy images.

Dermoscopy: CNNs are trained to detect subtle changes in skin lesions, including asymmetry, border irregularities, color variations, and size changes—factors associated with melanoma and other types of skin cancer (Faghihi et al., 2024).

Smartphone Applications: Some CNN-based models have been integrated into smartphone apps that allow users to take photos of skin lesions for an initial diagnosis.

3.1.4. Alzheimer's Disease Detection

CNNs are being used to detect early signs of Alzheimer's disease from medical imaging techniques such as MRI and PET scans.

MRI and PET Scans: In Alzheimer's detection, CNNs are trained to analyze brain scans, identifying structural and functional changes such as cortical thinning, hippocampal atrophy, and abnormal protein accumulation (e.g., amyloid plaques) (Alsubaie, et al., 2024).

3.1.5. Diabetic Retinopathy Detection

CNNs have been widely applied to detect diabetic retinopathy from retinal fundus images. Diabetic retinopathy is a complication of diabetes that affects the blood vessels in the retina and can lead to blindness if not treated early.

Retinal Fundus Images: CNNs are trained on large datasets of retinal images to detect microaneurysms, hemorrhages, and exudates, which are indicative of diabetic retinopathy. (Asia et al., 2022)

Example: Google's AI model for diabetic retinopathy detection achieved accuracy comparable to that of human ophthalmologists, helping to bring affordable screening to underserved populations.

3.1.6. Heart Condition Detection

CNNs are also being utilized in the detection of heart conditions, such as arrhythmias and coronary artery disease, from medical imaging and electrocardiogram (ECG) data.

Echocardiograms: CNNs analyze echocardiograms (ultrasound images of the heart) to detect structural abnormalities such as valvular defects, septal defects, and cardiomyopathies. They can identify changes in the heart's chambers, walls, and valves, enabling early diagnosis of heart diseases (Ghorbani et al., 2020).

ECG Analysis: CNNs are employed to detect arrhythmias by analyzing ECG signals. They can identify abnormal heart rhythms that may indicate conditions such as atrial fibrillation or ventricular tachycardia (Liu et al., 2021).

CT Coronary Angiography: CNNs can analyze CT coronary angiograms to detect plaque build-up in the arteries, assessing the risk of coronary artery disease and helping in the early detection of heart attacks (Alskaf et al., 2022).Bottom of Form

3.2 Image Segmentation and Localization:

Precise segmentation is a key step in medical image analysis, enabling accurate localization and assessment of diseased areas, which is vital for diagnosis, treatment planning, and monitoring disease progression. Convolutional Neural Networks (CNNs) have become a critical tool in radiology for the segmentation of organs, tumors, and other anatomical structures.

3.2.1. Segmentation in Radiology

Segmentation refers to the process of dividing a medical image into different regions, typically corresponding to various anatomical structures or regions of interest, such as organs or tumors. CNNs have proven particularly effective in medical image segmentation tasks, largely due to their ability to learn hierarchical feature representations and their capability to handle complex patterns and textures within images.

Fully Convolutional Networks (FCNs): A variant of CNNs used specifically for segmentation, FCNs eliminate the fully connected layers, enabling the network to make pixel-wise predictions. This is crucial for creating fine-grained segmentations of organs and tumors (Sultana et al., 2020).

U-Net: One of the most popular CNN architectures for medical image segmentation is the U-Net, which combines convolutional and deconvolutional layers to provide high-resolution segmentations. U-Nets are particularly effective because they capture both local and global context, which is important for medical images where small tumors may be located within large organs (Siddique et al., 2021).

a) Organ Segmentation

Accurately segmenting organs is crucial for understanding their structure, identifying abnormalities, and performing volumetric analysis, particularly in conditions like organ hypertrophy or atrophy. CNNs can precisely delineate organ boundaries, even when the contrast between different tissues is subtle.

- **Liver Segmentation**: In liver imaging, CNNs are used to automatically segment the liver and distinguish between healthy and diseased liver tissues. This aids in evaluating conditions such as liver cirrhosis or detecting liver tumors.
- **Heart Segmentation**: For cardiac imaging, CNNs can segment the heart's chambers (e.g., left ventricle, right atrium) from MRI or echocardiography data. Accurate heart segmentation helps assess cardiac function, detect structural heart diseases, and plan surgeries like valve replacements.
- **Kidney and Brain Segmentation**: Similarly, CNNs are applied in segmenting kidneys in CT scans and brains in MRI, aiding in conditions like chronic kidney disease and neurodegenerative disorders, respectively.

b) Tumor Segmentation

One of the most significant uses of CNNs in radiology is the segmentation of tumors, which is essential for planning surgeries, radiation therapy, and monitoring the growth or shrinkage of tumors during treatment.

- **Brain Tumors**: CNNs are widely used to segment brain tumors from MRI scans, where they can differentiate between different tumor regions (e.g., tumor core, necrosis, and edema). Precise segmentation is critical for radiation therapy planning and monitoring treatment outcomes.
    - o **Gliomas**: For example, in the segmentation of gliomas, one of the most common brain tumors, CNNs help delineate the tumor boundaries and assess the tumor's progression over time.
- **Lung Tumors**: In lung cancer, CNNs are used to segment nodules and tumors in CT scans. Accurate segmentation helps radiologists measure tumor size, assess its stage, and monitor the response to therapies like chemotherapy or radiation.
- **Breast Tumors**: In mammograms, CNNs assist in segmenting breast masses, differentiating between benign and malignant tumors, and aiding in biopsy planning.

3.3 Image Classification

Convolutional Neural Networks (CNNs) are at the forefront of medical image classification. Their ability to distinguish between abnormal and normal scans has revolutionized diagnostic processes across various medical fields. Image classification is the process of assigning a label or category to an input image based on its content. CNNs are especially well-suited to this task because they automatically learn to extract features from images, progressively identifying patterns that correlate with specific diagnostic categories. Below is an explanation of how CNNs classify images into diagnostic categories and their role in detecting abnormalities.

- **Training Process**: CNNs are trained using large datasets of labeled medical images, where each image is annotated as either normal or showing signs of a specific condition (e.g., cancer, lesions, organ malformations). The CNN learns to associate the pixel-level patterns in these images with their corresponding labels.

- **Feature Extraction**: The early layers of a CNN detect simple patterns like edges and textures, while deeper layers recognize more complex features such as shapes and high-level anatomical structures.
- **Classification Layer**: At the end of the CNN architecture, a fully connected layer or softmax layer assigns a probability score to each possible diagnostic category, ultimately classifying the image into a specific category (e.g., normal or abnormal).

3.3.1 Distinguishing Between Normal and Abnormal Scans

CNNs excel at differentiating normal from abnormal scans. Abnormalities may include the presence of tumors, tissue degradation, fluid build-up, or vascular irregularities. For instance, in brain MRIs, CNNs can distinguish normal brain tissue from areas affected by tumors, strokes, or neurodegenerative diseases. CNNs can be fine-tuned for sensitivity, ensuring they detect even the most subtle abnormalities, reducing the risk of false negatives. However, balancing sensitivity with specificity is critical to avoid excessive false positives, which could lead to unnecessary follow-up procedures.

3.3.2 Diagnostic Categories in Medical Imaging

CNNs may be used to classify images into multiple diagnostic categories, not just normal versus abnormal. For example, in the detection of specific diseases, a CNN might classify an image into one of several categories:

- **Cancer Detection**: CNNs are commonly used in diagnosing cancer from medical images. In breast cancer screening, for instance, a CNN can classify mammogram images into categories like "benign," "malignant," or "normal." Similarly, in lung cancer screening, CNNs analyze CT scans to classify nodules as "benign" or "cancerous."
- **Lung Diseases**: In chest X-rays or CT scans, CNNs are trained to classify scans into categories such as "normal," "pneumonia," "COVID-19," or "lung cancer," depending on the features present in the lungs.
- **Diabetic Retinopathy**: CNNs are used to classify retinal images into categories like "normal," "mild retinopathy," "moderate retinopathy," or "severe retinopathy." These classifications help ophthalmologists identify the stage of the disease and determine appropriate treatments.
- **Brain Disorders**: CNNs analyze brain MRI scans and classify them based on diagnostic categories like "normal," "tumor," "Alzheimer's disease," or "stroke." These classifications help in the early detection and intervention of neurodegenerative diseases.

3.3.3 End-to-End Diagnostic Aid

One of the major advantages of CNNs in image classification is their ability to provide an end-to-end solution, where the input (e.g., a medical image) is processed through the CNN, and the output is a diagnostic prediction or category. This helps radiologists, doctors, and healthcare providers in the following ways:

- **Early Detection**: CNNs can identify abnormalities in scans that may not be easily detectable by the human eye, allowing for early diagnosis of diseases such as cancer or Alzheimer's. Early detection is critical in improving patient outcomes.
- **Automated Diagnosis**: CNNs help automate routine diagnostic tasks, such as screening large volumes of medical images, thus reducing the burden on radiologists and improving the speed of diagnosis.
- **Decision Support**: While CNNs are not meant to replace human radiologists, they act as decision support systems. CNNs can flag abnormal scans for further review, offering a second opinion and reducing the likelihood of human error.

3.3.4 Post-Classification Steps

Once a CNN has classified an image into a diagnostic category, the results can be further utilized in a clinical setting. Typically, the classification outcome is not the end of the process but serves as a basis for further clinical decisions:

- **Referral for Additional Tests**: For scans classified as abnormal, further diagnostic tests such as biopsies, follow-up imaging, or blood tests may be recommended.
- **Treatment Planning**: In cases where CNNs classify an image as showing a specific disease (e.g., lung cancer or brain tumors), the results are used to tailor treatment plans, including surgery, radiation, or chemotherapy.
- **Progress Monitoring**: CNNs can also classify follow-up scans to monitor disease progression, determining whether a tumor is shrinking in response to treatment or if a disease like diabetic retinopathy is worsening.

3.4 3D Imaging and CNNs:

Convolutional Neural Networks (CNNs) have been pivotal in analyzing 2D medical images, but their application in 3D medical imaging modalities such as CT and MRI are an emerging frontier with transformative potential. 3D medical imaging provides rich volumetric data that enables deeper insights into the structure and function of organs and tissues, and CNNs adapted for 3D data play a crucial role in leveraging this information. These advancements are particularly impactful in the context of surgical planning, where precise localization and visualization of anatomical structures are critical (Singh et al., 2020).

3.4.1 3D Medical Imaging and Volumetric Scans

3D medical imaging, such as Computed Tomography (CT) and Magnetic Resonance Imaging (MRI), generates volumetric data by capturing multiple 2D slices of an anatomical region, which are then combined to create a 3D representation of the area of interest.

- **CT Scans**: CT scanning combines multiple X-ray images taken from different angles to create cross-sectional images of bones, blood vessels, and soft tissues. It is particularly useful in detecting bone injuries, tumors, and internal bleeding.

- **MRI Scans**: MRI uses magnetic fields and radio waves to produce detailed images of organs and tissues, especially soft tissues like the brain, spinal cord, and joints. It is ideal for diagnosing neurological, muscular, and skeletal disorders.

3.4.2 3D CNNs: Architecture and Functionality

3D CNNs extend traditional CNNs by applying 3D convolution operations on volumetric data, allowing them to analyze depth in addition to height and width.

- **3D Convolutions**: In 3D CNNs, the convolutional filters move through the data volume in three dimensions (height, width, depth), enabling the model to learn spatial patterns across multiple layers of the scan.
- **3D Pooling**: Similar to 2D pooling in traditional CNNs, 3D pooling layers reduce the dimensionality of the data while retaining important spatial features, thus reducing the computational load while preserving crucial information for classification or segmentation.
- **3D U-Nets and FCNs**: Variations of CNN architectures, like 3D U-Nets, have been developed specifically for tasks such as organ segmentation in 3D. These architectures are especially useful in processing complex volumetric data and generating detailed 3D segmentations.

3.4.3. Applications of 3D CNNs in Volumetric Imaging

3D CNNs are widely used for a variety of tasks in volumetric imaging, from detection and segmentation to classification and surgical planning.

- **Tumor Detection and Segmentation**: 3D CNNs are used to identify and segment tumors in organs like the brain, liver, and lungs from MRI or CT scans. Because tumors may span multiple slices, 3D CNNs are more effective in delineating their boundaries and understanding their volumetric shape compared to 2D methods.
    - **Brain Tumors**: In brain MRIs, 3D CNNs can segment brain tumors across multiple slices, enabling radiologists to better visualize the tumor's structure, location, and relationship with surrounding tissues.
    - **Lung Nodules**: In chest CT scans, 3D CNNs detect and segment lung nodules, providing a 3D view of the tumor that aids in diagnosis and treatment planning.
- **Organ Segmentation**: 3D CNNs are effective in segmenting organs from volumetric scans, which is essential for understanding anatomical variations and disease progression. For instance, 3D CNNs can segment the liver, kidneys, or heart in CT or MRI, aiding in the diagnosis of conditions like liver cirrhosis, kidney disease, or heart disease.
    - **Heart Imaging**: 3D CNNs are used to analyze cardiac MRI scans, segmenting the heart's chambers and vessels in 3D. This helps cardiologists assess heart function and plan interventions like valve repairs or stent placements.
- **Disease Classification**: 3D CNNs classify volumetric data into diagnostic categories. For example, in brain MRIs, 3D CNNs classify images based on the presence of tumors, neurodegenerative conditions like Alzheimer's, or abnormalities like brain bleeds.

3.4.4. Surgical Planning with 3D CNNs

One of the most impactful applications of 3D CNNs in healthcare is surgical planning. Accurate 3D segmentation and analysis of anatomical structures enable surgeons to visualize the target area in detail before performing complex procedures.

- **Pre-Surgical Mapping**: 3D CNNs provide detailed maps of the patient's anatomy, allowing surgeons to plan incisions, resections, and other interventions with precision. In neurosurgery, for instance, 3D CNNs help map the location of a brain tumor relative to critical areas, such as motor or speech centers, reducing the risk of damage during surgery.
- **Brain Surgery**: In brain tumor surgeries, 3D CNNs provide 3D reconstructions of the tumor's boundaries, allowing neurosurgeons to plan the optimal approach and minimize damage to surrounding healthy brain tissue.
- **Orthopedic Surgery**: In orthopedic surgeries, like joint replacements or fracture repairs, 3D CNNs help surgeons plan the precise placement of prosthetics or screws by providing detailed 3D models of the bone and surrounding tissues.
- **Augmented Reality and 3D Visualizations**: 3D CNNs enable the creation of detailed 3D models that can be used in augmented reality (AR) systems, allowing surgeons to visualize the patient's anatomy in real-time during surgery. This integration of 3D CNN-based models with AR helps guide the surgeon's hand, enhancing precision and safety.
    - **Liver Resection**: In liver surgeries, where it is critical to avoid damaging blood vessels and other structures, 3D CNNs segment the liver and its vascular network, enabling surgeons to plan the resection in a way that maximizes tumor removal while preserving healthy tissue.
- **Radiation Therapy Planning**: In radiation therapy for cancer, 3D CNNs help delineate both the tumor and nearby organs to ensure that radiation is accurately targeted at the tumor while sparing healthy tissues. Accurate 3D segmentation is critical to minimizing side effects and maximizing the efficacy of the treatment.

3.5 CNNs for Real-Time Imaging:

Convolutional Neural Networks (CNNs) are increasingly being integrated into real-time imaging devices for intraoperative guidance and real-time monitoring, transforming surgical procedures and enhancing precision. These advanced neural networks, combined with modern imaging technologies, provide real-time analysis of medical images during surgeries, enabling surgeons to make informed decisions on the spot. Below is a detailed discussion of how CNNs are used in intraoperative guidance and monitoring.

3.5.1 Real-Time Imaging and Intraoperative Guidance

Intraoperative imaging involves using imaging technologies such as ultrasound, MRI, or CT during surgical procedures to provide real-time visualization of internal structures.

- **Real-Time Image Analysis**: CNNs process incoming imaging data (e.g., from ultrasound or fluoroscopy) and instantly identify relevant features, such as the boundaries of tumors or the location of critical blood vessels. This is especially useful in delicate surgeries, like brain tumor removal, where precise delineation of the tumor is essential to avoid damaging healthy tissue (Ruan et al., 2020).

- **Intraoperative Ultrasound**: CNNs integrated with ultrasound devices can analyze real-time ultrasound images to provide continuous updates on the position of organs or tumors. This is crucial in procedures like liver or kidney surgery, where organ movement due to respiration can complicate the surgery.
- **Intraoperative MRI (iMRI)**: MRI provides high-resolution, soft-tissue imaging during surgery. CNNs can analyze iMRI images to update surgeons on the current status of a procedure. For example, in brain surgery, iMRI combined with CNNs helps ensure that the surgeon has removed the entire tumor without leaving any remnants behind.

3.5.2. CNN-Based Segmentation for Intraoperative Precision

A critical application of CNNs during surgery is real-time segmentation of anatomical structures. CNNs automatically identify and segment organs, tissues, or abnormalities (such as tumors) from intraoperative images, providing precise visualizations that guide surgical actions.

- **Tumor Segmentation**: CNNs can segment tumors in real-time during cancer surgeries, providing a clear boundary between healthy and abnormal tissues. This helps surgeons resect the tumor accurately while sparing healthy tissue, reducing the likelihood of complications or recurrence.
- **Organ and Vessel Segmentation**: In vascular surgeries or organ transplants, CNNs can segment critical structures like blood vessels and organs in real time, providing surgeons with clear guidance on where to cut or avoid. This improves surgical outcomes, especially in complex procedures involving intricate vascular networks.
- **Real-Time Feedback**: CNNs continuously analyze the imaging data and provide immediate feedback on the success of the intervention. For instance, if a surgeon is excising a tumor, the CNN can offer real-time updates on whether the resection is complete or if any tumor tissue remains. This minimizes the need for additional surgeries and enhances precision.

3.5.3. CNNs in Robotic-Assisted Surgery

Robotic-assisted surgery is another area where CNNs are playing a transformative role. In robotic surgery, a surgeon controls robotic instruments that perform delicate tasks, often using real-time imaging to guide the procedure. CNNs enhance these systems by providing real-time image analysis that informs the robot's actions.

- **Augmented Vision**: In robotic surgeries, CNNs enhance the real-time imaging feed, providing surgeons with augmented visual cues, such as highlighting critical areas (e.g., tumor margins, blood vessels). This improves the accuracy of robotic maneuvers.
- **Autonomous Actions**: Advanced robotic systems, integrated with CNNs, are capable of performing semi-autonomous tasks based on real-time image analysis. For example, during a kidney transplant, a CNN-guided robotic system could autonomously suture blood vessels with precision, reducing the risk of human error.

3.5.4. CNNs and Augmented Reality in Surgery

CNNs are also driving advancements in augmented reality (AR) for surgery. By integrating CNNs with AR systems, surgeons can overlay real-time 3D visualizations of the patient's anatomy onto their field of view during surgery.

- **AR Overlays**: CNNs segment and analyze real-time imaging data, which is then projected onto the surgeon's AR headset or screen. This provides the surgeon with enhanced visual guidance, such as showing the exact location of a tumor or highlighting critical areas to avoid. For example, in liver surgery, an AR system powered by CNNs can show the surgeon where to make incisions while avoiding major blood vessels.
- **Enhanced Precision**: By combining CNN-powered segmentation with AR, surgeons can operate with unprecedented precision, ensuring that they accurately target the area of interest while preserving healthy tissue.

4. ADVANCES IN CNN ARCHITECTURES FOR MEDICAL IMAGING

4.1 Transfer Learning and Pre-trained Networks

Transfer learning is a machine learning approach that leverages pre-trained models to solve new but related tasks. Instead of training a model from scratch, transfer learning utilizes knowledge from a previously trained model, often on a large dataset, and applies it to a smaller, task-specific dataset. This technique is particularly beneficial in scenarios with limited labeled data, as it reduces the need for extensive computational resources and time.

4.1.1 Technical Details of Transfer Learning

- **Pre-Trained Models**

Transfer learning starts with a model pre-trained on a large, general-purpose dataset (e.g., ImageNet for computer vision or GPT for natural language processing). These pre-trained models capture generic features or patterns, such as edges in images or linguistic structures in text.

- **Fine-Tuning**

The pre-trained model is then fine-tuned on a target task. Depending on the similarity between the pre-training and target domains, fine-tuning involves one of the following approaches:

✓ **Feature Extraction:** The pre-trained model's layers are frozen, and only the final classification or task-specific layers are re-trained on the new dataset.

✓ **Full Model Tuning:** All layers, including the pre-trained ones, are updated using the new dataset, allowing the model to adapt to task-specific nuances.

  - **Layer Transfer**

In some cases, only certain layers of the pre-trained model are reused, depending on their relevance to the new task. Early layers, which capture low-level features, are often more generalizable than deeper layers, which tend to be task-specific.

4.1.2 Hyperparameter Tuning in Transfer Learning

Hyperparameter tuning plays a pivotal role in optimizing the performance of models, particularly in transfer learning. Hyperparameters are external configurations that control the training process and model behavior. Fine-tuning these parameters ensures that the pre-trained model adapts effectively to the target task.

Key Hyperparameters in Transfer Learning

Learning Rate:

A critical parameter, the learning rate determines how quickly the model updates its weights during training. In transfer learning, the learning rate for the pre-trained layers is typically lower than that for task-specific layers to avoid catastrophic forgetting of pre-trained knowledge.

Batch Size:

Controls the number of samples used to update the model in each iteration. Smaller batch sizes often improve generalization but may lead to noisy gradient updates, requiring a balance.

Dropout Rate:

Regularization parameter that prevents overfitting by randomly dropping neurons during training.

Appropriate tuning ensures the model generalizes well without under-utilizing its capacity.

Weight Decay:

Helps prevent overfitting by penalizing large weights in the model. Particularly useful when fine-tuning on small datasets.

Number of Frozen Layers:

Determines which layers of the pre-trained model remain unchanged during fine-tuning. Freezing too many layers may limit task-specific learning, while fine-tuning all layers can lead to overfitting on small datasets.

Impact on Performance

Improved Accuracy:

Well-tuned hyperparameters ensure the model efficiently adapts to the new task, improving accuracy without overfitting or underfitting.

Efficient Training:

Optimal learning rates and batch sizes reduce training time, allowing for faster experimentation and deployment.

Generalization:

Properly tuned regularization parameters, such as dropout and weight decay, enhance the model's ability to generalize to unseen data, ensuring robust performance.

Reduced Overfitting:

Fine-tuning strategies and hyperparameter optimization help balance the use of pre-trained knowledge with task-specific learning, reducing the likelihood of overfitting, especially on smaller datasets.

4.1.3 Benefits of Transfer Learning for Medical Imaging

a) **Reducing Training Time:** One of the major advantages of using pre-trained CNN models is the significant reduction in training time. Training a CNN from scratch requires large datasets and considerable computational resources to adjust millions of parameters. In medical tasks, where labeled data is scarce, training from scratch is impractical.

b) **Overcoming Data Scarcity** Medical imaging datasets are typically small due to the difficulty of collecting and labeling data, as well as privacy concerns. Transfer learning helps address this issue by allowing models trained on large non-medical datasets to be applied to medical tasks.

4.2 U-Net, ResNet, and Advanced Architectures

General-purpose CNN architecture often needs to be adapted or extended to meet the unique challenges of medical applications, such as segmentation, classification, and detection. Specialized CNN architectures like **U-Net** and **ResNet** have emerged as top performers, offering enhanced accuracy and performance for specific tasks in medical imaging. Here's an overview of these specialized CNN architectures and how they excel in medical applications:

4.2.1. U-Net for Segmentation

U-Net is a CNN architecture specifically designed for medical image segmentation. It was introduced in 2015 and is widely used for segmenting organs, tumors, and other anatomical structures in medical images like MRI, CT, and ultrasound scans. The U-Net architecture is particularly effective in scenarios where precise pixel-wise segmentation is required, such as in cancerous tumor delineation or organ boundary detection.

Architecture

- **Encoder-Decoder Structure**: U-Net has a symmetric encoder-decoder structure. The **encoder** (left side) is responsible for extracting hierarchical features from the input image, while the **decoder** (right side) reconstructs the high-resolution output from these features.
- **Skip Connections**: One of the key innovations in U-Net is the use of **skip connections** that directly link corresponding layers in the encoder and decoder. These connections allow the model to transfer high-resolution features from the early layers of the encoder to the later stages of the decoder, which helps in recovering spatial information that is often lost during down sampling.

Enhanced Performance in Medical Applications

- **Accurate Segmentation**: U-Net excels at segmenting small and irregularly shaped structures, which is essential in tasks like tumor detection or vessel segmentation. The architecture's ability to capture fine details makes it particularly useful for delineating tumor boundaries in brain MRI scans or identifying polyps in endoscopy images.

- **High Efficiency with Limited Data**: U-Net performs well even on small medical datasets. Its design allows for accurate segmentation with fewer labeled examples, which is crucial in medical imaging, where acquiring large annotated datasets can be challenging.
- **Versatility Across Modalities**: U-Net is widely used across different imaging modalities, including MRI, CT, and ultrasound, for tasks such as liver, brain, and cardiac segmentation.

Applications

- **Tumor Segmentation**: U-Net is commonly used to segment tumors in brain MRI scans, breast cancer mammograms, and lung cancer CT scans.
- **Organ Segmentation**: It is applied to segment organs like the liver, kidneys, and lungs in CT and MRI scans for surgical planning or volumetric analysis.
- **Vessel Segmentation**: U-Net is used to segment blood vessels in retina images for diabetic retinopathy diagnosis or in brain images to analyze cerebrovascular diseases.

4.2.2. ResNet for Improved Accuracy

ResNet (Residual Network), introduced in 2015, is another specialized CNN architecture that has achieved remarkable success in medical image classification tasks. Its key innovation is the introduction of **residual connections**, which help mitigate the problem of vanishing gradients in deep networks, allowing the model to be trained more efficiently while achieving higher accuracy Abdou, M. A. (2022).

Architecture

- **Residual Blocks**: ResNet consists of residual blocks, which include **skip connections** that bypass one or more layers. These connections allow the model to learn identity mappings, making it easier to train very deep networks without performance degradation.
- **Deep Architecture**: ResNet can have hundreds or even thousands of layers due to its residual design, which prevents the network from suffering from vanishing gradients, a common issue in very deep networks.

Enhanced Performance in Medical Applications

- **Improved Classification Accuracy**: ResNet's deep architecture allows it to capture complex features in medical images, leading to improved classification accuracy. This is particularly useful in tasks like identifying subtle differences between healthy and abnormal tissues in histopathology images or classifying diseases from radiology scans.
- **Reduced Overfitting**: ResNet's ability to prevent overfitting makes it ideal for medical datasets, which are often limited in size. The residual connections help the network generalize better, even with a smaller number of training examples.
- **Transfer Learning**: ResNet is widely used in transfer learning, where pre-trained models on large datasets (such as ImageNet) are fine-tuned for medical imaging tasks. This significantly reduces training time while maintaining high performance.

Applications

- **Disease Classification**: ResNet is used in tasks such as classifying chest X-rays for pneumonia, tuberculosis, and COVID-19 detection. Its high accuracy makes it suitable for identifying diseases with subtle visual cues.
- **Pathology Image Analysis**: In digital pathology, ResNet is applied to classify histopathology images, distinguishing between cancerous and non-cancerous cells. It is particularly effective in detecting breast cancer, lung cancer, and colon cancer from pathology slides.
- **Retinal Image Classification**: ResNet is used to detect diabetic retinopathy from retinal fundus images, helping to classify images into different severity levels of the disease.

4.2.3. Other Notable CNN Architectures in Medical Applications

VGG (Visual Geometry Group Network)

VGG is another popular CNN architecture used in medical imaging, particularly for classification tasks. It consists of a simple, sequential structure with multiple convolutional layers, followed by fully connected layers.

- **Significance in Medical Imaging**: VGG is used for tasks like classifying skin lesions in dermatoscopic images, detecting lung diseases from chest X-rays, and identifying different stages of diabetic retinopathy.
- **Limitations**: While VGG achieves good performance, it requires more computational resources and memory compared to ResNet, making it less efficient for very deep networks.

DenseNet (Densely Connected Convolutional Network)

DenseNet introduces dense connections between layers, where each layer receives input from all preceding layers, enhancing feature reuse and improving gradient flow.

- **Advantages in Medical Imaging**: DenseNet's densely connected layers allow it to learn complex representations, making it highly effective for medical tasks like segmentation and classification. DenseNet has been used to detect abnormalities in brain MRI scans and classify breast cancer in mammograms.
- **Improved Efficiency**: DenseNet achieves better performance with fewer parameters than ResNet, making it more efficient in terms of memory and computation.

4.3 Explainable AI in CNNs

As the adoption of Convolutional Neural Networks (CNNs) and other deep learning models in medical applications continues to rise, the need for explainable AI (XAI) has become increasingly critical. The opaque nature of CNNs—often referred to as "black boxes"—poses significant challenges, particularly in high-stakes fields like healthcare. The importance of interpretability in medical AI systems cannot be overstated, as it directly impacts clinical decision-making, trust in AI systems, and patient safety (Van der Velden et al.,2022).

4.3.1. The Importance of Interpretability in Medical AI Systems

a) Trust and Acceptance
   - **Building Trust**: Clinicians must trust AI systems to integrate them effectively into clinical workflows. If healthcare professionals cannot understand how a model arrived at a specific conclusion or diagnosis, their willingness to rely on these systems diminishes.
   - **Enhancing Acceptance**: The interpretability of CNN decisions fosters greater acceptance of AI tools among healthcare providers. Clinicians are more likely to adopt AI systems that provide clear reasoning behind their recommendations.

b) Clinical Decision Support
   - **Supporting Clinical Judgments**: Explainable AI aids clinicians in understanding the rationale behind model predictions, enabling them to make informed decisions. When a CNN suggests a diagnosis based on an image, clinicians need insights into which features influenced that decision.
   - **Augmenting Human Expertise**: Interpretability helps integrate AI insights with human expertise, allowing clinicians to validate and contextualize AI recommendations. This synergy can lead to more accurate diagnoses and treatment plans.

c) Compliance and Accountability
   - **Regulatory Requirements**: The growing use of AI in healthcare brings scrutiny from regulatory bodies. Many regulatory frameworks demand a level of transparency in AI systems. Demonstrating how a model makes decisions is essential for compliance with ethical and legal standards.
   - **Accountability**: In the event of a misdiagnosis or adverse outcome, understanding the decision-making process of an AI system is crucial for accountability. Explainable AI helps delineate responsibilities between AI systems and healthcare providers.

4.3.2. Ongoing Research into Making CNN Decisions Explainable

Recognizing the challenges posed by the black-box nature of CNNs, researchers are actively exploring various methodologies to enhance the interpretability of these models in medical applications. Here are some key areas of focus:

a) Visualization Techniques
   - **Saliency Maps**: Techniques like saliency maps and gradient-weighted class activation mapping (Grad-CAM) visualize the areas of an image that most influence a model's prediction. By highlighting important regions in medical images, such as tumors in radiology scans, clinicians can better understand the basis for a CNN's decision.
   - **Feature Visualization**: Researchers are developing methods to visualize the features learned by CNN layers. By examining the features that contribute to certain predictions, clinicians can gain insights into the underlying processes of the model.

b) Model-Agnostic Approaches
   - **Local Interpretable Model-Agnostic Explanations (LIME)**: LIME is a technique that generates interpretable models around individual predictions. By perturbing input data and

observing changes in predictions, LIME helps to create a local model that explains the behavior of complex models like CNNs.

- **SHapley Additive exPlanations (SHAP)**: SHAP values provide a unified measure of feature importance by quantifying the contribution of each feature to the model's predictions. This approach aids clinicians in understanding which aspects of medical images are pivotal for diagnoses.

c) Integration of Clinical Knowledge

- **Incorporating Domain Expertise**: Research is exploring the integration of clinical knowledge into AI models to enhance interpretability. By aligning model predictions with established medical guidelines and expert opinions, systems can offer more interpretable outputs.
- **Symbolic AI and Logic-Based Approaches**: Combining CNNs with symbolic AI can facilitate the creation of more interpretable models. These approaches can provide human-readable rules and explanations based on the model's decisions.

d) Human-Computer Interaction

- **User-Centric Interfaces**: Developing user-friendly interfaces that present model predictions alongside interpretive information can enhance clinicians' understanding of AI decisions. Effective visualization and communication of AI insights are crucial for seamless integration into clinical practice.

5. CHALLENGES AND LIMITATIONS OF CNNS IN MEDICAL IMAGING

Convolutional Neural Networks (CNNs) have become a transformative tool in medical imaging, improving diagnostic accuracy and aiding treatment decisions. However, despite these advancements, there are several challenges and limitations associated with using CNNs in this domain.

5.1. Data Availability and Quality

Medical imaging datasets are often limited in size due to privacy concerns, the need for expert labeling, and complex regulatory requirements. CNNs are typically data-hungry, requiring vast amounts of labeled images for effective training. This lack of large, annotated datasets can lead to poor model performance, particularly in rare diseases where data scarcity is common. Moreover, data quality and consistency vary across institutions, affecting model generalizability. Differences in imaging equipment, protocols, and patient demographics introduce variabilities that CNNs struggle to handle without extensive domain-specific adjustments.

5.2. High Computational Costs

Training CNNs, especially deep networks with multiple layers, demands substantial computational resources. High-performance GPUs, specialized hardware, and significant energy consumption are necessary, making CNN implementation costly and inaccessible to resource-limited healthcare facilities. This computational complexity also makes real-time processing challenging, which is critical in clinical settings where timely diagnosis is crucial.

5.3. Interpretability and Trust

CNNs are often described as "black boxes" because they learn abstract representations that are not easily interpretable. In medical imaging, where trust and accountability are paramount, this lack of transparency poses a significant challenge. Clinicians and radiologists may be hesitant to adopt CNN-based systems if they cannot understand or explain the model's decisions, which can hinder integration into healthcare practices. Efforts to enhance model interpretability, such as using heatmaps to visualize areas of focus, only partially address this issue and do not provide complete insights into the decision-making process.

5.4. Risk of Overfitting and Generalization

Medical imaging datasets are often diverse in imaging modalities (e.g., MRI, CT, X-rays), and overfitting is a common problem when training CNNs on specific datasets. A model trained on data from a single hospital or demographic may not generalize well to other populations or imaging systems. Overfitting also limits the model's adaptability to new cases, especially those involving subtle variations or rare conditions that were underrepresented in the training data.

5.5. Ethical and Privacy Concerns

CNN models in medical imaging often require patient data, raising ethical and privacy issues. In some cases, the data used for training cannot be adequately anonymized, posing risks of data leakage and compromising patient confidentiality. Ethical considerations also arise regarding the use of AI in medical decision-making; questions around liability, accountability, and fairness remain largely unresolved.

5.6. Regulatory and Legal Barriers

Deploying CNN-based tools in clinical settings requires regulatory approval to ensure they meet safety and efficacy standards. However, the evolving nature of CNN models makes it difficult to standardize and gain approval, as any change or update may require a new round of evaluation and certification. This regulatory burden slows down innovation and integration into healthcare systems.

In summary, while CNNs have shown great potential in medical imaging, challenges such as limited data availability, high computational costs, interpretability issues, risks of overfitting, privacy concerns, and regulatory barriers hinder their widespread adoption. Addressing these limitations requires interdisciplinary efforts, combining advances in AI with improvements in data access, ethical frameworks, computational resources, and healthcare policies

6. FUTURE DIRECTIONS FOR CNNS IN MEDICAL IMAGING

The future of Convolutional Neural Networks (CNNs) in medical imaging promises significant advancements, with ongoing research aimed at overcoming current limitations and expanding CNN applications in healthcare. Several future directions hold potential for transforming CNNs into more robust, accessible, and effective tools in clinical environments.

6.1. Improved Data Availability and Synthetic Data Generation

One of the primary limitations in CNN-based medical imaging is the scarcity of large, labeled datasets due to privacy concerns and the need for expert annotations. A promising future direction is the use of synthetic data generation techniques, such as Generative Adversarial Networks (GANs), which can create realistic medical images to augment limited datasets. Synthetic data can be used to address data imbalance and improve model training for rare diseases, enhancing CNN performance without the ethical concerns associated with real patient data.

6.2. Transfer Learning and Pre-trained Models

Transfer learning has shown promise in medical imaging by allowing CNNs pre-trained on large general datasets to adapt to specific medical imaging tasks. This approach reduces the data requirements and training time, making it suitable for smaller datasets typical in healthcare. The development of dedicated pre-trained models specific to medical domains could further enhance the efficiency and accuracy of CNNs across various imaging modalities and diagnostic tasks.

6.3. Explainable AI (XAI) for Interpretability

Enhancing interpretability is essential for clinical acceptance, as clinicians need to understand CNN outputs to trust the technology. The future of CNNs in medical imaging includes integrating Explainable AI (XAI) methods to provide clear visualizations and explanations for predictions. Techniques such as attention maps, saliency maps, and Grad-CAM can help visualize which areas of an image influenced a CNN's decision, increasing transparency. More advanced interpretability tools that break down complex decision-making into understandable insights could bridge the trust gap between clinicians and AI systems.

6.4. Multimodal and Hybrid Models

Many medical diagnoses rely on information from multiple sources, such as imaging, clinical notes, and laboratory tests. CNNs could be combined with other AI models to analyze multimodal data, creating hybrid models that integrate various data types. This approach could improve diagnostic accuracy and enable a more holistic understanding of a patient's health status. Future models may blend CNNs with natural language processing (NLP) for clinical notes or reinforcement learning for adaptive decision-making, paving the way for comprehensive diagnostic tools.

6.5. Real-time and Edge Computing Applications

As CNNs become more efficient, they can be implemented on smaller, more localized devices, enabling real-time analysis at the point of care. Future CNN models optimized for edge computing could process medical images directly on devices, such as portable ultrasound machines or smartphone-based diagnostic tools. This development could bring advanced diagnostic capabilities to remote or resource-limited settings, facilitating quicker diagnoses and broader healthcare accessibility.

6.6. Federated Learning for Data Privacy

Privacy concerns are significant in healthcare, making federated learning a promising direction. This approach allows CNN models to train on decentralized data across multiple hospitals or institutions without moving data off-site, preserving patient privacy while still providing high-quality training data. By using federated learning, CNNs could learn from diverse patient populations, increasing their generalizability without compromising data security.

6.7. Integration with Clinical Workflows and Regulatory Support

For CNNs to have a transformative impact on healthcare, they must be integrated into existing clinical workflows. Future CNN development will likely focus on seamless compatibility with clinical software and electronic health record (EHR) systems, ensuring that CNN outputs can be accessed and utilized easily by healthcare professionals. Additionally, advancements in regulatory frameworks specific to AI-driven healthcare tools could streamline the approval process, making it easier to bring CNN-based medical imaging solutions to clinical settings.

In summary, the future of CNNs in medical imaging is directed toward creating more accurate, interpretable, and accessible models through synthetic data, transfer learning, explainable AI, and privacy-preserving methods like federated learning. By addressing these areas, CNNs could play an increasingly vital role in global healthcare, making sophisticated diagnostic tools available in diverse clinical environments.

7. COMPARISON BETWEEN CNNS AND TRADITIONAL IMAGE ANALYSIS METHODS

Convolutional Neural Networks (CNNs) have revolutionized image analysis, outperforming traditional methods in numerous applications. The key differences lie in their approach to feature extraction, scalability, and adaptability.

7.1. Feature Extraction

Traditional Methods:

Traditional image analysis relies on hand-crafted features, such as edges, textures, or shapes, extracted using techniques like SIFT, HOG, or wavelet transforms. These methods require domain expertise to design effective features and are often limited to capturing low-level patterns.

CNNs:

CNNs automatically learn features from data through convolutional layers. They extract hierarchical features, from edges in early layers to complex patterns in deeper layers, without manual intervention. This adaptability eliminates the need for domain-specific feature engineering.

7.2. Scalability and Performance

Traditional Methods:

Traditional algorithms struggle with large datasets and complex patterns due to their fixed feature sets and computational constraints. Their performance often plateaus as data complexity increases.

CNNs:

CNNs scale effectively with larger datasets, improving performance as more data becomes available. Techniques like transfer learning allow CNNs to leverage pre-trained models, enhancing efficiency for new tasks.

7.3. Adaptability

Traditional Methods:

Customization for different tasks often requires redesigning features and algorithms, making traditional methods less flexible.

CNNs:

CNNs are highly adaptable, capable of fine-tuning for specific tasks with minimal reconfiguration. This makes them suitable for diverse applications, from medical imaging to autonomous driving.

While traditional methods offer simplicity and interpretability, CNNs provide superior accuracy, scalability, and adaptability, making them the dominant choice for modern image analysis tasks

8. CONCLUSION

In conclusion, Convolutional Neural Networks (CNNs) have significantly transformed the landscape of medical imaging, offering remarkable advancements in the diagnosis and treatment of various diseases. Their ability to automatically extract hierarchical features from complex medical images has made CNNs indispensable in tasks such as detecting tumors, classifying diseases, and segmenting anatomical structures. By leveraging large datasets and deep learning techniques, CNNs can outperform traditional diagnostic methods, delivering faster, more accurate, and sometimes even earlier detection of abnormalities.

The integration of CNNs into clinical workflows enhances not only diagnostic precision but also treatment planning, improving patient outcomes. As CNN models evolve with more sophisticated architectures and the availability of diverse medical imaging data, their potential continues to grow. However, challenges remain, such as the need for interpretability, regulatory approval, and addressing ethical concerns related to data privacy and bias.

Moving forward, collaboration between AI researchers, clinicians, and healthcare professionals will be crucial to ensuring the successful and responsible deployment of CNNs in medical imaging. With ongoing advancements, CNN-based systems are poised to revolutionize healthcare, empowering practitioners with more accurate tools for personalized medicine and ultimately transforming patient care on a global scale.

REFERENCES

Aamir, M., Bazai, S., Bhatti, U. A., Dayo, Z. A., Liu, J., & Zhang, K. (2023, January). Applications of machine learning in medicine: Current trends and prospects. In *2023 Global Conference on Wireless and Optical Technologies (GCWOT)* (pp. 1-4). IEEE. DOI: 10.1109/GCWOT57803.2023.10064665

Aamir, M., Rahman, Z., Abro, W. A., Bhatti, U. A., Dayo, Z. A., & Ishfaq, M. (2023). Brain tumor classification utilizing deep features derived from high-quality regions in MRI images. *Biomedical Signal Processing and Control*, *85*, 104988. DOI: 10.1016/j.bspc.2023.104988

Aamir, M., Rahman, Z., Abro, W. A., Tahir, M., & Ahmed, S. M. (2019). An optimized architecture of image classification using convolutional neural network. *International Journal of Image. Graphics and Signal Processing*, *11*(10), 30–39. DOI: 10.5815/ijigsp.2019.10.05

Aamir, M., Rahman, Z., Dayo, Z. A., Abro, W. A., Uddin, M. I., Khan, I., Imran, A. S., Ali, Z., Ishfaq, M., Guan, Y., & Hu, Z. (2022). A deep learning approach for brain tumor classification using MRI images. *Computers & Electrical Engineering*, *101*, 108105. DOI: 10.1016/j.compeleceng.2022.108105

Abdou, M. A. (2022). Literature review: Efficient deep neural networks techniques for medical image analysis. *Neural Computing & Applications*, *34*(8), 5791–5812. DOI: 10.1007/s00521-022-06960-9

Aljuaid, A., & Anwar, M. (2022). Survey of supervised learning for medical image processing. *SN Computer Science*, *3*(4), 292. DOI: 10.1007/s42979-022-01166-1 PMID: 35602289

Alskaf, E., Dutta, U., Scannell, C. M., & Chiribiri, A. (2022). Deep learning applications in coronary anatomy imaging: A systematic review and meta-analysis. *Journal of Medical Artificial Intelligence*, *5*, 11. DOI: 10.21037/jmai-22-36 PMID: 36861064

Alsubaie, M. G., Luo, S., & Shaukat, K. (2024). Alzheimer's Disease Detection Using Deep Learning on Neuroimaging: A Systematic Review. *Machine Learning and Knowledge Extraction*, *6*(1), 464–505. DOI: 10.3390/make6010024

Asia, A. O., Zhu, C. Z., Althubiti, S. A., Al-Alimi, D., Xiao, Y. L., Ouyang, P. B., & Al-Qaness, M. A. (2022). Detection of diabetic retinopathy in retinal fundus images using CNN classification models. *Electronics (Basel)*, *11*(17), 2740. DOI: 10.3390/electronics11172740

Cantatore, A., & Müller, P. (2011). Introduction to computed tomography.

Chattopadhyay, A., & Maitra, M. (2022). MRI-based brain tumour image detection using CNN based deep learning method. *Neuroscience informatics, 2*(4), 100060. https://doi.org/DOI: 10.1016/j.neuri.2022.100060

Cui, N. (2018, April). Applying gradient descent in convolutional neural networks. In *Journal of Physics: Conference Series* (Vol. 1004, p. 012027). IOP Publishing. https://doi.org DOI: 10.1088/1742-6596/1004/1/012027

Faghihi, A., Fathollahi, M., & Rajabi, R. (2024). Diagnosis of skin cancer using VGG16 and VGG19 based transfer learning models. *Multimedia Tools and Applications*, *83*(19), 57495–57510. DOI: 10.1007/s11042-023-17735-2

Ghorbani, A., Ouyang, D., Abid, A., He, B., Chen, J. H., Harrington, R. A., Liang, D. H., Ashley, E. A., & Zou, J. Y. (2020). Deep learning interpretation of echocardiograms. *NPJ Digital Medicine*, *3*(1), 10. DOI: 10.1038/s41746-019-0216-8 PMID: 31993508

Guan, Y., Aamir, M., Rahman, Z., Ali, A., Abro, W. A., Dayo, Z. A., ... & Hu, Z. (2021). A framework for efficient brain tumor classification using MRI images.

Ibrahim, A. U., Ozsoz, M., Serte, S., Al-Turjman, F., & Yakoi, P. S. (2024). Pneumonia classification using deep learning from chest X-ray images during COVID-19. *Cognitive Computation*, *16*(4), 1589–1601. DOI: 10.1007/s12559-020-09787-5 PMID: 33425044

Javed, R., Abbas, T., Khan, A. H., Daud, A., Bukhari, A., & Alharbey, R. (2024). Deep learning for lungs cancer detection: A review. *Artificial Intelligence Review*, *57*(8), 197. DOI: 10.1007/s10462-024-10807-1

Kumar, R., Kumbharkar, P., Vanam, S., & Sharma, S. (2024). Medical images classification using deep learning: A survey. *Multimedia Tools and Applications*, *83*(7), 19683–19728. DOI: 10.1007/s11042-023-15576-7

Liu, X., Wang, H., Li, Z., & Qin, L. (2021). Deep learning in ECG diagnosis: A review. *Knowledge-Based Systems*, *227*, 107187. DOI: 10.1016/j.knosys.2021.107187

McKinney, S. M., Sieniek, M., Godbole, V., Godwin, J., Antropova, N., Ashrafian, H., Back, T., Chesus, M., Corrado, G. S., Darzi, A., Etemadi, M., Garcia-Vicente, F., Gilbert, F. J., Halling-Brown, M., Hassabis, D., Jansen, S., Karthikesalingam, A., Kelly, C. J., King, D., & Shetty, S. (2020, January). International evaluation of an AI system for breast cancer screening. *Nature*, *577*(7788), 89–94. DOI: 10.1038/s41586-019-1799-6 PMID: 31894144

Mizutani, H. (1994, May). The back propagation method for CNN. In *Proceedings of IEEE International Symposium on Circuits and Systems-ISCAS'94* (Vol. 6, pp. 463-466). IEEE. DOI: 10.1109/ISCAS.1994.409626

Muchuchuti, S., & Viriri, S. (2023). Retinal disease detection using deep learning techniques: A comprehensive review. *Journal of Imaging*, *9*(4), 84. DOI: 10.3390/jimaging9040084 PMID: 37103235

Muhammad, K., Ullah, A., Lloret, J., Del Ser, J., & de Albuquerque, V. H. C. (2020). Deep learning for safe autonomous driving: Current challenges and future directions. *IEEE Transactions on Intelligent Transportation Systems*, *22*(7), 4316–4336. DOI: 10.1109/TITS.2020.3032227

Pasveer, B. (1989). Knowledge of shadows: The introduction of X-ray images in medicine. *Sociology of Health & Illness*, *11*(4), 360–381. DOI: 10.1111/1467-9566.ep11373066 PMID: 29363814

Powers, J., & Kremkau, F. (2011). Medical ultrasound systems. *Interface Focus*, *1*(4), 477–489. DOI: 10.1098/rsfs.2011.0027 PMID: 22866226

Ruan, F., Zhang, X., Zhu, D., Xu, Z., Wan, S., & Qi, L. (2020). Deep learning for real-time image steganalysis: A survey. *Journal of Real-Time Image Processing*, *17*(1), 149–160. DOI: 10.1007/s11554-019-00915-5

Salehi, A. W., Khan, S., Gupta, G., Alabduallah, B. I., Almjally, A., Alsolai, H., Siddiqui, T., & Mellit, A. (2023). A study of CNN and transfer learning in medical imaging: Advantages, challenges, future scope. *Sustainability (Basel)*, *15*(7), 5930. DOI: 10.3390/su15075930

Siddique, N., Paheding, S., Elkin, C. P., & Devabhaktuni, V. (2021). U-net and its variants for medical image segmentation: A review of theory and applications. *IEEE Access : Practical Innovations, Open Solutions*, *9*, 82031–82057. DOI: 10.1109/ACCESS.2021.3086020

Singh, S. P., Wang, L., Gupta, S., Goli, H., Padmanabhan, P., & Gulyás, B. (2020). 3D deep learning on medical images: A review. *Sensors (Basel)*, *20*(18), 5097. DOI: 10.3390/s20185097 PMID: 32906819

Sohail, M., Shoukat, I. A., Fatima, H., Jafri, M. R., Yaqub, M. A., & Liotta, A. (2024). Deep Learning Based Multi Pose Human Face Matching System. *IEEE Access : Practical Innovations, Open Solutions*, *12*, 26046–26061. DOI: 10.1109/ACCESS.2024.3366451

Sultana, F., Sufian, A., & Dutta, P. (2020). Evolution of image segmentation using deep convolutional neural network: A survey. *Knowledge-Based Systems*, *201*, 106062. DOI: 10.1016/j.knosys.2020.106062

Talagala, S. L., & Lowe, I. J. (1991). Introduction to magnetic resonance imaging. *Concepts in Magnetic Resonance*, *3*(3), 145–159. DOI: 10.1002/cmr.1820030303

Van der Velden, B. H., Kuijf, H. J., Gilhuijs, K. G., & Viergever, M. A. (2022). Explainable artificial intelligence (XAI) in deep learning-based medical image analysis. *Medical Image Analysis*, *79*, 102470. DOI: 10.1016/j.media.2022.102470 PMID: 35576821

Wang, M., & Deng, W. (2021). Deep face recognition: A survey. *Neurocomputing*, *429*, 215–244. DOI: 10.1016/j.neucom.2020.10.081

Chapter 10
Data Augmentation Techniques in Deep Image Processing

Fikriye Ataman
https://orcid.org/0000-0002-0257-7730
Van Yüzüncü Yıl University, Turkey

ABSTRACT

Image data augmentation is a technique for artificially expanding and diversifying existing image datasets. This method is beneficial when training data is insufficient for machine learning and deep learning models. It allows models to generalize better during training and reduces overfitting. The main techniques include geometric transformations, color and light changes, noise addition, optical distortions, and modern blending methods. These methods expose the model to more diversity by simulating real-world variations. Thus, data collection and labeling costs are reduced while the model's performance and generalization capacity increase. Data augmentation plays a role in the basis of success, especially in studies where medical images are processed. This study explains the techniques used for image augmentation in detail. It also reveals the performance results of the methods used on data sets and their effects on deep models. The study includes the most frequently used methods and provides a detailed literature review.

1. INTRODUCTION

The relationship between artificial intelligence (AI) and medical imaging has become much more substantial. Medical imaging visualizes the body's internal structures to diagnose and treat disease. This process allows physicians to more accurately diagnose disease, personalize treatment plans, and track patient recovery (Aamir et al.,2023). Many diseases can be treated more successfully if they are diagnosed early (Carrasco Ramírez, 2024; Khalifa et al., 2024; Mahesh Batra & Reche, 2023; Pinto-Coelho, 2023; Rana & Shuford, 2024; Zatloukal et al., 2020). Medical imaging can detect disease earlier, allowing treatment to begin sooner (Guan et al., 2021). Medical images also give doctors detailed information about disease type, size, and location. This reduces the risk of misdiagnosis and allows the proper treatment to be chosen(Carrasco Ramírez, 2024; Khalifa et al., 2024; Mahesh Batra & Reche, 2023; Pinto-Coelho, 2023; Rana & Shuford, 2024). This is especially important for rare diseases (D. He et al., 2024; Zheng et al., 2024). In addition, imaging results can enable detailed preoperative planning for surgical procedures. This can shorten surgery time and reduce the risk of complications. During the treatment

DOI: 10.4018/979-8-3693-9816-6.ch010

process, medical imaging also helps evaluate the treatment's effectiveness and modify the treatment plan if necessary. Medical imaging can perform many procedures with more minor or even no incisions. This means less pain, faster recovery, and fewer complications for patients (Carrasco Ramírez, 2024; Khalifa et al., 2024; Rana & Shuford, 2024). Many different techniques are used to produce medical images. Standard imaging techniques include positron emission tomography, x-ray, magnetic resonance imaging, computed tomography, and ultrasound (Aamir et al., 2022). The processing of medical images, which impact people's lives, is naturally of great importance.

Medical image processing faces numerous challenges, including the complex nature of images (Zheng et al., 2024), the scarcity of high-quality data for specific diseases, the cost of accurately labeling medical images, and ethical concerns about data privacy and security (Jalal et al., 2021; Koohi-Moghadam & Bae, 2023; Sen et al., 2020; Tripathi & Musiolik, 2022). The reliability and transparency of AI models are crucial, and the distribution of data used for model training affects their ability to generalize to real-world data. The lack of data also negatively impacts model performance, as it can lead to overfitting and impairing the model's ability to generalize to new data. To address these challenges, research is being conducted to develop more extensive data sets, advanced algorithms, and powerful computational approaches (Jalal et al., 2021; Koohi-Moghadam & Bae, 2023; Sen et al., 2020; Tripathi & Musiolik, 2022).

Regardless of how big the problems are, the power of the advancement of medical image processing is straightforward (Jalal et al., 2021; Koohi-Moghadam & Bae, 2023). In recent years, the impact of deep neural networks on medical image processing has increased significantly. However, it is well known that medical data is often under-observed by nature, and the low volume of image data is a significant constraint on model training and performance. One important approach to address this is to increase the data sample size using image data augmentation (DA) methods. This study provides in-depth information on DA techniques developed in recent years. It also provides a detailed comparison of experimental results obtained by applying the models to state-of-the-art datasets. This study will provide researchers in the field with detailed information about DA techniques. By comparing the experimental results, it will help researchers to decide which technique or model is more appropriate for their data.

1.1. Image Data Augmentation (IDA)

IDA is a technique that increases the size and diversity of image data by creating new images from an existing dataset (Gao et al., 2019; C. Zhang et al., 2023; Zhao et al., 2023). It is used in computer vision fields like object recognition, classification, model training (Goodfellow et al., 2020), abstract visual reasoning (S. Hu et al., 2021), and segmentation(Lee et al., 2023). IDA methods improve classification performance in limited training data and can prevent overfitting by learning about statistical noise in the training data. It also enhances generalization performance in object detection and makes models more robust to changes in input data. DA is also used in abstract visual reasoning to create new models consistent with task rules(Goodfellow et al., 2020).

1.2. The Importance of Data Augmentation

DA is important because ML models contribute to performing several image processing tasks, including segmentation, object detection, and classification.

DA is used in an abstract visual reasoning task to create new visual models consistent with the underlying rules. Thanks to the DA technique, the model learns the task's rules more efficiently and adapts to new data at a more acceptable rate (W. He et al., 2023)

Situations may arise where the available data is missing, making it necessary to take action against rare events and run ML models. DA is a preferred technique for filling the data gaps in rare events and effectively utilizing ML algorithms (Min et al., 2023).

Deformations and variations in the data can hinder the desired result in object detection problems. The DA technique can solve these obstacles (H. Lee et al., 2023).

DL has achieved significant success in various computer vision tasks, such as segmentation, object identification, and image classification. However, inadequate datasets are utilized to train DL models, which can result in overfitting and poor generalization. Increasing the data sample size is an important measure to counter these problems.

There are many areas, like abstract visual reasoning (C. Zhang et al., 2023), image-to-image translation, hyperspectral image classification (Gao et al., 2019), where DA is applied(Xu et al., 2023).

Image classification is challenging because natural images have high intra-class and low inter-class diversity (Aamir et al., 2019). Cross-class learning aims to improve classification performance by learning the features that distinguish different classes. DA is a common approach used to improve the performance of cross-class learning. DA generates new data points that are consistent with the task's ground rules. DA will help the model learn features that distinguish between different classes more effectively (Tokozume et al., 2018; Zhu et al., 2017).

Another application area where DA is effective is Federated Learning (FL). FL and DA are two complementary technologies. FL is a collaborative ML method where user data never leaves users' devices, and the training process is distributed among many users (Hao et al., 2021; B. Hu et al., 2023; H. Zhang et al., 2023; J. Zhang & Jiang, 2022).

FL prevents sensitive data from being collected on a central server. DA methods can be integrated with FL and applied on local devices, and the model can be updated with augmented data from local data. The model is trained without sending data to a central server, and data privacy is protected(Hao et al., 2021; B. Hu et al., 2023; J. Zhang & Jiang, 2022).

FL brings together heterogeneous data sources from different institutions or devices. DA increases diversity by being applied to each of these heterogeneous data sets and makes the model more generalizable than DA alone. For example, DA performed with data from different demographic groups can reduce the model's biases(Hao et al., 2021; B. Hu et al., 2023; Menegatti et al., 2023; H. Zhang et al., 2023; J. Zhang & Jiang, 2022).

In some institutions, DA may have limited data sources. DA can be used locally to expand these small data sets and allow FL to benefit from these devices. For example, a few images on a mobile device can be used to train the model by augmenting them with augmentation methods(Hao et al., 2021; Menegatti et al., 2023; J. Zhang & Jiang, 2022).

DA can be included in FL processes by creating synthetic data with generative models. Using this synthetic data, FL can increase the performance of models without accessing sensitive data.

DA can increase anonymity in FL, especially in sensitive data scenarios. For example, anonymizing images with geometric transformations increases data privacy. FL trains the model securely with this anonymized augmented data. For example, FL and DA can be used together on medical images from different hospitals. Each hospital increases the overall success of the model by augmenting local data. However, there may be some disadvantages. DA and FL processes may require high computational resources on local devices. Some devices or institutions may have less or low-quality data, this data imbalance situation may limit the effect of FL. Also, in FL, each device should perform DA operations synchronously. FL and DA form a strong collaboration, especially in scenarios with sensitive and small data sets. FL and DA improve model performance while ensuring data privacy. Further integration of these technologies may provide more effective healthcare, finance, and mobile application solutions(Hao et al., 2021; B. Hu et al., 2023; Koohi-Moghadam & Bae, 2023; Menegatti et al., 2023; H. Zhang et al., 2023; J. Zhang & Jiang, 2022).

Deep neural networks (DNNs) have attained considerable success in image classification, object detection, and many other diverse computer vision tasks. DNNs often struggle to provide accurate uncertainty estimates, which can be important for jobs such as diagnosing disease and autonomous driving(D. He et al., 2024; Jalal et al., 2021; Koohi-Moghadam & Bae, 2023; Sen et al., 2020). DA is a common approach used to improve the robustness and uncertainty estimates of DNNs. It helps the DNN learn to generalize to new data, including competing examples. DA encourages the DNN to learn more informative features, allowing the model to make more accurate uncertainty estimates (Hendrycks et al., 2020).

DL is vital in computer vision and represents state-of-the-art results in many tasks, such as object detection, segmentation, and classification (Aamir et al., 2023). DL models need enormous amounts and various training data. DA can help fulfill this need by generating new instances from current data sets. Collecting enough diverse images for DL models could be difficult and expensive. Generating artificial image data creates an excellent comfort zone.

Table 1 includes the results of experimental-related studies conducted with state-of-the-art data sets.

Table 1. Overall performance of DA algorithms

Algorithm	Data Set	Accuracy %	Reference
Mixup	MNIST	%99.7	(H. Zhang et al., 2018)
GAN	MNIST CIFAR-10 CelebA	%98 %70 %80	(I. Goodfellow et al., 2020)
CycleGAN	Plant Village	%95	(Zhu et al., 2017)
RDAGAN	PASCAL VOC2007	%84.1	(Lee et al., 2023)
PatchGAN (Pix2Pix)	CelebA(a->b) CelebA(b->a)	%99 %98.7	(Isola et al., 2018)
PRAN	Indian Pines Pavia University	%99.5 %98.2	(Gao et al., 2019)
BCLearning	CIFAR-10	%93.7	(Tokozume et al., 2018)
CutMix	CIFAR-10	%95.2	(Yun et al., 2019)
AugMix	CIFAR-10	%96.4	(Hendrycks et al., 2020)
PuzzleMix	CIFAR-100	%77.1	(J.-H. Kim et al., 2020)

continued on following page

Table 1. Continued

Algorithm	Data Set	Accuracy %	Reference
Co-Mixup	CIFAR-10	%96.3	(J. H. Kim et al., 2021)
SuperMix	CIFAR-10	%97.2	(Dabouei et al., 2021)

1.3. The Challenges of Data Augmentation

The accountability of the model to be used plays a critical role in the diagnosis and treatment processes. It is necessary to explain why and how the models' outputs are formed. Otherwise, making a wrong diagnosis can have fatal risks (Altaf et al., 2019; Chlap et al., 2021; Hesamian et al., 2019; Razzak et al., 2018; Wei et al., 2023).

The model's decision-making processes should be transparent. That is, model errors should be traceable, and in the event of an error, the problem should be more easily detected and corrected. Ethically, applications must comply with international standards. Therefore, accountability is also a necessity for legal compliance(Chlap et al., 2021; Garcea et al., 2023; Razzak et al., 2018; Wei et al., 2023).

Patient image data is anonymized during augmentation, but certain image features can reveal the patient's identity. When synthetic data is produced, a sample like the original data can be created, leading to privacy violations(Koohi-Moghadam & Bae, 2023; Tripathi & Musiolik, 2022).

Black box models can create ethical problems in clinical decisions. For example: A model may classify a tumor as benign but ignore the presence of an abnormality in a certain area. In this case, it becomes difficult for physicians to question or verify model decisions.

In addition, if DA processes are based on incorrect or biased data, models can make biased decisions (Carrasco Ramírez, 2024; Khalifa et al., 2024; Koohi-Moghadam & Bae, 2023; Rana & Shuford, 2024; Tripathi & Musiolik, 2022).

Patients should be informed whether their medical images will be used for augmentation or synthetic data production. Explaining data use processes and obtaining patient consent are ethically imperative. The lack of accountability and transparency in the models on which medical decisions are based can reduce physician and patient trust (Koohi-Moghadam & Bae, 2023; Tripathi & Musiolik, 2022)

Despite all these limitations, explainable AI methods should be used. Quality control mechanisms should be implemented in DA processes. Legal regulations regarding data privacy should be considered in augmentation processes. Ethics committees should play an active role in clinical AI projects. In addition, clinical teams should be trained on the advantages, risks, and limitations of augmented data and AI models.

2. RELATED DATA AUGMENTATION METHODS

2.1. Mixup

Mixup is a DA technique used to improve performance in image classification tasks. It seeks to improve the model's capacity for generalization and robustness by generating random mixtures of images belonging to different classes (H. Zhang et al., 2018a).

When it is desired to combine an image pair such as (x_i,y_i) and (x_j,y_j), where the one-hot labels in an image data are denoted by y and the data itself is denoted by x, Equation 1, also called Vanilla Mixup and Mixup, is used (H. Zhang et al., 2018b). Here, λ is a hyper-parameter determining how to mix the two images. The blended images assist ML models in steadily improving their performance by understanding certain hidden relationships in the uncharted search area.

$$\tilde{x} = \lambda x_i + \left(1 - \lambda\right) x_j$$

$$\tilde{y} = \lambda y_i + \left(1 - \lambda\right) y_j$$

$$\mu\left(\tilde{x},\tilde{y}|x_i,y_i\right) = \frac{1}{n}\sum_j^n \underset{\lambda}{E}[\delta(\tilde{x},\tilde{y})], \lambda \sim Beta\left(\alpha,\alpha\right), \alpha \in \left(0,\infty\right) \tag{1}$$

2.2. CAM-Mix

The CAM-Mix algorithm is a new method designed to improve DA and model generalization for images (He et al., 2023). The algorithm consists of two main components. First, CAM uses a DL model to identify the most important regions and objects of the image. This allows the model to focus its attention on meaningful visual information and ignore background noise. Secondly, Mixup is a DA technique used to create new synthetic images by randomly mixing two images (He et al., 2023). CAM-Mix integrates Mixup with CAM modules to focus the mixing process on visually important regions.

CAM-Mix blends the visual attributes of two images without specifically extracting the visual attributes, unlike Mixup, which creates images with new visual attribute values outside the current limited set. This is accomplished by using Equation 2 and Equation 3 to define the following grey-level morphological procedures for a pair of grey-scale pictures I1 and I2 of size n×m. No new visual feature values are generated during the proposed image mixing process. The characteristics of the generated images are taken from each of the two original photos without the attributes being explicitly removed, and new images are created without the need for extra scalars or interpolation functions like vanilla mixup. By varying the candidate responses, the goal is to expand the training data. For this purpose, $A = \{a_c\} \cup A_N$, where a_c is the set containing correct answers, Q is the set to be eliminated, and A_N is the set containing incorrect (negative) answers. The main goal of the model is to use the suggested grey-level morphological processes to provide more negative candidate replies $\widehat{A}_N$. For this purpose, extra training data is generated with $\widehat{A} = \{a_c\} \cup \widehat{A}_N$. The procedures used to generate extra training data are shown in Equation 4 and Equation 5. Thus, the data produced by mixing negative candidate answers with positive candidate answers contains partial information about the real answers. As a result, the space of valid solutions can have a sharper decision boundary defined by the newly created $\widehat{A}_N$. The CAM-Mix architecture is given in Figure 1.

$$\mathrm{OR}\left(I_1, \mathrm{I}_2\right) = \min_{\mathrm{i}\in \mathrm{n}, \mathrm{j}\in m}\left\{ I_1\left(\mathrm{i}, \mathrm{j}\right), \mathrm{I}_2\left(\mathrm{i}, \mathrm{j}\right)\right\} \quad (2)$$

$$\mathrm{AND}\left(I_1, \mathrm{I}_2\right) = \max_{\mathrm{i}\in \mathrm{n}, \mathrm{j}\in m}\left\{ I_1\left(\mathrm{i}, \mathrm{j}\right), \mathrm{I}_2\left(\mathrm{i}, \mathrm{j}\right)\right\} \quad (3)$$

$$\forall a_i \in A_N, \hat{\mathrm{a}}_i = \mathrm{OR}\left(a_i, \mathrm{a}_c\right) \in \hat{A}_N \quad (4)$$

$$\forall a_i \in A_N, \hat{\mathrm{a}}_i = \mathrm{AND}\left(a_i, \mathrm{a}_c\right) \in \hat{A}_N \quad (5)$$

Figure 1. CAM-Mix Model Architecture

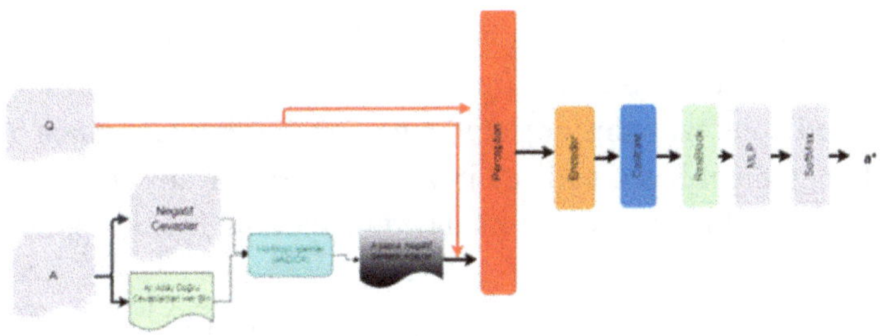

2.3. Generative Adversarial Networks (GAN)

Generative Adversarial Networks (GANs) is a DL algorithm consisting of two neural networks (Chen & Chan, 2023; I. Goodfellow et al., 2020; I. J. Goodfellow et al., 2014; Stankovic et al., 2024). The GAN model tries to generate new data by giving the training data set to the deep network, training the network, estimating a probability distribution for this data, and generating new data based on this distribution. In general, they are game-theoretic models based on optimization-based generative modeling. They are best known for their success in image data generation. In a competitive setup, two models are developed simultaneously: a discriminative D and a generative G. The generative model G learns the data distribution. In contrast, model D assesses the likelihood that a given sample comes from the training dataset. The goal of G is to maximize the chances that D will incorrectly classify the samples. This framework corresponds to a minimax two-player game. G and D are MLPs, and the whole system is trained by back-propagation. The proposed G and D networks are opposing networks. A discriminative network is designed to determine whether a sample originates from an actual data distribution or a generated model distribution, and it is compared to the generator network G. In this analogy, the discriminative network resembles law enforcement attempting to identify counterfeit currency. In contrast, the generative network represents a group of counterfeiters striving to produce fake currency and use it discreetly. The competitive nature of this "game" compels both sides to continuously improve their strategies until the generated data becomes indistinguishable from authentic data as shown in Figure 2. The model's algorithmic steps explain how the model operates with Algorithm 1 is shown in Figure 3.

The input noise variables $p_z(z)$ are pre-defined to learn the generator's distribution p_g over the data x. $G(z; \theta_g)$ is a mapping function to be applied to the data domain. In this case, an MLP with parameters θ_g represents the differentiable function G. The second MLP that produces a single scalar is the discriminant network D. $D(x; \theta_d)$ is the definition. The probability that x originates from the training data rather than the p_g distribution is given by D(x). The training process is not a one-time event but an iterative one when continuously optimizing the likelihood of correctly labeling training and G instances. When D is trained, G is trained to minimize log(1 - D(G(z))) at the same time. Equation 6 provides the two-player minimax game D and G play with value function V(G, D).

In reality, there might not be enough slope in Equation 6 for G to learn effectively. Since the samples differ from the training data, D may reject them with high confidence in the early stages of learning, while G is weak. Log(1 - D(G(z))) is saturated in this instance. It is suggested that G be trained to maximize logD(G(z)) rather than to minimize log(1 - D(G(z))) (I. J. Goodfellow et al., 2014). The dynamics of G and D reach the same fixed point with this objective function, but it offers much larger gradients at the beginning of learning. For gradient-based updates, it was proposed that any other common gradient-based learning rule might be applied; In the model, a momentum learning rule is applied.

$$\min_G \max_D V(D, G) = E_{x \sim p_{\text{data}}(x)}\left[\log D(x)\right] + E_{z \sim pz(z)}\left[\log\left(1 - D\left(G(z)\right)\right)\right] \tag{6}$$

$$D^*_G(x) = \frac{p_{\text{data}}(x)}{p_{\text{data}}(x) + p_g(x)} \tag{7}$$

$$E_{x \sim p_{\text{data}}}\left[\log D^*_G(x)\right] + E_{x \sim p_g}\left[\log\left(1 - D^*_G(x)\right)\right] \tag{8}$$

Figure 2. GAN Structure

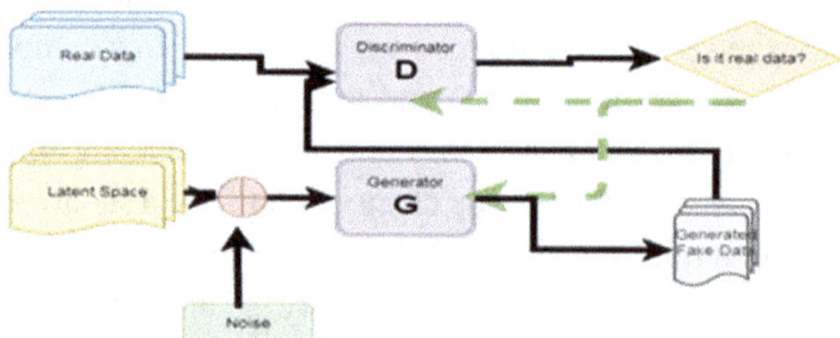

Figure 3. Pseudo-code for GAN Algorithm

Algorithm 1: GAN

Minibatch SGD training of GAN.
k: k is the number of steps to apply to the separator.
In the original work k = 1 was used (I. J. Goodfellow et al., 2014).

Initialize input: $x^{(i)}$:Real Data, z(i): noise vector, output: $G(z^{(i)})$, k:hyper-parameter
for the number of training iterations do
  for k steps do
    Sample minibatch of m noise samples $\{z^{(1)},\ldots,z^{(m)}\}$ from noise prior $p_g(z)$
    Sample minibatch of m examples $\{x^{(1)},\ldots,x^{(m)}\}$from data-generating distribution $p_{data}(x)$.
    Update the discriminator by ascending its stochastic gradient:
    $\nabla_{\theta d} \frac{1}{m}\sum_{i=1}^{m}[logD(x^{(i)}) + log(1 - D(G(z^{(i)})))]$
  end for
  Sample minibatch of m noise samples $\{z^{(1)},\ldots,z^{(m)}\}$from noise prior $p_g(z)$
  Update the generator by descending its stochastic gradient:$\nabla_{\theta g} \frac{1}{m}\sum_{i=1}^{m}[log(1 - D(G(z^{(i)})))]$
end for

2.4. CycleGAN

CycleGAN is a DL algorithm for visual style transfer between two different datasets (Zhu et al., 2017). It can work especially on mismatched datasets. It has two GANs (Goodfellow et al., 2020) and two discriminators, one for each GAN, and uses a cycle consistency loss function to transfer visual style from one image to another (Zhu et al., 2017). CycleGAN is given two datasets consisting of images from two different areas. The images in these sets do not need to match each other. It contains two generative layers, denoted by F and G. The first generating layer, G, transforms an image from one domain into another domain, while the second generating layer, F, tries to reverse this transformation. There is a separator for each area. These discriminators aim to differentiate between authentic images and fake ones the generators produce. An image is first transformed into the other domain with G and then returned to the first domain with F. The distance of the resulting image from the original image is called the cyclic coherence loss. The model is trained to minimize these losses. Thus, producers learn how to produce realistic images and, at the same time, reconstruct back to the original image.

In the model, $X = \{x_1,\ldots,x_N\}$ and $Y = \{y_1,\ldots,y_M\}$ are training data, and the variables x and y come from the same distribution. There are two distribution functions in the model, F and G which are defined as $F: X \rightarrow Y$ and $G: Y \rightarrow X$. In addition, two contrasting discriminators, D_x and D_y are defined. D_x learns the difference between {x} and {F(y)}, which is the result transformed to Y, while D_y learns the difference between {y} and {G(x)}. Basically, two losses are calculated here. The first is the loss in each transformation, called the opposite loss, and the second is the loss between the generated data and the actual data when the functions F and G complete a full cycle. Here, the counter loss is calculated using Equation 9 for function G and Equation 10 for function F. The loss of cyclic consistency at the end of the loop is calculated by Equation 11. The total loss of the model is considered the sum of these losses. The total loss is calculated with Equation 12, with the hyper-parameter λ of the G and F function losses representing the relative importance of the two models. The objective is to minimize the total loss.

$$L_{GAN}(G, D_Y, X, Y) = E_{y\sim p_{data}}(y)\left[\log D_Y(y)\right] + E_{x\sim p_{data}}(x)\left[\log\left(1 - D_Y(G(x))\right)\right] \quad (9)$$

$$L_{GAN}(F, D_X, Y, X) = E_{x\sim p_{data}}(x)\left[\log D_X(x)\right] + E_{y\sim p_{data}}(y)\left[\log\left(1 - D_X(G(y))\right)\right] \quad (10)$$

$$L_{cyc}(G, F) = E_{x\sim p_{data}}(x)\left[\|F(G(x)) - x\|1\right] + E_{y\sim p_{data}}(y)\left[\|G(F(y)) - y\|1\right]. \quad (11)$$

$$L(G, F, D_X, D_Y) = L_{GAN}(G, D_Y, X, Y) + L_{GAN}(F, D_X, Y, X) + \lambda L_{cyc}(G, F) \quad (12)$$

The algorithm of CycleGAN is shown with Algorithm 2 in Figure 4.

Figure 4. Pseudo-code for CycleGAN Algorithm

Algorithm 2: CycleGAN Algorithm

input: $y^{(i)}, x^{(i)}$: Data Sets

for the number of epochs **do**
  for the number of batches **do**
    sample minibatch← $\{x^{(i)}\}_{i=1}^{m}$ =∈ X
    sample minibatch← $\{y^{(j)}\}_{j=1}^{m}$ =∈ Y
    Generate m sample of G(x) and F(y)
    Generate m sample of F(G(x)) and G(F(y))
    X→ G(x)
    Y→ F(y)
    Update the Discriminator D_x and D_y
    $\max_{D_X} L_{GAN}(F, D_X, Y, X)$
    $\max_{D_y} L_{GAN}(G, D_y, X, Y)$
    Update the Generators G and F
    $\min_{G,F} L(G, F, D_X, D_y)$
  end for
end for

2.5. Robust Data Augmentation GAN (RDAGAN)

RDAGAN is a variant of GAN developed to increase the diversity of data and strengthen the generalization capability of the model. This model is particularly robust to limited data sets and changes in data distribution. It is used for tasks such as image synthesis, image translation and image editing (H. Lee et al., 2023).

The model is essentially based on the GAN model. Differently, it consists of two separate networks. The first one is the image object generator network and the second one is the image transformation network. The object generating network model uses the InfoGAN (X. Chen et al., 2016) architecture. The images produced by the object generating network model are given as input to the object transforming network and a loss function is calculated. Since the InfoGAN architecture has Info and GAN modules, which are the information layer, it calculates two different loss values. While the loss in the GAN module is calculated with Equation 13, the loss value of the Info module is calculated with Equation 14. The total loss of the producer network module is the sum of the losses of these two modules and is given by Equation 15. Equation 16 shows the total loss function of the model.

$$L^{obj}_{GAN} = \mathrm{E}_{R(i_t)\sim \mathrm{T}} \log \mathrm{D}_{\mathrm{obj}}\left(R\left(\mathrm{it}\right)\right) + \mathrm{E}_{R(i_c)\sim \mathrm{C}} \log\left(1 - \mathrm{D}_{\mathrm{obj}}\left(G_{\mathrm{obj}}\left(\mathrm{z}, \mathrm{c}\right)\right)\right) \tag{13}$$

$$L^{obj}_{Info} = \mathrm{E}_{c\sim N(0,1), c'\sim D_{\mathrm{obj}}\left(G_{\mathrm{obj}}\left(\mathrm{z}, \mathrm{c}\right)\right)}\left(\| c - c' \| 2\right) \tag{14}$$

$$L^{obj} = \lambda L^{obj}_{\mathrm{info}} + L^{obj}_{GAN} \tag{15}$$

$$L\left(\mathrm{G,F,D}_{X}, \mathrm{D}_{Y}\right) = \mathrm{L}_{\mathrm{GAN}}\left(\mathrm{G,D}_{Y}, \mathrm{X, Y}\right) + \mathrm{L}_{\mathrm{GAN}}\left(\mathrm{F,D}_{X}, \mathrm{Y,X}\right) + \lambda L_{\mathrm{cyc}}\left(\mathrm{G,F}\right) \tag{16}$$

L:loss, D: discriminator, z: noise, c: latentcode, G:generator, R(ic) clean images, it target Images, λ :power of information loss

The image transformation network combines clean images ($i_c \in C$) with target parts $G_{obj}(z,c)$ generated from the InfoGan model. It is very similar to the CycleGAN architecture. It is an encoder-decoder architecture containing ResNet blocks. The difference is that the generator keeps the sampling frequency flexible. Therefore, it provides flexibility to the size variance of the images. This generator module has two different discriminators, local(D^{local}_{tr}) and global(D^{global}_{tr}), which calculate the loss value of the module. The global allocator evaluates the image produced by the generating network. It does not use the whole image, but only a patchy part of it. Equation 17 gives a measure of how similar the image is to the target area image. The loss of the Info layer is calculated by Equation 18. The loss between the input image (i_c) and the generated image ($G_{tr}(i_p, i_c)$) is considered as the background loss and is calculated by Equation 19. Here L is loss, D is Discriminator, z is noise, G is generator, $\mathrm{m_b}$ is the mask, $\mathrm{i_c}$ is clean image, $\mathrm{i_t}$ is target image and λ is power of information loss.

The structure of RDGAN converter module is shown in Figure 5.

$$L^{tr}_{GAN} = \mathrm{E}_{i_t\sim p_T} \log \mathrm{D}^{global}_{tr}\left(i_t\right) + \mathrm{E}_{i_p\sim Gen(z,c), i_c\sim p_c} \log \mathrm{D}^{global}_{tr}\left(G_{\mathrm{rt}}\left(i_p, \mathrm{i}_c\right)\right)$$

$$+ \mathrm{E}_{i_t\sim p_T} \log\left(1 - \mathrm{D}^{global}_{tr}\left(R\left(i_t\right)\right)\right) + \mathrm{E}_{i_p\sim Gen(z,c), i_c\sim p_c} \log\left(1 - \mathrm{D}^{global}_{tr}\left(R\left(G_{\mathrm{tr}}\left(i_p, \mathrm{i}_c\right)\right)\right)\right) \tag{17}$$

$$L_{info}^{tr} = E_{c\sim N(0,1),i_p\sim G_{gen}(z,c),i_c\sim P_C}\left(\left\| c - D_{tr}^{local}\left(G_{tr}\left(i_p, i_c\right)\right)\right\| 2\right)$$

$$= E_{c\sim N(0,1),c'\sim D_{tr}^{local}\left(G_{gen}\left(i_p, i_c\right)\right)}\left(\left\| c - c' \right\| 2\right) \quad (18)$$

$$L_{BG}^{tr}\ E_{i_c\sim C,m_b\sim Pm_b,i_p\sim G_{gen}(z,c)}\left(\left\|\left(i_c * \left(1 - m_b\right)\right) - \left(G_{tr}\left(i_c, i_p\right) * \left(1 - m_b\right)\right)\right\| 1\right) \quad (19)$$

Figure 5. RDGAN Converter Module Structure

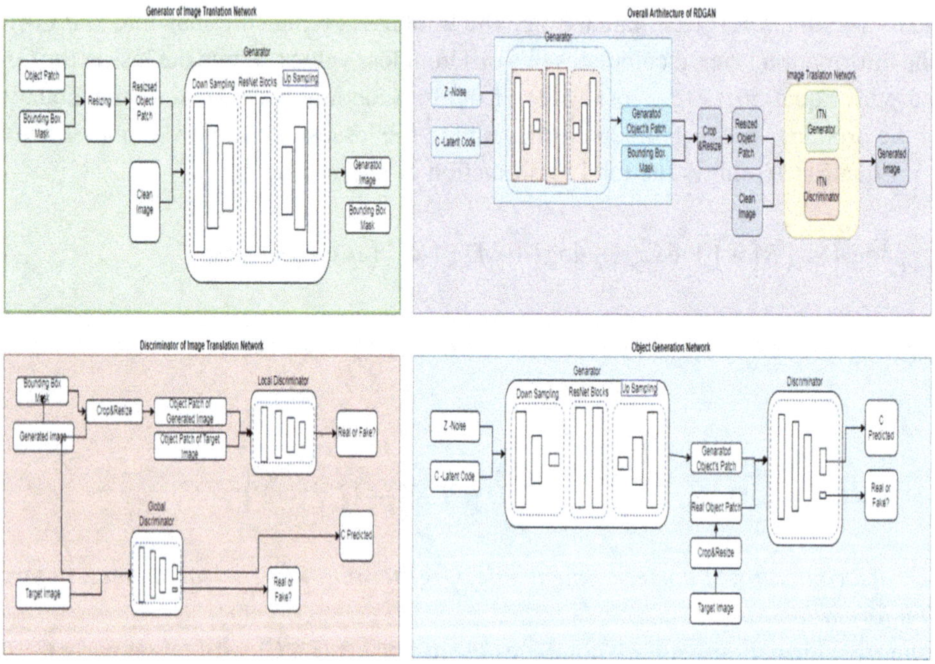

2.6. Pix2Pix (PatchGAN)

The Pix2Pix algorithm is a model proposed by (Isola et al., 2018). A similar model is given in another study (Wang et al., 2021) under the name PatchGAN. Since the two models are the same, they are given under one title. PatchGAN is a DL algorithm for tasks such as image synthesis, translation, and editing. It is a discriminative architecture used when generating data with GAN. It divides images into small pieces called patches and processes each patch separately. In this way, it can produce higher quality and more realistic images (Isola et al., 2018). While in classical classification problems, the whole image is reduced to one class, in patchGAN, each patch of the image is classified. Then, the average value of all the classified results is taken or combined by applying maximum pooling and given as a result. GANs are generative models that learn by minimizing a loss function and are designed to classify whether the output image is real or fake. Blurry images are unacceptable, as they can appear fraudulent. GANs are utilized for various tasks that typically require different loss functions since the loss function, they train with can adapt based on the data. In contrast, conditional GAN models have been produced in which an image is given as input as a condition (Goodfellow* et al., 2014). The conditional GAN model differs in that it learns a structural loss value. This structural loss penalizes the joint reconstruction of the output. Conditional GAN models provide a suitable architecture for picture-to-picture transformation. In the work by Isola et al. for PatchGAN, a U-Net and Encoder-Decoder architecture are used separately in the generator part. As a discriminator, it uses a convolutional network model and a classification model that penalizes image fragments rather than the whole image. GAN models here are generative models that create a new image from an image. G represents the generator and D the discriminator, cap G: z goes to y where z is the noisy input image vector, and y is the output image. The conditional GAN model is different because it tries to produce an outcome with the observation vector x and the noisy input image vector z. Therefore, the production function in the conditional GAN model is defined as $G: \{z,x\} \rightarrow y$. The generator G's goal is to create phony images that are identical to authentic ones. To assess the degree of difference between these phony and authentic photos, discriminator D is trained. Equation 20 provides the conditional GAN model's objective function. Equation 21 shows the total loss. While G tries to minimize the objective function, discriminator D discriminates by trying to maximize it. When x is not given as a condition, this loss is calculated as shown in Equation 22. In previous studies, these loss functions have been tested by adding the loss of L1 (Isola et al., 2018) and L2 (Pathak et al., 2016). (Isola et al., 2018) calculated the total loss by adding the L1 norm shown in Equation 23 as in Equation 24. What is essentially done in this model is that instead of training the generator G to minimize the error log(1 - D(x,G(x, z)), the network is trained to maximize the error logD(x, G(x, z)). This means the discriminative network (D) has a lower learning rate than the generative network (G). The model uses SGD as the activation function, learning rate 0.0002, ADAM as the optimization function, and $\beta 1 = 0.5$, $\beta 2 = 0.999$ as momentum parameters (Isola et al., 2018). PatchGAN's algorithm is shown in Figure 6. The Pix2Pix architecture is shown in Figure 7.

$$L_{cGAN}(G,D) = E_{x,y}\left[\log D(x,y)\right] + E_{x,z}\left[\log\left(1-D(x,G(x,z))\right)\right] \tag{20}$$

$$G^* = \arg\min_G \max_D L_{cGAN}(G,D) \tag{21}$$

$$L_{GAN}(G,D) = E_y\left[\log D(y)\right] + E_{x,z}\left[\log\left(1-D(G(x,z))\right)\right] \tag{22}$$

$$L_{L1}(G) = E_{x,y,z}\left[\|y - G(x,z)\|1\right] \tag{23}$$

$$G^* = \arg\min_G \max_D L_{cGAN}(G,D) + \lambda L_{L1}(G) \tag{24}$$

L: loss, *D*: separator, noise, *c*: latent code, *G*: Producer $R(i_c)$, $i_c \in$ Clean Images, $i_t \in$ Target Images, λ: power of information loss, m_b: mask

Figure 6. Pseudo-code for PatchGAN

Algorithm 3 : PatchGAN

Input: $y \sim P_{data}(y)$, $x \sim P_{data}(x)$, *sample size n*

Output: $G(x)$, $D(y,x)$

1: ***for*** *epoch − size* ***do***

2: *Sampling from the distribution of input images,*
with a sample size of n,result in the set $X = (x^1, x^2, x^3, \ldots, x^n)$

3: *Sampling from the distribution of target domain images,*
with a sample size of n,result in the set $Y = (y^1, y^2, y^3, \ldots, y^n)$

4: *Update the parameter weights of the discriminator using the following gradients*

$$\nabla \theta_d \frac{1}{n} \sum_{i=1}^{n} [\log D(y^i, x^i) + \log(1 - D(G(x^i), x^i))]$$

5: *Update the parameter weights of the generator using the following gradients*

$$\nabla \theta_g \frac{1}{n} \sum_{i=1}^{n} [\log(1 - D(G(x^i), x^i)) + \| y^i - G(x^i) \|_1]$$

6: ***end for***

7: ***return*** $G(x)$, $D(y,x)$

Figure 7. Conditional PatchGAN Structure (Wang et al., 2021)

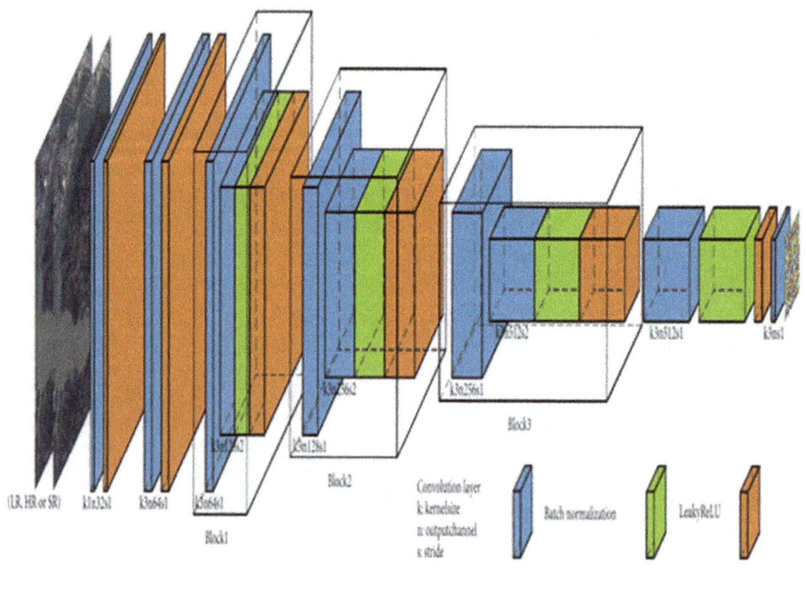

2.7. Pre-Activation Residual Attention Network (PRAN)

PRAN is a DL algorithm combining residual network principles and attention mechanisms. It is built to perform well on tasks like object detection, image reconstruction, and classification (Gao et al., 2019). The model was developed to classify hyperspectral images. A set of hyperspectral images is represented as $D \in R^{HxWxB}$ where H is the height, W is the width, and B is the hyperspectral bandwidth. Images are given to the model in segments. Each image is composed of SxS neighborhoods woven around the central label pixel. Therefore, a segmented image is of size SxSxB. Assuming that an image contains N label pixels, the dataset of fragment images will be $X=\{ x_1,\ldots,x_n\} \in R^{SxSxB}$. Their corresponding actual classes are defined as $Y= \{y_1,\ldots,y_n\} \in \{1,2,\ldots,Q\}$. Q here represents the classes of interest. What is emphasized in the model are the residual blocks that are replaced. The residue blocks are supplemented by two convolutional and a residue network, also called a hopping layer. This is called pre-activated residue. The modified residue block and the normal residue block used in the model are shown in the following Figure 8.

Figure 8. Normal residual block(a), pre-activated residual block (b)(Gao et al., 2019)

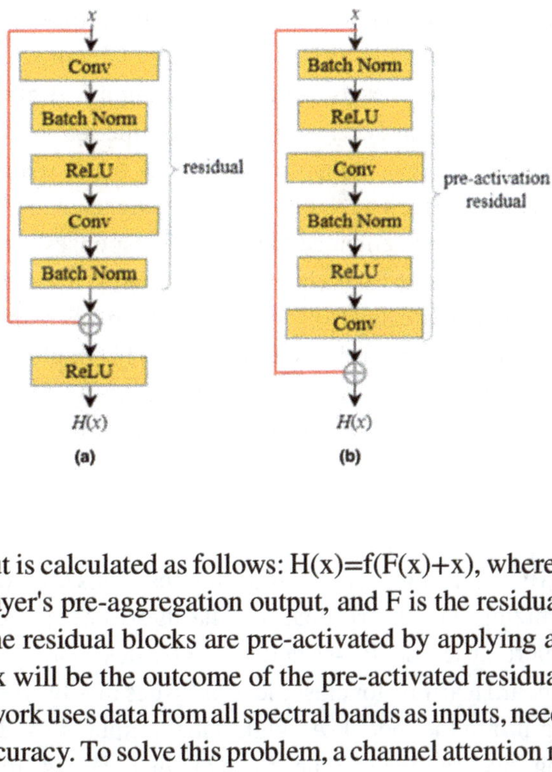

A residual block's output is calculated as follows: H(x)=f(F(x)+x), where f is the activation function, F(x) is the convolutional layer's pre-aggregation output, and F is the residual learning function. Before the convolutional layers, the residual blocks are pre-activated by applying a batch norm and RELU. In this instance, H(x)=F(x)+x will be the outcome of the pre-activated residual blocks.

Since the suggested network uses data from all spectral bands as inputs, needless redundant information lowers the classification accuracy. To solve this problem, a channel attention mechanism for recalibration is incorporated into the pre-activation residual block shown in Figure 9, comprised of the PRAN model.

Figure 9. Pre-activated residual attention block (PRAB) architecture (Gao et al., 2019)

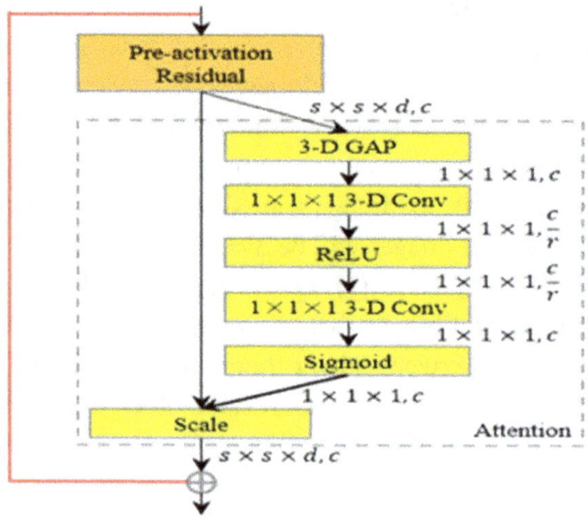

Assume that the attention mechanism has s × s × d and c input feature maps, where c and d represent the channel and depth dimensions, respectively. C 1×1×1 channel feature tensors are produced by compressing the global spatial information in each feature map using a 3-B global average pooling (GAP) layer. The channel dimensionality is then decreased by feeding the feature tensors as input to a 1×1×1 3-B convolutional layer. Specifically, the channel dimension of the feature tensor becomes c/r during convolution, where r is a reduction ratio. The value of r in the suggested network is 4.

After that, a ReLU function is used to enhance the channel responses' nonlinearity, a second 1×1×1 3-D convolutional layer is used to expand the channel's size, and c feature tensors are produced. The attention mechanism's final output is rescaled to cs × s × d feature maps by multiplying the output by the pre-activation residual's feature maps using a sigmoid function. This implementation allows each feature map to be adaptively recalibrated by assigning it a channel weight. Additionally, the $2*c^2/r$ parameters obtained from the two 3-D convolutional layers inside provide an attention mechanism.

2.8. BC Learning

Between-class learning (BC Learning) is a DL algorithm that aims to improve performance in image classification tasks by maximizing class discrimination. The algorithm focuses on learning the differences between images belonging to different classes and thus provides more accurate classification results (Tokozume et al., 2018). Standard learning for classification issues involves selecting one training sample from the dataset and feeding it into the model. A single-label output is used to train the model. On the other hand, with BC learning, two training samples from distinct classes are chosen randomly from the dataset and combined. After that, the model is trained to provide the mixing ratio for each class using the mixed data fed into it. The typical loss function, as opposed to cross-entropy loss, is the difference between the model's outputs and the ratio labels. Mixing is not performed in the test phase. In the model, let $\{x_1,t_1\}$ and $\{x_2,t_2\}$ be datasets belonging to two different classes labeled from the training data. $\tau \sim U(0,1)$ being a random variable from a uniform distribution, the image datasets are shuffled by this random rate. Labels are shuffled as $\tau t_1+(1-\tau)t_2$. The data are similarly shuffled simply as $\tau x_1+(1-\tau)x_2$. However, to make the data more appropriate, it was divided by a coefficient, and as a result, the confused data was corrected to $\frac{\tau.x_1+(1-\tau).x_2}{\sqrt{\tau^2+(1-\tau^2)}}$. In order to make the model more appropriate, the data is assumed to be a mixture of two separate image intensities, G1 and G2. A corresponding value of p is calculated, which is calculated as $P=\frac{1}{1+10^{\frac{G_1-G_2}{20}.\frac{1-\tau}{\tau}}}$. Depending on the variable p, the data combination $\frac{p.x_1+(1-p).x_2}{\sqrt{p^2+(1-p^2)}}$ will change. In the study with audio data, it was taken in this way. However, in the study with image data, the normal simple blending formula, Equation 29, was used. A new form for mixing was sought and this deficiency was overcome by converting the image data into wave data. The mean (μ) and standard deviation (σ) values were calculated for the red, green and blue colour channels in the image data. Thus, each image, $x_i=\mu_1+d_i$, was converted into waveform. Here the variable d is the wave component. If Equation 25 is substituted for the new x values, Equation 26 appears as a new blending formula. However, if we take the data in wave form, the wave component (d1 and d2) is the determinant. In addition, the static component may adversely affect the model. Because, in principle, it is assumed that the static components are the same for the mixing of two waves. Therefore, in this study, in order to remove the static component, the mean value is subtracted from each image and recalculated as Equation 27. In this case, the final form of the mixing will be as in Equation 28. In addition, the second thing that is done in the study is to determine the perception of the scrambled image x_1: x_2 = r: (1-r), the difference of image energies is taken into account. A coefficient p is calculated for this. It essentially gives the amplitude ratio $\rho.\sigma_1$: $(1-\rho).\sigma_2$=r:(1-r). In this case, the p coefficient is calculated as in Equation 29, taking into account the standard deviation of the images. Accordingly, the blending method is finalised by Equation 30. The main difference of this study from previous studies is that the standard deviation of each image is used instead of the sound pressure level by averaging the images.

$$\tau.x_1+(1-\tau).x_2 \tag{25}$$

$$\tau.(\mu_1+d_1)+(1-\tau).(\mu_2+d_2) \tag{26}$$

$$\tau.(x_1-\mu_1)+(1-\tau).(x_2-\mu_2) \tag{27}$$

$$\frac{\tau.(x_1-\mu_1)+(1-\tau).(x_2-\mu_2)}{\sqrt{\tau^2+(1-\tau^2)}} \tag{28}$$

$$p=\frac{1}{1+\frac{\sigma_1}{\sigma_2}.\frac{1-\tau}{\tau}} \tag{29}$$

$$\frac{p.(x_1-\mu_1)+(1-p).(x_2-\mu_2)}{\sqrt{p^2+(1-p^2)}} \tag{30}$$

2.9. CutMix

CutMix is a DA technique used to improve performance in image classification tasks. It aims to increase the generalization ability and robustness of the model by combining random fragments of images belonging to different classes (Yun et al., 2019). It is pretty similar to the Mixup model. In Mixup, data and labels of two images are mixed for all pixels, while in Cutmix, patches of two different images are mixed. This allows the model to produce more natural images. Where $x\in R^{WxHxC}$ is the training data and y is the label of the data, the aim is to generate the image $(\tilde{x}, \tilde{y})$ from two different training data (x_A, y_A) and (x_B, y_B). A combination process for this generation is given by Equation 31. Here $M \in \{0, 1\}^{W \times H}$ is a binary mask with ones denoting the mask filled with ones indicating the place to be extracted and filled from the two images. ⊙ is element-wise multiplication. λ is a sample taken from the beta distribution that represents the combination ratio between two data points ($\lambda \sim \beta(\alpha,\alpha)$). In the original study, α=1 in all experiments. In other words, λ is sampled from a uniform distribution (0, 1). Compared to Mixup, CutMix can create a locally natural image by substituting a patch from another training image for the image region. To take a sample of M, first, a boundary box $Boundary=(r_x, r_y, r_W, r_H)$ is defined, which determines the size of the image to be copied from image A to image B. The box coordinates are set as in Equation 32. The samples are taken as rectangles in accordance with the original dimensions of the images (Yun et al., 2019).

$$\tilde{x} = M \odot x_A + (1 - M) \odot x_B, M \in \{0,1\}^{WxH} \text{ and } \tilde{y} = \lambda y_A + (1 - \lambda) y_B \tag{31}$$

$$r_x \sim U(0, W), r_w = W\sqrt{1 - \lambda} \text{ and } r_y \sim U(0, H), r_h = H\sqrt{1 - \lambda} \tag{32}$$

The computational steps of CutMix are shown in Figure 10.

Figure 10. Pseudo-code of CutMix method

```
Algorithm 4: Pseudo-code of CutMix
Input: D = {(x_i, y_i) | i = 1,2,...,N}, b batchsize, model parameter θ, learning rate δ, height H and weight W of X_i image, c
Output: L(θ), θ
initialize the model parameters θ random
while θ is not converged do
    B = {(x_i, y_i)}_b ← sample b pairs from D
    B̃ = {}
    for i = 1 to b do
        (x_b, y_b) ← fetch a background image (x_i, y_i)
        (x_f, y_f) ← fetch a foreground image from D_{y_b}
        sample λ ~ Uniform(0,1)
        M ← Generate mask with H,W, λ
        x̃ ← CutMix x_b and x_f with M
        λ' ← Adjust weight λ with τ,κ,μ
        ỹ ← Mix label with y_b, y_f, λ'
        B̃ ← B̃ ∪ (x̃, ỹ)
    end for
    ℒ(θ) ← (1/b) Σ_{(x̃,ỹ)∈B̃} L((x̃, ỹ); θ)
    θ ← θ − δ ∇_θ L(θ)
end while
```

2.10. AugMix

Augmix is a simple yet effective data processing method designed to make image classification models more robust and resilient to uncertainty. Basically, it works by mixing versions of an image augmented in different ways (Hendrycks et al., 2020b). It creates augmented versions of the original images by various methods such as rotating, cropping, adding noise, and changing color. Thus, these augmented versions make the model more sensitive to different visual variations. Then, the augmented version images are mixed with a certain ratio. This blending process allows the model to focus on more general and abstract features. The blended images are given the same labeling as the original image. In this way, the model learns to correctly classify both different visual variations and their mixtures. In this way, the model gains robustness by becoming more resilient to unexpected changes in real-world images, such as lighting conditions. The model can better predict how confidently it classifies an image. This helps to reduce the risk of misclassification. This emphasizes the uncertainty estimation feature of the model. The model is a generalizing model that performs better on different data sets by focusing on more general and abstract visual features. The model is processed by data pre-augmentation, composite data generation from augmented data, and error calculation using Jensen-Shannon Divergence Consistency Loss. In data pre-augmentation, the data is augmented with three consecutive chains of 3 randomly selected operations. These augmentation results are then merged. The model is then trained by minimizing the Jensen-Shannon divergence between the original image x_{orig} and the posterior distributions of its augmented variants. Where $p_{orig} = \hat{p}(y|x_{orig})$, $p_{augmix1} = \hat{p}(y|x_{augmix1})$ and $p_{augmix2} = \hat{p}(y|x_{augmix2})$ the loss of the model is calculated by Equation 33. This loss represents an average estimate of the two augmented images together with the original image. We first take the error as the average error as in Equation 34 and then the Jensen-Shannon discrimination error for the 3 images is calculated from this average error value as in Equation 35.

$$L(p_{\text{orig}}, \text{y}) + \lambda\text{JS}(p_{\text{orig}}; \text{p}_{\text{augmix1}}; \text{p}_{\text{augmix2}}) \tag{33}$$

$$M = (p_{orig} + p_{augmix1} p_{augmix2})/3 \tag{34}$$

$$JS(p_{orig}; p_{augmix1}; p_{augmix2})$$

$$= \tfrac{1}{3}(KL[p_{orig} \| M] + KL[p_{augmix1} \| M] + KL[p_{augmix2} \| M]) \tag{35}$$

The Augmix algorithm is shown below in Figure 11.

Figure 11. Pseudo-code of CutMix method

Algorithm 5: Pseudo-code of AUGMIX

```
Input: Model p̂, Classification Loss L, Processes O = {rotate,...,posterize}
function AugmentAndMix(x_orig, k = 3, α = 1)
    Fill x_aug with zeros
    Sample mixing weights (w1, w2, . . . , wk) ~ Dirichlet(α, α, . . . , α)
    for i = 1, . . . , k do
        Sample operations op1, op2, op3 ~ O
        Compose operations with varying depth op12 = op2 ∘ op1 and op123 = op3 ∘ op2 ∘ op1
        Sample uniformly from one of these operations chain ~ {op1, op12, op123}
        x_aug += wi · chain(x_orig) . Addition is elementwise
    end for
    Sample weight m ~ Beta(α, α)
    Interpolate with rule x_augmix = m x_orig + (1 −m) x_aug
return x_augmix
end function
x_augmix1 = AugmentAndMix(x_orig), x_augmix1 is stochastically generated
x_augmix2 = AugmentAndMix(x_orig), x_augmix1 ≠ x_augmix2
        Loss        Output:        L(p̂(y | x_orig), y) + λ Jensen −
Shannon (p̂(y | x_orig); p̂(y|x_augmix1); p̂(y|x_augmix2))
```

2.11. PuzzleMix

PuzzleMix is a DA technique that uses saliency information and statistics of the underlying features of natural examples to improve performance in image classification tasks. It aims to increase the generalization ability and robustness of the model by randomly combining parts of images belonging to different classes (J.-H. Kim et al., 2020).

In the model, where $x \in X$ is the input data and $y \in Y$ is the label of this data, the data $\vee (x,y) \sim D (XxY)$ is each (x,y) image label pair will come from the distribution D. The blending process is given by the function g given by Equation 36 for the labels, the function h given by Equation 37 for the data itself, and the additive blending of the two is given by Equation 38. The loss value l given by Equation 39 is tried to be minimized. In the model, the mixing function is modified as in Equation 40. Here, Z is a mask consisting of $z_{ij} \in [0,1]$ and $\prod_0^T$ and $\prod_1^T$ are the n x n dimensional transport parts of the images to be blended. λ is the blending ratio and is calculated as $\lambda = \frac{1}{n}\sum_{ij} b_{ij}$. $\prod_{ij}^T$ is the binary transport fragment that gives information about how many images are moved from location i to location j after the transport. The aim here is to find the optimum blending mask z and the optimum transport plans Π. This is because the optimum values allow the data to maximize the saliency information of each input.

$$g(y_0, y_1) = (1 - \lambda) y_0 + \lambda y_1 \tag{36}$$

$$h(x_0, x_1) = (1 - \lambda) x_0 + \lambda x_1 \tag{37}$$

$$h(x_0, x_1) = (1 - \lambda) f(x_0) + \lambda f(x_1) \tag{38}$$

$$\underset{\theta}{\text{minimize}} \; \underset{(x_0,y_0),(x_1,y_1)\in D}{E} \; \underset{\lambda \sim q}{E} \; \ell\left(h\left(x_0, x_1\right), g\left(y_0, y_1\right); \theta\right) \tag{39}$$

$$h\left(x_0, x_1\right) = \left(1 - z\right) \odot \prod_0^T x_0 + z \odot \prod_1^T x_1, \lambda = \frac{1}{n}\sum_i z_i \tag{40}$$

The saliency information can be noisy, leading to a sub-optimal solution. Therefore, spatial regularisation terms ψ and $\varphi_{i,j}$ are used to control the smoothness of the mask and the local smoothness of the resulting mixed sample.

The transport cost Cij is defined as the distance between locations i and j. Care is taken to ensure that the structural integrity of each data is preserved in general, taking Cij into account and that the local salient structure of the data is preserved without dissipation after the transport. For this purpose, optimization is performed for binary transport plans. After subsampling, we optimize the main destination using mean pooling and saliency information s(x) to support multi-scale migration and masking. The downsampling size is n. In practice, randomly choosing the downsampling resolution for each mini-batch.

To optimize the Z mask, the range of the mask value is first decomposed. Let this decomposition interval $L = \left\{\frac{t}{m} \middle| t = 0,1,\dots,m\right\}$. Furthermore, to control the mixing ratio of the given inputs, we add the prior term $p(z_i)$ following a binomial distribution. Accordingly, the objective function will be shaped as in Equation 40. Optimizing Equation 40 leads to Equation 41.

$$\underset{z \in L^n, \prod_0, \prod_1 \in \{0,1\}^{nxn}}{\text{minimize}} - \left\|(1-z) \odot \prod_0^T s(x_0)\right\|_1 - \left\|z \odot \prod_1^T s(x_1)\right\|_1$$

$$+\beta \sum_{(i,j)\in N} \psi(z_i, z_j) + \gamma \sum_{(i,j)\in N} \phi_{i,j}(z_i, z_j) - \eta \sum_i \log p(z_i) + \xi \sum_{k=0,1} \left\langle \prod_k, C \right\rangle \tag{41}$$

Puzzle-Mix focuses on two main objectives. The first is to minimize Z and the second is to optimize $\prod_0^T$ and $\prod_1^T$ simultaneously. Puzzle Mix (J.-H. Kim et al., 2020) requires significantly more computational resources than previous studies. However, Puzzle Mix achieved higher accuracy than other methods in the same experimental setup.

In summary, the algorithm of PuzzleMix consists of the following steps as shown in Figure 12 with Algorithm 6:

Figure 12. Pseudo-code of PuzzleMix method

Algorithm 6: Pseudo-code of PuzzleMix

```
Input: data x_1, x_2, attack ball ∈, step r, probability p
x_{i,clean} = x_i for i = 1,2
Sample v_i ~ B(1,p) for i = 1,2
for i = 1,2 do
    if v_i == 1 then
        k_i ~ Uniform(−∈, ∈)
        x_i ← x_i + k_i
    end if
end for
calculate gradient ∇_x ℓ(x_i) for i = 1,2
optimize z· and Π_i· for i = 1,2
Sample δ ~ Uniform(0,1)
for i = 1,2 do
    if v_i == 1 then
        k_i ← k_i + r sign(∇_x ℓ(x_i))
        k_i ← clip(k_i, −∈, ∈)
        x_i ← x_{i,clean} + δ k_i
    end if
end for
Return z· ⊙ Π_1·^T x_1 + (1 − z·) ⊙ Π_2·^T x_2
```

3. CONCLUSION AND DISCUSSION

This study focuses on DA methods based on deep network models. It aims to examine new approaches that can deeply overcome the shortcomings of classical DA models. Image processing is widely used in medical data. Especially in medical data, it is vital for early diagnosis and early intervention in critical areas such as rare diseases. However, the low sample size of medical images is one of the most important limitations of this field. DA is one of the solutions that can be taken as a precaution. There are many methods used for DA. However, which of these methods should be preferred is usually a big question mark for researchers. In this study, current methods are explained in detail, and the comparison of the experimental results of the models with the state-of-the-art datasets to give researchers an idea is given in Table 1. In addition, model performances on the datasets are shown in Table 2. When we look at the literature, while a 99.7% success rate was achieved for Mixup in the studies conducted on the MNIST dataset, the GAN model reached a 98% success rate. Therefore, it is seen that Mixup is more successful than the GAN model in DA. As a result, it can be said that CAM-Mix has also contributed to the success of the CoPINET model. In the experimental results with CIFAR10, one of the frequently preferred current data sets, SuperMix comes with 97.2%, AugMix 96.4%, Co-Mixup 96.3%, CutMix 95.2%, BCLearning 93.7% and GAN 70% accuracy. Similarly, in the studies conducted with the Celeb-A data set, it is clear that the PatchGAN algorithm gives better results than the GAN model. In general, it is seen that the size and structure of the dataset directly affects DA performance and model training performance. Therefore, selecting the model to be used in DA is very important. However, although accepted datasets are used, whether real-life datasets will show the same success can only be revealed through experimental studies. Therefore, it should be known that there is still a significant gap in the field of medical image processing. This study gives a detailed framework of current and frequently used DA models.

3.1. Discussion of Ethical Issues

Augmented image data in clinical settings is a powerful tool for improving the performance of AI and ML models, especially in areas such as medical image analysis. DA techniques increase model performance in cases where medical image data is limited, prevent over-learning, and contribute to the model's generalization ability. Provides better representation in rare cases. In addition, imbalances in image data belonging to different age groups, genders, or ethnic groups can be eliminated with augmentation techniques, reducing model bias. However, besides these positive effects, there are ethical problems and risks related to model accountability, data privacy, and model transparency. For example, augmented image data may not fully reflect the characteristics of real-world clinical images. This can lead to misleading and pose great risks. Applications must be carefully designed to solve ethical issues such as data privacy, model transparency, and accountability. If this balance is achieved, DA can be used safely, ethically, and effectively in clinical decision-support systems.

3.2. Conclusion with Future Directions

The use of augmented data in medical imaging and AI is rapidly developing as a critical area shaping the future of clinical decision support systems. Potential developments in this area and the adoption of new technologies and emerging trends promise a major transformation in medical practices. It can provide more interactive diagnostic and medical education methods by integrating with Augmented Reality and Virtual Reality. In addition, more holistic clinical decision support can be provided by developing multimodal systems by combining them with large language models. Advanced models such as diffusion can create data that is almost indistinguishable from real medical images. This offers a significant opportunity, especially for simulating rare diseases, protecting data privacy, and reducing anonymity risks. With Federated Learning, model training can be done from many different sources without violating patient privacy, thus complying with data privacy regulations. It can enable the customization of medical models in the future. In the future, personalized diagnostic algorithms that consider individual risk factors for each patient can be created. More accurate results can be obtained by integrating the patient's genetic structure, lifestyle, and past medical images. Moreover, it will significantly contribute to algorithmic justice by reducing bias. Another contribution of DA will be to real-time continuous medical systems. It will help provide fast and effective model adaptation and make more accurate decisions in emergencies such as epidemics. Medical use of augmented data and AI models will be supported by stricter standards and regulations. This will ensure that the technology is used ethically and safely. The future of augmented data use in medical imaging offers multifaceted opportunities and challenges, both technologically and ethically. Advanced algorithms can potentially provide better diagnostic tools and personalized health solutions. However, the progress of these processes within the framework of reliable, transparent, and ethical principles will be critical for successfully adopting these technologies in the healthcare sector. Ongoing research will continue to add value to human health while expanding the boundaries of medical AI. Comparison of models according to features *and* specifications is shown in Table 3.

Table 2. Model performances based on state-of-the-art datasets

Data Set	Methods & Accuracy
MNIST	Mixup %99.7 GAN %98
CIFAR-10	SuperMix %97.2 AugMix %96.4 Co-Mixup %96.3 CutMix %95.2 BCLearning %93.7 GAN %70
CIFAR-100	PuzzleMix %77.1
Celeb-A	(a->b) PatchGAN %99 (b->a) PatchGAN %98.7 GAN %80
Plant Village	CycleGAN %95
PASCAL VOC2007	RDAGAN %84.1
Indian Pines Pavia University	PRAN %99.5 %98.2

Table 3. Comparison of models according to features and specifications

Model	Advantages	Disadvantages	Limitations	Practical Aspects
Mixup	- Simple to implement. - Reduces overfitting. - Diversifies data.	- Cannot learn more complex data relationships.	- May cause incorrect labels in image annotations.	- Easily integrates into many deep learning models with minimal computational cost.
GAN	- Highly effective in generating realistic data. - Widely used in creative applications.	- Training process is unstable. - Risk of mode collapse.	- Requires very large models and datasets. - Slow for real-time applications.	- Commonly used for data augmentation and synthesis. - Ideal for improving visual quality.
CycleGAN	- Performs bidirectional translation between two datasets.	- Success in visual transformation depends on specific data types.	- No need for labeled data, but can fail in specific scenarios.	- A powerful tool for style transfer and data transformation projects.
RDAGAN	- Advanced performance in generating and synthesizing random data.	- Long training times due to its complexity.	- Risk of mode collapse and data balance issues.	- Suitable for realistic image and data generation.
PatchGAN (Pix2Pix)	- Learns local details in high-resolution images. - Supports bidirectional translation.	- Requires large datasets. - Training can take a long time.	- Limited performance on small datasets.	- Used in image transformation and data augmentation tasks.

continued on following page

Table 3. Continued

Model	Advantages	Disadvantages	Limitations	Practical Aspects
PRAN	- Enriched with attention mechanisms. - Performs well in visual tasks.	- High hardware requirements. - Multi-parameter optimization may be needed.	- Requires robust infrastructure for high-resolution performance.	- A strong model for projects involving visual analysis and attention mechanisms.
BCLearning	- Integrates learning approaches tailored to network architecture.	- Effective only in specific scenarios.	- Dependent on architecture. - May require specialized data preparation.	- Can be used in small-scale tasks and niche projects.
CutMix	- Effective in data diversification and improving overall accuracy.	- Label distribution changes may cause erroneous learning.	- Weak performance in tasks requiring visual attention.	- Quick and effective for diverse datasets.
AugMix	- Effective in handling visual noise and distortions. - Improves model stability.	- Limited augmentation effect in some tasks.	- Dependent on data type. - Requires specialized application.	- Commonly used as a general solution for data augmentation.
PuzzleMix	- Advanced in data diversification. - Improves model generalization.	- High computational cost. - Complex to implement.	- More effective on large datasets. - May create excessive diversity on small datasets.	- Particularly useful for large-scale projects.
Co-Mix	- Shows strong performance with mixed data types. - Provides robust generalization.	- High computational requirements. - Complexity increases error rates.	- Limited impact on small datasets. - Difficult to optimize.	- Very powerful for large datasets and deep learning scenarios.

Table 4. List of abbreviations

Abbreviation	Context
ADAM	Adaptive Moment Estimation
AI	Artificial Intelligence
AN	Answer Network
AND	Logical AND
BC	Between-Class
CAM	Candidate Answer Morphological
CIFAR10	Canadian Institute For Advanced Research 10-class dataset
DA	Data Augmentation
DL	Deep Learning
DNN	Deep Neural Network
FL	Federated Learning
G1	Generator 1

continued on following page

Table 4. Continued

Abbreviation	Context
G2	Generator 2
GAN	Generative Adversarial Network
GAP	Global Average Pooling
IDA	Image Data Augmentation
L1/L2	Loss Functions
MLP	Multi-Layer Perceptron
MNIST	Modified National Institute of Standards and Technology dataset
OR	Logical OR
PRAB	Pre-Activation Residual Attention Block
PRAN	Pre-Activation Residual Attention Network
RDAGAN	Robust Data Augmentation GAN
RDGAN	Robust Data GAN
RELU	Rectified Linear Unit
SGD	Stochastic Gradient Descent
SRAN	Stratified Rule-Aware Network

Table 5. Models' Code Sources

Model	Source Code Link	
SuperMix	https://github.com/alldbi/SuperMix	(Dabouei et al., 2021)
SRAN	https://github.com/husheng12345/SRAN/blob/master/SRAN/	(Lee et al., 2023)
Co-Mixup	https://github.com/snu-mllab/Co-Mixup	(J. H. Kim et al., 2021)
BCLearning	https://github.com/mil-tokyo/bc_learning_sound	(Tokozume et al., 2018)
PatchGAN	https://github.com/He-jerry/PatchGAN/blob/master/README.md	(Isola et al., 2018)
PuzzleMix	https://github.com/snu-mllab/PuzzleMix/	(J.-H. Kim et al., 2020)

REFERENCES

Aamir, M., Bazai, S., Bhatti, U. A., Dayo, Z. A., Liu, J., & Zhang, K. (2023, January). Applications of machine learning in medicine: Current trends and prospects. In *2023 Global Conference on Wireless and Optical Technologies (GCWOT)* (pp. 1-4). IEEE. DOI: 10.1109/GCWOT57803.2023.10064665

Aamir, M., Rahman, Z., Abro, W. A., Bhatti, U. A., Dayo, Z. A., & Ishfaq, M. (2023). Brain tumor classification utilizing deep features derived from high-quality regions in MRI images. *Biomedical Signal Processing and Control, 85*, 104988. DOI: 10.1016/j.bspc.2023.104988

Aamir, M., Rahman, Z., Abro, W. A., Tahir, M., & Ahmed, S. M. (2019). An optimized architecture of image classification using convolutional neural network. *International Journal of Image. Graphics and Signal Processing, 11*(10), 30–39. DOI: 10.5815/ijigsp.2019.10.05

Aamir, M., Rahman, Z., Dayo, Z. A., Abro, W. A., Uddin, M. I., Khan, I., Imran, A. S., Ali, Z., Ishfaq, M., Guan, Y., & Hu, Z. (2022). A deep learning approach for brain tumor classification using MRI images. *Computers & Electrical Engineering, 101*, 108105. DOI: 10.1016/j.compeleceng.2022.108105

Altaf, F., Islam, S. M. S., Akhtar, N., & Janjua, N. K. (2019). Going deep in medical image analysis: Concepts, methods, challenges, and future directions. In *IEEE Access* (Vol. 7). DOI: 10.1109/ACCESS.2019.2929365

Carrasco Ramírez, J. G. (2024). AI in Healthcare: Revolutionizing Patient Care with Predictive Analytics and Decision Support Systems. *Journal of Artificial Intelligence General Science (JAIGS) ISSN:3006-4023, 1*(1). DOI: 10.60087/jaigs.v1i1.p37

Chen, L., & Chan, H. Y. (2023). Generative Adversarial Networks with Data Augmentation and Multiple Penalty Areas for Image Synthesis. *The International Arab Journal of Information Technology, 20*(3), 428–434. DOI: 10.34028/iajit/20/3/15

Chlap, P., Min, H., Vandenberg, N., Dowling, J., Holloway, L., & Haworth, A. (2021). A review of medical image data augmentation techniques for deep learning applications. In *Journal of Medical Imaging and Radiation Oncology* (Vol. 65, Issue 5). DOI: 10.1111/1754-9485.13261

Dabouei, A., Soleymani, S., Taherkhani, F., & Nasrabadi, N. M. (2021). SuperMix: Supervising the mixing data augmentation. *Proceedings of the IEEE Computer Society Conference on Computer Vision and Pattern Recognition*, 13789–13798. DOI: 10.1109/CVPR46437.2021.01358

Gao, H., Yang, Y., Yao, D., & Li, C. (2019). Hyperspectral Image Classification with Pre-Activation Residual Attention Network. *IEEE Access : Practical Innovations, Open Solutions, 7*(23), 176587–176599. DOI: 10.1109/ACCESS.2019.2957163

Garcea, F., Serra, A., Lamberti, F., & Morra, L. (2023). Data augmentation for medical imaging: A systematic literature review. In *Computers in Biology and Medicine* (Vol. 152). DOI: 10.1016/j.compbiomed.2022.106391

Goodfellow, I., Pouget-Abadie, J., Mirza, M., Xu, B., Warde-Farley, D., Ozair, S., Courville, A., & Bengio, Y. (2020). Generative adversarial networks. *Communications of the ACM, 63*(11), 139–144. DOI: 10.1145/3422622

Goodfellow, I. J., Pouget-Abadie†, J., Mirza, M., Xu, B., Warde-Farley, D., Ozair, S., Courville, A., & Bengio, Y. (2014). NIPS'14: Proceedings of the 27th International Conference on Neural Information Processing Systems - Volume 2. *Generative Adversarial Nets*, 2672–2680. DOI: 10.1109/ICCVW.2019.00369

Guan, Y., Aamir, M., Rahman, Z., Ali, A., Abro, W. A., Dayo, Z. A., ... & Hu, Z. (2021). A framework for efficient brain tumor classification using MRI images.

Hao, W., El-Khamy, M., Lee, J., Zhang, J., Liang, K. J., Chen, C., & Carin, L. (2021). Towards fair federated learning with zero-shot data augmentation. *IEEE Computer Society Conference on Computer Vision and Pattern Recognition Workshops*. DOI: 10.1109/CVPRW53098.2021.00369

He, D., Wang, R., Xu, Z., Wang, J., Song, P., Wang, H., & Su, J. (2024). The use of artificial intelligence in the treatment of rare diseases: A scoping review. In *Intractable and Rare Diseases Research* (Vol. 13, Issue 1). DOI: 10.5582/irdr.2023.01111

He, W., Ren, J., & Bai, R. (2023). Data augmentation by morphological mixup for solving Raven's progressive matrices. *The Visual Computer*. Advance online publication. DOI: 10.1007/s00371-023-02930-x

Hendrycks, D., Mu, N., Cubuk Google, E. D., Zoph Google, B., Gilmer Google, J., & Lakshminarayanan, B. (2020). AUGMIX: A SIMPLE DATA PROCESSING METHOD TO IMPROVE ROBUSTNESS AND UNCERTAINTY. *ICLR 2020: The Eighth International Conference on Learning Representations*, 1–13.

Hesamian, M. H., Jia, W., He, X., & Kennedy, P. (2019). Deep Learning Techniques for Medical Image Segmentation: Achievements and Challenges. *Journal of Digital Imaging*, *32*(4), 582–596. Advance online publication. DOI: 10.1007/s10278-019-00227-x PMID: 31144149

Hu, B., Zhang, M., Liu, K., Li, X., & Wang, Y. (2023). Federated Data Augmentation Algorithm based on Heterogeneity Assessment. *2023 2nd International Conference on Cloud Computing, Big Data Application and Software Engineering, CBASE 2023*. DOI: 10.1109/CBASE60015.2023.10439080

Hu, S., Ma, Y., Liu, X., Wei, Y., & Bai, S. (2021). Stratified Rule-Aware Network for Abstract Visual Reasoning. *35th AAAI Conference on Artificial Intelligence, AAAI 2021, 2B*, 1567–1574. DOI: 10.1609/aaai.v35i2.16248

Isola, P., Zhu, J.-Y., Zhou, T., & Efros, A. A. (2018). Image-to-Image Translation with Conditional Adversarial Networks. *Proceedings of 2023 IEEE 9th International Women in Engineering (WIE) Conference on Electrical and Computer Engineering, WIECON-ECE 2023*, 468–472. DOI: 10.1109/WIECON-ECE60392.2023.10456447

Jalal, S., Parker, W., Ferguson, D., & Nicolaou, S. (2021). Exploring the Role of Artificial Intelligence in an Emergency and Trauma Radiology Department. In *Canadian Association of Radiologists Journal* (Vol. 72, Issue 1). DOI: 10.1177/0846537120918338

Khalifa, M., Albadawy, M., & Iqbal, U. (2024). Advancing clinical decision support: The role of artificial intelligence across six domains. In *Computer Methods and Programs in Biomedicine Update* (Vol. 5). DOI: 10.1016/j.cmpbup.2024.100142

Kim, J. H., Choo, W., Jeong, H., & Song, H. O. (2021). Co-Mixup: Saliency Guided Joint Mixup with Supermodular Diversity. *ICLR 2021 - 9th International Conference on Learning Representations*, 1–21. http://arxiv.org/abs/2102.03065

Kim, J.-H., Choo, W., & Song, H. O. (2020). Puzzle Mix: Exploiting Saliency and Local Statistics for Optimal Mixup. *Proceedings of the 37th International Conference on Machine Learning*, 119.

Koohi-Moghadam, M., & Bae, K. T. (2023). Generative AI in Medical Imaging: Applications, Challenges, and Ethics. In *Journal of Medical Systems* (Vol. 47, Issue 1). DOI: 10.1007/s10916-023-01987-4

Lee, H., Kang, S., & Chung, K. (2023). Robust Data Augmentation Generative Adversarial Network for Object Detection. *Sensors (Basel), 23*(1), 157. Advance online publication. DOI: 10.3390/s23010157 PMID: 36616754

Mahesh Batra, A., & Reche, A. (2023). A New Era of Dental Care: Harnessing Artificial Intelligence for Better Diagnosis and Treatment. *Cureus*. Advance online publication. DOI: 10.7759/cureus.49319 PMID: 38143639

Menegatti, D., Giuseppi, A., Delli Priscoli, F., Pietrabissa, A., Di Giorgio, A., Baldisseri, F., Mattioni, M., Monaco, S., Lanari, L., Panfili, M., & Suraci, V. (2023). CADUCEO: A Platform to Support Federated Healthcare Facilities through Artificial Intelligence. *Healthcare (Basel), 11*(15), 2199. Advance online publication. DOI: 10.3390/healthcare11152199 PMID: 37570439

Min, B., Kim, T., Shin, D., & Shin, D. (2023). Data Augmentation Method for Plant Leaf Disease Recognition. *Applied Sciences (Basel, Switzerland), 13*(3), 1465. Advance online publication. DOI: 10.3390/app13031465

Pinto-Coelho, L. (2023). How Artificial Intelligence Is Shaping Medical Imaging Technology: A Survey of Innovations and Applications. In *Bioengineering* (Vol. 10, Issue 12). DOI: 10.3390/bioengineering10121435

Rana, Md. S., & Shuford, J. (2024). AI in Healthcare: Transforming Patient Care through Predictive Analytics and Decision Support Systems. *Journal of Artificial Intelligence General Science (JAIGS) ISSN:3006-4023, 1*(1). DOI: 10.60087/jaigs.v1i1.30

Razzak, M. I., Naz, S., & Zaib, A. (2018). Deep learning for medical image processing: Overview, challenges and the future. In *Lecture Notes in Computational Vision and Biomechanics* (Vol. 26). DOI: 10.1007/978-3-319-65981-7_12

Sen, D., Chakrabarti, R., Chatterjee, S., Grewal, D. S., & Manrai, K. (2020). Artificial intelligence and the radiologist: The future in the Armed Forces Medical Services. *Journal of the Royal Army Medical Corps, 166*(4), 254–256. Advance online publication. DOI: 10.1136/jramc-2018-001055 PMID: 30709922

Stankovic, M., Bacanin, N., Zivkovic, M., Jovanovic, L., Sarac, M., & Antonijevic, M. (2024). Generative Adversarial Network for Data Augmentation and Substitution. *2024 IEEE Zooming Innovation in Consumer Technologies Conference. ZINC, 2024*, 7–12. DOI: 10.1109/ZINC61849.2024.10579362

Tokozume, Y., Ushiku, Y., & Harada, T. (2018). Between-class Learning for Image Classification. *2018 IEEE/CVF CONFERENCE ON COMPUTER VISION AND PATTERN RECOGNITION (CVPR)*, 5486–5494. https://doi.org/DOI10.1109/CVPR.2018.00575

Tripathi, S., & Musiolik, T. H. (2022). Fairness and ethics in artificial intelligence-based medical imaging. In *Research Anthology on Improving Medical Imaging Techniques for Analysis and Intervention*. DOI: 10.4018/978-1-6684-7544-7.ch005

Wang, J., Gao, K., Zhang, Z., Ni, C., Hu, Z., Chen, D., & Wu, Q. (2021). Multisensor Remote Sensing Imagery Super-Resolution with Conditional GAN. *Journal of Remote Sensing (United States), 2021*, 2021/9829706. Advance online publication. DOI: 10.34133/2021/9829706

Wei, J., Wang, Q., Song, X., & Zhao, Z. (2023). The Status and Challenges of Image Data Augmentation Algorithms. *Journal of Physics: Conference Series, 2456*(1), 012041. Advance online publication. DOI: 10.1088/1742-6596/2456/1/012041

Xu, M., Yoon, S., Fuentes, A., & Park, D. S. (2023). A Comprehensive Survey of Image Augmentation Techniques for Deep Learning. *Pattern Recognition, 137*, 109347. Advance online publication. DOI: 10.1016/j.patcog.2023.109347

Yun, S., Han, D., Chun, S., Oh, S. J., Choe, J., & Yoo, Y. (2019). CutMix: Regularization strategy to train strong classifiers with localizable features. *Proceedings of the IEEE International Conference on Computer Vision, 2019-Octob*, 6022–6031. DOI: 10.1109/ICCV.2019.00612

Zatloukal, J., Brat, K., Neumannova, K., Volakova, E., Hejduk, K., Kocova, E., Kudela, O., Kopecky, M., Plutinsky, M., & Koblizek, V. (2020). Chronic obstructive pulmonary disease – diagnosis and management of stable disease; a personalized approach to care, using the treatable traits concept based on clinical phenotypes. Position paper of the czech pneumological and phthisiological society. *Biomedical Papers of the Medical Faculty of the University Palacky, Olomouc, Czechoslovakia, 164*(4), 325–356. Advance online publication. DOI: 10.5507/bp.2020.056 PMID: 33325455

Zhang, C., Zhong, W., Li, C., & Deng, H. (2023). Random walk-based erasing data augmentation for deep learning. *Signal, Image and Video Processing, 17*(5), 2447–2454. DOI: 10.1007/s11760-022-02461-3

Zhang, H., Cisse, M., Dauphin, Y. N., & Lopez-Paz, D. (2018). mixup: BEYOND EMPIRICAL RISK MINIMIZATION. *The Sixth International Conference on Learning Representations*, 78–92. https://doi.org/https://doi.org/10.48550/arXiv.1710.09412

Zhang, H., Hou, Q., Wu, T., Cheng, S., & Liu, J. (2023). Data-Augmentation-Based Federated Learning. *IEEE Internet of Things Journal, 10*(24), 22530–22541. Advance online publication. DOI: 10.1109/JIOT.2023.3303889

Zhang, J., & Jiang, Y. (2022). A Data Augmentation Method for Vertical Federated Learning. *Wireless Communications and Mobile Computing, 2022*, 1–16. Advance online publication. DOI: 10.1155/2022/6596925

Zhao, G., Cai, Z., Wang, X., & Dang, X. (2023). GAN Data Augmentation Methods in Rock Classification. *Applied Sciences (Basel, Switzerland), 13*(9), 5316. Advance online publication. DOI: 10.3390/app13095316

Zheng, Y., Sun, X., Feng, B., Kang, K., Yang, Y., Zhao, A., & Wu, Y. (2024). Rare and complex diseases in focus: ChatGPT's role in improving diagnosis and treatment. *Frontiers in Artificial Intelligence*, *7*, 1338433. Advance online publication. DOI: 10.3389/frai.2024.1338433 PMID: 38283995

Chapter 11
Convolutional Neural Networks (CNNs) for Medical Imaging:
Revolutionizing Diagnostic Accuracy and Treatment Planning

S. Aishwarya
https://orcid.org/0009-0001-3731-2062
Sri Eshwar College of Engineering, India

C. Selvamurugan
https://orcid.org/0000-0003-3447-1970
Dhaanish Ahmed Institute of Technology, India

K. G. Parthiban
Dhaanish Ahmed institute of Technology, India

J. Manoj Prabhakar
Dhaanish Ahmed institute of Technology, India

K. K. Lakshmikandhan
CMS College of Engineering and Technology, India

J. Tharik Raja
Dhaanish Ahmed Institute of Technology, India

ABSTRACT

The chapter delves into the transformative impact of Convolutional Neural Networks (CNNs) on medical imaging, highlighting their ability to enhance diagnostic accuracy, streamline workflows, and enable real-time image analysis. It provides a comprehensive overview of CNN architectures, their principles, and their integration into diverse medical imaging modalities, such as X-rays, MRIs, and CT scans. Through case studies, the chapter explores CNN applications in detecting brain tumours, pneumonia, and skin cancer, while addressing advanced techniques like transfer learning, GAN-based data augmentation, and hybrid models. The discussion emphasizes the role of Explainable AI (XAI) in overcoming challenges related to model interpretability and ethical considerations, such as patient confidentiality and bias. With a focus on future advancements, including personalized medicine and seamless integration into clinical workflows, the chapter underscores CNNs' potential to redefine diagnostic imaging, improving patient outcomes and revolutionizing healthcare.

DOI: 10.4018/979-8-3693-9816-6.ch011

INTRODUCTION

Saving lives and lessening the psychological and physical toll of illnesses and injuries depend on the early and precise detection of medical abnormalities. Advanced analysis of medical images obtained using a variety of modalities, including X-rays, magnetic resonance imaging (MRI), computed tomography (CT), positron emission tomography (PET), ultrasound scanning, and diagnostic imaging, is frequently required for conditions like glaucoma, diabetic retinopathy, tumours, interstitial lung diseases, cardiovascular disorders, and tuberculosis. Identifying abnormalities, defining their boundaries, estimating their sizes, and determining their severity are all necessary for effective picture interpretation. However, there are many obstacles in the way of conventional image analysis techniques. Diagnostic delays or mistakes may result from the variety of anomaly shapes, locations, and structures as well as the scarcity of skilled diagnosticians (Aamir et al., 2023).

The necessity for intelligent, automated technologies to improve medical imaging workflows is further highlighted by the subjective nature of manual interpretation, the possibility of expert weariness in humans, and the high expense of professional consultations (Sarvamangala & Kulkarni, 2022). Medical imaging has seen a significant transformation thanks to Convolutional Neural Networks (CNNs), which have made it possible to analyse and understand complex medical data in previously unheard-of ways. CNNs, a subtype of deep learning, are especially useful for applications like automated illness diagnosis, picture segmentation, and classification because of their ability to automatically learn hierarchical features from images. Because of their architecture, which is modelled after the human visual system, complex patterns and details that are frequently too subtle for conventional methods can be extracted from medical images.

This chapter begins with an overview of medical imaging, tracing its evolution and highlighting its significance in modern healthcare through various modalities such as X-rays, MRI, and CT scans. It then introduces Convolutional Neural Networks (CNNs), explaining their architecture and core components while emphasizing their transformative role in medical imaging. Subsequently, the chapter explores advancements in CNN frameworks, such as LeNet, VGGNet, and ResNet, showcasing their specific applications and advantages. Real-world examples and case studies demonstrate the use of CNNs in diagnosing conditions like brain tumours and pneumonia. Advanced learning techniques, including pretrained networks, transfer learning, and hybrid models, are discussed to address challenges posed by limited datasets. The chapter also examines critical challenges and ethical considerations, such as model interpretability and patient confidentiality, proposing solutions like Explainable AI (XAI). Finally, it highlights future directions, including real-time diagnostic tools and the integration of CNNs into clinical workflows, underscoring their potential to revolutionize healthcare.

MEDICAL IMAGING

Medical imaging is an indispensable cornerstone of modern healthcare, providing physicians with a powerful diagnostic and treatment tool that allows unprecedented visualization of internal body structures (Aamir et al. 2023). By utilizing advanced technologies like X-rays, CT scans, MRI, and ultrasound as shown in Figure 1, medical professionals can accurately diagnose diseases, detect abnormalities, and monitor treatment progress without invasive procedures. These imaging techniques enable early detection of critical conditions such as tumors, fractures, cardiovascular issues, and neurological disorders, significantly improving patient outcomes and survival rates. Beyond diagnosis, medical imaging guides surgical interventions, helps track disease progression, and supports personalized treatment strategies across multiple medical specialties. The non-invasive nature of these technologies reduces patient risk, minimizes healthcare costs, and provides detailed insights that physical examinations cannot reveal. From identifying microscopic changes in tissue to creating comprehensive 3D reconstructions (Ilesanmi et al., 2024) of complex anatomical structures, medical imaging represents a revolutionary approach to understanding human health, transforming medical practice by offering precise, real-time insights into the human body's intricate systems and potential health challenges.

TIMELINE OF MEDICAL IMAGING DEVELOPMENTS

Early Beginnings

- **1895**: Wilhelm Röntgen discovers X-rays
- **1896**: First widespread medical use of X-rays globally

Mid-20th Century Innovations

- **1955**: Ian Donald begins investigating ultrasound for medical diagnosis
- **1957**: First fiber-optic semi-flexible gastroscope developed
- **1967**: Godfrey Hounsfield conceives CT scanning technology
- **1971**: First CT scanner installed, performing the first patient brain scan
- **1973**: First Magnetic Resonance Imaging (MRI) images produced
- **1974**: First Positron Emission Tomography (PET) camera developed
- **1977**: First complete human body MRI scan performed

Modern Era

- **1979**: Hounsfield and Cormack win Nobel Prize for CT technology
- **1980s**: MRI scanners installed in hospitals
- **1990s**: Ultrasound becomes routine for prenatal monitoring
- **2000**: PET/CT scanner named medical invention of the year by TIME Magazine
- **2003**: Nobel Prize awarded to Lauterbur and Mansfield for MRI work
- **2014**: University of Canterbury begins developing the world's first human colour X-ray scanner

Recent Developments

- Ongoing integration of AI and machine learning in medical imaging
- Advanced 3D and 4D imaging techniques
- Increased focus on molecular and functional imaging
- Development of more precise, less invasive imaging technologies

This timeline showcases the remarkable evolution of medical imaging from a simple X-ray to sophisticated, AI-enhanced diagnostic tools that continue to revolutionize healthcare.

Figure 1. Medical imaging

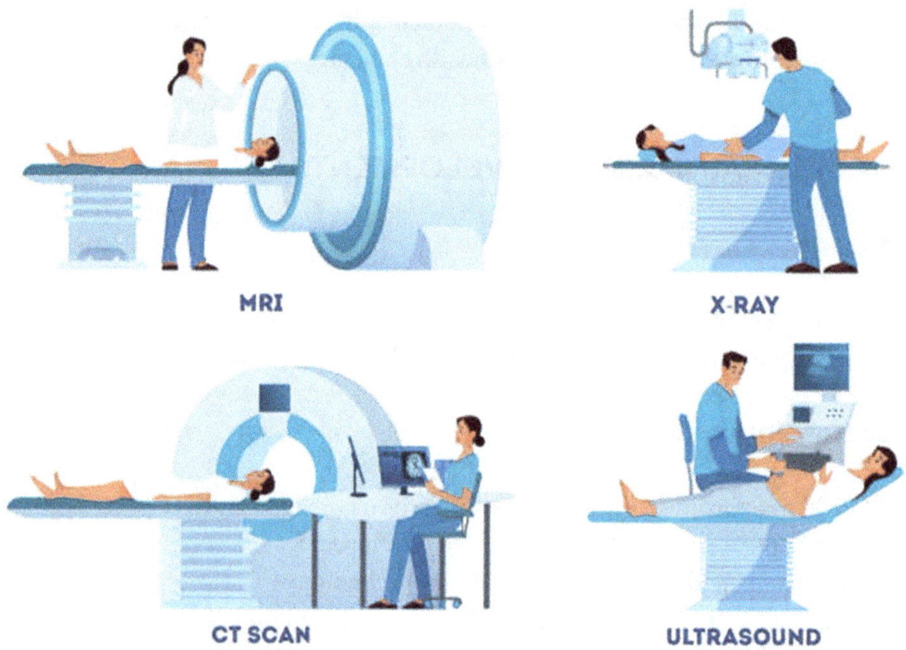

CORE PRINCIPLES OF MEDICAL IMAGING

Medical imaging relies on different types of "invisible" waves, including electromagnetic radiation, magnetic fields, and sound waves. These waves travel through the body, interact with tissues differently, and are captured by specialized detectors to create comprehensive images.

X-Ray

X-ray imaging represents a groundbreaking medical diagnostic technology that utilizes electromagnetic radiation to create detailed internal body images as shown in Figure 2. This technique generates high-energy electromagnetic waves through electron collisions with metal plates, typically tungsten, producing radiation capable of penetrating human tissues and creating visual representations of internal structures. (Ou et al., 2021) When X-ray beams pass through the body, different tissues absorb radiation uniquely - dense materials like bones absorb more radiation and appear white, soft tissues appear grey, and air-filled spaces like lungs appear black, enabling physicians to visualize intricate internal anatomical details with remarkable precision. Medical professionals utilize X-ray technology for diverse examinations including chest imaging, bone and joint assessments, dental diagnostics, abdominal surveys, and urological investigations.

Figure 2. X-ray of human body

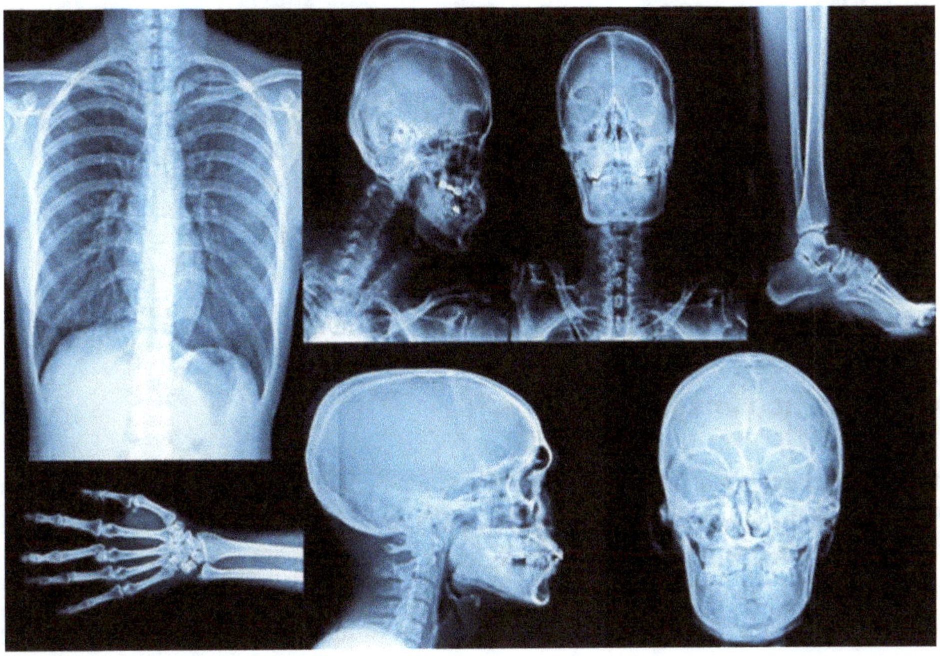

Computed Tomography (CT) Scanning

Computed Tomography (CT) scanning is a cutting-edge medical imaging method that produces finely detailed cross-sectional images of the human body using complex X-ray technology as shown in Figure 3. In order to create several X-ray beams that penetrate bodily tissues at various angles, the method revolves an X-ray tube and detectors around the patient. CT scans, in contrast to conventional X-rays, provide exceptional detail, enabling doctors to precisely inspect blood arteries, soft tissues, and bones all at once. The scanning process is quick, painless, and non-invasive (Mishra et al., 2021). Each CT scan generates multiple images that can be reformatted, printed, or transferred digitally, providing healthcare professionals with versatile diagnostic tools. Modern multi-slice CT scanners can obtain thinner image slices in less time, further enhancing diagnostic capabilities and reducing examination duration.

Figure 3. CT scan

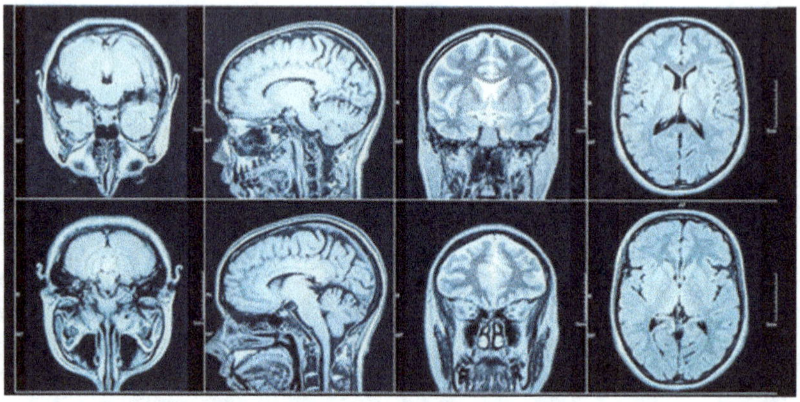

Magnetic Resonance Imaging (MRI)

Magnetic Resonance Imaging (MRI) is an advanced medical diagnostic technique that uses powerful magnetic fields and radio waves to create highly detailed internal body images without using ionizing radiation (Aamir et al., 2022). The technology works by aligning hydrogen protons within water molecules throughout the body, then applying radio frequency pulses that cause these protons to shift and emit signals when returning to their original state. These emitted signals are captured by specialized receivers and processed by computer algorithms to generate comprehensive cross-sectional images of organs, tissues, and structures with exceptional clarity. Unlike X-rays or CT scans, MRI provides exquisite soft tissue detail as shown in Figure 4, making it particularly valuable for examining the brain, spinal cord, muscles, and complex internal organs, while offering the significant advantage of being radiation-free.

Figure 4. MRI Scan of brain

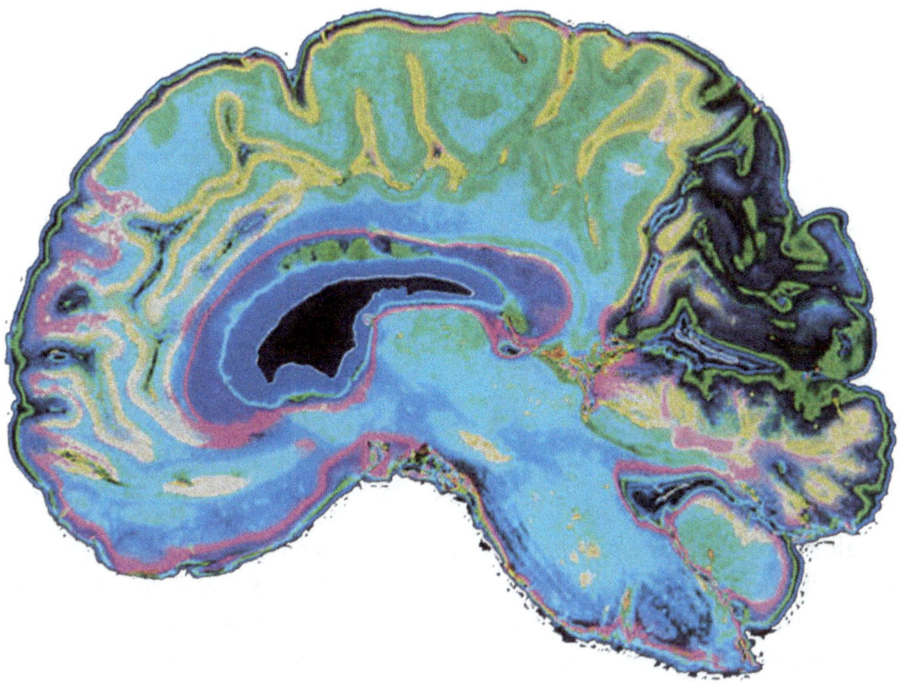

Nuclear Medicine Imaging

Nuclear Medicine Imaging is an innovative medical diagnostic technique that uses small amounts of radioactive materials called radiotracers to create detailed images of internal body processes at a cellular level. Unlike traditional imaging methods that focus on structural anatomy, nuclear medicine provides unique insights into organ function and metabolic activities by tracking how radiotracers interact with specific tissues.

Figure 5. Different types of Medical Imaging

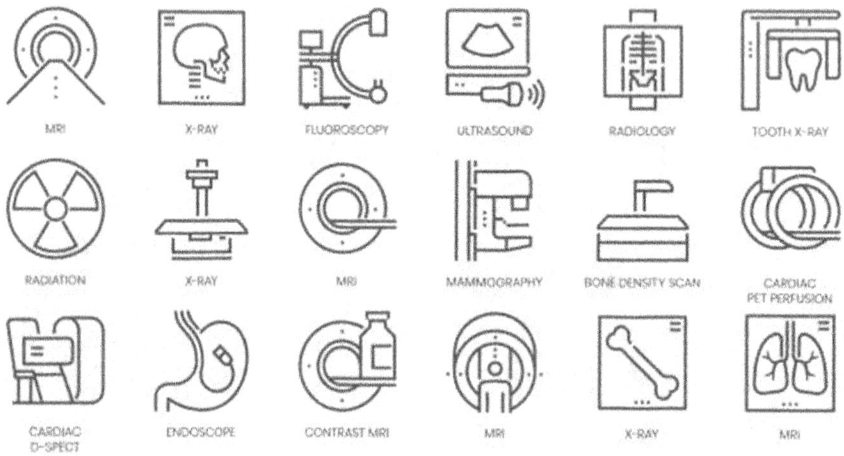

Medical imaging has undergone a profound transformation since its inception, marked by exponential technological advancements and remarkable market growth. Figure 5 shows different types of medical imaging. From the rudimentary X-ray machines of the late 19th century to today's sophisticated AI-integrated diagnostic tools, the field has experienced unprecedented evolution. The global medical imaging market has expanded dramatically, growing from a modest USD 29.2 billion in 2022 to a projected USD 48.8 billion by 2032, representing a consistent compound annual growth rate of approximately 5.40%. Modern CT scanners can now capture 128 image slices in less than a second, compared to just a few slices decades ago. MRI technology has advanced from 1.5 Tesla to 3 Tesla field-strength magnets, enabling unprecedented internal body visualization. Digital image acquisition has completely replaced traditional film, reducing processing time and increasing image clarity by nearly 70%. Artificial intelligence has revolutionized medical imaging, with AI-enabled solutions expected to grow from USD 1.35 billion in 2021 to an astounding USD 18.36 billion by 2032.

INTRODUCTION TO CONVOLUTIONAL NEURAL NETWORKS (CNNS)

A Convolutional Neural Network (CNN) is a sophisticated deep learning algorithm designed for processing visual data by mimicking the human visual cortex's hierarchical information processing (Aamir et al., 2019). These networks have achieved remarkable near-human level performance across diverse domains, demonstrating extraordinary capabilities in complex recognition tasks. In human activity recognition, CNNs have reached an impressive 97.20% accuracy in classifying movements, while autonomous vehicle object detection systems now match human perception in real-time tracking and identification. Medical imaging applications leverage CNN technologies to detect intricate patterns in radiology images, sometimes outperforming human experts in cancer detection and diagnostic interpretation. Facial recognition systems can now break down and analyse facial components with unprecedented precision, separating unique features from external variations like lighting and pose (Niranjani et al., 2023). Document analysis technologies powered by CNNs have reduced character-level error rates to an astonishing 0.4%, approaching near-perfect recognition. This revolutionary approach has transformed computer vision, extending beyond traditional image processing to applications in autonomous vehicles, medical diagnostics, natural language processing, and speech recognition, consistently pushing the boundaries of machine learning capabilities.

Figure 6. CNN Architecture

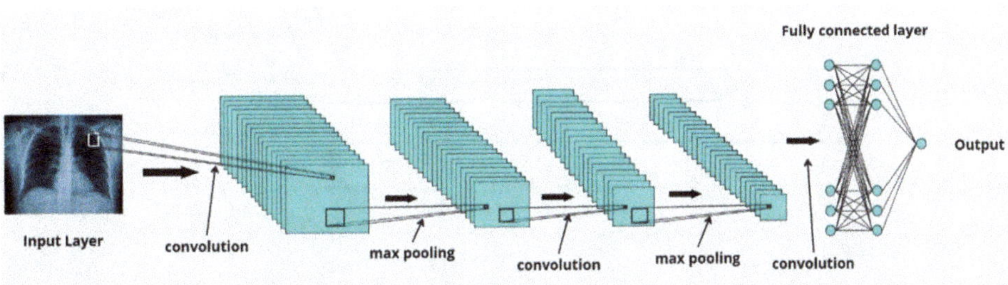

The figure 6 demonstrates the workflow of a convolutional neural network (CNN), starting from the input layer, followed by feature extraction and dimensionality reduction, and concluding with a fully connected layer for final predictions.

Input Layer

The input layer of a Convolutional Neural Network (CNN) serves as the entry point for the raw data, typically an image or a similar structured dataset. Images are represented as tensors, which consist of three dimensions: height (H), width (W), and the number of channels (C), where channels refer to the color components (e.g., RGB or grayscale) as shown in Figure 7. For instance, an RGB image of size 64×64 has a shape of 64×64x3. The input layer simply passes this data into the subsequent layers without applying any transformations. This layer is crucial as it ensures the data format aligns with the expectations of the network's architecture.

$$X \in R^{H \times W \times C}$$

Where:

- H: Height of the image.
- W: Width of the image.
- C : Number of channels (e.g., 3 for RGB, 1 for grayscale).

Figure 7. Input Layer

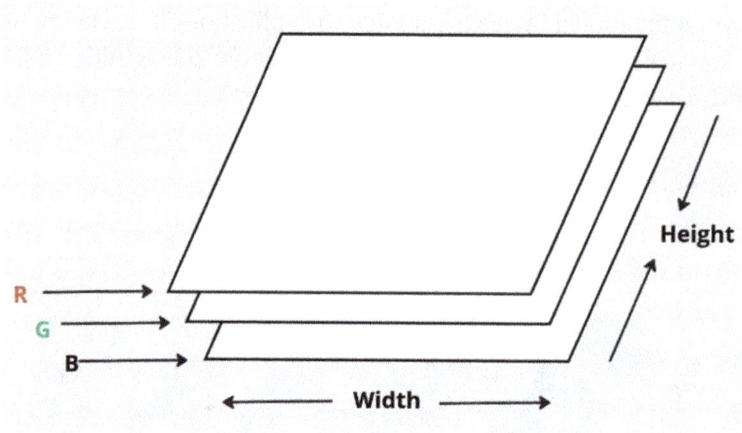

Convolutional Layers

The fundamental building blocks of a CNN are convolutional layers, which are made to automatically and adaptively extract spatial characteristics from the input data (Yamashita, Nishio, Do, & et al., 2018; Selvamurugan et al., 2024). These layers make use of a collection of filters, also known as kernels, which are tiny matrices with sizes like 2 by 2 or 5 by 5. The dot product between each filter's weights and the appropriate input sub-regions is calculated as each filter slides (or convolves) over the input. This process creates feature maps that draw attention to particular patterns, including corners, edges, or textures. Two important parameters govern how the filter moves across the input: padding, which controls how borders are handled, and stride, which establishes the step size as shown in Figure 8. CNNs are particularly useful for image and spatial data because of their ability to concentrate on local information thanks to convolutional layers.

Figure 8. Padding and Stride

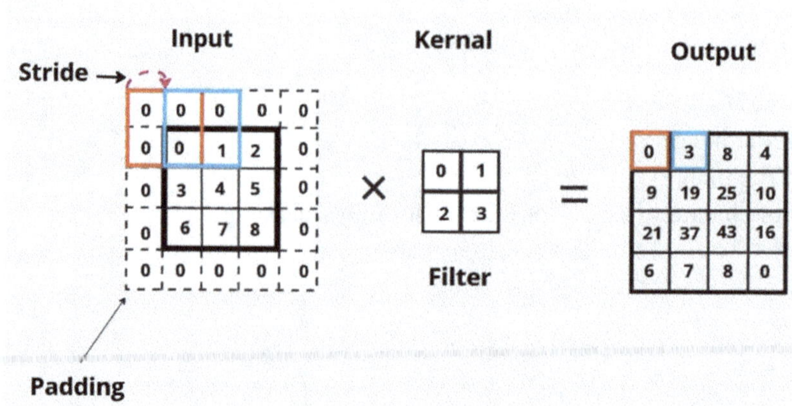

$$Y[i,j] = \sum_{m=0}^{k_h-1}\sum_{n=0}^{k_w-1}\sum_{c=0}^{C-1} K[m,n,c].\, X[i+m, j+n, c] + b$$

Where:

- $Y[i,j]$: The output at position (i,j)in the feature map.
- k_h, k_w: Height and width of the filter.
- C: Number of channels in the input.
- K: Convolutional filter (kernel).
- b: Bias term added after convolution.

This operation slides the filter over the input tensor with a defined **stride** and optionally applies **padding** to maintain the output dimensions.

The output feature map size is determined by:

$$H_{out} = \frac{H - k_h + 2P}{S} + 1$$

$$W_{out} = \frac{W - k_w + 2P}{S} + 1$$

Where:

- P: Padding size.
- S: Stride.

Activation Layers

Activation layers are deployed following each convolutional operation to add non-linearity to the network. In the absence of these, CNN would operate as a linear model, which would restrict its capacity to understand intricate linkages. The Rectified Linear Unit (ReLU), the most often employed activation function in CNNs, substitutes zero for negative values (f(x)=max(0,x)). This straightforward process solves the vanishing gradient issue while guaranteeing computational efficiency. In situations when characteristics may have negative relevance, variants like Leaky ReLU and Parametric ReLU may also be used. The network can represent complex patterns in the data thanks to these activation functions.

For each output value $Y[i,j]$ from the convolutional layer

$$Z[i,j] = f(Y[i,j])$$

Pooling Layers

Pooling layers are a crucial component in neural networks, designed to reduce the dimensionality of feature maps, enhance the network's resilience to minor input variations, and lower computational costs. Among the various types, **max pooling** is the most widely used. It extracts the most prominent feature within a specified window, such as a 2×2 region, by selecting the maximum value. Another less common option is **average pooling**, which computes the average value within the window.

For example, consider a 4×4 matrix in Figure 9, divided into 4 submatrices. In **max pooling**, the maximum value in the first submatrix (red-highlighted 2×2 submatrices) is 32, which becomes the first entry in the resulting 2×2 matrix. The same process applies to other submatrices. Conversely, in **average pooling**, the first submatrix's average value, 15, becomes the first entry in the output matrix, and the process is repeated for the other submatrices.

Pooling layers are simple yet powerful tools for dimensionality reduction. They operate independently on each feature map and do not rely on learnable parameters, making them computationally efficient while preserving key spatial features.

Figure 9. Pooling

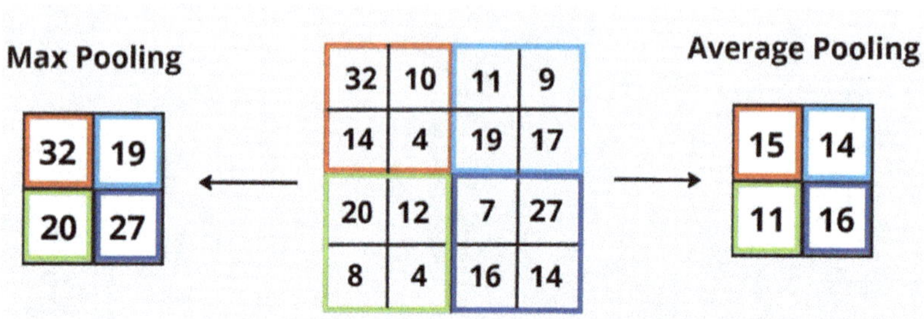

For **Max Pooling**:

$$Z[i,j] = \max\{Y[m,n] | m \in W_p, n \in H_p\}$$

Where $W_p \times H_p$ is the pooling window size.
For **Average Pooling**:

$$Z[i,j] = \frac{1}{[W_p]\cdot[H_p]} \sum_{m\in W_p, n\in H_p} Y[m,n]$$

The output size is calculated similarly to the convolutional layer:

$$H_{out} = \frac{H - k_p}{S} + 1$$

$$W_{out} = \frac{W - k_p}{S} + 1$$

Where k_p is the pooling kernel size.

Fully Connected (Dense) Layers

The convolutional and pooling layers extract high-level information, which are then merged for decision-making in the fully connected layer, the last stage of a CNN. First, a one-dimensional vector is created by flattening the feature maps. Every neuron is coupled to every input as this vector is then transferred through numerous layers. The model can incorporate the spatial hierarchies of features learned in previous layers thanks to this extensive link. For applications involving regression or classification, fully connected layers are usually employed. The final dense layer in an image classification task, for instance, can produce probabilities corresponding to various classes using a softmax activation function.

$$Z = W.X + b$$

Where:

- W: Weight matrix.
- X: Input vector (flattened feature map).
- b: Bias vector.
- Z: Output vector.

Output Layer

The output layer, which is the CNN's last layer, offers the predictions made by the network. The work at hand determines how it is structured. A softmax activation function, which generates a probability distribution across all classes, is commonly used by the layer for multi-class classification. A sigmoid activation function, which provides a single probability value for one class, is frequently used for binary classification. The output layer of regression tasks generates a continuous value by using a linear activation function. The output layer makes sure that the predictions made by the network can be understood and fit the specifications of the challenge.

For Classification (using Softmax activation):

$$\hat{y}_k = \frac{e^{z_k}}{\sum_{j=1}^{K} e^{z_j}}$$

Where:

- z_k: The k^{th}logit (output before activation).
- $\hat{y}_k$: Probability of the kth class.
- K: Number of classes.

For Binary Classification (using Sigmoid activation):

$$\hat{y} = \frac{1}{1 + e^{-z}}$$

Where z is the single logit for binary classification.

For Regression: The output is linear

$$\hat{y} = z$$

Batch Normalization and Dropout

Optional layers like batch normalization and dropout are frequently added to CNNs to enhance their generalization and performance. By normalizing the activations in every layer, batch normalization expedites training and lessens initialization sensitivity. In contrast, dropout forces the network to acquire more resilient properties by randomly deactivating a portion of neurons during training. In a variety of applications, these layers improve the model's adaptability and dependability.

***Batch Normalization*:** Batch normalization normalizes the input to a layer:

$$\hat{x} = \frac{x - \mu}{\sqrt{\sigma^2 + \epsilon}}, y = \gamma\hat{x} + \beta$$

Where:

- μ: Mean of the input batch.
- σ^2: Variance of the input batch.
- ϵ: Small constant for numerical stability.
- γ, β: Learnable scale and shift parameters.

***Dropout*:** Dropout randomly sets a fraction of neurons to zero during training:

$$z_i = \begin{cases} x_i, & \textit{with probability } p, \\ 0, & \textit{with probability } 1 - p. \end{cases}$$

Where p is the retention probability.

CNN FRAMEWORKS: A COMPREHENSIVE OVERVIEW

LeNet

LeNet was the first successful Convolutional Neural Network architecture developed in 1998. Created by Yann LeCun, this groundbreaking framework was initially designed for handwritten digit recognition. It introduced fundamental concepts of convolutional layers, pooling layers, and feature extraction that would become cornerstone principles in modern computer vision.

AlexNet

An important advancement in deep learning for image classification was made with AlexNet. This architecture, created by Alex Krizhevsky, showed off the capabilities of deep convolutional neural networks in 2012 when it achieved outstanding results on the ImageNet Large Scale Visual Recognition Challenge (ILSVRC). It made use of several convolutional and fully linked layers as well as cutting-edge methods including dropout and ReLU activation.

VGGNet

Created by the Visual Geometry Group at Oxford University, VGGNet is characterized by its uniform architecture with multiple convolutional layers. This framework significantly increased network depth, utilizing up to 16-19 layers and demonstrating that deeper networks could capture more complex visual features. VGGNet became a fundamental reference point for subsequent CNN architectures.

ResNet

ResNet, developed by Kaiming He and colleagues, introduced the revolutionary concept of residual connections. This innovation solved the vanishing gradient problem in very deep neural networks, allowing for the creation of networks with unprecedented depth. ResNet's architecture enables training of networks with over 100 layers, dramatically improving performance in image recognition tasks.

GoogleNet (Inception)

GoogleNet, also known as Inception, revolutionized CNN design by introducing the inception module. This innovative approach allows the network to choose between different convolution sizes within the same layer, creating a more flexible and efficient architecture. The framework significantly reduced computational complexity while maintaining high accuracy.

MobileNet

Specifically designed for mobile and embedded vision applications, MobileNet focuses on creating lightweight, efficient neural networks. By using depth wise separable convolutions, this framework achieves impressive performance with minimal computational resources, making it ideal for deployment on smartphones and IoT devices.

Specific advantages of CNNs in medical image analysis

Convolutional Neural Networks (CNNs) offer several critical advantages in medical image analysis:

Superior Diagnostic Performance

CNNs have demonstrated remarkable performance, frequently outperforming human experts in various medical diagnostic tasks. For instance:

- GoogleNet achieved 89% accuracy in cancer detection, compared to human pathologists' 70%.
- CheXNet outperformed four radiologists in pneumonia diagnosis using over 100,000 chest X-rays (Yadav & Jadhav, 2019)
- A study utilizing multi-modal medical images achieved an impressive 98.61% classification accuracy

Enhanced Diagnostic Workflow

CNNs promise to optimize healthcare processes by:

- Streamlining diagnostic workflows
- Providing faster image interpretation
- Enabling personalized treatment planning
- Assisting in early disease detection
- Supporting radiologists' decision-making

By leveraging large annotated datasets, CNNs can learn intricate patterns and relationships within medical images, ultimately contributing to more precise and efficient healthcare diagnostics.

ADVANCED LEARNING STRATEGIES: PRETRAINED NETWORKS AND TRANSFER LEARNING FOR MEDICAL IMAGING

Pretrained models are neural networks trained on large datasets to learn generalized features, enabling them to be fine-tuned for specific tasks across diverse domains (Guan et al., 2021). The core mechanism of pretrained networks involves a hierarchical learning approach where neural architectures progressively extract increasingly complex features across multiple computational layers. Initial network layers capture fundamental elements like basic geometric shapes and elementary patterns, while deeper layers develop increasingly nuanced capabilities to recognize sophisticated semantic representations and intricate contextual relationships. This architectural design enables models to develop remarkable computational intelligence that can be transferred across diverse domains.

Transfer learning emerges as a critical technique within this framework, enabling developers to repurpose existing neural network models from one domain to address challenges in related computational contexts (Salehi et al., 2023). By strategically retaining learned features and selectively adjusting final network layers, researchers can dramatically reduce training time, minimize computational resource requirements, and achieve superior performance levels even when working with relatively limited datasets.

Pretrained networks have emerged as a critical innovation in medical imaging, offering sophisticated solutions to the challenges of limited medical datasets and complex diagnostic requirements. Researchers have developed specialized approaches like RadImageNet and MedNet to address the unique complexities of medical image analysis, recognizing that traditional ImageNet-trained models often fail to capture the nuanced characteristics of medical imaging.

RadImageNet: A Groundbreaking Medical Imaging Dataset

RadImageNet (Mei et al., 2022) represents a significant advancement in medical imaging datasets, distinguished by its unprecedented scale and comprehensive approach to medical image analysis. The dataset comprises 1.35 million annotated medical images from 131,872 patients, covering multiple imaging modalities including CT, MRI, and ultrasound across 11 anatomical regions and 165 pathologic labels.

Performance Across Different Applications The dataset demonstrated significant performance gains across various medical imaging tasks:

- Thyroid nodule classification: 9.4% improvement
- Breast mass detection: 4.0% improvement
- Anterior cruciate ligament injuries: 4.8% improvement
- Meniscal tears: 4.5% improvement
- Pneumonia detection: 1.9% improvement
- COVID-19 classification: 6.1% improvement

Innovative Pretrained Model Architectures

Researchers have developed specialized pretrained networks tailored specifically for medical imaging, including:

- ResNet50
- DenseNet121
- InceptionResNetV2
- InceptionV3
- ConvNeXtBase
- EfficientNetB7

These models are designed to overcome the limitations of general-purpose image recognition networks by training exclusively on medical imaging datasets, enabling more accurate and contextually relevant feature extraction.

MEDICAL IMAGING MODALITIES AND APPLICATIONS

MRI (Magnetic Resonance Imaging): Using CNNs for tumor detection

The neural network architectures deployed in brain tumour detection represent complex, multi-layered computational systems designed to mimic human visual processing.

```
import os


import tensorflow as tf
```

```
from tensorflow.keras.preprocessing.image import ImageDataGenerator

from tensorflow.keras.models import Sequential, Model

from tensorflow.keras.layers import Conv2D, MaxPooling2D, Flatten, Dense, Dropout, Input

from sklearn.metrics import classification_report, confusion_matrix

import numpy as np
```

These imports set the stage for constructing a deep learning pipeline for classifying brain tumour images. With the necessary tools and libraries at hand, the code proceeds to define paths, preprocess data, build the CNN, and train and evaluate it, ensuring a comprehensive workflow.

```
# Dataset Path

dataset_path = '/kaggle/input/brian-tumor-dataset/Brain Tumor Data Set/Brain Tumor Data Set'

# Parameters

batch_size = 32

img_height = 224

img_width = 224

epochs = 10
```

Dataset Path:The variable dataset_path holds the file path to the dataset directory. This path points to the folder containing two subdirectories, "Brain Tumor" and "Healthy," each representing a class of images.

Batch Size:The batch_size parameter is set to 32, meaning the model will process 32 images at a time during training and validation. Using batches improves computational efficiency by dividing the dataset into manageable chunks.

Image Dimensions:img_height and img_width are set to 224 pixels each.

Epochs:The epochs parameter determines the number of complete passes through the entire training dataset. Here, it is set to 10, meaning the model will train for 10 iterations to minimize the loss function.

Data Augmentation and Preprocessing

```
# Data Augmentation and Preprocessing

train_datagen = ImageDataGenerator(

rescale=1.0/255,

validation_split=0.2, # 80% train, 20% validation

rotation_range=15,

width_shift_range=0.1,

height_shift_range=0.1,

horizontal_flip=True

)



# Train and Validation Data Loaders

train_generator = train_datagen.flow_from_directory(
```

```
dataset_path,

target_size=(img_height, img_width),

batch_size=batch_size,

class_mode='binary',

subset='training'

)



validation_generator = train_datagen.flow_from_directory(

dataset_path,

target_size=(img_height, img_width),

batch_size=batch_size,

class_mode='binary',

subset='validation'

)
```

The ImageDataGenerator class is used to create an instance named train_datagen for augmenting and preprocessing images. Key aspects of the configuration include:

1. ***rescale=1.0/255***:This normalizes pixel values of the images from the range [0, 255] to [0, 1], improving model performance by standardizing the data.
2. ***validation_split=0.2***:Two subsets of the dataset are separated: 20% for validation and 80% for training. This guarantees that throughout training, the model is assessed on unseen data, giving an early indication of its capacity for generalization.
3. **Augmentation Parameters**:
   - rotation_range=15: To make the model resilient to various orientations, photos are randomly rotated by up to 15 degrees.
   - To simulate real-world fluctuations, photos are randomly shifted horizontally and vertically by up to 10% of their width or height using width_shift_range=0.1 and height_shift_range=0.1.
   - horizontal_flip=True: To increase resilience against mirrored inputs, images are randomly flipped horizontally.

Only the training data subset is subjected to data augmentation, which increases diversity and avoids overfitting.

Train and Validation Data Loaders

1. ***Training Data Loader***:The flow_from_directory method is used to load images from the dataset directory.
   - **target_size=(img_height, img_width)**: Resizes all images to 224x224 pixels to match the input dimensions required by the CNN.
   - **batch_size=batch_size**: Loads images in batches of 32 for efficient training.
   - **class_mode='binary'**: Specifies binary classification (Brain Tumour or Healthy).
   - **subset='training'**: Selects the training portion of the dataset based on the validation_split.
2. ***Validation Data Loader***: A similar flow_from_directory call is made to load validation images with the same parameters. However, **subset='validation'** ensures this loader contains the validation split.

The train_generator and validation_generator objects serve as efficient data pipelines, providing batches of augmented or raw images along with their corresponding labels during training. This approach not only automates image preprocessing but also ensures consistent data handling across different experiments.

```
import matplotlib.pyplot as plt

import numpy as np

# Get a batch of training data

data_batch, labels_batch = next(train_generator)
```

```
# Define a function to plot images with labels

def plot_images_with_labels(images, labels, class_indices):

class_names = {v: k for k, v in class_indices.items()} # Reverse the dictio-
nary

plt.figure(figsize=(12, 12))

for i in range(min(9, len(images))): # Display up to 9 images

plt.subplot(3, 3, i + 1)

plt.imshow(images[i])

plt.title(class_names[int(labels[i])])

plt.axis('off')

plt.tight_layout()

plt.show()

# Call the function

plot_images_with_labels(data_batch, labels_batch, train_generator.class_in-
dices)
```

The code provided is designed to visually inspect a batch of training images along with their corresponding labels, helping to ensure the data generator is working correctly and to better understand the dataset. First, the script retrieves a batch of images and labels using the train_generator. This generator fetches a batch of preprocessed images from the dataset, and the next(train_generator) call provides access to these images and their associated binary labels (e.g., 0 for one class and 1 for another).

Finally, the function is called with the batch of data fetched earlier, along with the class index mapping from the generator. The resulting output is a grid of images, each annotated with its correct label, such as "Brain Tumor" or "Healthy." This visualization step is crucial in verifying that the images are correctly loaded and that the labels correspond accurately to the data. It also provides an opportunity to observe the variations and augmentations in the training images, offering insights into how the model will perceive the data during training as shown in Figure 10.

Figure 10. Image with labels

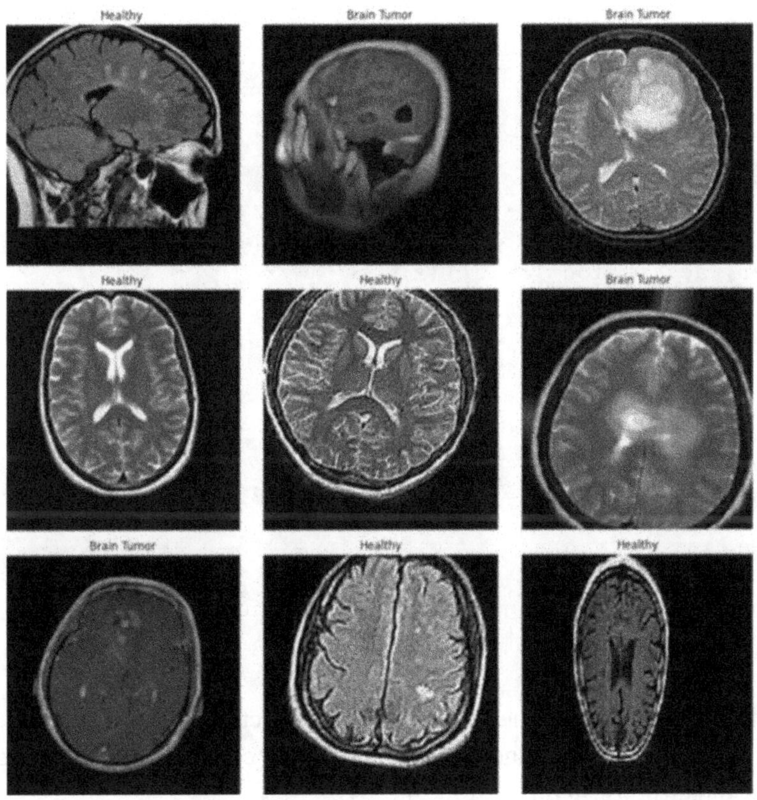


```
# Define CNN Model

model_input = Input(shape=(img_height, img_width, 3)) # Define input shape

x = Conv2D(32, (3, 3), activation='relu')(model_input)
```

```
x = MaxPooling2D(pool_size=(2, 2))(x)

x = Conv2D(64, (3, 3), activation='relu')(x)

x = MaxPooling2D(pool_size=(2, 2))(x)

x = Conv2D(128, (3, 3), activation='relu')(x)

x = MaxPooling2D(pool_size=(2, 2))(x)

x = Flatten()(x)

x = Dense(128, activation='relu')(x)

x = Dropout(0.5)(x)

output = Dense(1, activation='sigmoid')(x) # Binary classification

model = Model(inputs=model_input, outputs=output)
```

Model Input:

With the help of the Input function, the input layer is constructed. The input images' shape is specified as (img_height, img_width, 3), where 3 indicates the RGB color channels and img_height and img_width indicate the images' dimensions (in this case, 224x224).

First Convolutional Block:

The input image is subjected to 32 convolutional filters of size (3, 3) in the network's first layer. The Conv2D layer is used to do this. By adding non-linearity, the ReLU activation function (relu) aids in the network's ability to recognize intricate patterns. A MaxPooling2D layer with a pool size of (2, 2) comes next, which effectively downsamples the data and lowers computing complexity by reducing the spatial dimensions of the feature maps.

Second Convolutional Block:There is an additional Conv2D layer added, with 64 filters of size (3, 3). It employs ReLU activation, just like the previous block, and further down-samples the feature maps with a MaxPooling2D layer.

Third Convolutional Block:128 filters of size (3,3) are added to the deeper convolutional layer. As previously, max-pooling is used for down-sampling after this layer.

Flattening the Feature Maps:The final convolutional layer's 2D feature maps are transformed into 1D vectors by the Flatten layer. To get from the network's convolutional to its fully linked sections, this is required.

Fully Connected Layer:A 128-unit dense layer with ReLU activation is introduced. By combining the features that the convolutional layers have extracted, this layer learns high-level representations of the data.

Dropout Layer:During training, 50% of the neurons are randomly turned off by a Dropout layer with a rate of 0.5. By adding regularization and strengthening the network, this helps avoid overfitting.

Output Layer:A single neuron with a sigmoid activation function makes up the last layer, which is a dense layer. A probability value between 0 and 1 is produced by the sigmoid function, which is appropriate for binary classification jobs such as this one (0 for "Healthy" and 1 for "Brain Tumor").

The input and output layers of the model are specified using the Model class from Keras. The input layer is represented by the model_input variable, and the final output layer is represented by the output variable.

```
# Compile the Model

model.compile(

optimizer='adam',

loss='binary_crossentropy',

metrics=['accuracy']

)

optimizer='adam'
```

Adam Optimizer: A well-liked optimization technique that combines the benefits of the Adamax and RMSprop optimizers is called Adam (Adaptive Moment Estimation). It works well with deep learning models and adjusts the learning rate during training. By adjusting weights according to the gradients calculated during backpropagation, this optimizer aids in effectively decreasing the loss function.

```
loss='binary_crossentropy'
```

Binary Crossentropy Loss: When the goal has only two possible outcomes—typically 0 (Healthy) or 1 (Brain Tumor)—this is employed for binary classification tasks. The difference between the actual label and the projected probability is measured by the loss. It has the following mathematical definition:

$$L(y,\hat{y}) = -[y\,.\log(\hat{y}) + (1 - y)\,.\log(1 - \hat{y})]$$

where y is the actual label (0 or 1) and $\hat{y}$ is the predicted probability.

```
metrics=['accuracy']
```

Accuracy:A straightforward indicator of the model's performance is accuracy. It determines the percentage of samples that were correctly classified out of all the samples.

During training and evaluation, the model will track this metric to understand its performance.

```
# Train the Model

history = model.fit(

train_generator,

validation_data=validation_generator,

epochs=epochs

)
```

The model must be trained using the fit approach. Along with the number of epochs, which establishes how many times the complete dataset is run through the model, it receives the training and validation data.

1. ***train_generator***:This is the data generator that supplies the training dataset in batches. It handles loading the images and labels for the training set.
2. ***validation_data=validation_generator***:This is the data generator for the validation set, which ensures the model is evaluated on unseen data during training.
3. ***epochs=epochs***:The number of times the model will iterate over the entire training dataset. More epochs typically improve the performance but can also lead to overfitting if the model is not regularized well.
4. ***history***:The output of fit contains the training history, which holds information such as loss, accuracy, and validation loss/accuracy for each epoch. These metrics are tracked and used to monitor the model's performance over time.

By modifying its weights with the Adam optimizer and binary crossentropy loss, the model begins learning in this step. Until the predetermined number of epochs is reached, it keeps updating these weights. The accuracy has increased on each epoch can be seen in Figure 11.

Figure 11. Training output

```
Epoch 1/10
116/116 ━━━━━━━━━━━━━━━━━━━━ 63s 492ms/step - accuracy: 0.5801 - loss: 0.71
84 - val_accuracy: 0.6148 - val_loss: 0.7138
Epoch 2/10
116/116 ━━━━━━━━━━━━━━━━━━━━ 54s 441ms/step - accuracy: 0.7109 - loss: 0.57
03 - val_accuracy: 0.6986 - val_loss: 0.5743
Epoch 3/10
116/116 ━━━━━━━━━━━━━━━━━━━━ 53s 431ms/step - accuracy: 0.7715 - loss: 0.48
79 - val_accuracy: 0.7236 - val_loss: 0.5433
Epoch 4/10
116/116 ━━━━━━━━━━━━━━━━━━━━ 52s 427ms/step - accuracy: 0.8016 - loss: 0.42
80 - val_accuracy: 0.7922 - val_loss: 0.4718
Epoch 5/10
116/116 ━━━━━━━━━━━━━━━━━━━━ 52s 428ms/step - accuracy: 0.7964 - loss: 0.44
09 - val_accuracy: 0.7933 - val_loss: 0.4671
Epoch 6/10
116/116 ━━━━━━━━━━━━━━━━━━━━ 52s 427ms/step - accuracy: 0.8077 - loss: 0.38
46 - val_accuracy: 0.8281 - val_loss: 0.3946
Epoch 7/10
116/116 ━━━━━━━━━━━━━━━━━━━━ 52s 425ms/step - accuracy: 0.8232 - loss: 0.37
84 - val_accuracy: 0.8085 - val_loss: 0.4055
Epoch 8/10
116/116 ━━━━━━━━━━━━━━━━━━━━ 51s 421ms/step - accuracy: 0.8265 - loss: 0.35
56 - val_accuracy: 0.8183 - val_loss: 0.3753
Epoch 9/10
116/116 ━━━━━━━━━━━━━━━━━━━━ 52s 429ms/step - accuracy: 0.8485 - loss: 0.34
03 - val_accuracy: 0.8020 - val_loss: 0.4144
Epoch 10/10
116/116 ━━━━━━━━━━━━━━━━━━━━ 52s 427ms/step - accuracy: 0.8529 - loss: 0.31
86 - val_accuracy: 0.8259 - val_loss: 0.3832
```

```
# Evaluate the Model on Validation Data

val_loss, val_accuracy = model.evaluate(validation_generator)

print(f"Validation Loss: {val_loss}")

print(f"Validation Accuracy: {val_accuracy}")

# Predictions and Metrics

# Predicting on validation data
```

```
val_generator = validation_generator

val_generator.reset() # Ensure generator starts from beginning

predictions = model.predict(val_generator)

predictions = (predictions > 0.5).astype(int).flatten() # Convert probabili-
ties to binary labels

# True labels

true_labels = val_generator.classes

# Confusion Matrix and Classification Report

conf_matrix = confusion_matrix(true_labels, predictions)

class_report = classification_report(true_labels, predictions, target_
names=train_generator.class_indices.keys())

print("\nConfusion Matrix:")

print(conf_matrix)

print("\nClassification Report:")

print(class_report)
```

1. **model.evaluate(validation_generator)**:
   - The model is assessed using the validation dataset in this line. The validation accuracy and validation loss are the two values that are returned.

- Loss: Shows the difference between the expected and actual numbers. Better model performance is implied by a lower loss.
- Accuracy: Indicates the percentage of accurate predictions made on the validation set.

2. **predictions = model.predict(val_generator)**:
   - The model makes predictions on the validation set. This step generates probability scores for each sample.
3. **predictions = (predictions > 0.5).astype(int).flatten()**:
   - Converts the continuous probability scores into binary predictions (i.e., tumor present or not) by thresholding at 0.5.
   - **0.5** is a common threshold in binary classification problems to determine the final class label.
4. **true_labels = val_generator.classes**:
   - Extracts the true class labels from the validation data generator.
5. **Confusion Matrix**:
   - The number of true positives, true negatives, false positives, and false negatives produced by the model is determined by the confusion_matrix(true_labels, predictions). It is an essential indicator for assessing the performance of the model.
6. **Classification Report**:
   - For every class, classification_report(true_labels, predictions) offers comprehensive performance data such as accuracy, precision, recall, and F1-score.
7. **Printing**:
   - To give information about the model's performance, including its capacity to accurately distinguish between photos with and without tumors, the confusion matrix and classification report are printed.

The output of the above code snippet is given in Figure 12 which shows the confusion matrix and Classification report.

Figure 12. Confusion Matrix

```
29/29 ──────────────────── 10s 356ms/step - accuracy: 0.8234 - loss: 0.3938
Validation Loss: 0.3916085660457611
Validation Accuracy: 0.8258976936340332
29/29 ──────────────────── 10s 353ms/step

Confusion Matrix:
[[277 225]
 [235 182]]

Classification Report:
              precision    recall  f1-score   support

 Brain Tumor       0.54      0.55      0.55       502
     Healthy       0.45      0.44      0.44       417

    accuracy                           0.50       919
   macro avg       0.49      0.49      0.49       919
weighted avg       0.50      0.50      0.50       919
```

```
# 5. Save the Model

model.save('brain_tumor_cnn_model.h5')
```

This line saves the trained model to a file named brain_tumor_cnn_model.h5

```
# 6. Visualize Training History

import matplotlib.pyplot as plt

# Plot accuracy

plt.plot(history.history['accuracy'], label='Train Accuracy')

plt.plot(history.history['val_accuracy'], label='Validation Accuracy')

plt.legend()

plt.title('Model Accuracy')

plt.xlabel('Epochs')

plt.ylabel('Accuracy')

plt.show()
```

Figure 13. Train Accuracy

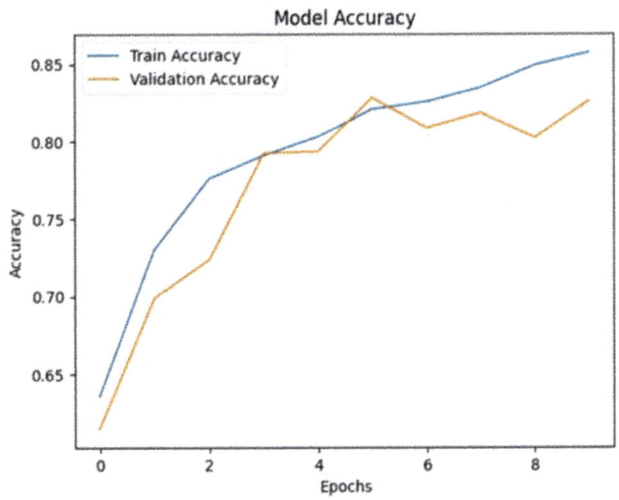


```
# Plot loss

plt.plot(history.history['loss'], label='Train Loss')

plt.plot(history.history['val_loss'], label='Validation Loss')

plt.legend()

plt.title('Model Loss')

plt.xlabel('Epochs')

plt.ylabel('Loss')

plt.show()
```

Figure 14. Test Accuracy

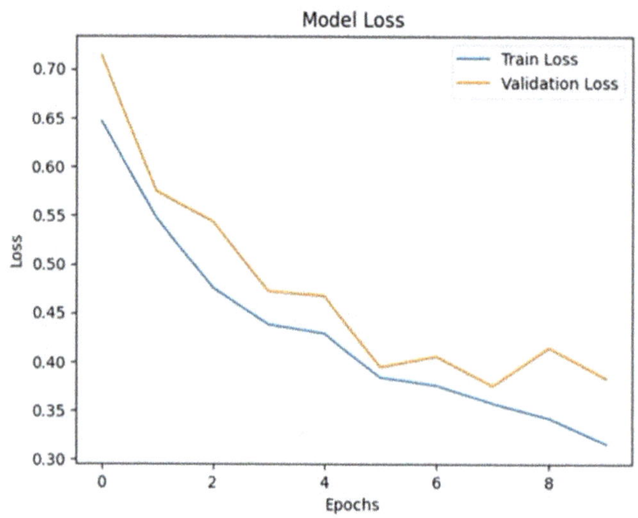

These charts illustrate how accuracy and loss vary throughout epochs, hence visualizing model performance. By comparing the training and validation accuracy on train and test datasets as shown in Figure 13 and Figure 14 respectively, the accuracy plot aids in the detection of overfitting. The model is learning efficiently, as evidenced by the loss map, which displays the decline in training and validation loss. We can evaluate the model's generalization and make any required modifications by examining these curves. In the end, they shed light on the model's development and functionality.

Medical Image Binary Classification with Convolutional Neural Networks

Pneumonia is a serious condition where the lungs get infected. Doctors often use X-rays to check if a patient has pneumonia or healthy lungs. Figure 15 and Figure 16 shows the image of normal lungs and lungs with pneumonia respectively. Our goal is to create a model that looks at chest X-rays and helps doctors quickly identify whether the X-ray shows normal lungs or lungs with pneumonia.

```
import tensorflow as tf

from tensorflow.keras.preprocessing.image import ImageDataGenerator

from tensorflow.keras.applications import VGG16

from tensorflow.keras import layers
```

```
from tensorflow.keras import Model

from tensorflow.keras.preprocessing import image

import numpy as np

# Set the paths to your dataset

train_dir = '/kaggle/input/chest-xray-pneumonia/chest_xray/train'

test_dir = '/kaggle/input/chest-xray-pneumonia/chest_xray/test'

val_dir = '/kaggle/input/chest-xray-pneumonia/chest_xray/val'

# Image dimensions and batch size

image_size = (224, 224)

batch_size = 32
```

Figure 15. Pneumonia

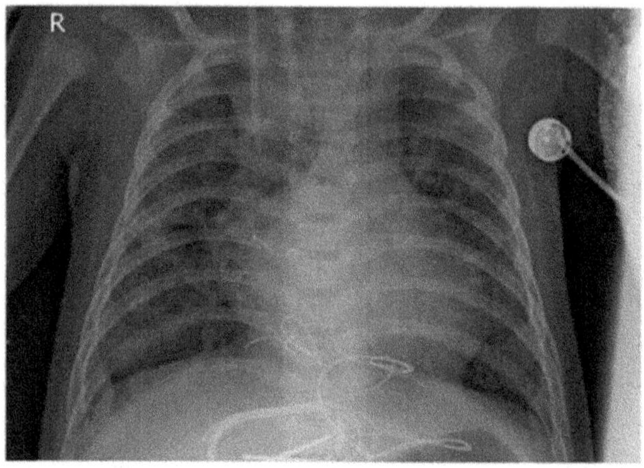

Figure 16. Normal

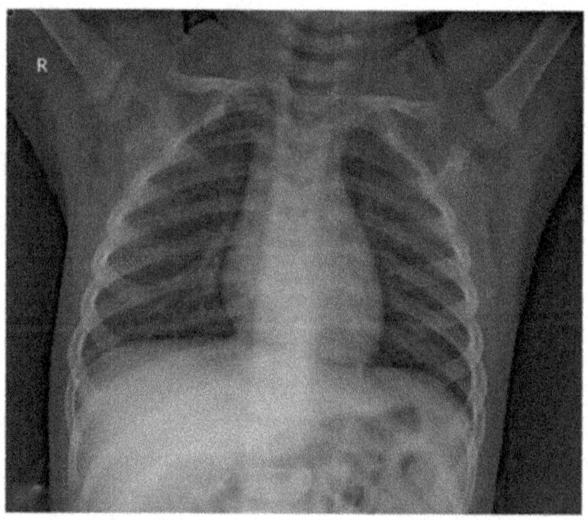

We use specific techniques on the training photos to strengthen our model. To ensure that the model can handle changes such as different angles, positions, or zoom levels, for instance, we rotate, shift, and zoom the photographs. This helps the model learn and generalize effectively when it encounters new data.

```
train_datagen = ImageDataGenerator(

rescale=1.0/255,
```

```
rotation_range=20,
width_shift_range=0.2,
height_shift_range=0.2,
shear_range=0.2,
zoom_range=0.2,
horizontal_flip=True,
fill_mode='nearest'
)
# Preprocess and augment the training data
train_generator = train_datagen.flow_from_directory(
train_dir,
target_size=image_size,
batch_size=batch_size,
class_mode='binary'
)
```

```
# Preprocess the test and validation data

test_datagen = ImageDataGenerator(rescale=1.0/255)

test_generator = test_datagen.flow_from_directory(

test_dir,

target_size=image_size,

batch_size=batch_size,

class_mode='binary'

)

val_generator = test_datagen.flow_from_directory(

val_dir,

target_size=image_size,

batch_size=batch_size,

class_mode='binary'

)
```

We use a powerful pre-trained model called **VGG16**, which is already trained to recognize common objects from billions of images. We "freeze" some of its earlier layers (to use its learned features) and then add a few custom layers on top to adjust it for our specific task of detecting pneumonia.

- We flatten the features from the pre-trained model.
- We add a **dense layer** with 512 neurons to learn complex features.
- We add **dropout** to reduce overfitting (which helps the model avoid relying too much on random noise in the data).
- Finally, we have a **sigmoid output layer** to predict whether the image is normal or pneumonia.

```
base_model = VGG16(include_top=False, weights='imagenet', input_shape=(224, 224, 3))

for layer in base_model.layers:

layer.trainable = False

x = layers.Flatten()(base_model.output)

x = layers.Dense(512, activation='relu')(x)

x = layers.Dropout(0.5)(x)

x = layers.Dense(1, activation='sigmoid')(x)

model = Model(base_model.input, x)
```

We train the model on our dataset, but instead of allowing it to train indefinitely, we implement a technique called **Early Stopping**. This approach halts training once the model ceases to show improvement, conserving both time and computational resources. For instance, as illustrated in Figure 17, training stopped at epoch 5 instead of continuing to epoch 10, as no further improvement was observed.

```
from tensorflow.keras.callbacks import EarlyStopping

# Define EarlyStopping callback

early_stopping = EarlyStopping(monitor='val_loss', patience=3, restore_best_weights=True)
```

```
# Compile the model

model.compile(optimizer=tf.keras.optimizers.Adam(lr=0.0001), loss='binary_
crossentropy', metrics=['accuracy'])

# Train the model with EarlyStopping

history = model.fit(

train_generator,

epochs=10,

validation_data=val_generator,

callbacks=[early_stopping] # Add the EarlyStopping callback

)
```

Figure 17. Training epoch output

```
Epoch 1/10
163/163 [==============================] - 139s 808ms/step - loss: 0.4604 -
accuracy: 0.8731 - val_loss: 0.3810 - val_accuracy: 0.7500
Epoch 2/10
163/163 [==============================] - 99s 606ms/step - loss: 0.2091 -
accuracy: 0.9168 - val_loss: 0.2438 - val_accuracy: 0.8750
Epoch 3/10
163/163 [==============================] - 95s 585ms/step - loss: 0.1904 -
accuracy: 0.9233 - val_loss: 0.3293 - val_accuracy: 0.7500
Epoch 4/10
163/163 [==============================] - 96s 590ms/step - loss: 0.1697 -
accuracy: 0.9352 - val_loss: 0.3747 - val_accuracy: 0.7500
Epoch 5/10
163/163 [==============================] - 97s 597ms/step - loss: 0.1787 -
accuracy: 0.9237 - val_loss: 0.4123 - val_accuracy: 0.8125
```

Once the model is trained, we evaluate it on the test set to check its accuracy. Figure 18 shows the output of evaluating the model on the test set which is 89.9%. After that, we show the model a new X-ray image (one that it hasn't seen before) and ask it to make a prediction. It's prediction is shown in Figure 19.

- If the model predicts a **low probability** (less than 0.5), it assumes the lungs are **normal**.
- If the probability is high, it predicts **pneumonia**.

```
# Evaluate the model on the test set

test_loss, test_accuracy = model.evaluate(test_generator)

print(f'Test accuracy: {test_accuracy * 100:.2f}%')
```

Figure 18. Test Accuracy Output

```
20/20 [==============================] - 9s 470ms/step - loss: 0.2449 - acc
uracy: 0.8990
Test accuracy: 89.90%
```

```
# Load an example image for prediction

image_path = '/kaggle/input/chest-xray-pneumonia/chest_xray/val/PNEUMONIA/
person1946_bacteria_4874.jpeg'

img = image.load_img(image_path, target_size=(224, 224))

img = image.img_to_array(img)

img = np.expand_dims(img, axis=0)

# Make prediction
```

```
predictions = model.predict(img)

# Interpret the prediction

if predictions[0] < 0.5:

print("The image is NORMAL.")

else:

print("The image indicates PNEUMONIA.")
```

Figure 19. Model Prediction

```
1/1 [==============================] - 0s 133ms/step
The image indicates PNEUMONIA.
```

This process helps doctors quickly diagnose pneumonia, saving time and potentially improving patient care.

TECHNIQUES FOR IMAGE PREPROCESSING AND AUGMENTATION

Use of GANs for Augmenting Limited Medical Datasets

Due to patient privacy issues, expensive data gathering costs, and ethical limitations, medical picture databases are frequently constrained. By producing artificial medical images that closely resemble the statistical characteristics of actual data, Generative Adversarial Networks (GANs) have become a potent remedy for this problem and have the ability to enhance existing datasets.

Two neural networks—a discriminator and a generator—that are simultaneously and competitively trained make up a GAN (Motamed et al., 2021; Makhlouf, Maayah, Abughanam, et al., 2023). By differentiating between generated and actual images, the discriminator assesses the authenticity of the artificial images produced by the generator. Through iterative training, the generator becomes proficient in producing realistic images that can supplement limited datasets.

In medical imaging, GANs have been successfully applied to a variety of tasks:

Data Augmentation: GANs can create synthetic variations of medical images by altering properties like orientation, contrast, or texture, enabling models to learn from diverse scenarios. For example, GANs have been used to generate MRI scans with varying tumor shapes and sizes to improve the robustness of tumor detection models.

Image-to-Image Translation: Conditional GANs (cGANs) can translate one type of medical image to another, such as converting CT scans to MRI-like images or enhancing low-resolution images. This is particularly useful for modalities where acquiring high-quality images is difficult or expensive.

Anomaly Detection: GANs can learn the distribution of normal medical images and identify anomalies by detecting deviations from this learned distribution. This is valuable in identifying rare or subtle pathological conditions.

Synthetic Minority Oversampling: GANs address class imbalance by generating additional samples for underrepresented categories, such as rare diseases, ensuring that models are trained on a more balanced dataset.

Notwithstanding their benefits, there are drawbacks to using GANs in medical imaging. Because badly generated data can add noise and impair model performance, it is crucial to ensure the authenticity and realism of synthetic images. Furthermore, GANs are computationally demanding and need to be carefully adjusted to prevent problems such as mode collapse, in which the generator only generates a small number of different images.

Case Studies: Recent breakthroughs in CNNs applied to radiology and pathology

Convolutional Neural Networks (CNNs) have significantly advanced medical imaging, particularly in radiology and pathology, by enhancing diagnostic accuracy and efficiency. Here are detailed case studies illustrating recent breakthroughs:

1. Brain Tumour Segmentation Using CNNs

Accurate segmentation of brain tumours in MRI scans is crucial for diagnosis and treatment planning. Traditional methods often struggle with variability in tumour shape, size, and location. CNNs have been employed to automate this process, learning complex features directly from imaging data. For instance, a study demonstrated the application of CNNs in segmenting brain tumours, achieving high accuracy and robustness across diverse datasets.

2. High-Resolution Class Activation Mapping (HR-CAM)

Localizing pathological regions within medical images is essential for precise diagnosis. Traditional Class Activation Mapping (CAM) techniques often produce coarse localization maps. The HR-CAM approach enhances this by aggregating feature maps from multiple CNN layers, providing detailed and high-resolution localization of abnormalities (Shinde et al., 2019). This method has been applied to classify ependymomas from glioblastomas in MRI and predict Parkinson's disease from neuromelanin-sensitive MRI, offering clinically interpretable, subject-specific localizations.

3. CNN Classification of Cancer Cytopathology Images

In cytopathology, distinguishing between benign and malignant cells is vital. CNNs have been utilized to automate this classification, reducing reliance on subjective human judgment. A study focusing on breast cancer cytopathology images employed an InceptionV3-based CNN model with transfer learning, achieving accuracy rates exceeding 92% across various magnification levels. This advancement underscores the potential of CNNs in enhancing diagnostic efficiency in cytopathology.

4. CNNs in Diagnosing Colon and Lung Cancer from Histopathological Images

Histopathological analysis is the gold standard for cancer diagnosis but is time-consuming and requires expert interpretation (Al-Jabbar et al., 2023). CNNs have been developed to classify histopathological images of lung and colon tissues, distinguishing between benign and malignant samples.A study utilizing a shallow CNN architecture reported diagnostic accuracies exceeding 97% for lung cancer and 96% for colon cancer, highlighting the efficacy of CNNs in supporting pathological diagnoses.

These case studies exemplify the transformative impact of CNNs in medical imaging, offering tools that enhance diagnostic precision and streamline workflows in radiology and pathology.

Examples of CNN models deployed in real-world diagnostic systems.

Convolutional Neural Networks (CNNs) have been instrumental in advancing medical diagnostics by automating and enhancing the accuracy of image analysis. Here are detailed examples of CNN models deployed in real-world diagnostic systems:

1. Pneumonia Detection in Chest X-Rays

CNN-based algorithms have been applied to classify pneumonia in chest X-ray images. By training on labeled datasets, these models can distinguish between normal and pneumonia-affected lungs, aiding in rapid diagnosis. Such systems have been integrated into clinical workflows to assist radiologists, especially in resource-limited settings.

2. Skin Cancer Diagnosis with Optimized CNN Architectures

Deep learning, particularly CNNs, has been explored to enhance the accuracy and efficiency of skin cancer diagnosis. By training CNN models on dermoscopic images, these systems can classify different types of skin lesions, assisting dermatologists in early detection and treatment planning.

3. COVID-19 Detection Using Quantum CNN (Q-CNN) Models

The Q-CNN model performs better than a number of benchmark models for COVID-19 diagnosis when noise is present. During the pandemic, this method has been used to analyze chest CT scans, offering a quick and non-invasive diagnosis tool (Song et al., 2024).

4. Lightweight CNNs for Disease Prediction in Healthcare Systems

A novel healthcare system integrating a lightweight CNN has been developed for swift disease prediction through artificial intelligence. This system is designed to operate efficiently with limited computational resources, making it suitable for deployment in various healthcare settings, including telemedicine platforms.

5. Ensemble CNN Models with Explainable AI for COVID-19 Diagnosis

In order to guarantee model interpretability prior to ensemble generation, research has combined several CNN models with explainable AI approaches. This method improves the dependability of AI-powered diagnostic tools by enabling physicians to comprehend and have faith in the model's judgment.

Challenges and Ethical Considerations

Convolutional Neural Networks (CNNs) have revolutionized medical imaging, particularly in diagnosing conditions like brain tumours. However, their complex architectures often render them "black boxes," making it challenging to interpret their decision-making processes. This opacity poses significant challenges and ethical considerations (Herington et al., 2023) in clinical settings.

- **Lack of Transparency:** CNNs process data through multiple layers, each extracting increasingly abstract features. This complexity makes it difficult to trace how specific input features influence the final output, leading to a lack of transparency in predictions. In medical contexts, this opacity can hinder clinicians' understanding of AI-driven diagnoses, potentially affecting clinical acceptance and ethical deployment.
- **Trust and Reliability:** Clinicians may hesitate to rely on CNN-based diagnoses without clear explanations, potentially hindering the integration of AI into medical practice. The inability to interpret model decisions can lead to skepticism and reduced trust in AI systems, limiting their adoption in healthcare.
- **Error Identification:** Without interpretability, identifying and correcting errors or biases within the model becomes challenging, which can perpetuate inaccuracies. This lack of insight into the model's workings can result in undetected flaws, leading to potential misdiagnoses or inappropriate treatment recommendations.
- **Bias and Fairness:** Opaque models may inadvertently perpetuate biases present in training data, leading to unfair treatment recommendations..
- **Post-Hoc Explanations:** Methods like saliency maps and Layer-wise Relevance Propagation (LRP) highlight which parts of an image influenced the model's decision, offering insights into the model's focus areas.
- **Patient Confidentiality Challenges:** Integration of AI and Big Data: New ethical conundrums are brought about in the healthcare industry by the confluence of AI, big data, and blockchain technologies. These developments provide obstacles to protecting patient anonymity even while they have the potential to completely transform patient care and the administration of medical information (Jia et al., 2024).
- **Regulatory Compliance**: It is crucial to follow laws like the General Data Protection Regulation (GDPR) and the Health Insurance Portability and Accountability Act (HIPAA). Legal ramifications and a decline in patient trust may result from noncompliance.

Mitigation Strategies:

- ***Enhanced Data Security Measures*:** Implementing robust cybersecurity protocols, including encryption and secure access controls, is vital to protect patient data from breaches.
- ***Effective Anonymization Techniques*:** Employing advanced anonymization methods can help prevent re-identification of patients, thereby safeguarding confidentiality.
- ***Clear Data Governance Policies*:** Establishing transparent policies regarding data ownership and obtaining explicit informed consent from patients ensures ethical use of their information.

Addressing these challenges is crucial to maintain patient trust and uphold ethical standards in the application of AI for brain tumour diagnostics.

Future Directions in CNNs for Medical Imaging

Despite the achievements of CNN in Medical Imaging, challenges persist, driving research into future directions. These include the integration of emerging architectures, such as Vision Transformers (ViTs), the use of hybrid models, federated learning for privacy preservation, explainable AI, and the development of robust datasets. Below are key areas of exploration supported by recent literature:

Integration of Vision Transformers (ViTs) in Medical Imaging

Vision Transformers (ViTs) have emerged as a revolutionary paradigm in computer vision, offering an alternative to Convolutional Neural Networks (CNNs) by utilizing self-attention mechanisms. Unlike CNNs, which rely on spatial hierarchies and local receptive fields, ViTs process images as sequences of patches, akin to words in natural language processing (Azad et al., 2023). This architecture excels at capturing global context, which is particularly valuable in medical imaging where fine-grained and large-scale patterns coexist. For instance, in tasks such as tumor detection or organ segmentation, ViTs can more effectively model long-range dependencies within the data, improving diagnostic precision. By integrating ViTs with CNNs, researchers aim to leverage the strengths of both architectures: CNNs' ability to extract detailed local features and ViTs' capacity for global understanding.

Hybrid models that combine CNNs and ViTs have shown promise in overcoming limitations inherent in standalone architectures. These models often employ CNNs as feature extractors, feeding the outputs into ViTs for enhanced contextual reasoning. This synergy is particularly advantageous for medical imaging applications that demand high accuracy, such as 3D imaging or multimodal data integration. For example, combining ViTs with CNNs has improved segmentation accuracy in complex medical images, like those from MRI or CT scans, where the global understanding of organ structure is critical. Additionally, the hybrid approach enhances model robustness against noise and variability in imaging conditions. This integration represents a significant step forward in addressing the challenges of medical image analysis, positioning ViTs as a critical component of next-generation diagnostic systems.

Explainable AI (XAI) Solutions for CNNs

The need for Explainable AI (XAI) (Van Der Velden et al., 2022) solutions is rising as convolutional neural networks (CNNs) play a bigger role in medical imaging. By offering tools to decipher and comprehend CNNs' decision-making processes, XAI resolves the "black-box" character of these systems and promotes accountability and trust in AI-powered healthcare systems.

1. ***Saliency Maps:*** Saliency maps show which areas of an input image are most important for influencing the model's predictions. Saliency maps assist physicians in confirming whether the model is concentrating on pertinent medical aspects, such a tumor or lesion, by emphasizing these regions.
    - Example: Identifying regions in an MRI scan that led to a diagnosis of brain tumor.
2. ***Grad-CAM (Gradient-weighted Class Activation Mapping):*** Grad-CAM creates heatmaps that are superimposed on the original image to show the areas that go into a model's classification. It is frequently employed in medical imaging to draw attention to particular characteristics, including aberrant growths in CT or X-ray scans.

    Example: Identifying lung nodules in a chest X-ray to identify pneumonia.

3. ***LIME (Local Interpretable Model-agnostic Explanations):*** By altering the input image and tracking variations in the model's predictions, LIME generates local explanations. It is appropriate for case-by-case medical analysis since it aids in the instance-level explanation of decisions.
    - Example: Explaining why a CNN diagnosed a particular mammogram as malignant by analyzing pixel-level importance.
4. ***SHAP (SHapley Additive exPlanations):*** SHAP utilizes game theory to assign importance scores to individual input features. In medical imaging, SHAP can explain how different image regions or features influence a prediction.
    - Example: Quantifying the contribution of specific pixels in an ultrasound image to a model's prediction of fetal health.
5. ***Attention Mechanisms:*** Attention-based models, such as those using self-attention, highlight image regions that significantly influence predictions. This approach is inherently interpretable and often used in segmentation tasks.
    - Example: Identifying the precise boundaries of a tumor in a PET scan.

Hybrid Architectures (CNNs and Transformers)

Table 1. Hybrid Models

Combination	Description	Example in Medical Imaging	Advantages
CNN + RNN (e.g., LSTM)	Combines CNNs for spatial feature extraction and RNNs for capturing temporal dependencies in sequential data.	Dynamic imaging like functional MRI or echocardiography for modeling disease progression over time.	Models both spatial and temporal patterns effectively.
CNN + Transformers	Uses CNNs for local feature extraction and Transformers for capturing global contextual relationships.	Diagnosing systemic conditions like sepsis by integrating local (e.g., X-ray) and global contexts.	Combines local precision with global attention mechanisms.
CNN + Autoencoders (AEs)	Uses AEs for denoising or dimensionality reduction before CNN analysis.	Preprocessing noisy CT or MRI scans before tumor detection.	Enhances feature quality and reduces noise in input data.
CNN + Graph Neural Networks	Combines CNNs for feature extraction and GNNs for modeling relationships between image regions or features.	Segmenting and classifying connected brain regions in MRI scans.	Captures complex spatial relationships between regions.
CNN + Attention Mechanisms	Adds attention layers to CNNs for focusing on significant regions of an image.	Identifying tumor boundaries in CT scans.	Improves accuracy by highlighting critical regions.
CNN + GANs	Uses GANs for synthetic image generation, super-resolution imaging, or anomaly detection, paired with CNNs for analysis.	Generating high-resolution mammograms for breast cancer detection.	Addresses data scarcity and improves image quality.
CNN + Reinforcement Learning	Applies RL to refine CNN outputs by learning optimal segmentation or object detection policies.	Refining tumor localization in MRI using RL policies.	Enhances precision through iterative policy optimization.
CNN + Variational Autoencoders (VAEs)	Combines CNNs with VAEs for generating probabilistic latent spaces, aiding in anomaly detection.	Learning normal anatomical structures and flagging deviations for rare disease detection.	Enables unsupervised learning and interpretable feature spaces.
CNN + Decision Trees	Uses CNN-extracted features for classification using methods like decision trees or random forests.	Classifying retinal diseases using CNN features and random forests for decision-making.	Enhances interpretability and diagnostic reliability.
CNN + Bayesian Neural Networks	Combines CNNs with BNNs for uncertainty estimation in predictions.	Diagnosing skin lesions with confidence metrics to guide further clinical investigations.	Provides confidence levels for critical decisions.
CNN + Multi-Modal Approaches	Integrates CNNs with other models to analyze additional data types, such as clinical records or genomic data.	Combining radiology images with patient demographics to predict cancer risk.	Enables holistic and personalized diagnostics.
CNN + Ensemble Learning	Uses multiple CNN architectures or blends CNNs with other classifiers to combine predictions.	Detecting diabetic retinopathy with CNN ensembles and gradient-boosted decision trees.	Improves robustness and reduces overfitting.

Potential for real-time image analysis and integration into clinical workflows

Convolutional Neural Networks (CNNs) have significantly advanced medical imaging, offering the potential for real-time analysis and seamless integration into clinical workflows. This integration can enhance diagnostic accuracy, streamline processes, and improve patient outcomes.

Real-Time Image Analysis with CNNs: CNNs are adept at processing complex imaging data, enabling real-time analysis in clinical settings. For instance, a study introduced a custom deep learning CNN architecture tailored for medical data analysis, demonstrating its capability in real-time medical image classification.

Integration with Clinical Workflows: Integrating CNNs these workflows involves embedding AI models into existing systems, such as Electronic Health Records (EHRs) and Picture Archiving and Communication Systems (PACS). This integration allows for immediate analysis of medical images, providing clinicians with timely insights. A comprehensive bibliometric overview highlighted the growing application of CNNs in medical imaging, emphasizing their role in automating tasks like image classification, segmentation, and detection.

Benefits of Integration

- **Enhanced Diagnostic Accuracy**: CNNs can recognize subtle patterns in medical images, leading to more accurate diagnoses.
- **Improved Workflow Efficiency**: Automating image analysis reduces manual workload, allowing clinicians to focus on patient care.
- **Timely Decision-Making**: Real-time analysis facilitates prompt clinical decisions, which is crucial in emergency situations.
- **Standardization of Assessments**: AI models provide consistent evaluations, reducing inter-observer variability.

Robustness and Real-World Applications in Medical Imaging

Robustness in medical imaging ensures AI models maintain consistent performance across diverse real-world conditions, such as varying imaging modalities, equipment, and patient demographics. Challenges like noisy or incomplete data and imaging artifacts require techniques such as data augmentation and domain adaptation to enhance reliability. These measures are crucial for applications like tumour detection, where accurate results are needed across different imaging conditions.

In practice, robustness also involves model interpretability and adaptability. Explainable AI (XAI) helps clinicians trust AI predictions, while scalable systems ensure models can adapt to new imaging protocols and computational environments. This focus ensures AI tools remain accurate, efficient, and practical for deployment in real-world clinical settings, enabling reliable support for critical medical decisions.

CONCLUSION

CNNs revolutionized medical imaging by providing unparalleled diagnostic accuracy and efficiency. This chapter has explored the foundational principles of CNNs, their architectures, and the transformative impact of their applications across various medical imaging modalities, including X-rays, MRIs, and CT scans. The ability of CNNs to automate complex tasks such as disease detection, image segmentation, and classification has enhanced diagnostic workflows, enabling earlier detection of diseases and more personalized treatment planning.

While the potential of CNNs in medical imaging is immense, challenges such as interpretability, ethical considerations, and data privacy must be addressed to ensure their reliable integration into clinical practice. Techniques such as Explainable AI (XAI) and advanced learning strategies like transfer learning and hybrid AI models provide promising pathways to overcoming these challenges.

Looking forward, the future of CNNs in medical imaging lies in the development of real-time diagnostic tools, seamless integration into clinical workflows, and further refinement of AI-driven solutions to ensure equitable and ethical healthcare delivery. By bridging the gap between technological advancements and medical needs, CNNs are set to redefine the landscape of diagnostic imaging, making healthcare more efficient, accurate, and accessible for all.

REFERENCES

Aamir, M., Bazai, S., Bhatti, U. A., Dayo, Z. A., Liu, J., & Zhang, K. (2023, January). Applications of machine learning in medicine: Current trends and prospects. In *2023 Global Conference on Wireless and Optical Technologies (GCWOT)* (pp. 1-4). IEEE. DOI: 10.1109/GCWOT57803.2023.10064665

Aamir, M., Rahman, Z., Abro, W. A., Bhatti, U. A., Dayo, Z. A., & Ishfaq, M. (2023). Brain tumor classification utilizing deep features derived from high-quality regions in MRI images. *Biomedical Signal Processing and Control*, *85*, 104988. DOI: 10.1016/j.bspc.2023.104988

Aamir, M., Rahman, Z., Abro, W. A., Tahir, M., & Ahmed, S. M. (2019). An optimized architecture of image classification using convolutional neural network. International Journal of Image. *Graphics and Signal Processing*, *11*(10), 30–39. DOI: 10.5815/ijigsp.2019.10.05

Aamir, M., Rahman, Z., Dayo, Z. A., Abro, W. A., Uddin, M. I., Khan, I., Imran, A. S., Ali, Z., Ishfaq, M., Guan, Y., & Hu, Z. (2022). A deep learning approach for brain tumor classification using MRI images. *Computers & Electrical Engineering*, *101*, 108105. DOI: 10.1016/j.compeleceng.2022.108105

Al-Jabbar, M., Alshahrani, M., Senan, E. M., & Ahmed, I. A. (2023). Histopathological Analysis for Detecting Lung and Colon Cancer Malignancies Using Hybrid Systems with Fused Features. *Bioengineering (Basel, Switzerland)*, *10*(3), 383. DOI: 10.3390/bioengineering10030383 PMID: 36978774

Azad, R., Kazerouni, A., Heidari, M., Aghdam, E. K., Molaei, A., Jia, Y., Jose, A., Roy, R., & Merhof, D. (2023, October). Advances in medical image analysis with vision Transformers: A comprehensive review. *Medical Image Analysis*, *91*, 103000. DOI: 10.1016/j.media.2023.103000 PMID: 37883822

Guan, Y., Aamir, M., Rahman, Z., Ali, A., Abro, W. A., Dayo, Z. A., ... & Hu, Z. (2021). A framework for efficient brain tumor classification using MRI images.

Herington, J., McCradden, M. D., Creel, K., Boellaard, R., Jones, E. C., Jha, A. K., Rahmim, A., Scott, P. J. H., Sunderland, J. J., Wahl, R. L., Zuehlsdorff, S., & Saboury, B. (2023, October). Ethical Considerations for Artificial intelligence in Medical Imaging: Data collection, development, and evaluation. *Journal of Nuclear Medicine*, *64*(12), 1848–1854. DOI: 10.2967/jnumed.123.266080 PMID: 37827839

Ilesanmi, A.E. et al. 2024. Reviewing 3D convolutional neural network approaches for medical image segmentation. Heliyon. 10, 6 (Mar. 2024), e27398. DOI:.DOI: 10.1016/j.heliyon.2024.e27398

Jia, H., Zhang, J., Ma, K., Qiao, X., Ren, L., & Shi, X. (2024, May 1). Application of convolutional neural networks in medical images: A bibliometric analysis. *Quantitative Imaging in Medicine and Surgery*, *14*(5), 3501–3518. DOI: 10.21037/qims-23-1600 PMID: 38720828

Makhlouf, A., Maayah, M., Abughanam, N., & Catal, C. (2023). The use of generative adversarial networks in medical image augmentation. *Neural Computing & Applications*, *35*(34), 24055–24068. DOI: 10.1007/s00521-023-09100-z

Mei, X., Liu, Z., Robson, P. M., Marinelli, B., Huang, M., Doshi, A., Jacobi, A., Cao, C., Link, K. E., Yang, T., Wang, Y., Greenspan, H., Deyer, T., Fayad, Z. A., & Yang, Y. (2022, July). RaDImageNet: An open radiologic deep learning research dataset for effective transfer learning. *Radiology. Artificial Intelligence*, *4*(5), 5. DOI: 10.1148/ryai.210315 PMID: 36204533

Mishra, L., Behera, R., Pattanaik, S., & Singh, N. R. (2022). Role of CT scan in medical and dental imaging. In *Biomedical Imaging Instrumentation* (pp. 13–32). Academic Press.

Motamed, S., Rogalla, P., & Khalvati, F. (2021, January). Data augmentation using Generative Adversarial Networks (GANs) for GAN-based detection of Pneumonia and COVID-19 in chest X-ray images. *Informatics in Medicine Unlocked*, *27*, 100779. DOI: 10.1016/j.imu.2021.100779 PMID: 34841040

Niranjani, V. et al. 2023. Deep Fake Detection: Unmasking the illusion using CNN and LSTM. IEEE. (Dec. 2023), 861–865. DOI:.DOI: 10.1109/ICIMIA60377.2023.10426523

Ou, X., Chen, X., Xu, X., Xie, L., Chen, X., Hong, Z., Bai, H., Liu, X., Chen, Q., Li, L., & Yang, H. (2021). Recent Development in X-Ray Imaging Technology. *Future and Challenges. Research (Washington, D.C.)*, *9892152*, 2021/9892152. Advance online publication. DOI: 10.34133/2021/9892152 PMID: 35028585

Salehi, A. W., Khan, S., Gupta, G., Alabduallah, B. I., Almjally, A., Alsolai, H., & Mellit, A. (2023). A study of CNN and transfer learning in medical imaging: Advantages, challenges, future scope. *Sustainability*, *15*(7), 5930.

Sarvamangala, D. R., & Kulkarni, R. V. (2022). Convolutional neural networks in medical image understanding: A survey. *Evolutionary Intelligence*, *15*(1), 1–22. DOI: 10.1007/s12065-020-00540-3 PMID: 33425040

Selvamurugan, A., Kunnathur Ganesan, P., Nayak, S. S., Simiyon, A., & Indiran, T. (2024, November). CNN-LSTM-Based Nonlinear Model Predictive controller for temperature trajectory tracking in a batch reactor. *ACS Omega*, *9*(47), 47203–47212. DOI: 10.1021/acsomega.4c07893 PMID: 39619559

Shinde, S., Chougule, T., Saini, J., & Ingalhalikar, M. (2019). HR-CAM: Precise localization of pathology using multi-level learning in CNNS. In Medical Image Computing and Computer Assisted Intervention–MICCAI 2019: 22nd International Conference, Shenzhen, China, October 13–17, 2019 [Springer International Publishing.]. *Proceedings*, *22*(Part IV), 298–306.

Song, K.-Y., Tiong, L. C. O., & Lee, Y. (2024, October). See through the noise: Revolutionizing medical image diagnosis with quadratic convolutional neural network (Q-CNN). *International Journal of Machine Learning and Cybernetics*. Advance online publication. DOI: 10.1007/s13042-024-02451-6

Van Der Velden, B. H. M., Kuijf, H. J., Gilhuijs, K. G. A., & Viergever, M. A. (2022, May). Explainable artificial intelligence (XAI) in deep learning-based medical image analysis. *Medical Image Analysis*, *79*, 102470. DOI: 10.1016/j.media.2022.102470 PMID: 35576821

Yadav, S. S., & Jadhav, S. M. (2019, December). Deep convolutional neural network based medical image classification for disease diagnosis. *Journal of Big Data*, *6*(1), 1. DOI: 10.1186/s40537-019-0276-2

Yamashita, R., Nishio, M., Do, R. K. G., & Togashi, K. (2018). Convolutional neural networks: An overview and application in radiology. *Insights Into Imaging*, *9*(4), 611–629. DOI: 10.1007/s13244-018-0639-9 PMID: 29934920

Chapter 12
Emerging Trends in Artificial Intelligence for Medical Application

Hari Shankar Punna
https://orcid.org/0009-0009-1142-6254
CVR College of Engineering, India

Law Kumar Singh
https://orcid.org/0000-0002-7073-6852
Amity University, Mohali, India

V. S. Veena
https://orcid.org/0009-0009-1125-1327
St. Peter's College of Engineering and Technology, India

P. Selvakumar
https://orcid.org/0000-0002-3650-4548
Department of Science and Humanities, Nehru Institute of Technology, Coimbatore, India

P. Mercy
https://orcid.org/0009-0006-9697-0774
Anand Institute of Higher Technology, India

T. C. Manjunath
https://orcid.org/0000-0003-2545-9160
Rajarajeswari College of Engineering, India

ABSTRACT

Is poised to transform the landscape, personalizing plans, and streamlining efficiencies. Emerges as a powerful ally in addressing these challenges. Quickly far beyond human capabilities presents unprecedented improvement. This brings us to diagnostics. In, have shown remarkable promise, diabetic retinopathy, and. By training on extensive datasets, AI models, and pathologists' abnormalities precision, thus the likelihood of misdiagnosis. For instance, systems experts interpret medical images, allowing for earlier intervention and better patient outcomes. AI also offers substantial advancements alongside, optimizing efficacy and minimizing side systems that can identify specific biomarkers that indicate how might medication, be prescribed. This shift toward personalized treatment not only enhances the effectiveness of therapies but also fosters patient engagement and satisfaction. Operational efficiencies in healthcare systems are. Predictive analytics can optimize scheduling and supply chain. AI systems manage staff resources more effectively.

DOI: 10.4018/979-8-3693-9816-6.ch012

INTRODUCTION TO ARTIFICIAL INTELLIGENCE IN HEALTHCARE: OPPORTUNITIES AND CHALLENGES

Is poised to transform the landscape, personalizing plans, and streamlining efficiencies. Emerges as a powerful ally in addressing these challenges. Quickly far beyond human capabilities presents unprecedented improvement. This brings us to diagnostics. In, have shown remarkable promise, diabetic retinopathy, and. By training on extensive datasets, AI models, and pathologists' abnormalities precision, thus the likelihood of misdiagnosis. For instance, systems experts interpret medical images, allowing for earlier intervention and better patient outcomes. AI also offers substantial advancements alongside, optimizing efficacy and minimizing side systems that can identify specific biomarkers that indicate how might medication, be prescribed. This shift toward personalized treatment not only enhances the effectiveness of therapies but also fosters patient engagement and satisfaction. Operational efficiencies in healthcare systems are. Predictive analytics can optimize scheduling and supply chain. AI systems manage staff resources more effectively. This leads to reduced wait times, improved patient care, and enhanced overall system performance. Furthermore, 24/7 for appointment scheduling, reminders, and general health inquiries, thus alleviating some of the administrative burdens on healthcare providers. However, alongside these opportunities, AI's in healthcare. One of the foremost concerns is the healthcare sector the integration necessitates to prevent breaches. Ensuring compliance with other the deployment of AI technologies.

Organizations must establish stringent protocols to safeguard data while utilizing it for AI training and model development. Bias in AI algorithms is another critical challenge that must be addressed. Care and health marginalized. To mitigate this risk, healthcare organizations must prioritize the use of diverse datasets and engage in data-driven decisions. Poses challenges related to acceptance and trust among healthcare professionals. This can stem from displacement, the reliability of AI recommendations, and the perceived complexity of integrating these tools into existing systems. Building trust requires comprehensive training, clear communication about AI's role, and evidence demonstrating AI applications. Regulatory hurdles present significant existing, creating uncertainty around the approval and oversight of AI applications in healthcare. Policymakers must work to establish clear guidelines that ensure safety, efficacy, and accountability while promoting innovation. Collaborative efforts between regulatory agencies, healthcare providers, and AI developers will be essential in shaping a regulatory landscape that fosters responsible AI use. In summary, the integration offers immense diagnostics, personalized treatment, and improved operational efficiencies. However, resistance from healthcare professionals, and regulatory uncertainties, sector. As stakeholders navigate this complex landscape, a collaborative approach that emphasizes ethical considerations, transparency, and ongoing education will be crucial. Head-on, industry transformative health.

MACHINE LEARNING AND DEEP LEARNING FUNDAMENTALS FOR MEDICAL APPLICATIONS

Have emerged as pivotal technologies, driving significant diagnostics, treatment personalization, and healthcare operational efficiency. At their core, As the sector increasingly turns to, understanding fundamentals and DL is essentially medical. Machine Learning Fundamentals: algorithms are datasets, paired correctly. For example, in a medical context, a supervised learning algorithm might analyze patient data using linear regression. These methods have proven effective in predicting readmission rates by classifying medical images. Algorithm systems must identify patterns or groupings by exploring complex datasets, identifying subtypes of diseases, or discovering new biomarkers (Sharifani K., et al, 2023). Techniques like clustering and dimensionality reduction help researchers uncover hidden structures in data, facilitating insights that can lead to new hypotheses in medical research. Focuses on, where agents learn to make decisions by receiving feedback from their environment. In healthcare, this approach can be applied to optimize treatment strategies or manage chronic diseases by adapting interventions based on patient responses over time. This dynamic learning process allows for personalized care that evolves with the patient's needs. Deep Learning Fundamentals: process complex datasets with multiple layers of abstraction. These Excel tasks speech recognition, well medical applications volumes of unstructured (hrs). The foundation consists of processing input data and generating outputs. Each layer of the network. Medical imaging, and textures, might, such as tumors' anatomical features. CNNs specialized in particularly effective processing utilized automatically, and significantly. In healthcare, have been successfully applied to interpret radiological images, dermatological assessments, and even pathology slides, achieving accuracy comparable to that of human experts (Castiglioni I., et al, 2021; Aamir et al., 2019). Processing in applications such as time-series analysis of patient vital signs or analyzing genomic sequences. These networks maintain internal memory, allowing them to learn dependencies over time, which is crucial for understanding patient histories and predicting disease progression.

Applications in Medicine: DL Medical is reshaping the landscape of healthcare (Aamir et al., 2023). Key areas of impact include Diagnostic Imaging: ML and DL algorithms success. By automating image analysis, radiologists detect, reducing diagnostic errors, expediting patient care (Aamir et al., 2023; Aamir et al., 2022; Guan et al., 2021). Can historical future health outcomes. For instance, algorithms can assess the likelihood of disease onset, patient readmissions, or treatment responses, allowing for early interventions and improved care strategies. Genomics and Personalized Medicine: Deep learning is instrumental in analyzing, and helping variants enable personalized efficacy while (Cui S., et al, 2020). Driven support in vast amounts of systems provides evidence-based recommendations, enhancing the quality of care. Considerations: potential ML and DL for. Data privacy security remains paramount, particularly given the such as HIPAA critical protection while enabling. Additionally, issue bias algorithms cannot be overlooked., the resulting models' predictions, potentially exacerbate health disparities. Fairness equity algorithm that patients receive appropriate care. Finally, technologies experience acceptance among healthcare professionals. Training and education are vital to build trust and ensure that practitioners feel confident in leveraging AI tools in their practice (Mahrishi M., et al, 2020). In conclusion, foundational are revolutionizing medical applications. Their actionable has the, to enhance diagnostics, and optimize the field continues to evolve, addressing associated user acceptance crucial harnessing transformative power. By fostering collaboration among researchers, clinicians, and technologists, the healthcare sector these technologies significantly.

DATA PREPROCESSING AND VISUALIZATION FOR MEDICAL AI APPLICATIONS

Data preprocessing and visualization are crucial steps in the development of applications. AI largely depends and relevance. Given medical data, robust preprocessing techniques are essential to prepare datasets for analysis. Moreover, effective visualization tools are vital for interpreting results, gaining insights, and facilitating communication among healthcare professionals. Data Preprocessing in Healthcare: Data preprocessing involves a series of steps that are designed, transformed, and organized suitable. This process is particularly important in healthcare, where datasets can be incomplete, noisy, and unstructured. Key stages of data preprocessing include Data Cleaning: This initial step addresses missing values, duplicates, and errors within the dataset. In healthcare, missing data can arise from various sources, such as incomplete patient records or failures in data entry (Diaz O., et al, 2021). Techniques such as imputation (filling in missing values using statistical methods) or deletion of incomplete records are commonly employed. Integrity is misleading and affects patient care. Visualization Techniques in Medical AI: Once data has been preprocessed, effective visualization plays a key role in understanding patterns and communicating findings (Obuchowicz R., et al, 2024). Visualization tools enable clinicians and researchers to explore complex datasets intuitively and to derive readily numerical alone. Key visualization techniques include: Descriptive Statistics: Basic statistical, box plots, provide an overview of the distribution and relationships among variables. For instance, histograms can illustrate the distribution of patient ages in a dataset, while scatter plots can reveal correlations between different clinical measures, such as blood pressure and cholesterol levels. Heatmaps: Heatmaps are particularly useful for visualizing correlation matrices, allowing practitioners to quickly identify relationships between multiple variables. In medical research, heatmaps can reveal associations between various clinical factors and patient outcomes, facilitating hypothesis generation and informing further analysis.

The Curve (AUC) is critical for evaluating the performance of classification models. These visualizations help assess how well a model distinguishes between different classes, such as healthy versus diseased patients. Clinicians can use these metrics to compare models one Model Interpretability Tools: visualization techniques that explain model predictions by highlighting the contribution of individual features. This transparency is essential in healthcare, where decisions can significantly impact patient outcomes. Dashboard Interfaces: Interactive dashboards enable clinicians to visualize and explore data in real-time (Vellido A., et al, 2020). The reliance on black box models can lead to skepticism among healthcare professionals regarding their use in clinical decision-making. This necessitates a concerted effort to develop user-friendly visualization tools that elucidate model behavior and results (Shi F., et al, 2020). Conclusion: Data preprocessing and visualization are foundational components in the successful implementation of applications in healthcare. Revolutionizing the medical landscape, the importance of high-quality, well-prepared datasets cannot be overstated. Effective preprocessing ensures that data is reliable and relevant, while robust visualization techniques facilitate understanding and communication of insights among healthcare professionals. Addressing heterogeneity, model interpretability AI in medicine. By prioritizing these aspects, diagnostics, personalize. As we advance, fostering collaboration among, clinicians, and create an ecosystem that supports innovation while safeguarding patient interests.

AI-DRIVEN MEDICAL IMAGE ANALYSIS: TECHNIQUES AND APPLICATIONS

AI-driven medical image analysis represents a transformative frontier in healthcare, leveraging advanced computational techniques from various modalities—artificial intelligence offers the capability to analyze these images efficiently and effectively, identifying elude. This is underpinned by a variety of techniques, each contributing to its widespread applications in clinical practice. Techniques in AI-Driven Image Analysis: Machine Learning Algorithms: Traditional, have been foundational in developing early AI applications in medical imaging. These algorithms require feature extraction from images, often necessitating expert input to identify relevant features. For example, in mammography, features such as mass shape, margin, and density can be extracted to help classify images as benign or malignant. While effective, these methods are generally limited by their reliance on and subjective (Dodda S., et al, 2024). Deep Learning Models: The advent of medical image analysis, are adept at processing visual data. CNNs automatically extract features through multiple layers, allowing them to capture complex patterns in images. Deep synthetic. In medical imaging, gans can be used to augment training datasets, creating variations of existing images to improve model robustness (Panayides A S., et al, 2020). They also facilitate the synthesis of medical images from non-image data, such as generating MRI scans from CT scans. Enhancing availability of rare pathological cases for training purposes. Applications in Medical Imaging. AI-driven image analysis medical, each demonstrating the potential: Radiology: In radiology, AI algorithms assist in the interpretation of various imaging modalities. For instance, AI systems can analyze chest X-rays for signs of pneumonia, tuberculosis, or lung nodules, significantly reducing radiologists' workloads and enabling faster diagnoses. Experts, leading to improved patient outcomes. Oncology: In oncology, vital cancer planning. Analyzing mammograms, CT scans, and MRIs, AI systems can identify tumors at earlier stages, when they are more treatable. Moreover, AI can assist in assessing tumor response to therapy by comparing sequential imaging studies, thereby enabling personalized treatment adjustments.

Cardiology: AI applications in cardiology include the analysis of echocardiograms, electrocardiograms (ECGs), and cardiac MRIs. For example, deep learning models can automatically identify arrhythmias from ECG data, providing timely alerts to clinicians. In echocardiography, AI can assist in measuring heart chamber sizes and function, enhancing the accuracy of diagnoses related to heart diseases. Pathology: Digital pathology has been transformed by AI-driven image analysis. Whole-slide imaging allows for the capture of high-resolution deep learning to identify cancerous cells. AI systems can also assist pathologists in quantifying tumor areas and assessing features associated with prognostic outcomes, ultimately supporting (Habuza T., et al, 2021). Additionally, presents logistical consider how to incorporate tools effectively into existing processes without disrupting patient care. Training staff to use these technologies and ensuring seamless integration with electronic health records are critical for successful implementation (Liu W., et al, 2023). Conclusion: AI-driven medical image analysis diagnostic accuracy, treatment planning, clinical workflows. Through techniques—ranging—AI offers powerful tools for analyzing complex medical images. The applications across various medical specialties, from radiology to oncology, demonstrate and streamline healthcare delivery. However, interpretability, and integration into clinical practice medical imaging. Clinicians, and technology developers in creating effective and trustworthy AI solutions. By prioritizing these considerations, the sector enhances patient care, drives innovation, and ultimately leads to efficiency and effectiveness.

DEEP LEARNING FOR MEDICAL IMAGE SEGMENTATION AND DETECTION

Groundbreaking segmentation and detection, significantly enhance the ability to analyze employing advanced algorithms, and deep learning effectively process and interpret medical imaging data, providing crucial insights to patients. Data-driven methodologies, the adoption is becoming essential. Understanding and Detection: involves partitioning an image to facilitate, such as organs, tissues, or tumors. Accurate segmentation is vital for quantifying anatomical features and understanding the spatial relationships within images. In contrast, detection refers to identifying and localizing specific abnormalities or conditions, such as tumors or lesions, within the imaging data. Both tasks were effective. Deep Learning Techniques for Segmentation: most approaches for medical analysis (Wang R., et al, 2022). This is particularly beneficial in medical imaging, where lesions or tumors may occupy a small portion. By enhancing the ability to concentrate on critical features, attention-based architectures improve segmentation precision. Transfer Learning: Given the challenges associated with acquiring large labeled datasets in medical imaging, transfer learning has become a valuable strategy. Pre-trained models, initially trained on approach enable models to leverage previously learned features, significantly improving performance in segmentation tasks even with limited medical data. Deep Learning Techniques for Detection: Object Detection Algorithms: Deep learning has revolutionized object detection in medical images, allowing for the identification and localization of abnormalities. Techniques such as been widely adopted for detecting lesions, tumors, and other critical features in medical images. These algorithms use bounding boxes to localize objects and classify them in a single pass, providing rapid and accurate detection (Liu X., et al, 2021). Region Proposal Networks (rpns): rpns are integral to models like Faster R-CNN, generating for an. Utilizing deep learning streamlines the detection process, improving advantageous time-sensitive clinical settings, where rapid detection can facilitate timely intervention. Hybrid Models: Combining segmentation and detection capabilities into a single model has gained traction in recent years. For instance, models that simultaneously segment and detect tumors can provide comprehensive insights from a single analysis, computational image analysis. Hybrid approaches enhance the efficiency of diagnostic workflows in clinical practice.

Applications in Healthcare: Deep learning-based segmentation and detection techniques have found numerous applications across various medical fields, showcasing their potential to transform healthcare. Oncology: In oncology, deep learning models are employed to detect and segment tumors in imaging modalities like CT and MRI. Accurate segmentation of tumors is critical for assessing their size, shape, and location, which directly influences treatment decisions. AI-driven tools are being developed to aid radiologists in identifying malignancies at earlier stages, improving the chances of successful intervention. Neurology: Medical imaging helps diagnose neurological conditions (Jha D., et al, 2020). Collaborative efforts among healthcare institutions to share annotated data could be AI. Interpretability is also a critical concern in deep learning applications (Chen X., et al, 2022). Remarkably, their complexity leads to a lack of transparency regarding how reasoning will be essential for fostering trust among clinicians and ensuring responsible use in clinical settings. Finally, integrating deep learning tools into clinical workflows presents logistical challenges. Healthcare providers must consider how to incorporate AI technologies seamlessly into existing processes without disrupting patient care. Training staff to use these tools effectively and ensuring compatibility with electronic health record systems will be vital for successful implementation. Conclusion: Deep learning has fundamentally changed the landscape of medical image segmentation and detection, providing that and. Through sophisticated architectures like CNN, U-Net, and hybrid models, deep learning enables precise, facilitating abnormalities in informed clinical decision-making. Embrace AI technologies, and addressing challenges related to data privacy, will be crucial. By prioritizing these considerations, can be fully realized, that AI is an integral healthcare delivery improving patient outcomes. Among healthcare professionals, and technologists, deep will continue to drive innovation in the medical imaging field, ultimately benefiting patients and clinicians alike.

COMPUTER-AIDED DIAGNOSIS: AI-DRIVEN DECISION SUPPORT SYSTEMS

Computer-aided (CAD) has technologies, leading to advanced decision support systems. These AI-driven systems utilize medical, aiding clinicians in interpreting complex information and making informed decisions. As healthcare increasingly relies on data-driven methodologies, understanding the components and applications of AI-driven CAD systems is essential for optimizing patient care. The Evolution of CAD Systems: Traditional CAD systems focused on specific imaging modalities, providing basic analysis tools that aided radiologists in interpreting X-rays, CT scans, and MRIs. These systems primarily used rule-based algorithms and manual feature extraction to identify abnormalities. While they represented a significant advancement in radiology, their limitations in adaptability and learning from new data often hindered their effectiveness. AI, particularly landscape CAD transformed. Modern AI-driven decisions support vast datasets and generalizability (Simegn G L., et al, 2022). This shift has enabled CAD systems to not only assist in image analysis but also integrate clinical data, providing comprehensive support for diagnostic and treatment decisions. Key Components: Data Integration: driven CAD systems their diverse data sources. These systems can analyze not only imaging data but also, laboratory results, and demographics. By synthesizing this information, AI models can provide a. CAD systems are sophisticated machine learning algorithms, effective for analyzing imaging, and automatically extracting features without the need for manual input. CAD systems play a critical role in oncology by providing decision support for tumor detection, staging, and treatment planning. AI models can analyze imaging data to assess tumor response to therapies, guiding oncologists in modifying treatment protocols based on results. Capability improves outcomes and facilitates personalized medicine approaches (Bagheri M., et al, 2024). Cardiology: In cardiology, evaluate echocardiograms, ECGs, and cardiac MRIs to detect conditions such as arrhythmias or heart failure. These systems are overlooked in traditional analyses. Additionally, they can assist in risk stratification, helping clinicians determine appropriate management strategies for risk. Pathology: applications of digital pathology involve analyzing whole-slide images to identify cancerous cells and other abnormalities. CAD systems can assist pathologists by providing quantitative assessments of tumor characteristics, streamlining the diagnostic process, and reducing variability among interpretations. Efficiency cancer. Primary Care: AI-driven CAD systems are increasingly being adopted in primary care settings to support clinicians in diagnosing common conditions. By analyzing patient symptoms, lab results, and history, these systems can provide differential diagnoses and recommend further investigations. This support helps primary care physicians make informed decisions while managing their patient populations effectively.

Significant advancements in driven CAD systems, particularly given the nature of health HIPAA for protecting patients while enabling AI-driven innovations. Algorithmic bias is another critical concern. Outcomes exacerbate health disparities. Ensuring diversity in training data and implementing fairness assessments are vital steps in developing equitable AI solutions. The interpretability of AI models also poses challenges in clinical practice. While AI systems can provide recommendations, understanding the rationale behind these suggestions is crucial for building clinician trust. Developing transparent algorithms and providing clear explanations for AI-driven recommendations will enhance acceptance among healthcare professionals (Yeasmin M N., et al, 2024). Additionally, CAD systems require careful planning. Clinicians must be, and systems must be designed to complement, rather than disrupt, existing processes. Ensuring seamless interoperability with this and other healthcare technologies will be essential in clinical settings. Future Directions: computer-aided diagnosis promising, in technology methodology. Machine learning techniques have greater accuracy and efficiency than CAD systems. Integration of more sophisticated algorithms, including those capable of multi-modal data analysis, will enhance decision support capabilities. Moreover, the development of real-time AI-driven systems will enable clinicians to access decision support immediate interventions, and comprehensive patient assessments. Big improvements in computational will further enhance the capabilities of AI-driven CAD systems. Collaboration among healthcare providers, data scientists, and regulatory bodies = essential ethical data security, and development implementing AI technologies. By fostering an environment of collaboration and innovation, full AI-driven CAD systems outcomes and revolutionize diagnostic practices (Niranjan K., et, 2023). Conclusion: AI-driven computer-aided diagnosis represents a significant advancement in healthcare, providing powerful decision support systems that enhance diagnostic accuracy and improve clinical workflows. Through sophisticated algorithms, data integration, and user-friendly interfaces, these systems empower healthcare professionals. Interpretability and practice will be crucial. By focusing on collaboration and ethical considerations, sector-driven CAD systems, AI is an integral diagnostic and optimizing patient management. With promise computer-aided diagnosis is set to become a cornerstone of modern healthcare, ultimately benefiting patients and clinicians alike.

AI-DRIVEN CLINICAL DECISION SUPPORT SYSTEMS: DESIGN AND IMPLEMENTATION

AI-driven (CDSS) have emerged as transformative tools in modern healthcare, for clinicians. Technologies these medical, provide assist diagnosing and treating patients. The design and implementation require careful consideration of several factors, including data integration, user interface design, and clinical workflow compatibility. Driven CDSS the analysis of unstructured relevant free-text entries, algorithms can enhance the system's ability to interpret patient histories and symptoms. This capability nuanced conditions, ultimately accurate recommendations. User Interface Design: The effectiveness of an AI-driven CDSS is heavily influenced by its user interface. A well-designed interface should present information clearly and concisely, minimizing the cognitive load on clinicians. And, can insights an easy format. Additionally, the system should allow for intuitive navigation, enabling clinicians to access the information they need without unnecessary delays. Feedback Mechanisms: Continuous learning is CDSS. Implementing feedback mechanisms allows the system clinician interactions to capture outcomes and clinician responses to recommendations, the system can refine its algorithms and enhance the relevance of its suggestions. CDSS clinical practices and evolving medical knowledge (Bleher H., et al, 2022). Implementation Strategies: Successful implementation strategies consider both technical and organizational factors. Here are key strategies for effective implementation: Stakeholder Engagement: Engaging stakeholders, including clinicians, administrators, and IT professionals, is critical for the successful implementation of AI-driven CDSS. The system aligns with existing workflows. Regular communication and collaboration can foster a sense of ownership among stakeholders, increasing the likelihood of adoption. In controlled environment allows healthcare organizations to evaluate the system's performance and usability. These tests can help identify potential issues and gather valuable feedback from clinicians, enabling necessary adjustments to be made before wider implementation.

Training and Support: Providing comprehensive training for clinicians is essential to facilitate thedriven CDSS Training sessions should cover the system's functionalities, how to interpret recommendations, and how to provide feedback. Ongoing support and resources, such as help desks or user manuals, can further enhance clinician confidence and comfort with the technology. Monitoring and Evaluation:

After implementation, continuous monitoring and evaluation of the AI-driven CDSS are crucial for assessing its impact on clinical practice. Key performance indicators (kpis) can include metrics such as diagnostic accuracy, time savings, and clinician satisfaction. Regular evaluations can help inform to system (Vasey B., et al, 2022). That the AI complies Organizations must consider, security, and recommendations. Critical protect patient information while utilizing AI technologies. Future Directions: The future methodology. As machine learning algorithms become more sophisticated, CDSS will likely offer even more accurate and personalized recommendations. Advanced reinforcement learning and, could enhance the system's (Braun M., et al, 2021). Moreover, a growing emphasis on personalized medicine will drive the development of CDSS that consider genetic, environmental, and lifestyle factors in their recommendations. By incorporating genomic data and other personalized factors, these systems can provide tailored insights that significantly improve patient care. Will address ethical and practical challenges associated with AI-driven CDSS. Establishing, implementing, and evaluating these systems will foster an environment conducive to innovation while ensuring patient safety and quality of care. Clinical power that enhances accuracy and streamlines clinical workflows. Through effective data integration, sophisticated machine learning algorithms, and user-friendly design, these systems empower healthcare professionals to patients. Quality, clinician acceptance, and regulatory compliance will be crucial as prioritizing collaboration, training, and continuous evaluation, healthcare organizations can harness CDSS, improving patient outcomes and revolutionizing clinical practice. With ongoing innovation and commitment to ethical standards, the future of AI in clinical decision support is set to make a lasting impact on healthcare delivery.

PREDICTIVE ANALYTICS FOR PATIENT OUTCOMES AND RISK STRATIFICATION

Predictive analytics is pivotal in modern, facilitating improved patient outcomes and effective risk stratification. By leveraging (EHRS), clinical trials, and even, predictive analytics employs sophisticated algorithms and statistical models to forecast future patient events, such as disease progression, hospital readmission, or complications. This capability not only enhances clinical decision-making but also improves overall healthcare delivery. Understanding: utilizes trends to inform decisions. Encompasses demographics and imaging. Advanced algorithms, particularly machine learning techniques, are then applied to this data to uncover insights that might be missed through traditional analysis. Goals stratify patient risk, allowing healthcare providers high adverse outcomes. Stratification enables targeted interventions, proactive management, and example, or monitored more closely, reducing the likelihood of severe complications. Key Components of Predictive Analytics: Effective. This includes not only clinical data from EHRS but also demographic information, socioeconomic factors, and behavioral health data. The ability to synthesize this information (Huang Y., et al, 2021). Essential in predictive analytics, and patterns. Common models used include logistic regression, these models can be trained to identify risk factors, improving their accuracy over time. Hospital Readmission Prevention: in reducing hospital readmissions (Irwin M S., et al, 2021). Predictive discharge summaries, comorbidities, and social, By intervening with post-discharge support, such as follow-up appointments and patient education, healthcare providers can significantly lower readmission rates and enhance patient satisfaction. Emergency Department (ED) Utilization: Predictive analytics can help manage and reduce unnecessary ED visits by identifying patients who frequently utilize emergency services. By analyzing their health records and underlying issues, healthcare providers can develop targeted outreach programs to address their specific needs, potentially diverting them to more appropriate care settings and alleviating pressure on emergency services.

Population Health Management: In population health initiatives, predictive analytics allows healthcare organizations to identify at-risk populations and implement preventative measures. By analyzing community health data, organizations can address social determinants of health, and deploy targeted health more across populations. Clinical Decision Support: Predictive analytics enhances (CDSS) by. For instance, predictive physicians' conditions presenting symptoms and history, or alerting them to potential drug interactions medication list. Predictive analytics in clinical workflows enhances the overall decision-making process. Is not without predictions and ineffective interventions. Ensuring that data collected from various sources is standardized and reliable is crucial for the success of predictive models. Issue interoperability between different (Champion M L., et al, 2024). Many healthcare organizations use disparate systems that may not communicate effectively, making it difficult to compile comprehensive datasets necessary for accurate predictions. Furthermore, the expansion of collaborative healthcare initiatives will foster data sharing and integration, enhancing the effectiveness of predictive analytics (Kanwal F., et al, 2021). By pooling data from various organizations, healthcare providers can develop more robust models that account for diverse patient populations and healthcare settings. Ultimately, the continued focus on driving the adoption of predictive analytics in healthcare. By emphasizing outcomes and cost-effectiveness, predictive analytics can help organizations, align with the overarching goal of improving patient care while reducing healthcare costs. Conclusion: Predictive analytics healthcare, facilitates effective risk stratification. Data, advanced algorithms, anticipate patient needs, prevent adverse events, and optimize resource allocation. Quality, interoperability, and clinician acceptance are essential to maximizing the benefits of predictive analytics. With ongoing innovations and a commitment to ethical data use, effective promise predictive analytics improving delivery outcomes is immense, data-driven patient care proactive rather than reactive.

NATURAL LANGUAGE PROCESSING FOR CLINICAL TEXT ANALYSIS AND DECISION SUPPORT

Has become an indispensable tool in healthcare, particularly for clinical text analysis and decision support. Technologies enhance meaningful information the unstructured text found, discharge summaries, and application in healthcare not only streamlines workflows but also facilitates. Understanding NLP in Healthcare: human in the clinical context, it involves the transformation of unstructured text into structured data that can be easily analyzed. Given that a significant portion of clinical information exists in text form, leveraging NLP is essential for harnessing this wealth of data. Text data, such as tokenization, lemmatization, and entity recognition. These steps help convert raw text into a format that can be analyzed, enabling the identification of key terms, concepts, and relationships. Key Components of NLP for Clinical Text Analysis Named Entity Recognition (NER): One of the foundational tasks in clinical NLP is named entity recognition, which is key to the medications, and symptoms, NER helps in creating structured datasets from unstructured clinical notes, enabling healthcare providers to retrieve pertinent information efficiently (Rajput A., 2020). For instance, when a clinician enters a patient's symptoms, an NLP-enabled the literature potential diagnoses, relevant guidelines, and appropriate treatment options (Patra B G., et al, 2021). Risk Stratification: By analyzing clinical notes, NLP can identify risk factors associated with patient populations. For example, NLP systems can analyze narratives to extract information on social determinants of health, comorbidities, and medication adherence, helping healthcare providers risk of readmissions. Quality Improvement: NLP can assist in quality improvement initiatives by identifying gaps in care. By analyzing clinical documentation, NLP systems can flag instances where care protocols are not followed or where documentation lacks essential information. This capability supports ongoing efforts to enhance care quality and patient safety.

Clinical Research: In clinical research, NLP is invaluable for extracting data from unstructured sources. Researchers can utilize NLP to mine clinical trial reports, medical literature, and ehrs for relevant data, facilitating systematic reviews and meta-analyses. This application accelerates the research process and enhances evidence-based practice. Patient Communication: NLP technologies are increasingly being used to improve patient-provider communication. For instance, powered by NLP. These tools enhance and improve access to care, particularly in underserved populations. Challenges in Implementing NLP in Healthcare: implementation NLP clinical settings. One significant hurdle is the variability in clinical language, including the use of abbreviations, jargon, and context-specific terms (Buchlak Q D., et al, 2020). Developing NLP models that accurately interpret this variability requires extensive training on diverse datasets, which resource-intensive. By analyzing patient feedback, sentiment, and communication patterns, NLP can help healthcare providers tailor their approaches to meet individual patient needs, fostering stronger provider-patient relationships (Eyre H., et al, 2022). Conclusion: Natural Language Processing is revolutionizing clinical text analysis and decision support, offering healthcare providers insights unstructured. By enabling efficient data processing, and enhancing improving engagement, NLP impacts patient outcomes and overall quality of care. Addressing challenges related to data variability, privacy, and benefits of NLP healthcare. With continued friendly applications, the future of NLP in clinical decision support appears bright. As healthcare increasingly becomes data-driven, the role of NLP will continue to expand, efficiently, By harnessing the power of language, NLP can ultimately transform how healthcare providers interact with information and their patients, leading to improved health outcomes for all.

AI-DRIVEN PERSONALIZED MEDICINE: GENOMICS AND PRECISION HEALTH

Personalized medicine groundbreaking evolution, particularly through the lenses of genomics and precision health. Characteristics, integrating to optimize therapeutic strategies., and clinicians' genomic sets, uncover complex and derive actionable insights that enhance patient care and outcomes. This transformative approach not only shifts the paradigm model framework revolutionizing prevention and treatment. Understanding Personalized Medicine and Genomics: Personalized medicine focuses on the customization of healthcare, with an emphasis on individual patient differences. At its core functions. Advances in genomic sequencing technologies, such as, having to sequence the genome, enable variations to contribute to. These variations can inform risk assessments for various conditions, guide treatment decisions, and facilitate early interventions (Johnson K B., et al, 2021). By analyzing large datasets from clinical trials and patient cohorts, AI algorithms can identify genetic variations outcomes, and new therapeutic target strategies. Driven tools can be based on individual patient data. These decision support systems analyze a patient's genomic profile in conjunction with clinical guidelines, helping physicians choose the most appropriate interventions and monitor patient responses more effectively. Adaptation: AI facilitates monitoring of. By continuously analyzing genomic and lifestyle data, AI systems can provide insights that allow for timely adjustments to treatment plans, ensuring optimal outcomes. Oncology: driven personalized medicine oncology. Genomic profiling of tumors enables the identification of specific mutations that drive cancer growth (Yogeshappa V G., et al, 2024). AI algorithms can analyze these profiles to match patients with targeted therapies, such as monoclonal antibodies or small molecule inhibitors, significantly improving treatment reduction. Pharmacogenomics: how and efficacy is a key aspect of personalized medicine. AI can analyze pharmacogenomic data to a certain, allowing the customization of drug selection and dosing. This approach enhances patient safety and treatment outcomes. Rare Disease Diagnosis: AI-driven genomics is particularly valuable in diagnosing rare diseases, where traditional diagnostic methods may fall short. Sequences pathogenic variants conditions, facilitating earlier more accurate diagnoses. This timely identification management strategies prognosis. Chronic Disease Management: In chronic disease management, AI can help identify at-risk populations by analyzing genetic predispositions and lifestyle factors. By stratifying patients based on their risk profiles, can target health. Preventive Health: AI-driven personalized medicine genomics preventive strategies. By identifying genetic, and hereditary cancers, healthcare providers can tailor screening programs and lifestyle interventions to mitigate risks before disease onset.

Challenges in AI-Driven Personalized Medicine: Despite the potential benefits, the promise of AI-driven personalized medicine. Genomic data is highly personal. Compliance with regulations such as HIPAA while utilizing large datasets for analysis safeguarding. Is needed for robust data quality and standardization. Variability in genomic data collection methods, reporting practices, and clinical annotations can hinder the effectiveness of AI algorithms. Establishing standards for genomic data management and sharing is essential for creating reliable datasets that can be effectively analyzed. Furthermore, there is the issue of clinician acceptance. Healthcare providers educated on the capabilities and limitations of AI-driven tools to foster trust and facilitate adoption (Taherdoost H., et al, 2024). Furthermore, as patient engagement becomes increasingly prioritized, AI-driven personalized medicine will likely involve more direct participation from patients. Empowering individuals to access and understand their genetic information will foster a proactive approach to health management, allowing for greater involvement in their care decisions (Kalusivalingam A K., et al, 2021). Conclusion: AI-driven personalized medicine represents a paradigm shift in healthcare, fundamentally transforming how we understand and treat diseases. By leveraging genomic data and sophisticated AI algorithms, can enhance the quality of care. While clinician acceptance remains, in technology collaborative efforts among stakeholders will become the standard of care. As we move toward this future, the potential of AI to unlock the complexities of human genetics and provide actionable insights holds immense promise for improving health and well-being globally. Embracing this transformation fosters equitable effectiveness that prioritizes precision and personalization.

GENOMIC ANALYSIS AND INTERPRETATION USING AI AND MACHINE LEARNING

Genomic analysis is transforming genomics, enabling researchers and clinicians to decode complex genetic information with unprecedented accuracy and speed. Genomic sequencing, the amount of genomic data generated is skyrocketing, necessitating advanced computational tools for effective analysis and interpretation. AI and ML techniques are at the forefront of this evolution, facilitating meaningful, improving our understanding of genetic variation, and guiding personalized medicine initiatives. The

Importance of Genomic Analysis: Genomic analysis involves examining sequence diseases, treatment responses, or other health-related traits. Traditional methods of genomic analysis, while valuable, often struggle to manage the produced next-generation (NGS) ML, intricate patterns in genomic data, and translate these patterns into actionable clinical insights (Quazi S., et al, 2022). AI and ML can be utilized at various stages of genomic analysis, from preprocessing raw sequencing data to identifying disease-associated variants and predicting phenotypic outcomes. The application of these technologies' interpretations, paving clinical. Establishing links between genotypes and phenotypes is a central goal of genomic research. Techniques, and models, alongside phenotypic information associations, may not be immediately evident (De La Vega F M., et al, 2021). These models can reveal how specific genetic variations. Predictive Modeling: AI and ML forecast disease risk based on an individual's genomic profile. By integrating genomic data with other factors, such as lifestyle and environmental exposures, these models' likelihood of developing can guide preventive measures and personalized treatment strategies. Future genomic analysis lies in, which encompasses. AI algorithms can analyze these diverse data types simultaneously, uncovering intricate biological networks and pathways that contribute to health and disease. This holistic approach enhances our understanding of the complexity and facilitates development comprehensive. Applications AI ML in Genomic Analysis: Cancer Genomics: and ML genomic analysis oncology. By analyzing tumor genomes, researchers can identify mutations that drive cancer progression and resistance to therapy. AI-driven tools help in the classification of tumors based on their genetic profiles, enabling oncologists to tailor treatment characteristics.

Rare Disease Diagnosis: AI and ML techniques are particularly valuable in diagnosing rare genetic disorders. By analyzing genomic data from affected individuals and their families, pathogenic variants are responsible for these conditions. In managing rare diseases, AI significantly accelerates this process. Pharmacogenomics: Understanding how genetic variations affect drug metabolism and efficacy is essential for personalized individual healthcare therapies and dosages based on a patient's genetic makeup. Public Health Genomics: AI-driven genomic analysis can also inform public health initiatives by identifying genetic risk factors associated with trends. Genomic researchers uncover links between genetic variants and common diseases, guiding preventive measures and resource allocation in healthcare. Gene Therapy and Editing: As gene therapies and CRISPR technology gain traction, AI targets gene editing. By analyzing genomic data, AI algorithms can predict potential off-target effects and optimize gene-editing strategies, enhancing the safety and efficacy of these innovative treatments (Nawaz M S., et al, 2021). Engaging diverse ethicists, policymakers, and patient advocates, will AI implement equity, transparency, and patient autonomy. Conclusion: genomic analysis interpretation, unlocking the potential of vast genomic datasets to inform personalized medicine and improve patient outcomes (Castaldo R., et al, 2021). By automating data preprocessing, enhancing variant calling, and establishing genotype-phenotype associations, these technologies are transforming how researchers and clinicians approach genomic information. While challenges related to data quality, privacy, and interpretability remain, AI genomic analysis. As we continue to embrace these innovations, the promise of a more precise, personalized, and effective healthcare system is within reach, ultimately improving the lives of patients through targeted therapies and informed health decisions. The synergy between AI and genomics will pave medicine, one prioritizes individual differences and harnesses the power of genetic information for better health outcomes.

PRECISION MEDICINE AND TARGETED THERAPIES: AI-DRIVEN APPROACHES

Focusing on tailored treatments that consider, environmental, and lifestyle patient care by delivering interventions specifically designed for each person's unique characteristics. Central to the advancement which our datasets, identify patient-specific biomarkers, and develop targeted therapies that improve. Understanding Precision Medicine: Precision medicine differs from traditional approaches that typically apply standardized treatments to large populations. Instead, it emphasizes the importance of understanding the underlying biological mechanisms that contribute to disease. By considering factors such as genetic variations, epigenetic modifications, and molecular profiles, precision medicine enables healthcare providers to develop more effective strategies. Targeted therapies and component molecular alterations drive disease progression (Raparthi M., et al, 2022). This continuous feedback loop enhances fosters. Powered by CDSS vast amounts of, clinical systems can recommend personalized treatment options to individuals. Applications of AI-Driven Precision Medicine: Oncology: oncology exemplifies potential precision medicine (Mendhe D., et al, 2024). Can analyze tumor genomics to identify mutations and alterations that drive cancer growth. By matching these profiles with targeted therapies, clinicians can select treatments that are more likely to succeed. For example, drugs targeting specific mutations, such as EGFR or ALK inhibitors in lung cancer, have revolutionized treatment outcomes for patients with those genetic profiles. Cardiovascular Disease: AI-driven approaches are also making strides in cardiovascular medicine. Genomic and clinical individuals are high for heart disease, guiding preventive measures and tailored interventions. Furthermore, AI can assist in cardiovascular conditions.

Rare Diseases: In the context of rare diseases, where traditional diagnostic methods often fall short, AI can aid in identifying genetic variants responsible for conditions that may otherwise go undiagnosed. Genomic-affected individuals, models can pinpoint pathogenic variants, leading to earlier and facilitating. Pharmacogenomics: field pharmacogenomics benefits significantly from AI-driven precision medicine. Understanding how genetic variations affect drug metabolism is essential for optimizing treatment. Genomic individuals' specific medications, for personalized drugs. Infectious Diseases: AI technologies are increasingly being applied to the field of infectious diseases. Genomic sequences of pathogens' resistance mechanisms inform treatment strategies (Mulukuntla S., et al, 2020). Ongoing research in the field of genomics will yield new insights into disease mechanisms, Furthermore, approaches—combining, proteomic, metabolomic, and other types of patient health (Peiris M S., et al, 2024). Algorithms will play analyzing dimensional, enabling informed personalized treatment strategies. Researchers will be vital for quality, and algorithm transparency. Building robust datasets and sharing best practices across institutions will enhance the reliability of AI-driven solutions in precision medicine. Additionally, as patient engagement becomes increasingly prioritized, AI-driven precision medicine will likely involve more direct participation from patients. Empowering individuals to access and understand their genetic information will foster a proactive approach to health management, allowing for greater involvement in their care decisions. Conclusion: AI-driven precision medicine and targeted therapies are revolutionizing the landscape of personalized treatment options.

AI-DRIVEN TELEMEDICINE AND REMOTE HEALTH MONITORING

Telemedicine and health are transforming the healthcare landscape, addressing patient care, accessibility, and efficiency. Telemedicine allows healthcare providers to deliver services remotely, leveraging digital communication technologies to connect with patients. This approach highlighted the need for safe and effective healthcare delivery models. AI-driven tools enhance telemedicine by providing advanced analytics and optimizing resource utilization. The Importance of Telemedicine: Telemedicine has emerged. It facilitates access to medical consultations, diagnoses, and follow-up visits, thereby overcoming and reducing wait times. The convenience of telemedicine empowers patients to seek care promptly and, with satisfaction (Talati D., et al, 2023). As telemedicine evolves, technologies offer further effectiveness by streamlining processes and personalizing patient interactions. Chronic Disease Management: AI-driven telemedicine is particularly effective in managing (Dogheim G M., et al, 2023). By continuously monitoring vital signs and lifestyle factors, AI systems can provide personalized recommendations and alerts, helping patients manage their conditions more effectively. Mental Health Services: The demand for mental health services has surged, and AI technologies can enhance teletherapy by providing tools for patient engagement and support. AI chatbots can facilitate initial assessments and ongoing check-ins, while AI analytics can help therapists track patient progress and adapt treatment strategies in real-time. Post-Operative Care: Telemedicine is increasingly used for post-operative follow-ups, enabling surgeons to monitor patients' recovery their systems analyze recovery, flagging any concerns that may require further evaluation, thus improving the efficiency of post-operative care and reducing unnecessary hospital visits.

Remote Consultations: AI-driven platforms enable specialists to conduct remote consultations with patients, regardless of their location. By analyzing patient data and symptoms, AI specialists and appropriate options, ensure that patients receive expert care even in rural or underserved areas. Emergency Response: In emergencies, AI can enhance telemedicine by rapidly analyzing patient data and providing healthcare professionals with critical information to inform treatment decisions. AI systems can prioritize cases based on urgency, and crises. Challenges in AI-Driven Telemedicine: Another, well-annotated datasets. Variability in data collection practices can lead to biases and inaccuracies in AI predictions, which can impact clinical decision-making. Establishing standardized collection-sharing critical to ensuring reliability-driven tools. Existing telemedicine experience. Healthcare providers must be trained in these tools designed to complement, rather than complicate, clinical practices. Ensuring that AI systems provide clear and actionable insights is crucial for fostering clinician adoption and maximizing their impact on patient care. Modal combining, environmental, and behavioral information—will more a view of patient health (Nwankwo E I., et al, 2024). Will develop tailored interventions that address the unique needs of each patient, ultimately improving outcomes. While clinician adoption remains, in technology and collaborative efforts among stakeholders' telemedicine becomes an integral part of healthcare delivery. As we embrace these innovations, the enhanced health outcomes and quality of care are immense and patient-centered. Through continued integration and telemedicine, we can foster a healthcare environment that is proactive, responsive, and equitable, for individuals when they need it.

EXPLAINABLE AI AND TRANSPARENCY IN MEDICAL DECISION-MAKING

Revolutionized medical decision-making, for diagnosis, and management. However, increasingly explainability and transparency of these technologies have become paramount. Approaches outputs, thereby fostering trust and facilitating the. This is particularly critical in healthcare, where decisions are well-being. Importance Explainability in Healthcare: In the medical field, healthcare professionals rely on judgment, established guidelines introduction of AI systems, and complex algorithms, resulting in outputs that resemble black boxes, where the reasoning behind predictions or recommendations is obscured. This lack of transparency poses several challenges. First, clinicians generated the conclusions that were reached. Second, regulatory bodies and patients alike demand accountability in healthcare decisions, necessitating that AI systems provide clear rationales for their recommendations. Explainability becomes even more crucial in high-stakes scenarios, such as diagnosing diseases or determining treatment options (Pillai V., et al, 2024). Contexts, incorrect decisions misdiagnosis, inappropriate treatments, and compromised patient safety. Providing metrics that rank the importance of various input features can help clinicians understand which factors the AI considers most relevant in making its recommendations. By highlighting these features, healthcare providers can better assess the validity of the AI's conclusions and determine whether they align with clinical knowledge and experience (Reddy S., et al, 2022). Bodies increasingly focused on establishing guidelines for the in healthcare. Adhere ethical standards provide explanations for their decisions is essential for promoting responsible AI use. Regulations may require healthcare organizations to disclose information about the AI systems they employ, ensuring that patients and providers are informed about how AI influences care.

Benefits of Explainable AI in Medical Decision-Making: Enhanced Collaboration: Explainable AI fosters collaboration between clinicians and AI systems by clinicians. This collaborative dynamic allows healthcare providers to leverage AI as a decision support, ultimately outcomes. Clinical: When healthcare providers can understand and trust AI recommendations, they are more likely to integrate these insights into their clinical workflows. This can lead to, optimized and improved management. Patient Empowerment: Transparency explainability in systems extends to patient interactions as well. When patients understand how AI contributes to their care decisions, actively process. Empowered patients make informed choices about their health, and satisfaction with care (Lötsch J., et al, 2021). Reduction of Bias and Errors: Explainable AI mitigates healthcare providing insights into how decisions are made, stakeholders can recognize potential disparities and ensure that AI systems promote equitable care for all patients. Collaboration between AI researchers, clinicians, ethicists, and policymakers will be vital in shaping the landscape of explainable AI (Amann J., et al, 2022). Furthermore, patient engagement in the development of explainable AI cannot be overlooked. Involving patients in discussions about AI-driven decision-making can provide their concerns and the creation of user-centered solutions. The future will also see an increased emphasis on regulatory frameworks that mandate explainability. Establishing guidelines for the ethical deployment of AI will that effective. Conclusion: Explainable AI medical technologies. By enhancing the interpretability of AI systems, we can foster alike, ultimately improving quality care. A transformative, prioritizing explainability will ensure that these technologies serve as effective tools for enhancing patient outcomes and promoting equitable healthcare practices. By embracing transparency and collaboration, the medical community AI fundamental patient-centered care.

FUTURE DIRECTIONS IN MEDICAL AI: ETHICS, REGULATIONS, AND EMERGING TECHNOLOGIES

As AI systems are designed to assist in clinical decision-making, ensuring that they operate fairly across diverse patient demographics is imperative. This necessitates a rigorous evaluation of strategies, such as using diverse training cohorts and conducting regular audits of AI systems (Kumar P., et al, 2023). Understanding how they arrive at conclusions becomes increasingly challenging. This involves demonstrating reliability their effectiveness in real-world settings. Regulatory agencies will need to develop frameworks that account for the dynamic nature of AI, allowing for ongoing assessment and updates as new data becomes available (Nadella G S., et al, 2023). Furthermore, the concept of algorithmic accountability is emerging as a critical component of regulatory discussions. This entails holding healthcare accountable for performance impact systems. Establishing clear responsibilities for data management, algorithmic transparency, and ethical considerations will be vital in fostering a culture of accountability within the AI healthcare ecosystem. Emerging Technologies in Medical AI: medical also a range of emerging technologies that promise to enhance healthcare delivery. One of the most exciting areas is the development of. Learn from complex, improving diagnostic accuracy and treatment personalization. For instance, great medical imaging allows for cancer through automated radiological.

(NLP) is another transforming healthcare providers' AI systems. More intuitive healthcare providers and AI tools. This can enhance clinical documentation, streamline patient interactions, and provide valuable, such as. Additionally, technologies are poised to revolutionize patient care. These devices can recommendations alerts. Supports proactive healthcare management, empowering patients. Telemedicine, augmented by AI, is also gaining traction, particularly driven telehealth solutions improve triage processes, facilitate remote diagnostics, and enhance patient engagement, individuals. Collaboration and Interdisciplinary Approaches: The future of medical AI will rely heavily on, policymakers, Interdisciplinary approaches that bring together expertise from medicine, computer science, ethics, and law will be healthcare (Jarvis T., et al, 2020). Collaborative research initiatives that involve academic institutions, industry leaders, and healthcare organizations can accelerate the development of AI solutions that address pressing healthcare challenges (Avacharmal R., et al, 2023).

CONCLUSION

Landscape application's profound, marked trends promise to reshape healthcare delivery and various facets of medicine—from diagnostics to treatment personalization. One of the most significant trends is the increasing adoption of algorithm models that vast unattainable. These capabilities are revolutionizing areas such as medical imaging, genomics, and patient monitoring while facilitating tailored that account for individual patient characteristics. As these technologies become more sophisticated, the potential to predict patient outcomes and intervene proactively is transforming how healthcare providers approach patient care. Another critical trend is the rise of, which is streamlining enhancing the between healthcare providers and AI systems. By converting unstructured data from electronic health records into actionable insights, NLP is not only improving efficiency but also allowing clinicians more rather than administrative. This trend is further enhanced by the development of, in real-time, thereby empowering swiftly. Moreover, integration with wearable technology and telemedicine is remote patient monitoring management. More patients utilize these tools, AI can analyze health timely and alerts empower patients and clinicians to be proactive particularly valuable in managing chronic conditions, as it enables continuous monitoring and timely interventions, patient. However, advancement, including bias and, the need for transparency, are paramount. Integral to, ensuring these technologies operate fairly and transparently among. Regulatory frameworks must evolve to address these issues, providing guidelines that foster innovation while safeguarding patient rights and safety. Crucial diverse stakeholders—ranging from clinicians and data scientists to ethicists and patients—ensure that AI applications are developed with a comprehensive understanding of their implications. This collaborative approach not only enhances the design and functionality of AI systems accountability of their deployment. Medical applications are both complex. As emerging trends continue to evolve, they quality care, streamline processes and empower in their health journeys. By, regulatory, and practical technologies, the healthcare community is effective, The journey ahead requires a commitment to innovation, collaboration, and ethical integrity, across all levels of healthcare. As we embrace these emerging trends, we must remain vigilant and proactive as a powerful ally in the pursuit of improved health and well-being for all.

REFERENCES

Aamir, M., Bazai, S., Bhatti, U. A., Dayo, Z. A., Liu, J., & Zhang, K. (2023, January). Applications of machine learning in medicine: Current trends and prospects. In *2023 Global Conference on Wireless and Optical Technologies (GCWOT)* (pp. 1-4). IEEE. DOI: 10.1109/GCWOT57803.2023.10064665

Aamir, M., Rahman, Z., Abro, W. A., Bhatti, U. A., Dayo, Z. A., & Ishfaq, M. (2023). Brain tumor classification utilizing deep features derived from high-quality regions in MRI images. *Biomedical Signal Processing and Control, 85*, 104988. DOI: 10.1016/j.bspc.2023.104988

Aamir, M., Rahman, Z., Abro, W. A., Tahir, M., & Ahmed, S. M. (2019). An optimized architecture of image classification using convolutional neural network. *International Journal of Image. Graphics and Signal Processing, 11*(10), 30–39. DOI: 10.5815/ijigsp.2019.10.05

Aamir, M., Rahman, Z., Dayo, Z. A., Abro, W. A., Uddin, M. I., Khan, I., Imran, A. S., Ali, Z., Ishfaq, M., Guan, Y., & Hu, Z. (2022). A deep learning approach for brain tumor classification using MRI images. *Computers & Electrical Engineering, 101*, 108105. DOI: 10.1016/j.compeleceng.2022.108105

Amann, J., Vetter, D., Blomberg, S. N., Christensen, H. C., Coffee, M., Gerke, S., Gilbert, T. K., Hagendorff, T., Holm, S., Livne, M., Spezzatti, A., Strümke, I., Zicari, R. V., & Madai, V. I. (2022). To Explain or Not to Explain?—Artificial Intelligence Explainability in Clinical Decision Support Systems. *PLOS Digital Health, 1*(2), 2022. DOI: 10.1371/journal.pdig.0000016 PMID: 36812545

Avacharmal R, Gudala L, (2023). "…: A Comprehensive Review of Emerging Artificial Intelligence Technologies, Ethical Considerations, And Global Governance Models in The Pursuit of Trustworthy AI". Learning Research and Applications, 2023.

Bagheri, M., Bagheritaba, M., Alizadeh, S., & Parizi, M. S. (2024). "AI-Driven Decision-Making in Healthcare Information Systems: A Comprehensive Review". *Preprints*, 2024.

Bleher, H., & Braun, M. (2022). Diffused Responsibility: Attributions of Responsibility in the Use of AI-Driven Clinical Decision Support Systems. *AI and Ethics, 2022*(4), 747–761. Advance online publication. DOI: 10.1007/s43681-022-00135-x PMID: 35098247

Braun, M., Hummel, P., Beck, S., & Dabrock, P. (2021). Primer on an Ethics of AI-Based Decision Support Systems in the Clinic. *Journal of Medical Ethics, 2021*(12), e3. Advance online publication. DOI: 10.1136/medethics-2019-105860 PMID: 32245804

Buchlak, Q. D., Esmaili, N., Leveque, J. C., Farrokhi, F., Bennett, C., Piccardi, M., & Sethi, R. K. (2020). Machine Learning Applications to Clinical Decision Support in Neurosurgery: An Artificial Intelligence Augmented Systematic Review. *Neurosurgical Review, 2020*(5), 1235–1253. Advance online publication. DOI: 10.1007/s10143-019-01163-8 PMID: 31422572

Castaldo, R., Cavaliere, C., Soricelli, A., Salvatore, M., Pecchia, L., & Franzese, M. (2021). Radiomic and Genomic Machine Learning Method Performance for Prostate Cancer Diagnosis: Systematic Literature Review. *Journal of Medical Internet Research, 2021*(4), e22394. Advance online publication. DOI: 10.2196/22394 PMID: 33792552

Castiglioni, I., Rundo, L., Codari, M., Di Leo, G., Salvatore, C., Interlenghi, M., Gallivanone, F., Cozzi, A., D'Amico, N. C., & Sardanelli, F. (2021). AI Applications to Medical Images: From Machine Learning to Deep Learning. *Physica Medica*, *80*, 2021. DOI: 10.1016/j.ejmp.2021.02.006 PMID: 33662856

Champion, M. L., Blanchard, C. T., Lu, M. Y., Shea, A. E., Lively, A. I., Jenkins, J. M., Howell, S. E., Lee, G. M., Casey, B. M., Battarbee, A. N., & Subramaniam, A. (2024). A More Selective vs a Standard Risk-Stratified, Heparin-Based, Obstetric Thromboprophylaxis Protocol. *Journal of the American Medical Association*, *2024*(4), 310. Advance online publication. DOI: 10.1001/jama.2024.8684 PMID: 38935391

Chen, X., Wang, X., Zhang, K., Fung, K. M., Thai, T. C., Moore, K., Mannel, R. S., Liu, H., Zheng, B., & Qiu, Y. (2022). Recent Advances and Clinical Applications of Deep Learning in Medical Image Analysis. *Medical Image Analysis*, *76*, 2022. DOI: 10.1016/j.media.2022.102444 PMID: 35472844

Cui, S., Tseng, H. H., Pakela, J., Ten Haken, R. K., & El Naqa, I. (2020). Introduction to Machine and Deep Learning for Medical Physicists. *Medical Physics*, *47*(7), 2020. DOI: 10.1002/mp.14140 PMID: 32418339

De La Vega, F. M., Chowdhury, S., Moore, B., Frise, E., McCarthy, J., Hernandez, E. J., Wong, T., James, K., Guidugli, L., Agrawal, P. B., Genetti, C. A., Brownstein, C. A., Beggs, A. H., Löscher, B.-S., Franke, A., Boone, B., Levy, S. E., Õunap, K., Pajusalu, S., & Kingsmore, S. F. (2021). Artificial Intelligence Enables Comprehensive Genome Interpretation and Nomination of Candidate Diagnoses for Rare Genetic Diseases. *Genome Medicine*, *2021*(1), 153. Advance online publication. DOI: 10.1186/s13073-021-00965-0 PMID: 34645491

Diaz, O., Kushibar, K., Osuala, R., Linardos, A., Garrucho, L., Igual, L., Radeva, P., Prior, F., Gkontra, P., & Lekadir, K. (2021). Data Preparation for Artificial Intelligence in Medical Imaging: A Comprehensive Guide to Open-Access Platforms and Tools. *Physica Medica*, *80*, 2021. DOI: 10.1016/j.ejmp.2021.02.007 PMID: 33684723

Dodda, S., Chintala, S., & Kanungo, S. (2024). Exploring AI-Driven Innovations in Image Communication Systems for Enhanced Medical Imaging Applications. *Journal of Electrical Engineering*, •••, 2024.

Dogheim G M, Hussain A, (2023). "Patient Care through AI-Driven Remote Monitoring: Analyzing the Role of Predictive Models and Intelligent Alerts in Preventive Medicine". Journal of Contemporary Healthcare, 2023.

Eyre, H., Chapman, A. B., & Peterson, K. S. (2022). "Launching into Clinical Space with MedspaCy: A New Clinical Text Processing Toolkit in Python". *AMIA Annual Symposium Proceedings*, 2022.

Guan, Y., Aamir, M., Rahman, Z., Ali, A., Abro, W. A., Dayo, Z. A., ... & Hu, Z. (2021). A framework for efficient brain tumor classification using MRI images.

Habuza, T., Navaz, A. N., Hashim, F., Alnajjar, F., Zaki, N., Serhani, M. A., & Statsenko, Y. (2021). AI Applications in Robotics, Diagnostic Image Analysis and Precision Medicine: Current Limitations, Future Trends, Guidelines on CAD Systems for Medicine. *Informatics in Medicine Unlocked*, *22*, 2021. DOI: 10.1016/j.imu.2021.100596

Huang, Y., Liu, Y., Steel, P A D., Axsom, K. M., Lee, J. R., Tummalapalli, S. L., Wang, F., Pathak, J., Subramanian, L., & Zhang, Y. (2021). Deep Significance Clustering: A Novel Approach for Identifying Risk-Stratified and Predictive Patient Subgroups. *Journal of the American Medical Informatics Association : JAMIA*, *2021*(12), 2641–2653. Advance online publication. DOI: 10.1093/jamia/ocab203 PMID: 34571540

Irwin, M. S., Naranjo, A., Zhang, F. F., Cohn, S. L., London, W. B., Gastier-Foster, J. M., Ramirez, N. C., Pfau, R., Reshmi, S., Wagner, E., Nuchtern, J., Asgharzadeh, S., Shimada, H., Maris, J. M., Bagatell, R., Park, J. R., & Hogarty, M. D. (2021). Revised Neuroblastoma Risk Classification System: A Report from the Children's Oncology Group. *Journal of Clinical Oncology*, *2021*(29), 3229–3241. Advance online publication. DOI: 10.1200/JCO.21.00278 PMID: 34319759

Jarvis, T., Thornburg, D., Rebecca, A. M., & Teven, C. M. (2020). Artificial Intelligence in Plastic Surgery: Current Applications, Future Directions, and Ethical Implications. *Plastic and Reconstructive Surgery. Global Open*, *8*(10), 2020. DOI: 10.1097/GOX.0000000000003200 PMID: 33173702

Jha, D., Riegler, M. A., & Johansen, D. (2020). DoubleU-Net: A Deep Convolutional Neural Network for Medical Image Segmentation. *IEEE Journal of Biomedical and Health Informatics*, *24*(10), 2020. DOI: 10.1109/JBHI.2020.3002733

Johnson, K. B., Wei, W. Q., Weeraratne, D., Frisse, M. E., Misulis, K., Rhee, K., Zhao, J., & Snowdon, J. L. (2021). Precision Medicine, AI, and the Future of Personalized Health Care. *Clinical and Translational Science*, *2021*(1), 86–93. Advance online publication. DOI: 10.1111/cts.12884 PMID: 32961010

Kalusivalingam A K, Sharma A, (2021). "Leveraging Deep Learning and Random Forest Algorithms for AI-Driven Genomics in Personalized Medicine". Cognitive Computing Journal, 2021.

Kanwal, F., Shubrook, J. H., Adams, L. A., Pfotenhauer, K., Wai-Sun Wong, V., Wright, E., Abdelmalek, M. F., Harrison, S. A., Loomba, R., Mantzoros, C. S., Bugianesi, E., Eckel, R. H., Kaplan, L. M., El-Serag, H. B., & Cusi, K. (2021). Clinical Care Pathway for the Risk Stratification and Management of Patients with Nonalcoholic Fatty Liver Disease. *Gastroenterology*, *2021*(5), 1657–1669. Advance online publication. DOI: 10.1053/j.gastro.2021.07.049 PMID: 34602251

Kumar, P., Chauhan, S., & Awasthi, L. K. (2023). Artificial Intelligence in Healthcare: Review, Ethics, Trust Challenges & Future Research Directions. *Applied Artificial Intelligence*, •••, 2023.

Liu, W., Zhao, F., Shankar, A., & Maple, C. (2023). Explainable AI for Medical Image Analysis in Medical Cyber-Physical Systems: Enhancing Transparency and Trustworthiness of IoMT. *IEEE Journal of Biomedical and Health Informatics*, *27*(4), 2023. DOI: 10.1109/JBHI.2023.3260715 PMID: 37027578

Liu, X., Song, L., Liu, S., & Zhang, Y. (2021). A Review of Deep-Learning-Based Medical Image Segmentation Methods. *Sustainability (Basel)*, *13*(11), 2021. DOI: 10.3390/su13031224

Lötsch, J., Kringel, D., & Ultsch, A. (2021). Explainable Artificial Intelligence (XAI) in Biomedicine: Making AI Decisions Trustworthy for Physicians and Patients. *BioMedInformatics*, *2*(1), 2021. DOI: 10.3390/biomedinformatics2010001

Mahrishi M, Hiran K K, Meena G, Sharma P, (2020). "Machine Learning and Deep Learning in Real-Time Applications". 2020.

Mendhe, D., Dogra, A., Nair, P. S., & Punitha, S. (2024). "AI-Enabled Data-Driven Approaches for Personalized Medicine and Healthcare Analytics". *Ninth International Conference on Advances in Computing, Communications and Informatics*, 2024, DOI: 10.1109/ICONSTEM60960.2024.10568722

Mulukuntla S, Venkata S P, (2020). "AI-Driven Personalized Medicine: Assessing the Impact of Federal Policies on Advancing Patient-Centric Care". EPH-International Journal of Medical and Health Sciences, 2020.

Nadella G S, Satish S, Meduri K, Meduri S S, (2023). "A Systematic Literature Review of Advancements, Challenges and Future Directions of AI And ML in Healthcare". International Journal of Scientific Development and Computational Sciences, 2023.

Nawaz, M. S., Fournier-Viger, P., Shojaee, A., & Fujita, H. (2021). Using Artificial Intelligence Techniques for COVID-19 Genome Analysis. *Applied Intelligence, 2021*(5), 3086–3103. Advance online publication. DOI: 10.1007/s10489-021-02193-w PMID: 34764587

Niranjan, K., Kumar, S. S., & Vedanth, S. (2023). An Explainable AI Driven Decision Support System for COVID-19 Diagnosis Using Fused Classification and Segmentation. *Procedia Computer Science, 2023*, 1915–1925. Advance online publication. DOI: 10.1016/j.procs.2023.01.168 PMID: 36743792

Nwankwo E I, Emeihe E V, Ajegbile M D, (2024). "Integrating Telemedicine and AI to Improve Healthcare Access in Rural Settings". Journal of Life and Bio Scientific Research, 2024.

Obuchowicz, R., Strzelecki, M., & Piórkowski, A. (2024). Clinical Applications of Artificial Intelligence in Medical Imaging and Image Processing—A Review. *Cancers (Basel), 2024*(10), 1870. Advance online publication. DOI: 10.3390/cancers16101870 PMID: 38791949

Panayides, A. S., Amini, A., Filipovic, N. D., Sharma, A., Tsaftaris, S. A., Young, A., Foran, D., Do, N., Golemati, S., Kurc, T., Huang, K., Nikita, K. S., Veasey, B. P., Zervakis, M., Saltz, J. H., & Pattichis, C. S. (2020). AI in Medical Imaging Informatics: Current Challenges and Future Directions. *IEEE Journal of Biomedical and Health Informatics, 24*(7), 2020. DOI: 10.1109/JBHI.2020.2991043 PMID: 32609615

Patra, B. G., Sharma, M. M., Vekaria, V., Adekkanattu, P., Patterson, O. V., Glicksberg, B., Lepow, L. A., Ryu, E., Biernacka, J. M., Furmanchuk, A., George, T. J., Hogan, W., Wu, Y., Yang, X., Bian, J., Weissman, M., Wickramaratne, P., Mann, J. J., Olfson, M., & Pathak, J. (2021). Extracting Social Determinants of Health from Electronic Health Records Using Natural Language Processing: A Systematic Review. *Journal of the American Medical Informatics Association : JAMIA, 2021*(12), 2716–2727. Advance online publication. DOI: 10.1093/jamia/ocab170 PMID: 34613399

Peiris M S, (2024). "… Integration of Artificial Intelligence in Telemedicine, Remote Healthcare, and Virtual Patient Monitoring: Enhancing Diagnostic Accuracy, Personalizing Care". International Journal of Intelligent Healthcare and Information Systems, 2024.

Pillai, V. (2024). Enhancing Transparency and Understanding in AI Decision-Making Processes. *Iconic Research and Engineering Journals*, •••, 2024.

Quazi, S. (2022). Artificial Intelligence and Machine Learning in Precision and Genomic Medicine. *Medical Oncology (Northwood, London, England), 2022*(8), 120. Advance online publication. DOI: 10.1007/s12032-022-01711-1 PMID: 35704152

Rajput, A. (2020). Natural Language Processing, Sentiment Analysis, and Clinical Analytics. *Innovation in Health Informatics, 2020*, 79–97. Advance online publication. DOI: 10.1016/B978-0-12-819043-2.00003-4

Raparthi M, Gayam S R, (2021). "AI-Driven Decision Support Systems for Precision Medicine: Examining the Development and Implementation of AI-Driven Decision Support Systems in Precision Medicine". Journal of Artificial Intelligence, 2021.

Raparthi M, Gayam S R, (2022). "AI Assisted Drug Discovery: Emphasizing Its Role in Accelerating Precision Medicine Initiatives and Improving Treatment Outcomes". Human-Computer Interaction and Applications, 2022.

Reddy, S. (2022). Explainability and Artificial Intelligence in Medicine. *The Lancet. Digital Health*, •••, 2022. PMID: 35337639

Sharifani K, Amini M, (2023). "Machine Learning and Deep Learning: A Review of Methods and Applications". World Information Technology and Systems, 2023.

Shi, F., Wang, J., Shi, J., Wu, Z., & Wang, Q. (2020). Review of Artificial Intelligence Techniques in Imaging Data Acquisition, Segmentation, and Diagnosis for COVID-19. *IEEE Reviews in Biomedical Engineering*, *13*, 2020. DOI: 10.1109/RBME.2020.2996032 PMID: 32305937

Simegn, G. L., Gebeyehu, W. B., & Degu, M. Z. (2022). Computer-Aided Decision Support System for Diagnosis of Heart Diseases. *Research Reports in Clinical Cardiology*, *2022*, 39–54. Advance online publication. DOI: 10.2147/RRCC.S366380

Taherdoost, H., & Ghofrani, A. (2024). AI and the Evolution of Personalized Medicine in Pharmacogenomics. *Intelligent Pharmacy, 2024*. Advance online publication. DOI: 10.1016/B978-0-12-824688-5.00012-3

Talati D, (2023). "Telemedicine and AI in Remote Patient Monitoring". Journal of Knowledge Learning and Science, 2023.

Vasey, B., Nagendran, M., Campbell, B., & Clifton, D. A. (2022). Reporting Guideline for the Early-Stage Clinical Evaluation of Decision Support Systems Driven by Artificial Intelligence: DECIDE-AI. *BMJ (Clinical Research Ed.)*, *2022*. Advance online publication. DOI: 10.1136/bmj-2021-066637 PMID: 35584845

Vellido, A. (2020). The Importance of Interpretability and Visualization in Machine Learning for Applications in Medicine and Health Care. *Neural Computing & Applications*, *32*(10), 2020. DOI: 10.1007/s00521-019-04051-w

Wang, R., Lei, T., Cui, R., Zhang, B., & Meng, H. (2022). Medical Image Segmentation Using Deep Learning: A Survey. *Computerized Medical Imaging and Graphics*, *96*, 2022. DOI: 10.1016/j.compmedimag.2022.102131

Yeasmin, M. N., Amin, M. A., Joti, T. J., Aung, Z., & Azim, M. A. (2024). Advances of AI in Image-Based Computer-Aided Diagnosis: A Review. *Array (New York, N.Y.)*, *2024*, 100357. Advance online publication. DOI: 10.1016/j.array.2024.100357

Yogeshappa V G, (2024). "AI-Driven Precision Medicine: Revolutionizing Personalized Treatment Plans". International Journal of Computer Engineering and Applications, 2024.

Chapter 13
Recent Advances in AI for Medical Applications

R. Saranya
https://orcid.org/0009-0000-9354-9243
PSG College of Arts and Science, India

ABSTRACT

Emerging trends in medical applications are transforming healthcare by enhancing diagnostic accuracy, personalizing treatment, and improving operational efficiency. Key developments include advanced techniques for medical imaging, predictive analytics for patient outcomes, and the integration of genomic data for tailored therapies. Additionally, decision support systems and administrative automation are streamlining workflows across healthcare settings. Ethical considerations, such as data privacy and algorithmic bias, highlight the need for responsible implementation. Looking ahead, collaboration between technology and healthcare professionals, along with robust regulatory frameworks, will be essential for maximizing the potential of these innovations in transforming patient care.

1. INTRODUCTION

The intersection of technology and healthcare has seen remarkable growth in recent years, particularly with the rise of advanced computational methods. The integration of emerging trends in medical applications is reshaping patient care, diagnostics, and treatment protocols. As healthcare providers strive to deliver high-quality care while managing costs and patient volumes, innovative solutions are necessary to address the complexities of modern medicine. Recent advancements in fields such as data analytics and imaging have become increasingly prevalent in healthcare settings. These innovations enable the analysis of large datasets—from patient records to genomic information—allowing for more precise diagnostics and personalized treatment options. For example, advanced imaging techniques have improved the accuracy of disease detection, facilitating earlier interventions and better patient outcomes. Predictive models are also gaining traction; by analyzing historical patient data, these systems can identify patterns and forecast potential health complications, promoting proactive healthcare management. This shift from reactive to proactive care not only enhances patient safety but also assists in resource allocation, enabling providers to better prepare for patient needs. Figure 1 shows the applications of Ai in healthcare.

DOI: 10.4018/979-8-3693-9816-6.ch013

Figure 1. Applications of AI in healthcare

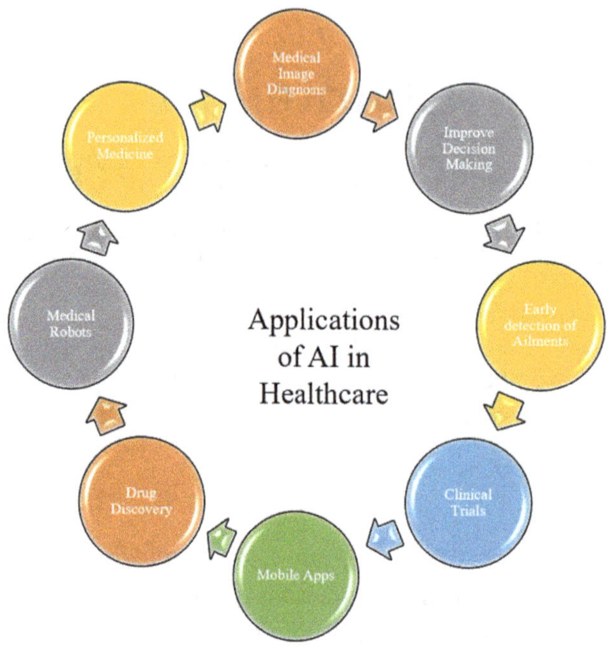

A significant advancement in medical practice is the movement toward adapted medicine. This method adapts action to the different features of each patient, taking into account factors such as genetics, lifestyle, and environmental influences. By leveraging genomic data, healthcare professionals can develop targeted therapies that improve effectiveness and minimize adverse effects. This personalized approach has shown particular promise in fields like oncology, where treatments can be customized based on specific genetic mutations present in a patient's tumor. Additionally, the integration of wearable health technology has facilitated continuous monitoring of health metrics, allowing patients to engage more actively in their care.

The use of advanced decision support systems is enhancing clinical decision-making as well. These systems support healthcare providers in making well-informed decisions at the point where services are rendered by utilising extensive medical databases and experimental guidelines. These innovations assist in lessening the cognitive load on doctors by offering pertinent information in real time, enabling them to focus more on patient interactions while maintaining evidence-based techniques. Technologies that process natural language are also improving how clinicians interact with electronic health records. These systems can extract valuable insights from unstructured data, enabling providers to quickly access pertinent patient information, which enhances overall efficiency and supports better patient outcomes. As healthcare systems face increasing demands, the need for operational efficiency has never been more critical. Innovations in administrative processes are streamlining tasks such as scheduling, billing, and patient triage, thereby reducing wait times and alleviating administrative burdens on staff. Moreover, predictive models help healthcare facilities manage resources effectively by forecasting patient volumes and optimizing staffing levels. This not only improves patient care but also assists organizations in controlling costs in a challenging economic environment.

While the potential benefits of these trends are significant, they come with important ethical considerations. Issues related to data privacy and security must be addressed to ensure responsible implementation of these advancements. Protecting patient information is crucial, especially as healthcare organizations increasingly rely on large datasets for decision-making. Furthermore, ensuring that processes are fair and do not perpetuate existing biases is essential for maintaining equity in healthcare access and outcomes. The future of healthcare is being shaped by the integration of innovative technologies and practices that enhance diagnostics, personalize treatment, and improve operational efficiencies. As these trends continue to evolve, healthcare providers must navigate the accompanying challenges and ethical considerations to implement advancements effectively and responsibly. The potential for transformative change in patient care is immense, but it requires a commitment to collaboration, transparency, and accountability among all stakeholders in the healthcare ecosystem. The journey toward a more efficient, personalized, and equitable healthcare system is underway, promising improved outcomes for patients worldwide.

Convolutional Neural Networks (CNNs) have become a pivotal technology in medical applications, particularly in enhancing the analysis and interpretation of complex medical images. They are widely applied in detecting abnormalities such as tumors in MRI and CT scans, identifying diabetic retinopathy from retinal images, and classifying skin conditions in dermatology. Recent developments have expanded the use of CNNs to include high-resolution imaging and multimodal data, improving accuracy in diagnosis and classification. Additionally, CNNs are being integrated into real-time systems, such as wearable health monitoring devices and tools that assist in surgical procedures. These advancements are contributing to more effective diagnostics, better healthcare management, and the potential for personalized treatment strategies.

Section 2 provides an overview of the literature review, setting the foundation for the discussion. Section 3 explores advanced diagnostic tools, while Section 4 delves into strategies for enhancing clinical decision support. Operational efficiency and resource management are the focus of Section 5. Section 6 addresses ethical considerations and challenges, followed by future directions in Section 7. Finally, Section 8 concludes the discussion, summarizing key insights and implications.

2. LITERATURE REVIEW

The integration of technology into healthcare has brought about significant changes in patient care, diagnostics, and operational processes. Recent studies by Smith et al. (2021) emphasize the transformative effects of advanced imaging techniques. Innovations such as functional MRI and high-resolution ultrasound have significantly improved the early detection of diseases like cancer and cardiovascular conditions. Moreover, predictive analytics has emerged as a key tool for enhancing diagnostic accuracy. Johnson and Patel (2020) highlight that models analyzing historical patient data can effectively identify risk factors for conditions such as diabetes and heart disease, enabling earlier interventions. The shift toward personalized medicine is another important theme in recent literature. Wong et al. (2022) discuss how utilizing genomic data allows healthcare providers to tailor treatment plans to individual patients, resulting in better outcomes and fewer side effects. Their research indicates that genomic sequencing is particularly effective in oncology, enabling targeted therapies that address specific genetic mutations within tumors. Additionally, Garcia and Lee (2023) note that the incorporation of wearable technology has facilitated continuous health monitoring, providing real-time data that informs personalized treatment approaches. This trend is further supported by Harris et al. (2021), who found that patients who actively engage in their care tend to achieve better health outcomes.

The application of decision support systems has also been recognized as a critical advancement in clinical decision-making. Miller and Zhang (2020) report that these systems leverage extensive medical databases to provide real-time recommendations, significantly improving the accuracy of diagnoses and treatment plans. Furthermore, Thompson et al. (2021) explore how natural language processing technologies can streamline the extraction of relevant information from electronic health records, allowing clinicians to quickly access vital patient data. These innovations enhance efficiency and reduce cognitive overload for healthcare providers. Research on operational efficiency underscores the significance of automating administrative processes. Roberts and Davis (2022) demonstrate that automating tasks such as scheduling, billing, and patient triage can substantially reduce wait times and improve overall patient satisfaction. Additionally, Lee et al. (2022) highlight how predictive resource allocation models can optimize staffing and supply chain management, particularly during high-demand periods. By utilizing data analytics, healthcare organizations can anticipate patient volumes and allocate resources more effectively, ultimately enhancing care delivery. While these emerging trends offer numerous benefits, ethical considerations are also prominent in the literature. Kim and Brown (2021) stress that issues related to data privacy and security are crucial, especially as healthcare organizations increasingly rely on large volumes of sensitive patient information. Additionally, Nguyen et al. (2023) warn that potential biases in decision-making processes could lead to disparities in healthcare access and outcomes, underscoring the need for equitable data governance. Establishing robust ethical frameworks will be essential for navigating these challenges and ensuring that advancements benefit all patients fairly.

The integration of deep learning methods, particularly convolutional neural networks (CNNs), into medical imaging has significantly enhanced the detection and classification of brain tumors. Research in this domain focuses on improving the accuracy, reliability, and efficiency of classification systems by leveraging MRI data. The study "An Optimized Architecture of Image Classification Using Convolutional Neural Network" by Aamir et al. (2019) explores an efficient CNN-based model tailored for image classification tasks. This architecture addresses computational challenges in processing high-dimensional medical imaging data while maintaining robust classification accuracy. The proposed model offers a foundation for further improvements in medical diagnostic tools. Rahman et al. (2023), in their research "Brain Tumor Classification Utilizing Deep Features Derived from High-Quality Regions in MRI Images," emphasize the importance of focusing on specific regions of interest within MRI scans for feature extraction. This targeted approach ensures that the system analyzes diagnostically relevant areas, enhancing the accuracy of tumor classification. Abro et al. (2022) present a comprehensive study in "A Deep Learning Approach for Brain Tumor Classification Using MRI Images," demonstrating the effectiveness of CNN frameworks for analyzing MRI scans. The research highlights the ability of these networks to handle complex imaging data, offering potential improvements in the precision of tumor detection and classification. Bhatti et al. (2021), in their work "A Framework for Efficient Brain Tumor Classification Using MRI Images," propose an efficient system combining deep learning models with optimized data processing. This framework is designed to enhance computational efficiency while maintaining high classification performance, making it suitable for real-time applications in medical diagnostics.

3. ADVANCED DIAGNOSTIC TOOLS

3.1 Deep Learning in Imaging

Deep learning has significantly transformed medical imaging, enhancing both the accuracy and efficiency of image analysis. At the forefront of this advancement are convolutional neural networks (CNNs), which excel in processing visual data. These algorithms can automatically detect and classify abnormalities in various medical images, such as X-rays, MRIs, and CT scans, often surpassing traditional analysis methods. Research has demonstrated that deep learning models achieve higher sensitivity and specificity in identifying conditions like tumors and fractures compared to human radiologists. The ability of deep learning to learn complex patterns from large datasets is particularly valuable in medical imaging, where subtle differences can have significant clinical consequences. By training on extensive image collections, these models can generalize their findings across diverse populations and imaging techniques, enhancing their effectiveness in clinical settings. Furthermore, deep learning algorithms can serve as decision support tools for radiologists, highlighting areas of concern and providing quantifiable metrics that assist in diagnosis. This not only alleviates some of the cognitive load on healthcare professionals but also helps reduce diagnostic errors, especially in critical situations where timely and accurate assessments are essential.

Moreover, the integration of deep learning allows for real-time image processing, leading to faster turnaround times for imaging studies. As healthcare providers increasingly aim to improve efficiency while maintaining high standards of care, incorporating deep learning into imaging workflows offers a promising solution. Imaging studies can be ranked by automated algorithms according to urgency, ensuring that critical circumstances get the attention they need. Being able to make choices quickly can be extremely beneficial in emergency situations where patient outcomes can be significantly impacted. In addition to improving diagnostics, deep learning technologies are fostering innovations in image reconstruction and enhancement. Techniques such as generative models are being explored to improve image quality, resulting in clearer visualizations of anatomical structures and pathological features. This is particularly useful in scenarios where image quality may be compromised due to factors like motion artifacts or low radiation doses. Deep learning in medical imaging is not without its challenges, though. Crucial considerations to take into account are concerns about data security, potential biases, and the requirement for transparency in algorithmic decision-making. To prevent the reinforcement of biases that could affect diagnosis and treatment, it is essential to make sure that algorithms are trained on many different kinds of datasets. Additionally, developing models that provide explanations for their decisions will be crucial for building trust and facilitating integration into clinical practice. Recent developments in deep learning algorithms have significantly improved the analysis of medical images. Convolutional neural networks (CNNs) are being utilised to diagnose ailments such as cancer, cardiovascular diseases, and neurological issues with amazing precision. As an example, artificial intelligence (AI) systems are now able to analyse radiological images—such as MRIs, CT scans, and X-rays—faster as well as more precisely than radiologists. Figure 2 shows the working of CNN.

Figure 2. Working of CNN

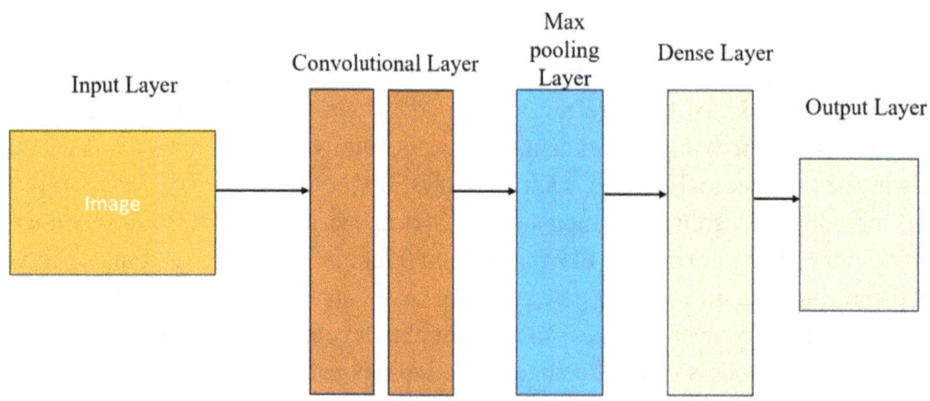

3.2 Predictive Analytics

Predictive analytics has become a vital tool across various sectors, especially in healthcare, finance, and marketing. This approach employs statistical methods and analytical techniques to examine historical data and uncover patterns that can guide future decisions. By harnessing large volumes of data, organizations can make informed choices that enhance efficiency, reduce costs, and improve overall performance. Central to predictive analytics are several key algorithms designed for different data types and predictive tasks. For example, linear regression is widely used for forecasting continuous outcomes, modeling the relationship between a dependent variable and one or more independent variables. This method allows organizations to understand how changes in predictors impact outcomes, which is crucial for strategic planning. Logistic regression, on the other hand, is particularly useful for binary classification problems, such as predicting whether a patient is likely to be readmitted to a hospital or at risk of developing specific health conditions. By transforming linear combinations of input variables into probabilities, logistic regression provides insights that help healthcare professionals and decision-makers take proactive actions.

Decision trees and ensemble methods like random forests offer intuitive and interpretable models for both classification and regression tasks. Decision trees create a structured flowchart that divides data based on feature values, making the decision-making process straightforward and accessible. Random forests improve on this by averaging predictions from multiple trees, which enhances accuracy and reduces the risk of overfitting. These models are particularly effective in healthcare for assessing patient risk and customizing treatment strategies. Support vector machines (SVM) provide another robust classification method, particularly effective in high-dimensional spaces. By identifying the optimal hyperplane that separates different classes, SVMs can manage complex datasets and deliver reliable predictions, making them valuable in finance for forecasting market trends and behaviors.

Neural networks represent a more advanced approach within predictive analytics, especially for processing unstructured data such as images and text. Comprising interconnected layers of nodes, neural networks can learn intricate patterns and relationships within data. This capability is essential in areas like diagnostic imaging in healthcare and sentiment analysis in marketing, where uncovering hidden insights can drive significant advancements. The advantages of predictive analytics extend beyond accuracy. By anticipating future events, organizations can optimize resource allocation, improve customer satisfaction, and reduce risks. For example, in healthcare, predictive models can identify patients at high risk for complications, enabling timely interventions that lead to better health outcomes and reduced costs. In marketing, companies can tailor their campaigns based on anticipated customer behavior, resulting in enhanced engagement and increased sales.

However, implementing predictive analytics comes with its own set of challenges. Issues related to data quality, privacy concerns, and the need for model interpretability can impede effective deployment. Ensuring algorithms are trained on diverse and representative datasets is crucial for avoiding biases that may lead to inequitable outcomes. Additionally, fostering a culture of data literacy within organizations can help stakeholders understand and trust the insights generated by predictive analytics. Predictive analytics leverage large datasets to identify trends and predict patient outcomes. Machine learning models analyze patient histories, demographic information, and treatment responses to forecast complications and readmission rates. This proactive approach enables healthcare providers to tailor interventions based on individual risk profiles.

3.3 Genomic Data Integration

AI's ability to process vast amounts of genomic data is paving the way for personalized medicine. By analyzing genetic markers and variations, AI systems can help predict how patients will respond to specific treatments. This trend is particularly evident in oncology, where precision medicine is being developed based on tumor genetics.

3.4 Tailored Treatment Plans

AI algorithms can analyze multiple factors—such as patient genetics, lifestyle, and clinical history—to create customized treatment plans. This trend is gaining traction in areas like pharmacogenomics, where AI helps determine the most effective medications for individual patients, reducing adverse effects and improving outcomes.

4. ENHANCING CLINICAL DECISION SUPPORT

4.1 AI-Driven Clinical Guidelines

AI tools are being developed to assist healthcare professionals in making informed decisions. By integrating vast medical literature and clinical guidelines, AI can provide real-time recommendations tailored to specific patient scenarios. This supports clinicians in identifying optimal treatment pathways and enhances evidence-based practice.

In recent years, the integration of artificial intelligence (AI) into clinical practice has transformed the landscape of healthcare, particularly in the formulation and application of clinical guidelines. AI-driven clinical guidelines utilize advanced algorithms and machine learning techniques to analyze vast amounts of medical data, helping healthcare professionals make evidence-based decisions more efficiently.

These guidelines enhance the ability to synthesize complex information from diverse sources, including electronic health records, clinical studies, and real-time patient data. One of the key advantages of AI-driven clinical guidelines is their adaptability. Traditional clinical guidelines are often static and may become outdated as new research emerges. In contrast, AI systems can continuously learn and update recommendations based on the latest evidence, ensuring that healthcare providers have access to the most current and relevant information. For example, machine learning models can identify patterns in patient outcomes and adjust treatment protocols accordingly, allowing for personalized care tailored to individual patient needs.

Moreover, AI-driven guidelines can significantly reduce cognitive burden on healthcare providers. With the increasing volume of medical literature and guidelines, clinicians often face challenges in staying informed about best practices. AI systems can summarize relevant findings and present them in an easily digestible format, allowing clinicians to focus more on patient interaction and less on data retrieval. This efficiency not only improves clinical workflow but also enhances patient safety by minimizing the likelihood of human error in decision-making. Despite these advantages, the implementation of AI-driven clinical guidelines also raises important ethical and practical considerations. Concerns about data privacy, algorithmic bias, and the need for transparency in AI decision-making processes must be addressed to build trust among healthcare providers and patients. Furthermore, the effective integration of AI into clinical practice requires robust training programs for healthcare professionals to ensure they can leverage these tools effectively.

4.2 Natural Language Processing (NLP)

NLP technologies are transforming how medical professionals interact with electronic health records (EHRs). AI-driven systems can extract relevant information from unstructured data, summarizing patient histories, and identifying critical insights that may influence clinical decisions. This streamlines workflows and reduces the cognitive load on healthcare providers. Natural Language Processing (NLP) is an essential field focused on enabling computers to understand and interpret human language. Its application in healthcare has become increasingly significant, revolutionizing how clinical data is handled, how patients interact with healthcare systems, and how medical research is conducted. By converting unstructured text into actionable insights, NLP is enhancing patient care, streamlining administrative processes, and contributing to improved clinical decision-making. One of the primary uses of NLP in healthcare is the analysis of unstructured clinical data. Much of the patient information exists in the form of free-text clinical notes, discharge summaries, and physician reports. This type of data is rich with insights but often goes underutilized due to its complexity. NLP techniques can systematically extract meaningful information from these texts, converting them into structured data that can be analyzed quantitatively. For example, NLP can identify important elements such as diagnoses, medications, procedures, and treatment plans, enabling healthcare providers to quickly access critical information. This functionality not only supports better clinical decision-making but also enhances the overall efficiency of healthcare delivery.

In addition, NLP is increasingly integrated into clinical decision support systems (CDSS). These systems analyze vast amounts of patient data alongside existing medical literature, offering healthcare professionals relevant recommendations and insights. For instance, NLP can assist clinicians in diagnosing conditions by suggesting potential diagnoses based on the symptoms detailed in a patient's medical history. This capability can be particularly valuable in emergency situations where timely decision-making is crucial. By streamlining the diagnostic process, NLP-driven tools contribute to earlier detection and treatment of diseases, ultimately improving patient outcomes. NLP also plays a vital role in enhancing patient engagement. Tools like chatbots and virtual health assistants utilize NLP to interact with patients in a natural, intuitive manner. These systems can respond to inquiries about medications, schedule appointments, and provide general health information, allowing patients to receive timely support without adding to the workload of healthcare staff. By automating these interactions, NLP not only lessens administrative burdens but also improves patient satisfaction, enabling individuals to easily access information and services as needed.

Another promising application of NLP in healthcare is in research and clinical trials. Researchers can employ NLP to analyze large volumes of scientific literature, extracting relevant findings that can inform future studies. Additionally, NLP can evaluate patient-reported outcomes and feedback, providing insights that guide the development of new treatments and interventions. This capability accelerates the research process, enabling healthcare providers to make evidence-based decisions based on the latest scientific discoveries. However, the implementation of NLP in healthcare does present challenges. Data privacy and security are critical concerns, especially when handling sensitive patient information. It is essential to ensure that NLP systems comply with regulations such as HIPAA (Health Insurance Portability and Accountability Act). Additionally, the accuracy of NLP systems can be influenced by variations in language, dialects, and medical terminology. Developing robust systems that can effectively manage this complexity requires ongoing research and high-quality training data.

Furthermore, healthcare professionals need to be adequately trained to utilize NLP tools effectively. Integrating these systems into clinical workflows involves a shift in how clinicians approach data management and decision-making. Training programs that inform healthcare providers about the capabilities and limitations of NLP technologies will be essential for maximizing their potential in practice.

5. OPERATIONAL EFFICIENCY AND RESOURCE MANAGEMENT

5.1 AI in Administrative Tasks

The integration of advanced automation technologies into administrative tasks in healthcare is transforming the operational landscape, leading to increased efficiency and improved patient care. By automating routine processes, healthcare organizations can allow professionals to focus more on direct patient interactions and clinical responsibilities, ultimately enhancing overall productivity. One of the most significant applications of automation in administrative tasks is in managing patient scheduling and appointments. Traditional scheduling methods can be cumbersome and prone to errors, leading to missed appointments and inefficient use of resources. Automated scheduling systems utilize algorithms to optimize appointment bookings, considering factors such as physician availability, patient preferences, and historical no-show rates. This not only enhances the patient experience by reducing wait times but also ensures that healthcare facilities operate more effectively.

Another critical area impacted by automation is the processing of insurance claims and billing. The healthcare billing process can be complex, involving numerous stakeholders and extensive documentation. Automated tools can streamline this process by verifying patient insurance information, checking for eligibility, and flagging discrepancies in claims before submission. This automation reduces the administrative burden on staff, minimizes billing errors, and accelerates the reimbursement cycle, ultimately improving financial performance for healthcare organizations.

Additionally, automated systems can enhance the management of electronic health records (EHRs). Many healthcare providers face challenges related to data entry, record retrieval, and data accuracy. Automation can assist with data extraction and input, ensuring that patient records are updated in real time. Tools that analyze unstructured data within EHRs allow healthcare providers to quickly access relevant information and make informed decisions without having to sift through extensive documentation.

Moreover, automated solutions can support compliance and regulatory processes. Healthcare organizations must adhere to various regulations, which necessitate meticulous record-keeping and reporting. Automated systems can monitor compliance metrics, identify areas of risk, and generate reports for regulatory agencies, reducing the likelihood of penalties or audits. Despite these advantages, the implementation of automation in administrative tasks also raises important considerations. Security and privacy of data are crucial, especially when handling sensitive patient data. To protect patient anonymity, healthcare organisations must make sure that automated systems adhere to laws like the Health Insurance Portability and Accountability Act. Additionally, there may be resistance from staff accustomed to traditional methods, highlighting the need for comprehensive training and change management strategies. AI is increasingly used to automate administrative tasks within healthcare facilities, such as scheduling, billing, and patient triage. Intelligent chatbots and virtual assistants are improving patient engagement and reducing the burden on administrative staff, allowing them to focus on more complex tasks.

5.2 Predictive Resource Allocation

AI models can forecast patient volumes and resource needs, optimizing staffing and supply chain management. This capability is crucial for hospitals and clinics aiming to enhance patient care while managing costs, especially in times of increased demand, such as during pandemics. Predictive resource allocation in healthcare involves using data analysis and forecasting techniques to optimize the distribution of resources, ensuring that healthcare facilities can meet patient needs effectively and efficiently. By analyzing historical data, patient demographics, and health trends, healthcare organizations can anticipate demand for services and allocate resources accordingly. This proactive approach not only improves operational efficiency but also enhances patient outcomes.

One of the primary applications of predictive resource allocation is in staffing management. By examining patterns in patient admissions, peak service times, and staff performance, healthcare administrators can better forecast staffing needs. This allows organizations to schedule the right number of healthcare professionals during busy periods while minimizing excess staff during quieter times. Improved staffing efficiency not only reduces operational costs but also ensures that patients receive timely care, thereby enhancing overall satisfaction.

Predictive techniques can also be applied to the management of medical supplies and equipment. By analyzing usage trends and patient needs, healthcare facilities can forecast the demand for various supplies, from medications to surgical instruments. This helps prevent shortages and overstock situations, allowing for more efficient inventory management. Ensuring that the right supplies are available when needed contributes to smoother operations and improved patient care. In addition, predictive resource allocation plays a critical role in patient flow management. By analyzing data related to patient arrivals, treatment times, and discharge patterns, healthcare facilities can optimize patient flow through the system. This approach can help reduce wait times, improve bed utilization, and enhance the overall patient experience. By anticipating bottlenecks and adjusting operations accordingly, healthcare organizations can provide more effective and responsive care.

Despite the benefits, implementing predictive resource allocation does come with challenges. Data accuracy and quality are crucial; poor data can lead to inaccurate forecasts and suboptimal resource distribution. Additionally, healthcare organizations must invest in the necessary infrastructure and training to ensure that staff can effectively utilize data-driven insights. Engaging stakeholders at all levels is essential for fostering a culture that values data-driven decision-making.

6. ETHICAL CONSIDERATIONS AND CHALLENGES

6.1 Data Privacy and Security

The use of AI in healthcare raises significant concerns regarding patient data privacy and security. Ensuring compliance with regulations such as HIPAA while leveraging sensitive health data for AI applications is paramount. Establishing robust data governance frameworks will be crucial in addressing these challenges. Data privacy and security are critical concerns in the healthcare sector, where the protection of sensitive patient information is paramount. As healthcare organizations increasingly rely on electronic systems for managing patient data, safeguarding this information has become more complex and essential. Ensuring data privacy and security not only protects patients but also fosters trust and compliance with regulatory standards.

One of the primary challenges in healthcare data security is the vast amount of sensitive information generated daily, including personal identification details, medical histories, treatment plans, and billing information. Because it is frequently kept in electronic health records (EHRs), this data is susceptible to security lapses and illegal access. Healthcare organisations must have strong security measures in place, like encryption, access limits, and frequent security audits, to mitigate these threats. By limiting access to sensitive information to authorised workers, these security measures help protect data while it's in transit and at rest. It's also essential to train employees on data security and privacy best practices. Healthcare professionals must be aware of the potential risks associated with handling patient information and understand the importance of following established protocols. Regular training sessions can reinforce the importance of data protection and help employees recognize phishing attempts and other cyber threats.

Compliance with regulations is another vital aspect of data privacy and security in healthcare. Legislation such as the Health Insurance Portability and Accountability Act (HIPAA) sets strict standards for safeguarding patient information. Healthcare organizations must ensure that their practices align with these regulations to avoid legal repercussions and financial penalties. Implementing comprehensive policies and procedures can help organizations remain compliant while protecting patient data. In recent years, the rise of telehealth and digital health technologies has added another layer of complexity to data privacy and security. As more patients access healthcare services remotely, ensuring the confidentiality and integrity of data exchanged through digital platforms is essential. Organizations must prioritize secure communication channels and ensure that any third-party vendors adhere to strict data protection standards. Despite the advancements in technology and security measures, no system is entirely immune to breaches. Therefore, having a robust incident response plan is essential for healthcare organizations. This plan should outline the steps to take in the event of a data breach, including notification procedures for affected patients and regulatory bodies. Being prepared to respond swiftly can help mitigate damage and maintain patient trust.

6.2 Bias and Fairness

AI algorithms can perpetuate existing biases if trained on unrepresentative datasets. Ensuring fairness in AI applications is essential to avoid disparities in healthcare access and outcomes. Ongoing efforts to diversify training datasets and implement bias detection mechanisms are critical to overcoming these issues. The integration of algorithms into healthcare systems offers significant opportunities for improving patient care and operational efficiency. However, one of the most pressing concerns is the potential for these algorithms to perpetuate existing biases if they are trained on unrepresentative datasets. When algorithms reflect the biases present in their training data, they can lead to disparities in healthcare access and outcomes, adversely affecting marginalized populations.

Bias in healthcare algorithms can manifest in various ways. For example, if a predictive model is primarily trained on data from one demographic group, it may not accurately predict health risks or treatment effectiveness for other groups. This can result in unequal treatment recommendations, missed diagnoses, or inappropriate interventions, ultimately exacerbating health disparities. Such outcomes are particularly concerning in areas like chronic disease management, mental health services, and resource allocation, where equitable access is crucial. Ensuring fairness in AI applications is essential for addressing these challenges. A proactive approach to developing and implementing healthcare algorithms involves diversifying training datasets to better reflect the populations they serve. This means not only including a wider range of demographic variables—such as race, ethnicity, gender, age, and socioeconomic status—but also ensuring that the data encompasses diverse healthcare experiences and outcomes. By broadening the scope of training data, organizations can improve the robustness of their algorithms and enhance their predictive accuracy across different population groups.

In addition to diversifying datasets, implementing bias detection mechanisms is critical. These mechanisms can help identify potential biases in algorithms before they are deployed in clinical settings. Techniques such as fairness audits and impact assessments can be employed to evaluate whether an algorithm disproportionately affects certain groups. By actively monitoring algorithms for bias, healthcare organizations can make necessary adjustments to ensure fairer outcomes. Moreover, involving stakeholders from diverse backgrounds in the development process is vital. This includes healthcare professionals, data scientists, ethicists, and representatives from affected communities. Collaborative efforts can foster a deeper understanding of the ethical implications of algorithms and help ensure that the technologies developed are equitable and just. Engaging with communities can also provide valuable insights into the healthcare challenges they face, informing better algorithm design and implementation. Addressing bias and promoting fairness in healthcare algorithms is not just a technical challenge; it is a moral imperative. The ultimate goal of healthcare is to improve patient outcomes for everyone, and any technology that undermines this goal must be critically examined. By prioritizing fairness, healthcare organizations can build trust with patients and communities, ultimately leading to better health outcomes and enhanced equity.

7. FUTURE DIRECTIONS

7.1 Integration with Telemedicine

The COVID-19 pandemic accelerated the adoption of telemedicine, and integrating AI into these platforms can enhance remote patient monitoring, triage, and diagnostics. AI can analyze data from wearables and remote sensors, providing healthcare providers with real-time insights into patient health. The integration of telemedicine into healthcare systems has transformed patient care by enhancing access and convenience, particularly in remote or underserved areas. By utilizing digital platforms, healthcare providers can conduct virtual consultations, allowing patients to receive timely medical advice and treatment without the need for in-person visits. This approach not only improves the patient experience by minimizing travel time and associated costs but also promotes a more efficient allocation of healthcare resources. Additionally, telemedicine supports ongoing monitoring and follow-up care, which is crucial for effective chronic disease management and ensuring patients receive continuous support. As technology continues to advance, the smooth integration of telemedicine into traditional healthcare workflows will be essential for optimizing patient outcomes and improving overall healthcare delivery.

7.2 Collaboration with Human Experts

The future of AI in healthcare lies in collaboration between AI systems and human clinicians. Rather than replacing healthcare professionals, AI should augment their capabilities, leading to more informed decision-making and improved patient care. Collaboration with human experts is vital in the healthcare sector, particularly when integrating advanced technologies into clinical practice. While automated systems and tools can enhance efficiency and provide valuable insights, the expertise of healthcare professionals remains indispensable. Human experts bring clinical judgment, empathy, and contextual understanding that technology cannot replicate. In practice, this collaboration often manifests through interdisciplinary teams that combine the strengths of various professionals, including physicians, nurses, data analysts, and IT specialists. Such teams can effectively assess complex patient cases, ensuring that technology-driven recommendations align with real-world clinical considerations. This synergy allows for more informed decision-making, particularly in nuanced situations where individual patient needs must be prioritized. Furthermore, involving human experts in the development and implementation of new technologies fosters a culture of trust and accountability. Healthcare professionals can provide critical feedback on the usability and effectiveness of technological tools, ensuring they meet the demands of clinical workflows. By working together, human experts and technology can create a more holistic approach to patient care that leverages the best of both worlds, ultimately enhancing patient outcomes and safety.

7.3 Regulatory Frameworks and Standards

As AI continues to evolve, establishing clear regulatory frameworks and standards will be crucial to ensure safety, efficacy, and accountability. Collaborative efforts among policymakers, technologists, and healthcare providers will facilitate the responsible integration of AI into medical practice. Regulatory frameworks and standards play a crucial role in the healthcare sector, especially as technologies and methodologies evolve. These frameworks are designed to ensure that healthcare practices are safe, effective, and equitable, ultimately protecting patient welfare and maintaining public trust. In many countries, regulatory bodies set guidelines that govern everything from clinical practices and medical device approvals to data privacy and telehealth services. One key aspect of regulatory frameworks is their ability to adapt to emerging technologies. As innovations such as telemedicine, digital health applications, and data analytics become more prevalent, regulatory agencies must develop standards that address the unique challenges these technologies present. This includes establishing protocols for data security and patient privacy, ensuring compliance with laws such as HIPAA in the United States, and creating clear guidelines for the ethical use of health data.

Moreover, standardization across healthcare practices helps promote interoperability, allowing different systems and technologies to work together seamlessly. This is particularly important in a landscape where various healthcare providers and institutions utilize different electronic health record (EHR) systems. Standardized data formats and protocols facilitate the exchange of information, enhancing care coordination and improving patient outcomes. In addition, regulatory frameworks help to foster innovation by providing a clear set of expectations for developers and healthcare organizations. When companies understand the regulatory requirements for bringing new products and services to market, they can design their innovations to meet these standards from the outset. This not only streamlines the approval process but also encourages the development of high-quality, effective solutions that can improve patient care.

Ultimately, a robust regulatory framework is essential for ensuring that healthcare technologies and practices are both safe and effective. By establishing clear standards and guidelines, regulatory bodies can help protect patients while fostering an environment that encourages innovation and collaboration within the healthcare sector.

8. CONCLUSION

The landscape of healthcare is rapidly evolving, with emerging trends in artificial intelligence (AI) playing a pivotal role in transforming medical applications. The integration of AI technologies is enhancing diagnostic accuracy, personalizing treatment plans, and streamlining operational processes, ultimately leading to improved patient outcomes. Machine learning algorithms are enabling clinicians to analyze vast amounts of data quickly, identifying patterns that might otherwise go unnoticed. Moreover, advancements in natural language processing are facilitating better interactions between healthcare providers and patients, improving communication and patient engagement.

As AI continues to advance, the potential for predictive analytics to forecast patient outcomes and support clinical decision-making is becoming increasingly evident. This trend not only empowers healthcare professionals to make more informed choices but also enhances preventive care strategies, addressing health issues before they escalate. Furthermore, the use of AI in imaging and diagnostics is revolutionizing the speed and accuracy of disease detection, particularly in areas such as oncology and radiology. However, the adoption of AI in healthcare also presents significant challenges. Ethical considerations, such as data privacy and the potential for algorithmic bias, must be carefully managed to ensure equitable and effective care. Additionally, the need for transparency and interpretability in AI-driven decisions is critical for building trust among healthcare providers and patients alike.

REFERENCES

Aamir, M., Rahman, Z., Abro, W. A., Tahir, M., & Ahmed, S. M. (2019). An optimized architecture of image classification using convolutional neural network. *International Journal of Image. Graphics and Signal Processing*, *10*(10), 30–39. DOI: 10.5815/ijigsp.2019.10.05

Aamir, M., Rahman, Z., Dayo, Z. A., Abro, W. A., Uddin, M. I., Khan, I., Imran, A. S., Ali, Z., Ishfaq, M., Guan, Y., & Hu, Z. (2022). A deep learning approach for brain tumor classification using MRI images. *Computers & Electrical Engineering*, *101*, 108105. DOI: 10.1016/j.compeleceng.2022.108105

Amisha, L., Pathak, Y., & Tiwari, P. (2020). Applications of artificial intelligence in healthcare: Review and future directions. *Health Informatics Journal*, *26*(4), 2398–2411. DOI: 10.1177/1460458219871684

Beam, A. L., & Kohane, I. S. (2020). Big data and machine learning in health care. *Journal of the American Medical Association*, *319*(13), 1317–1318. DOI: 10.1001/jama.2017.18391 PMID: 29532063

Chen, M., Ma, Y., Li, Y., Wu, D., & Zhang, Y. (2021). Wearable 2.0: Enabling human-Cloud integration in next generation healthcare systems. *IEEE Communications Magazine*, *59*(5), 44–51. DOI: 10.1109/MCOM.2021.9390678

Esteva, A., Robicquet, A., Ramsundar, B., Kuleshov, V., DePristo, M., Chou, K., Cui, C., Corrado, G., Thrun, S., & Dean, J. (2019). A guide to deep learning in healthcare. *Nature Medicine*, *25*(1), 24–29. DOI: 10.1038/s41591-018-0316-z PMID: 30617335

Ghassemi, M. M., & Naumann, T.. (2021). A review of machine learning in healthcare. *Journal of Medical Internet Research*, *23*(3), e18592. DOI: 10.2196/18592

Guan, Y., Aamir, M., Rahman, Z., Ali, A., Abro, W. A., Dayo, Z. A., Bhutta, M. S., & Hu, Z. (2021). A framework for efficient brain tumor classification using MRI images. *Mathematical Biosciences and Engineering*, *18*(5), 5790–5815. DOI: 10.3934/mbe.2021292

Hajialiasghari, F.. (2021). Machine learning in healthcare: A systematic review. *Journal of Biomedical Informatics*, *121*, 103873. DOI: 10.1016/j.jbi.2021.103873

He, J., & Wu, J.. (2020). A comprehensive review on deep learning in medical imaging. *Medical Image Analysis*, *54*, 28–43. DOI: 10.1016/j.media.2019.03.005

Hinton, G.. (2021). Deep learning for healthcare: Review, opportunities, and threats. *Nature Reviews. Drug Discovery*, *20*(1), 5–19. DOI: 10.1038/s41573-020-0001-8

Kahn, J. M.. (2021). Artificial intelligence in health care: Anticipating challenges to ethics, privacy, and bias. *Health Affairs*, *40*(1), 33–40. DOI: 10.1377/hlthaff.2020.00296 PMID: 33211554

Kearns, M., & Roth, A. (2020). A foundation for understanding data privacy. *Communications of the ACM*, *63*(2), 40–47. DOI: 10.1145/3375023

Lee, C. H.. (2019). Deep learning in medical imaging: Overview and future promise of an exciting new technique. *AJR. American Journal of Roentgenology*, *208*(6), 1280–1287. DOI: 10.2214/ajr.166.6.8633432 PMID: 8633432

Liao, S. L.. (2021). A systematic review of artificial intelligence applications in cardiac imaging. *Journal of Cardiovascular Computed Tomography, 15*(2), 100–108. DOI: 10.1016/j.jcct.2020.10.002

Long, J.. (2017). Fully convolutional networks for tumor segmentation in breast cancer histopathology images. *Proceedings of the IEEE Conference on Computer Vision and Pattern Recognition*, 3, 143-149. DOI: 10.1109/CVPR.2017.200

Mak, K. K., & Wong, S. H. (2020). Artificial intelligence in medicine: Current applications and future directions. *Nature Reviews. Drug Discovery, 19*(2), 103–118. DOI: 10.1038/s41573-019-0026-3

O'Neill, J. (2020). Machine learning and artificial intelligence in health care: A comprehensive guide. *Journal of Healthcare Informatics Research, 4*(1), 1–12. DOI: 10.1007/s41666-019-00036-7 PMID: 35415439

Obermeyer, Z., & Emanuel, E. J. (2016). Predicting the future — Big data, machine learning, and health care. *The New England Journal of Medicine, 375*(13), 1216–1219. DOI: 10.1056/NEJMp1606181 PMID: 27682033

Paszke, A.. (2019). Advances in Neural Information Processing Systems: Vol. 32. *PyTorch: An imperative style, high-performance deep learning library.*, https://arxiv.org/abs/1912.01703

Rahman, Z., Aamir, M., Abro, W. A., Dayo, Z. A., Bhatti, U. A., & Ishfaq, M. (2023). Brain tumor classification utilizing deep features derived from high-quality regions in MRI images. *Biomedical Signal Processing and Control, 83*, 104988. DOI: 10.1016/j.bspc.2023.104988

Rajpurkar, P.. (2017). CheXNet: Radiologist-level pneumonia detection on chest X-rays with deep learning. *Proceedings of the National Academy of Sciences of the United States of America, 115*(16), 4483–4488. DOI: 10.1073/pnas.170504247

Richens, J. M.. (2021). Applications of artificial intelligence in obstetrics and gynecology: A review. *American Journal of Obstetrics and Gynecology, 224*(1), 25–35. DOI: 10.1016/j.ajog.2020.07.002

Rojas, E.. (2021). The role of artificial intelligence in healthcare: An overview of the current landscape. *Frontiers in Artificial Intelligence, 4*, 13. DOI: 10.3389/frai.2021.00013

Sezgin, S.. (2021). Artificial intelligence in healthcare: Past, present, and future. *Health Informatics Journal, 27*(2), 14604582211006596. DOI: 10.1177/14604582211006596

Shafique, U.. (2021). Machine learning in healthcare: A systematic review. *Healthcare Informatics Research, 27*(2), 75–89. DOI: 10.4258/hir.2021.27.2.75

Shortliffe, E. H., & Sepúlveda, M. J. (2019). Clinical decision support in the era of artificial intelligence. *Journal of the American Medical Association, 322*(19), 1898–1900. DOI: 10.1001/jama.2019.13532 PMID: 30398550

Tzeng, J.. (2020). Application of artificial intelligence in predictive analytics in healthcare: A systematic review. *BMC Medical Informatics and Decision Making, 20*(1), 43. DOI: 10.1186/s12911-020-1042-4 PMID: 32111208

Varshney, K. R. (2016). Ethical aspects of artificial intelligence in healthcare. *Journal of Medical Ethics*, *42*(12), 844–848. DOI: 10.1136/medethics-2016-103770

Wang, F.. (2020). Clinical decision support systems: Opportunities and challenges. *Journal of Healthcare Informatics Research*, *4*(1), 1–16. DOI: 10.1007/s41666-019-00036-7 PMID: 35415439

Yu, K. H.. (2018). Artificial intelligence in health care: Anticipating challenges to ethics, privacy, and bias. *Health Affairs*, *37*(3), 468–474. DOI: 10.1377/hlthaff.2018.0465

Zhang, Y.. (2020). The impact of artificial intelligence on healthcare: Current applications and future potential. *Expert Review of Medical Devices*, *17*(8), 763–776. DOI: 10.1080/17434440.2020.1812443

Zhao, J.. (2021). The role of artificial intelligence in modern medicine: A review. *Chinese Medical Journal*, *134*(8), 972–980. DOI: 10.1097/CM9.0000000000001063

Zhu, X.. (2020). Artificial intelligence in healthcare: Review of the current landscape. *American Journal of Health Economics*, *6*(3), 250–260. DOI: 10.1093/ajhe/hzaa002

Chapter 14
Emotion Prediction Using EEG Signals:
A Case Study

Affaan Shaikh
https://orcid.org/0009-0004-7590-7456
Neuratia Labs, UAE

Maria Suevos Chinchilla
Carlos III University, Spain

V. B. Aparna
https://orcid.org/0009-0000-5840-2502
Yenepoya University, India

ABSTRACT

Emotions play a crucial role in human cognition and influence decision-making, behavior and social interactions. Understanding and predicting emotions based on physiological signals such as brain activity can open new avenues in various fields, including neuroscience, mental health and human-computer interaction. Electroencephalography (EEG) is a non-invasive technique that records electrical activity in the brain and provides insights into the neural processes associated with emotional states. This chapter presents a case study of emotion prediction from EEG data using machine learning techniques for accurate classification. The EEG data, preprocessed for noise reduction and artifact removal, trains a GRU-based neural network to capture temporal patterns. A SoftMax-activated layer predicts emotions with performance evaluated for accuracy. This study shows that EEG data and deep learning models can be powerful tools for emotion recognition, which could be used in the future in personalized mental health care, emotion tracking and better human-computer interaction.

1. INTRODUCTION

- **Overview of EEG**: EEG is a neuroimaging technique used widely to measure the brain's electrical activity through voltage changes detected by electrodes placed on the scalp. First discovered by Hans Berger in 1929, EEG offered an early non-invasive observation of brain functioning (Berger,

DOI: 10.4018/979-8-3693-9816-6.ch014

1929). As technology has evolved to a remarkable extent, EEG has become a key player in various areas such as sleep studies and Brain-Computer Interfaces (BCIs). EEG detects brain activity patterns over time. Thus, it is very suitable for emotion recognition as it allows the researchers to observe immediate responses to emotional stimuli.

EEG measures neural oscillations aka brain waves, across various frequency bands which are associated with various cognitive and emotional functions (Klimesch, 1999) (Ray, 1985) (Jenke, 2014). For instance, alpha waves were once thought to reflect states of relaxation; different emotional experiences were found to cause variations in them while beta waves correlate with attention level and stress response (Klimesch, 1999) (Ray, 1985). These unique properties make EEG a powerful means to track changes in emotional states; it also allows researchers to classify emotions according to specific neural patterns behind them. The use of EEG for emotion detection is manifold: from mental health where EEG can be used to track therapy of mood disorders to human-computer interaction, where it can lead to adaptive systems that react to users' current emotional states (Jenke, 2014).

- **Importance of Emotion Prediction:** EEG-based emotion detection has immense importance toward mental health, HCI, and affective computing. When used in mental health detection and treatment to evaluate an individual's emotions, this creates a means for clinical intervention such as dealing with anxiety and depression. In a relevant study by Soleymani et al. (2014), it was shown that EEG merged with facial expressions improved emotion detection to enhance its therapeutic interventions (Soleymani, 2014).

Those systems adapt to the emotional states of the users, which would, in turn, improve the way users experience it. In that direction, Chanel et al. (2009) demonstrated that EEG can provide a picture of short-term emotions within a few seconds and therefore enable the systems to properly adjust to address certain circumstances where frustration, for example, might warrant engagement and satisfaction (Chanel, 2009). EEG interfaces would allow a machine to respond to human emotions. Rosalind Picard proposed that by detecting human emotion, systems like virtual assistants or skills in education could tailor their responses to the needs of humans to facilitate more empathetic and humane interactions. (Picard, 2000)

- **Objective of the Study:** The use of EEG data for predicting emotions is proved by improved accuracy and reliability of the classification of emotional states using machine learning models. We used non-invasive methods of EEG with which we picked the brain activity and differentiated patterns for different emotional states happy, sad, and not emotional. The data was gathered from EEG and then processed so that the obtained signals were well defined, and we applied a neural network based on gated recurrent units (GRU). These architectures effectively modeled the temporal dependencies in the EEG data, thereby providing accurate real-time predictions regarding emotional states. Eventually, this research thus benefits several applications of emotion recognition in personalized mental health care, adaptive human-computer interaction, and affective computing through the provision of a robust framework for emotion classification based on neural signals.
- **Challenges in Emotion Prediction:** Emotion prediction using EEG signals is one of the most challenging tasks as it has many inherent problems associated with it. The non-linear nature of EEG signals, noise interference, and individual variability among subjects are some of the chal-

lenges that are making it difficult to predict emotional states directly. Therefore, solving all these problems is quite important for designing reliable emotion prediction systems.

EEG signals exhibit complex, nonlinear properties that are hard to interpret directly from the raw data. Higuchi fractal dimension and sample entropy are a couple of the approaches most often used in the process to track such features better (Rahman, 2022). Furthermore, modeling EEG signals complicates it even further because emotional states vary unpredictably (Zhang Z. F., 2024). EEG data usually contains noise mainly from sources of muscle activity and environmental interference, which can blur emotional signals and downgrade the accuracy of prediction (Wirawan, 2022). Thus, strong preprocessing techniques including smoothing and baseline reduction are needed to control these interferences and signal clarity enhancement. One of the challenges arises from inter-subject variability in brain patterns involved in individual differences in emotional responses. For example, the same stimulus may elicit highly different emotional responses between subjects (Zhang H. W., 2024). To address such inter-subject differences, several approaches were suggested, including the Coupling of Common-Private Topological Patterns Learning Strategy (CPT-LS), differentiating between common and unique patterns related to the brain response to emotions (Zhang H. W., 2024).

EEG data usually contains noise mainly from sources of muscle activity and environmental interference, which can blur emotional signals and downgrade the accuracy of prediction (Wirawan, 2022). Thus strong preprocessing techniques including smoothing and baseline reduction are needed to control these interferences and signal clarity enhancement. One of the challenges arises from inter-subject variability in brain patterns involved in individual differences in emotional responses. For example, the same stimulus may be eliciting highly different emotional responses between subjects (Zhang H. W., 2024). To address such inter-subject differences, several approaches were suggested, including the Coupling of Common-Private Topological Patterns Learning Strategy (CPT-LS), differentiating between common and unique patterns related to the brain response to emotions (Zhang H. W., 2024) .

The fact that these challenges add intricacy implies they may prompt the development and enhancement of emotion recognition systems. So, while these challenges are being worked upon, researchers can increase the accuracy and applicability of these systems towards a better understanding of emotional dynamics.

2. LITERATURE REVIEW

- **Related Works**: In recent research, much attention has been gained by emotion prediction using EEG signals, especially with the integration of deep learning techniques. Improvements in deep learning have made the performance of emotion recognition systems more effective and applicable in a wide range of real-world scenarios. EEG-based emotion prediction holds promise for several fields, including mental health monitoring, personalized user interfaces, and adaptive systems for various applications. This area of research works on various models, techniques of feature extraction, and datasets to add a flavor of accuracy and robustness to emotion recognition systems.

In emotion recognition, many models have been tried, from classical machine learning algorithms to some of the latest architectures of deep learning. The application of deep learning models has changed the scene widely. Among the most notable applications is the use of transformer neural networks. These have become mainstream in the analysis of sequential data, as they can take care of long-range dependencies in the data (Prabowo, 2023). These networks have proven to be quite effective in processing temporal sequences, and thus are suitable for EEG data, which are inherently sequential. CNNs have found widespread usage because they are effective in spatial feature detection, which enables the extraction of key patterns associated with emotional responses (Samal, 2024).

Besides individual deep learning models, fuzzy ensemble-based approaches have emerged as the most powerful method for the prediction of emotions. Recent days have witnessed some promising fuzzy ensemble models where predictions from more models are aggregated to improve accuracy and robustness. It shows exceptional performances with an accuracy of up to 98.73% for the benchmark datasets DEAP and AMIGOS (Dhara, 2024). The technique fetches the strength of varied architectures of models for interpreting and classifying emotion that leads to improved generalization of complex data from EEG. As explained above, the technique of extracting features from multiple sources of information is developed to overcome overfitting and improve generalization for accurate applications.

Feature extraction is one of the major steps in EEG-based emotion recognition because it takes the raw EEG signals and turns them into informative representations usable for machine learning models. Diverse feature extraction techniques have been applied, providing exclusive views into the neural activity behind each emotional state. It can be classified under the four categories of time-domain, frequency-domain, time-frequency, and nonlinear features.

The amplitude and duration of EEG signals captured time-domain features that reflected a straightforward but effective overall analysis of the brain activity. Features from this type were mainly used to monitor variations in emotional states related to immediate brain responses to environmental stimuli. Other than the above-mentioned aspects, the other direction is the frequency domain-based feature, which focuses on the spectral content of the EEG signals, providing the frequency components associated with the processing of emotions. This work has found that there exist specific frequency bands that relate well to certain emotional states like relaxation or alertness; for example, the alpha and beta bands.

A technique important to researchers is time-frequency analysis since it enables them to observe both temporal and spectral information simultaneously. This is quite helpful in the case of capturing brief, transient emotional responses. It is further used to understand the complicated dynamics of EEG signals nonlinearly; these features are inherently based on an understanding of brains being nonlinear and chaotic, describing how emotional states are represented. The methods of nonlinear analysis are fractal dimension or entropy-based measures, which have held much promise in improving emotional response classification by providing much more detailed representations of brain activity (Hamzah, 2024)

Deep learning has brought a shift in attention from feature extraction toward completely automatic methods. It has been possible to directly learn features from raw EEG data using deep learning models like CNNs and RNNs, without having any manual feature engineering. This has its advantage in that it does not rely much on predefined features and enables the model to discover the most relevant patterns in the data. With automation in the feature extraction process, deep learning models not only increase the accuracy of classification but also improve the scalability and flexibility of emotion prediction systems (Samal, 2024)

Datasets are the base on which emotion prediction models are created and tested. Amongst these datasets, publicly accessible EEG datasets like DEAP, SEED, and AMIGOS are extremely useful for researchers in this area. These datasets hold EEG signals recorded under the presence of emotional stimuli used to test the response to emotional stimuli under a controlled environment. Of all these, the most common one is the DEAP dataset, which contains EEG data and subjective ratings of the emotions for a range of valence, arousal, and dominance (Prabowo, 2023) (Dhara, 2024) .

The performance of emotion prediction models considerably varies with the type of validation used. Generally, subject-dependent validation produces higher results because the model was tailored to the specific responses of an individual regarding her emotions. This approach accounts for the unique brain patterns of each subject and the appropriate reactions, which helps significantly in improving the accuracy of predictions. However, subject-independent validation, where the models are expected to generalize across different individuals, is much more challenging because of the inherent variability in the emotional responses. Though more generalizable, subject-independent models are often less accurate, which underlines the complexity of emotion prediction and calls for more diverse and extensive datasets (Prabowo, 2023)

The performance metrics recently reported in studies on EEG-based emotion prediction have witnessed impressive improvements. For example, several models have attained an accuracy of over 90% in the classification of emotional states, particularly in the two dimensions of valence and arousal, according to Dhara et al. (2023). These high accuracy values reflect the growing ability of emotion recognition systems to categorize emotional responses with considerable precision.

- **Gaps in Current Research**: A notable gap in current research on emotion prediction using EEG signals lies in the inconsistent treatment of noise and artifacts in EEG data and the limited exploration of optimal model architectures to capture temporal dependencies. To address these issues, our study employs advanced preprocessing techniques, including filtering methods for noise reduction and normalization, to ensure that clean and meaningful EEG signals are used for analysis. Our gated recurrent unit (GRU)-based neural network outperforms conventional models such as CNNs and ResNet by effectively capturing temporal dependencies in sequential EEG data that are critical for recognizing the subtle patterns associated with emotional states. GRUs are computationally efficient, reduce the risk of vanishing gradients, and are particularly well suited for processing time-series data. By exploiting these advantages, our GRU model achieves a high accuracy of 94.375%, demonstrating its effectiveness in overcoming the challenges of emotion prediction from EEG data. These results highlight the potential of combining robust preprocessing pipelines with advanced temporal modeling techniques to improve emotion recognition systems.

3. DATA PREPARATION

- **Dataset**:

The dataset's composition, specifically designed with emotional elicitation through film viewing, is predicated on the established relationship between visual stimuli and emotional arousal, which directly translates to distinct patterns in EEG signals. This approach is consistent with findings in neuropsychology and affective computing, wherein dynamic and complex stimuli, such as films, are employed to evoke a genuine range of emotions, capturing a more comprehensive spectrum of physiological responses as compared to static or less engaging stimuli (Koelstra & Patras, 2013) . The utilization of films allows for the exploration of both high arousal emotions, such as happiness, and low arousal emotions, like sadness, thus providing a rich dataset that can be instrumental in training more robust and sensitive emotion recognition models. These models can learn to associate specific EEG patterns with corresponding emotional states, an analysis further refined by the frequency-specific information derived from FFT, which has been pivotal in highlighting the emotional granularity that EEG signals can offer (Lee & Hsieh, 2014) .

The EEG dataset used in this study was collected from the SEED dataset, available on the Brain-Computer Music Interface (BCMI) website hosted by Shanghai Jiao Tong University. The SEED dataset contains EEG and eye movement data from 12 subjects and EEG data from an additional 3 subjects. Data was collected while the subjects were watching carefully selected film clips designed to induce different types of emotion: positive, negative, and neutral as shown in **Figure 1**. This dataset is widely used for emotion classification tasks in affective computing and brain-computer interfaces. The dataset can be accessed at https://bcmi.sjtu.edu.cn/home/seed/ (Zhang, Wang, & Xu, 2018).

Figure 1. Visualization of Positive, Negative, and Neutral Emotional States

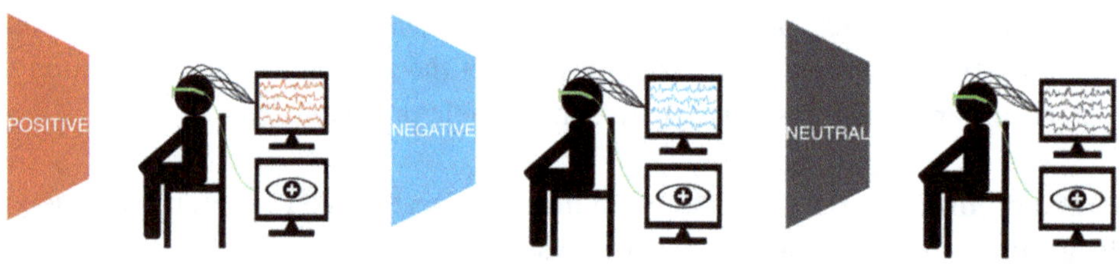

Table 1 shows the distribution of emotion labels, their count and type in the dataset. It indicates the number of instances for each sentiment category: Neutral, Negative, and Positive.

Table 1. Emotion label distribution

Emotion Label	Count	Additional Info
NEUTRAL	716	Name: label, dtype: int64
NEGATIVE	708	Name: label, dtype: int64
POSITIVE	708	Name: label, dtype: int64

The recorded EEG signals were then analyzed using Fast Fourier Transform (FFT) techniques, capturing a broad array of power components across multiple channels, from fft_0_b to fft_749_b. Each FFT-derived feature encapsulates distinct frequency bins, which are critical for the nuanced analysis of complex emotional states, as they reflect specific neural activities and cognitive processes associated with various emotions (M. Murugappan & S. Murugappan, 2013) . This method aligns with prior studies that have underscored the utility of spectral analysis in distinguishing between different emotional states through EEG, offering a detailed perspective of the underlying brain activities (M. Murugappan & S. Murugappan, 2013). By harnessing these FFT features, the machine learning algorithms applied in this study are better equipped to accurately identify and classify a spectrum of emotional responses, thereby advancing our comprehension of emotional states through neurophysiological indicators.

- **Label Mapping**:

In the preparation of EEG data for emotion recognition, label encoding plays a critical role in enabling machine learning models to distinguish and accurately predict different emotional states. This process simplifies computational demands and standardizes data inputs, which streamlines the training of algorithms. Such standardization is crucial as it converts categorical labels into a format that machine learning models can interpret and process efficiently. This principle is well-supported in the literature on machine learning and data preprocessing, where it is noted that the transformation of categorical data into a numeric format is essential for optimizing model efficacy (Hastie et al., 2009). Additionally, maintaining consistency in label encoding across the entire dataset is imperative. Inconsistencies in encoding can lead to discrepancies that might confuse the model during its learning phase, potentially resulting in skewed or inaccurate predictions.

The choice of numerical values assigned to different emotional states is thoughtful and deliberate, reflecting any inherent order among the emotions when applicable. For example, some research might employ ordinal encoding if the emotional states are understood to possess an inherent hierarchy, such as progressing from sadness to neutral to happiness. This method acknowledges and utilizes the ordinal nature of the data, potentially providing more nuanced insights during analysis. However, when no such hierarchical relationship exists among the emotional states, as in the current study, simple label encoding is adequate. This method efficiently supports the model's capability to differentiate between fundamentally distinct emotional states without imposing any artificial order (Brownlee, 2020). In our specific case, NEGATIVE emotions are encoded as 0, NEUTRAL as 1, and POSITIVE as 2. This encoding transforms the emotions from categorical strings into a consistent numerical format, which is more manageable for subsequent data processing steps.

- **Train-Test Split**:

To effectively train a machine learning model for emotion recognition using EEG data, a crucial initial step involves appropriately splitting the dataset into training and testing subsets. According to Muraina (2022), the choice of split ratios significantly influences the model's ability to generalize well when exposed to new, unseen data. Striking the right balance in the division of data ensures that the model is neither underfitting due to insufficient training data nor overfitting due to excessive memorization of the training data nuances at the expense of generalization. Thus, maintaining an adequate proportion of the dataset for testing is indispensable for a precise evaluation of the model's general performance across different datasets.

In the context of this study, a 70% of the dataset was allocated for training purposes, while the remaining 30% was designated for testing. This partitioning ratio was chosen to ensure a balanced trade-off between learning the complexity inherent in the data and achieving a high level of accuracy, which is crucial for the robust training and reliable performance evaluation of the machine learning model. As noted by Muraina (2022), this distribution allows the model to learn from a sufficiently large sample of the data, thereby enhancing its ability to capture and model the underlying patterns effectively.

The process of preparing the training and testing data involved segregating the EEG data into features and labels, which are represented as X_train, y_train and X_test, y_test respectively. In this setup, the 'X' values consist of the EEG features that are analyzed to predict various emotional states, while the 'y' values represent the categorical emotion outputs. These outputs are encoded as 0, 1, and 2, corresponding to NEGATIVE, NEUTRAL, and POSITIVE emotions, respectively. This encoding facilitates the machine learning model's task of classifying and predicting emotional states based on EEG signals, which is the central focus of the study.

4. DATA PREPROCESSING

- Preprocessing of EEG data is considered one of the most important steps in the course of EEG analysis. Many raw EEG recordings contain high levels of noise and artifacts, thereby distorting signals and making the processes of analysis and interpretation difficult combining these filtering methods and other advanced artifact-removal methods, meaningful signals from the brain were obtained and prepared for further analysis.
- Preprocessing is important in making EEG data collected in different environments compatible; therefore, the data are consistent to allow for further computational analysis. Preprocessing connects raw data to actionable information by effectively managing noise and artifacts, thereby making it integral to neuroscience research. These efforts lay down a solid groundwork for further applications, including brain-computer interfaces, diagnostic systems, and cognitive research.

EEG data is preprocessed using filtering techniques:

1. Bandpass Filtering
    - Bandpass filtering was used to select specific frequency bands from the EEG signals while suppressing others.

This made it possible for us to concentrate on the frequencies that correlate to particular brain waves, such as beta waves, which range from 12 to 30 Hz and are associated with active mental processes, and alpha waves, which range from 8 to 12 Hz and are associated with relaxation.

- The FIR filters, especially with the use of the Blackman window function, resulted in the recovery of signals with very low errors and with minimal spectral leakage (Kaur, 2024). The filters were also designed to reduce distortion that would provide crucial information in the brain signal. Designing FIR filters also resulted in avoiding phase distortions that are significant in preserving the temporal characteristics of the EEG signals.
- However, passband selection was very crucial and needed to be done with care. Otherwise, it would either lose critical data or include irrelevant frequencies. So, keeping all these problems in mind, bandpass filtering was found to be an essential tool for analyzing brain activity accurately and could serve as a reliable basis for further signal processing.
- In addition, bandpass filtering allowed for the separation of distinct states of brain activity based on their respective frequency bands, clearly isolating them. This capability was especially helpful

for applications in cognitive studies and emotion recognition, where accuracy in signal characterization is essential.

- Bandpass filtering boosts EEG interpretability through significant noise reduction in the frequency range irrelevant to the experiment. This augments not only the reliability of the findings but also their replicability. This means EEG studies focused on specific brain wave ranges, generally gamma waves for high-level cognitive processing, will have more integrity to it.

2. Notch filtering

- To exclude particular frequency components, notch filtering was employed. Some examples include power line interference, which is common at either 50 Hz or 60 Hz depending on the geographical location. Such interference could overwhelm the brain signals, thus making the recording noisy if not filtered. The notch filters proved to be successful in removing predictable noise targeted at narrow bands of frequencies with minimal effects on surrounding frequencies (Sen, 2023).
- Even though successful, notch filtering was far from being a panacea to all sources of noise. It was most useful when eradicating narrow-band interference but less effective against artifacts from muscle movements or other board-spectrum noises. In addition, when applied improperly, the filter degraded the frequencies nearby slightly. Tus, the quality of the data was reduced by it.
- Even though notch filtering had limitations, it was still one reliable means of excluding types of noise associated with EEG recording. Since it was sensitive in detecting small frequency bands to be excluded, that created the commodity for this type of filtering in its pursuit for clear data, specifically in controlled environments where considerations were in regard to power line noise. Aside from utility for noise removal, notch filtering also generally made pipelines stronger. Power line interference being consistently removed systematically meant the downstream analysis could be made almost undistorted in those signals and made the dependability of our result to a good extent stronger.
- Adaptive notch filters have also been investigated in modern installations to adjust in real-time to varying noise frequencies, especially in electrically noisy environments that are subject to fluctuation. The adaptive technique allows for better data quality without an ongoing need to retrain the notch filters.

3. Independent Component Analysis (ICA) for Artifact Removal

- To achieve the separation of mixed EEG signals, Independent Component Analysis (ICA) was carried out so that neural activities could be distinguished from other artifacts such as eyeball movements or muscle twitching. Statistical analysis indeed filtered off some artifacts; hence it significantly helped in improving the clarity of EEG signals (Ansari, 2023).
- For instance, ICA effectively removed the artifacts of eye blinks from the signal such that only neural activity was analyzed. This was especially crucial because, for studies that needed multiple eye movements, traditional filtering often could not distinguish between brain activity and ocular artifact. Although ICA has proven to be very effective the downside is that when they do overlap useful neural signal may be removed with an artifact. Overlap is somewhat of a problem in guaranteeing the fidelity of the data.

- The ANC method was indeed more reliable because it canceled noise without depressing neural signals (Ansari, 2023) . The combined approach thus provided a well-rounded solution to artifact removal for better accuracy and reliability in processed EEG. With all this flexibility, it's possible to tailor the preprocessing pipeline to every experiment's need. For instance, while doing motor imagery, ICA worked best while catching signals from the motor cortex and eliminating noise signals, such as ones that were irrelevant to the former. Such adaptability will ensure that preprocessing steps are in tune with all purposes of every study with maximum usage of EEG data. This has actually enabled us to overcome most issues with the raw EEG data as the preprocessing techniques combined proved. It gave a firm foundation for meaningful and accurate analysis in the sense that we were systematically getting rid of the noise and artifacts.
- The results of the studies have already demonstrated that the integration of ICA with machine learning algorithms for automatically detecting and removing artifacts produces better results by reducing the need for manual intervention and providing a standardized preprocessing scheme across large-scale studies. Such integration greatly enhances the efficiency of preprocessing pipelines and gives them necessary scalability for collaborations in multi-site research.

In the code, the function preprocess_inputs(df) prepares the input data for machine learning. It starts by creating a copy of the input data frame df to avoid changing the original data. The 'label' column is then mapped to new values using a predefined label_mapping. The labels (y) are then separated from the features (x) by extracting the 'label' column and saving the remaining columns as features. The data set is then split into a training and a test data set using train_test_split (70% for training and 30% for testing), using train_test_split with a fixed random value is used for reproducibility. Finally, the function returns the training and testing sets for both the features and the labels.

5. FEATURE VISUALIZATION

- **Plotting EEG Features**:

The extraction and visualization of EEG features, particularly in the frequency domain, play a crucial role in deciphering the intricate relationship between emotional states and brain activity. In our study, we meticulously plotted the frequency domain features ranging from fft_0_b to fft_749_b. Each plot was designed to distinctly display the amplitude of frequency components, systematically arranged with frequency bins labeled on the x-axis (from fft_0_b to fft_749_b) and their corresponding amplitudes noted on the y-axis. This structured and methodical representation of data not only facilitated the clear identification of unique frequency patterns but also linked these patterns to various emotional states as depicted in the EEG data. The ability to visually trace and differentiate these patterns is instrumental in understanding how specific frequencies correlate with emotional responses.

The importance of such visual plots is further emphasized by existing literature and studies, which highlight that particular frequency bands are intricately linked with distinct psychological states. For example, as noted by Wolfgang and others, the alpha frequency band, typically ranging from 8 to 12 Hz, is often associated with states of relaxation and calmness, possibly indicating a 'NEUTRAL' emotional state in our study. Conversely, the beta band, which ranges approximately from 12 to 30 Hz, is frequently linked to heightened states of alertness, active thinking, and attentiveness, characteristics that might correlate with 'POS-

ITIVE' emotional states. By visually mapping these frequencies, our research was able to delve deeper into a nuanced exploration of how specific emotional states categorized as 'POSITIVE', 'NEGATIVE', or 'NEUTRAL' are reflected in or influence the brain's electrical activity. These insights are pivotal in enhancing our understanding of the neurological underpinnings of emotions.

Matplotlib, the library used for these visualizations, is a widely used plotting library in the Python programming ecosystem. Renowned for its extensive functionality, Matplotlib provides a broad range of versatile and robust plotting capabilities, establishing it as an indispensable tool for data visualization in scientific computing. As noted by Barrett et al. (2005), Matplotlib not only facilitates the creation of high-quality plots but does so efficiently, utilizing minimal lines of code. This feature is particularly advantageous during exploratory data analysis, where rapid and clear visual insights are essential. The ability to generate intuitive and informative visualizations quickly allows researchers to make informed decisions and interpretations with visual representation of complex data sets, such as those involved in EEG analysis.

Figure 2. Visualization of FFT Features (fft_0_b to fft_749_b) for a Selected Sample

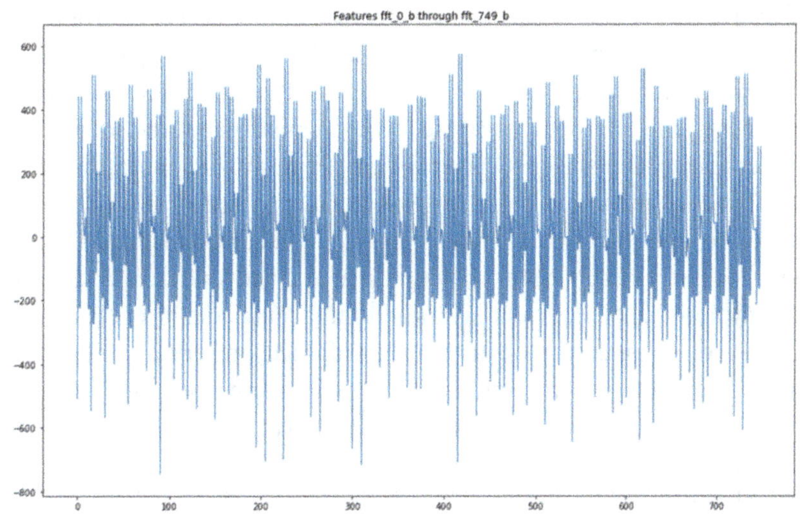

The plot in **Figure 2** visualizes 750 FFT (Fast Fourier Transform) features extracted from the dataset, covering the range from **fft_0_b** to **fft_749_b**. The x-axis represents the indices of these features, while the y-axis shows their corresponding values. The values oscillate significantly, ranging approximately between -800 and 600, indicating a waveform-like pattern. This plot helps analyze the distribution and variation of FFT-transformed features, providing insights into the frequency-domain characteristics of the data for the selected sample.

6. MODEL ARCHITECTURE

The architecture of the model consists on several layers with the objective of handling effectively the sequential and complex nature of EEG data. The initial layer was responsible for inputting EEG features, followed by a GRU layer to process the temporal sequences. This was succeeded by a flattening process and concluded with a dense output layer equipped with a softmax function for classification into three emotional states: Negative, Neutral, and Positive.

The input layer functioned as the initial stage where preprocessed EEG features were introduced. These features, encapsulating the brain's electrical dynamics related to emotional states, were derived from the data preprocessing steps detailed earlier. Through these techniques, the data was rendered suitable for neural network model input, ensuring an optimized foundation for emotion recognition analysis.

Following the input layer, a GRU (Gated Recurrent Unit) layer with two hundred fifty-six units processes the sequential data. GRUs are a variant of recurrent neural networks (RNN) optimized to handle sequences by maintaining information over time and addressing the vanishing gradient problem that plagues traditional RNNs. This problem, where gradients either vanish or explode, making it difficult to learn long-range dependencies within data sequences, is effectively mitigated by the unique architecture of GRUs as they utilize update and reset gates that regulate the flow of information, allowing them to retain or forget data selectively, thus enhancing their ability to model temporal sequences with better precision (Zargar, 2021) This capability makes GRUs particularly well-suited for EEG data, which inherently contains dynamic and temporal information critical for distinguishing between different emotional states.

The flattened layer comes after the GRU layer, where it converts the multi-dimensional output from the GRU into a one-dimensional array. This transformation is essential as it prepares the data to meet the input specifications of the subsequent dense layer, which requires a flat vector for processing. The process of flattening is a standard and critical practice in neural network architectures, particularly when bridging between convolutional or recurrent layers and fully connected layers (Calin, 2020) . It ensures that the spatial hierarchy of the input data is effectively condensed, preserving essential information while transforming it into a format that is more suitable for classification tasks. It is important to understand that this layer maintains the integrity of the data's underlying patterns, which are crucial for the accurate classification of emotional states based on EEG signals.

Finally, the output layer of the model consists of a dense layer with a softmax activation function. This layer is designed to classify the input EEG features into one of three emotional states: Negative, Neutral, and Positive. The softmax function is particularly useful in multi-class classification tasks as it outputs the probabilities of each class, providing a clear indication of the model's decision-making process. Duan et al. (2003) highlights the efficacy of softmax in neural networks for classifying inputs into mutually exclusive classes, which is essential for the clarity and accuracy in the prediction of emotional states.

In the final stage of our model, the output layer employs a dense layer with three layers and a softmax activation function, chosen for its proficiency in classifying the processed EEG features into one of three predefined emotional states: Negative, Neutral, and Positive. The softmax function is particularly well-suited for our case, as it computes the probabilities of each class possibility based on the input processed by the preceding layers of the neural network (Duan et al., 2003) . This function is adept at handling inputs requiring classification into exclusive categories, making it an optimal choice for our purposes. Hence, the output layer generates a probability distribution across the three emotional states, indicating the likelihood that a specific EEG reading aligns with each state.

The model, named **"functional_1"**, is a neural network designed for a classification task with 3 output classes. It starts with an input layer that accepts data with 2548 features. The input is then expanded into a 3D shape using the **ExpandDims** layer, transforming the data from **(None, 2548)** to **(None, 2548, 1)**. Following this, a **GRU (Gated Recurrent Unit)** layer processes the sequential data, outputting a sequence of 256-dimensional vectors with a shape of **(None, 2548, 256)**. The output from the GRU layer is flattened into a 1D vector with 652,288 elements by the **Flatten** layer. Finally, a **Dense** layer produces 3 output units, likely for classification. The model has a total of 2,155,779 parameters, all of which are trainable, meaning all the weights and biases are updated during training. No non-trainable parameters are present in the model. **Table 2** shows the summary of the model architecture, including the layers, their output shapes, and the corresponding number of parameters for each layer.

Table 2. Model Architecture Summary

Layer (type)	**Output Shape**	**Param #**
input_1 (InputLayer)	(None, 2548)	0
tf_op_layer_ExpandDims	(None, 2548, 1)	0
gru (GRU)	(None, 2548, 256)	198,912
flatten (Flatten)	(None, 652288)	0
dense (Dense)	(None, 3)	1,956,867
Total params		**2,155,779**
Trainable params		**2,155,779**
Non-trainable params		0

7. MODEL COMPILATION

Model compilation for this research involved designing a compilation process for efficient training and strong performance for the multi-class classification task. In this regard, the selection of the optimizer, loss function, and evaluation metric played crucial roles towards effective model convergence and reduced resource usage to achieve high accuracy with optimal model performance. Every component was handpicked to fit the challenge presented by the task at hand.

- **Optimizer**: In this experiment, the Adam optimizer was selected, with the capability to adapt the learning rate, and performed efficiently and stably during the training process. Specifically, Adam is a new optimizer that combines AdaGrad and RMSProp, which are two of the most popular adaptation-based optimization algorithms. It adapts the learning rate through the properties of the gradient. This makes each update more efficient for any parameter (Kingma & Ba, 2015). This adaptive shift of learning rates ensures that the optimizer functions sensibly with noisy gradients and differential magnitudes of updates, a feature that is extremely useful in deep learning tasks involving large datasets and intricate models.

One of the greatest merits of Adam is its individual learning rate adaptation to each parameter, which speeds up the training very significantly. This, in turn, makes the optimizer less likely to experience slow convergence and overshooting, which are significant drawbacks found when applying a standard optimization algorithm, like SGD. Indeed, experiments have been conducted, and it has been witnessed that Adam frequently is better than the classic SGD, especially when applied to deep learning tasks in a series of CNN applications (Barakat, 2021) (Cong, 2018) . In this experiment, Adam gave better performance both in terms of computational efficiency and decrease in memory usage. It also reduced overfitting requiring many hyperparameter settings that are usually needed by other optimizers such as SGD.

The impact of weight decay Adam was investigated as a measure to minimize overfitting and guarantee strong generalization performance. This technique is in line with the contemporary research which found that weight decay can enhance Adam's stability in complex neural networks, particularly in Multinomial classification tasks.

- **Loss Function**: To tackle the multi-class classification efficiently, a sparse categorical cross-entropy loss function was selected. It is diffezrent from other loss functions since it directly accepts integer-encoded labels, without needing any one-hot encoding, which simplifies the training process and consequently reduces computational overhead. This was a critical property within the context of this work since simplifying the pipeline of data preprocessing was imperative for reducing computational overhead and speeding up the training process.

Sparse categorical cross entropy applies the logarithm of the likelihood of the correct class for each input and penalizes the wrong predictions. That reduces the noise in the model by assigning greater probabilities to the correct class, thus improving its performance in classification. Apart from that, sparse categorical cross entropy is also known to be good when classes have imbalances. Of course, that was a concern in this study because the categories are unevenly distributed. From previous studies, sparse categorical cross entropy can improve the model's accuracy and time to convergence, most significantly for large, imbalanced datasets (Ghosh, 2023) .

In addition to the above, techniques that help reducing overfitting were also used by modifying the loss function. Here, dropout layers are known to be an important part in helping the model get trained on strong features without getting too much biased towards the training data. This additional strategy further led to enhancement of learning models capability of generalization to novel scenarios.

- **Metrics**: The primary evaluation metric used in this research was accuracy, which is commonly employed in classification tasks. Accuracy provides a straightforward and understandable evaluation of model performance by calculating the percentage of accurate predictions compared to all forecasts. By tracking accuracy throughout the training process, the model's progress could be easily monitored, and any potential issues, such as underfitting or overfitting, could be quickly identified.

An accuracy of 94.375% clearly demonstrates the model's strong performance, allowing for direct comparisons between different models. Accuracy was monitored during each epoch, which indicates the model's learning progress. This approach allows for timely adjustments, if necessary, to ensure the model stays on track towards achieving optimal performance.

Even though accuracy was sufficiently indicative of the general performance of the model, it is important to indicate that precision, recall, and F1-score metrics could have been considered as further appropriate in the determination of a more perfect validation, especially for imbalanced datasets (Mohan, 2024), (Agarwal, 2024). These metrics would yield much more detailed analysis about the ability of the model to correctly classify positive and negative instances, making its sense of performance more nuanced.

Finally, we applied early stopping criteria during training to halt the process once validation performance plateaued, thereby preventing unnecessary overfitting and allowing for efficient use of computational resources. This adaptability in the approach allowed the model to achieve optimal performance without undue stress on the training process, thus demonstrating an effective compilation strategy well-suited to the particular task at hand.

8. MODEL TRAINING & TESTING

Model training:

During the model training phase, we adopted an structured approach to optimize the machine learning model for recognizing emotions from EEG data. The initial step involved feeding a substantial volume of labeled EEG data into the model, which facilitated the model's learning process by allowing it to identify and associate specific patterns and features in the data with corresponding emotional states. To further refine the model's accuracy, we engaged in a rigorous process of hyperparameter tuning. This important step involved adjusting parameters such as learning rate, batch size, and number of layers, among others, to minimize the discrepancy between the predicted outcomes and the actual labels, thereby significantly boosting the model's predictive performance as noted by Uçar et al., 2020.

Fine-tuning hyperparameters is crucial for enhancing the efficacy of a machine learning model. The learning rate is a pivotal parameter that regulates the extent to which the model updates its weights based on the observed error. Lower learning rates might result in slower convergence, while higher rates could overshoot optimal solutions. The batch size has a major impact on model training as it is the number of training samples used to compute the gradient in each iteration. Smaller batch sizes might update the model more frequently but can introduce noise into the updates, whereas larger batch sizes offer more stable gradient estimates but consume more computational power. Additionally, the model's ability to learn complex patterns is significantly affected by the number of layers within a neural network. Increasing the number of layers allows the model to learn more detailed features, but it also raises the risk of overfitting and complicates the training process. Furthermore, number of layers within a neural network affects substantially the capacity of a model to learn complex patterns. Adding more layers to the model has the advantage of allowing it to capture more intricate features; however, it also introduces the downside of increasing the risk of overfitting and making the training process more complex. Properly managing these hyperparameters is essential for boosting the model's precision and ability to generalize across different datasets.

A pivotal technique employed during this phase was the implementation of Early Stopping. As noted by Dietterich in 1995, overfitting is a common challenge in model training, where the model becomes excessively tailored to the training data, compromising its performance on new, unseen data. To counteract this, we meticulously monitored the validation loss throughout the training process. Should the validation loss fail to improve for a continuous span of five epochs, the training process was promptly halted. This approach is vital as it indicates that the model is no longer extracting beneficial, generalizable insights from the training data, thereby averting the risk of overfitting. By instituting early stopping and reverting to the best set of weights at the point where the validation loss was at its minimum, we effectively safeguarded the model's ability to generalize effectively to new datasets, a strategy underscored by Prechelt in 2002.

Furthermore, the model's training was strategically set to run for a predefined total of 50 epochs, with the data inputted in batches of 32. This batch size was selected not only to optimize memory usage during the training process but also to foster a more stable and effective convergence of the model's weights. By averaging the gradients over multiple samples before proceeding with a weight update, we were able to enhance the stability and reliability of the learning process, thereby improving the overall robustness of the model. This structured and strategic approach to model training ensured that the machine learning model developed was both efficient and powerful in recognizing emotional states from EEG data, setting a strong foundation for accurate and reliable predictions.

Testing:

Finally, predictions were made on the test set using the fully trained model. These predictions involved the model outputting the emotional state it inferred from the EEG data, which were then compared against the actual labels to assess accuracy. This step was an essential phase in the development of machine learning models where we can evaluate the model's ability to generalize beyond the data on which it was trained. This testing phase offers an unbiased assessment of the model's effectiveness by measuring its performance on a separate dataset that was not used during the training phase determining the model's robustness and accuracy in predicting new, unseen data (Uçar et al., 2020). This evaluation helps in identifying potential overfitting issues, where a model might perform exceptionally well on training data but poorly on data it hasn't seen before.

In our research, we specifically reserved 30% of the EEG dataset during the data preprocessing stage for the testing phase which served as a final benchmark for evaluating our model's performance. By applying the trained model to this reserved test set, we could directly compare the predicted emotional states against the actual labels, providing a clear measure of the model's accuracy in real-world conditions. This testing procedure not only demonstrated the model's ability to learn and apply complex relationships from the training data to new, unseen examples but also highlighted its potential in practical applications within the field of emotion recognition from EEG signals. The achieved accuracy of 94.375%, reflects the effectiveness of our training process and confirmed the model's capability in accurately classifying emotional states, thereby underscoring the model's overall utility and its potential to contribute significantly to advancements in affective computing and neuroscience research.

9. RESULTS VISUALIZATION

Following the extensive data processing, feature extraction, and modeling phases, the machine learning model demonstrated promising results in emotion prediction from EEG signals. The effectiveness of the model can be clearly observed in the confusion matrix and a detailed classification report containing various metrics.

A confusion matrix is a powerful graphic tool used to examine the performance of classification models. It presents the actual versus predicted classifications in a matrix format, allowing for a straightforward assessment of the accuracy of the model's predictions. The rows of the matrix represent the actual classes, also known as the ground truth, while the columns represent the classes as predicted by the model. This layout facilitates a direct comparison between what the model predicted and what was actually true (Naidu et al., 2023).

Each cell in the matrix shows the count of predictions made by the model for a given actual-predicted pair, providing clear insight into how many predictions were correct (diagonal cells where predicted classes match the actual classes) and how many were errors (off-diagonal cells where there is a mismatch between predicted and actual classes) (Naidu et al., 2023) . This setup is particularly useful in identifying not just the overall accuracy but also specific areas where the model might be confusing one class for another. For instance, a high number of off-diagonal entries in rows and columns corresponding to two different emotions would suggest that the model frequently misclassifies between these emotions (Beauxis-Aussalet & Hardman, 2014).

The classification report generated in this study includes several key components: precision, recall, and F1-score for each emotional state classified (happiness, sadness, and neutral). Each metric gives a different perspective on the performance of the model and is crucial for a comprehensive evaluation.

P Precision measures a classification model's ability to make accurate positive predictions. It is defined as the ratio of true positive predictions (properly predicted positive cases) to total predicted positives (true positives + false positives). This metric is particularly insightful as it helps in understanding the proportion of correct predictions among those classified as a specific emotion, providing a clear indication of the model's reliability in predicting positive instances correctly. Precision is essential in scenarios where the costs of false positives are high, ensuring that the model's positive predictions are trustworthy (Naidu et al., 2023; Rainio et al., 2024) (Lab, n.d.)

Recall, also known as sensitivity, is a measure that assesses the model's capability to correctly identify all relevant instances of a particular class. It is calculated by dividing the number of true positive predictions by the actual positives (sum of true positives and false negatives). This ratio indicates how well the model can detect all samples of a specific emotion, emphasizing the model's effectiveness in capturing all positive cases without missing any. High recall is essential in situations where missing a positive instance (false negative) could have severe implications, ensuring comprehensive coverage of positive cases (Naidu et al., 2023; Rainio et al., 2024) .

The F1-score is a strong measure that balances precision and recall by calculating their harmonic mean. This metric is particularly useful as it maintains a balance between the model's precision and recall, ensuring that neither metric is disproportionately favored. The F1 score is a valuable indicator of the model's overall accuracy, especially in scenarios where both false positives and false negatives carry significant consequences. By harmonizing precision and recall, the F1 score offers a single metric that encapsulates the model's performance in terms of both reliability and completeness (Naidu et al., 2023; Rainio et al., 2024)

The confusion matrix presented in **Figure 3** provides insights into the performance of the emotion classification model, which achieved an overall accuracy of 94.37%. The matrix reveals that the NEUTRAL class achieved the highest accuracy, with 228 out of 231 samples correctly classified and only 3 misclassified as POSITIVE. For the NEGATIVE class, 187 out of 201 samples were correctly classified, with 14 misclassified as POSITIVE. Similarly, the POSITIVE class had 189 correct predictions out of 208 samples, with 17 misclassified as NEGATIVE and 2 as NEUTRAL.

Figure 3. Confusion Matrix Visualizing Model Performance Across Three Classes (NEGATIVE, NEUTRAL, POSITIVE)

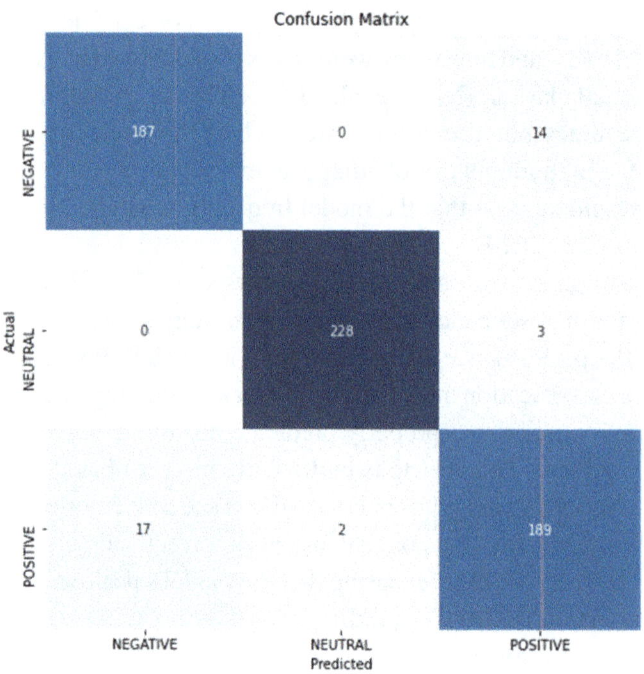

These results underscore the model's effectiveness, particularly in distinguishing NEUTRAL emotions with minimal error. However, moderate misclassifications between the NEGATIVE and POSITIVE classes suggest areas for further refinement. Overall, the model demonstrates reliable performance, highlighting its potential utility in emotion classification tasks within affective computing and neuroscience applications.

Table 3. shows the classification performance of the model, including precision, recall, F1-score, and support for each class (Negative, Neutral, Positive). Additionally, it provides the overall accuracy along with the macro and weighted averages of the performance metrics across all classes.

Table 3. Classification Report of the Model

Class	**Precision**	**Recall**	**F1-Score**	**Support**
NEGATIVE	0.92	0.93	0.92	201
NEUTRAL	0.99	0.99	0.99	231
POSITIVE	0.92	0.91	0.91	208
Accuracy			0.94	640
Macro Avg	0.94	0.94	0.94	640
Weighted Avg	0.94	0.94	0.94	640

10. LIMITATIONS OF EMOTION PREDICTION USING EEG

Emotion prediction using EEG faces several challenges that illustrate the complexity of this field. EEG signals are highly individual and are influenced by factors such as age, gender and mental state, which makes it difficult to generalize results for different populations. In addition, EEG recordings are prone to noise and artifacts due to muscle movement and external electrical interference, which can affect data quality. The small sample sizes often used in studies further limit the ability to capture variability in emotional responses. While EEG offers high temporal resolution, its low spatial resolution limits the ability to pinpoint specific brain regions associated with emotions. Furthermore, emotions are complex and multidimensional and are influenced by cultural, environmental and contextual factors, making accurate categorization a major challenge. Many studies are conducted in controlled laboratory settings that may not reflect the real-world conditions where emotions are dynamic.

11. ETHICAL CONSIDERATIONS

The use of EEG to predict emotions raises important ethical issues that need to be carefully considered to ensure responsible development and application of this technology. One important issue is the protection of privacy, as EEG data contains sensitive information about a person's mental and emotional state. Unauthorized access or misuse of such data could lead to a violation of an individual's privacy. To protect users' neural data, secure data storage and robust encryption methods are essential.

Another concern is the potential misuse of emotion prediction technologies, e.g. in surveillance, marketing or manipulative practices that exploit people's emotional vulnerability. To stop unethical applications, clear rules and restrictions are required. Additionally, people must be fully informed about the collection, processing, and use of their EEG data in order to give their informed consent.

The accuracy and reliability of emotion prediction models must also be taken into account. Inaccurate predictions could lead to unintended consequences, especially in critical applications like mental health diagnostics. Developers need to make sure the technology minimizes biases and has scientific validation. To guarantee that the technology is used responsibly and serves society as a whole, ethical issues should continue to be the primary focus.

12. FUTURE RESEARCH DIRECTIONS

The field of emotion prediction using EEG offers numerous opportunities for future exploration to address existing limitations and expand its applications. Developing robust methods to handle variability in EEG signals across diverse populations is essential for creating generalized and inclusive models. Improving artifact removal techniques and employing advanced signal processing methods can enhance the quality and reliability of EEG data. Increasing sample sizes and incorporating data from diverse demographic groups would provide more comprehensive insights into emotional responses.

Future studies should focus on combining EEG data with other modalities, such as facial expressions, voice analysis, or physiological signals, to develop multimodal systems that improve the accuracy and robustness of emotion prediction. Real-world validation of models in dynamic, non-laboratory settings is also critical to ensure practical applicability.

13. CONCLUSION

The research conducted in this study fully investigates EEG-based emotion prediction and successfully proves the efficiency of the developed model in decoding neural activity. The findings of our research also reflect the supremacy of GRU models that achieved an accuracy of **94.375%,** with the effective capture of the temporal patterns within EEG signals. The findings also emphasize the importance of frequency-specific features, particularly from the delta, theta, and alpha bands, for differentiating emotional states. So, the performance of the model was successful because of the robust preprocessing techniques such as band-pass filtering, Independent Component Analysis, and feature extraction such as Fast Fourier Transform.

The real-world applicability of the model was further validated through a case study. It was demonstrated to have good predictability of emotional states with high reliability in various scenarios. It was established that well-optimized pipelines for machine learning led to better efficiency as well as accuracy. It was also a very important phenomenon of showing possible application in all healthcare, educational, and entertainment sectors where emotion recognition is gaining more importance these days.

Presently, several promising areas of future research are discussed here. Some possible directions toward further steps to capture spatial and temporal features of EEG dynamics include integration with such complex models as transformers. Real-time integration of EEG data along with multimodal approaches, such as incorporating it with facial expression analysis or physiological sensors, might significantly enhance both model performance and applicability. Ethics, for example, data privacy and inclusivity, and more datasets to be able to generalize across various populations, were also very significant mentions in the development of this field.

In successfully demonstrating the utility of our model by finishing up this research, it thus contributes toward the growing field of emotion recognition based on EEG signals and opens avenues for making smarter and more responsive systems. The understanding thus generated provides a very strong platform for further study and innovations in decoding human emotions through their neural activity.

REFERENCES

Agarwal, M. G. (2024). Analysing Digits with Sequential Convolutional Neural Networks and Adam Optimizer. *In2024 IEEE International Conference on Information Technology, Electronics and Intelligent Communication Systems (ICITEICS)*, 1-4. DOI: 10.1109/ICITEICS61368.2024.10625453

Ansari, N. K. (2023). Automatic removal of ocular and cardiac artifacts and retention of embedded EEG information via adaptive noise cancellation. *In2023 International Conference on Recent Advances in Electrical, Electronics & Digital Healthcare Technologies (REEDCON)* (pp. 133-138). IEEE. DOI: 10.1109/REEDCON57544.2023.10151101

Barakat, A., & Bianchi, P. (2021). Convergence and Dynamical Behavior of the ADAM Algorithm for Nonconvex Stochastic Optimization. *SIAM Journal on Optimization*, *31*(1), 244–274. DOI: 10.1137/19M1263443

Barrett, P., Hunter, J., Miller, J. T., Hsu, J., & Greenfield, P. (2005). matplotlib--A Portable Python Plotting Package. Paper presented at the Astronomical Data Analysis Software and Systems XIV, 347 91.

Beauxis-Aussalet, E., & Hardman, L. (2014). Visualization of confusion matrix for non-expert users. Paper presented at the IEEE Conference on Visual Analytics Science and Technology (VAST)-Poster Proceedings, 1–2.

Berger, H. (1929). Über das elektroenkephalogramm des menschen. *Archiv für psychiatrie und nervenkrankheite*, 527-570.

Brownlee, J. (2020). *Data preparation for machine learning: data cleaning, feature selection, and data transforms in Python. Machine Learning Mastery. Calin, O. (2020). Deep learning architectures*. Springer.

Chanel, G. K., Kierkels, J. J. M., Soleymani, M., & Pun, T. (2009). Short-term emotion assessment in a recall paradigm. *International Journal of Human-Computer Studies*, *67*(8), 607–627. DOI: 10.1016/j.ijhcs.2009.03.005

Cong, G. (2018). *On Adam Trained Models and a Parallel Method to Improve the Generalization Performance. In 2018 IEEE/ACM Machine Learning in HPC Environments (MLHPC)*. IEEE.

Dhara, T. S., Singh, P. K., & Mahmud, M. (2024). A Fuzzy Ensemble-Based Deep learning Model for EEG-Based Emotion Recognition. *Cognitive Computation*, *16*(3), 1364–1378. DOI: 10.1007/s12559-023-10171-2

Dietterich, T. (1995). Overfitting and undercomputing in machine learning. *ACM Computing Surveys*, *27*(3), 326–327. DOI: 10.1145/212094.212114

Duan, K., Keerthi, S. S., Chu, W., Shevade, S. K., & Poo, A. N. (2003). Multi-category classification by soft-max combination of binary classifiers. Paper presented at the *Multiple Classifier Systems:4th International Workshop, MCS 2003 Guildford,UK,June 11–13, 2003Proceedings 4,* 125–134. DOI: 10.1007/3-540-44938-8_13

Ghosh, J. &. (2023). ADAM Optimizer and CATEGORICAL Loss Function-Based CNN Method for Diagnosing Colorectal Cancer. In *In2023 International Conference on Computational Intelligence and Sustainable Engineering Solutions* (pp. 470-474). IEEE. DOI: 10.1109/CISES58720.2023.10183491

Hamzah, H. A., & Abdalla, K. K. (2024). EEG-based emotion recognition systems; Comprehensive study. *Heliyon, 10*(10), e31485. DOI: 10.1016/j.heliyon.2024.e31485 PMID: 38818173

Jenke, R. P., Peer, A., & Buss, M. (2014). Feature extraction and selection for emotion recognition from EEG. *IEEE Transactions on Affective Computing, 5*(3), 327–339. DOI: 10.1109/TAFFC.2014.2339834

Kaur, G. A. (2024). An Insightful Analysis of Preprocessing Methods Used in EEG Signals for Computer-Assisted Cognitive Domain. In *Congress on Intelligent System* (pp. 53–65). Springer. DOI: 10.1007/978-981-99-9043-6_5

Klimesch, W. (1999). EEG alpha and theta oscillations reflect cognitive and memory performance: A review and analysis. *Brain Research. Brain Research Reviews, 29*(2-3), 169–195. DOI: 10.1016/S0165-0173(98)00056-3 PMID: 10209231

Koelstra, S., & Patras, I. (2013). Fusion of facial expressions and EEG for implicit affective tagging. *Image and Vision Computing, 31*(2), 164–174.

Lab, M. M. (n.d.). *Affective Computing*. Retrieved 12 1, 2024, from https://www.media.mit.edu/research/groups/affective-computing

Lee, Y. Y., & Hsieh, S. (2014). Classifying different emotional states by means of EEG-based functional connectivity patterns. *PLoS One, 9*(4), e95415. DOI: 10.1371/journal.pone.0095415 PMID: 24743695

Mohan, A. a. (2024). Classification of Sign Language Gestures using CNN with Adam Optimizer. *024 2nd International Conference on Disruptive Technologies (ICDT)*, 430--433.

Muraina, I. (2022). Ideal dataset splitting ratios in machine learning algorithms: general concerns for data scientists and data analysts. Paper presented at the *7th International Mardin Artuklu Scientific Research Conference,* 496–504.

Muraina, I. (2022). Ideal dataset splitting ratios in machine learning algorithms: general concerns for data scientists and data analysts. Paper presented at the 7th International Mardin Artuklu Scientific Research Conference, 496–504.

Murugappan, M., & Murugappan, S. (2013). Human emotion recognition through short time Electro-encephalogram (EEG) signals using Fast Fourier Transform (FFT). Paper presented at the *2013 IEEE 9th International Colloquium on Signal Processing and its Applications,* 289–294. https://doi.org/DOI: 10.1109/CSPA.2013.6530058

Naidu, G., Zuva, T., & Sibanda, E. M. (2023). A rview of evaluation metrics in machine learning algorithms. Paper presented at the *Computer Science on-Line Conference,* 15–25.

Picard, R. W. (2000). *Affective computing*. MIT press. DOI: 10.7551/mitpress/1140.003.0008

Prabowo, D. W., Nugroho, H. A., Setiawan, N. A., & Debayle, J. (2023). A systematic literature review of emotion recognition using EEG signals. *Cognitive Systems Research, 82*, 101152. DOI: 10.1016/j.cogsys.2023.101152

Prechelt, L. (2002). *Early stopping-but when? Neural Networks: Tricks of the trade*. Springer.

Rahman, M. M., Sarkar, A. K., Hossain, M. A., & Moni, M. A. (2022). EEG-based emotion analysis using non-linear features and ensemble learning approache. *Expert Systems with Applications, 207*, 207. DOI: 10.1016/j.eswa.2022.118025

Rainio, O., Teuho, J., & Klén, R. (2024). Evaluation metrics and statistical tests for machine learning. *Scientific Reports, 14*(1), 6086. DOI: 10.1038/s41598-024-56706-x PMID: 38480847

Ray, W. J., & Cole, H. W. (1985). EEG alpha activity reflects attentional demands, and beta activity reflects emotional and cognitive processes. *Science, 228*(4700), 750–752. DOI: 10.1126/science.3992243 PMID: 3992243

Samal, P., & Hashmi, M. F. (2024). Role of machine learning and deep learning techniques in EEG-based BCI emotion recognition system: A review. *Artificial Intelligence Review, 57*(3), 50. DOI: 10.1007/s10462-023-10690-2

Sen, D. M. (2023). A Review of the Filtering Techniques used in EEG Signal Processing. *In 2023 7th International Conference on Trends in Electronics and Informatics (ICOEI)* (pp. 270-277). IEEE.

Soleymani, M. A.-E. (2014). Continuous emotion detection using EEG signals and facial expressions. *IEEE international conference on multimedia and expo (ICME)*, 1-6.

Tuba, E., Bačanin, N., Strumberger, I., & Tuba, M. (2021). Convolutional neural networks hyperparameters tuning. In *Artificial intelligence: theory and applications* (pp. 65–84). Springer International Publishing. DOI: 10.1007/978-3-030-72711-6_4

Uçar, M. K., Nour, M., Sindi, H., & Polat, K. (2020). The effect of training and testing process on machine learning in biomedical datasets. *Mathematical Problems in Engineering, 2020*(1), 2836236.

Wirawan, I. M. (2022). The challenges of emotion recognition methods based on electroencephalogram signals: A literature review. *International Journal of Electrical and Computer Engineering, 12*(2), 1508–1519. DOI: 10.11591/ijece.v12i2.pp1508-1519

Zargar, S. (2021). *Introduction to sequence learning models: RNN, LSTM, GRU*. Department of Mechanical and Aerospace Engineering, North Carolina State University.

Zhang, H. W. (2024). A Coupling of Common-Private Topological Patterns Learning Strategy to Eliminate Individual Differences for Eeg Emotion Recognition. *SSRN*. DOI: 10.2139/ssrn.4714931

Zhang, Y., Wang, S., & Xu, S. (2018). SEED: A Large-Scale EEG Dataset for Emotion Recognition. Brain-Computer Music Interface, Shanghai Jiao Tong University. Retrieved from https://bcmi.sjtu.edu.cn/home/seed/

Zhang, Z., Fort, J. M., & Giménez Mateu, L. (2024). Mini review: Challenges in EEG emotion recognition. *Frontiers in Psychology*, 14. 1289816.

Chapter 15
Enhancing Clinical Diagnostics and Patient Monitoring With Recurrent Neural Networks:
A Comparative Study of LSTM and GRU Architectures

S. Dhivya
PSG College of Arts and Science, India

R. Saranya
https://orcid.org/0009-0000-9354-9243
PSG College of Arts and Science, India

ABSTRACT

Recurrent Neural Networks (RNNs), particularly Long Short-Term Memory (LSTM) and Gated Recurrent Unit (GRU) architectures, are powerful tools for modeling clinical time-series data where sequential information is essential. This paper explores the effectiveness of RNNs in analyzing patient vital signs, electrocardiogram (ECG) readings, and other time-sensitive health data. The recurrent design of these networks enables the capture of short- and long-term dependencies, vital for predicting patient outcomes, anomaly detection, and aiding in diagnostic decisions. We review recent advancements in RNN applications for healthcare, addressing challenges like irregular sampling, missing data, and the need for interpretability in clinical settings. Through experiments with real-world clinical datasets, we demonstrate that RNNs outperform traditional machine learning models, enhancing diagnostics, patient monitoring, and personalized treatment planning. Our results highlight the significant potential of RNNs in advancing healthcare analytics and supporting data-driven decision-making.

DOI: 10.4018/979-8-3693-9816-6.ch015

1. INTRODUCTION

1.1 Overview of Medical Time-Series Data

Definition and Significance in Healthcare

The term "medical time-series data" describes a set of data points that are usually captured sequentially across time. These data points are essential to the healthcare industry because they help clinicians make well-informed judgments and offer insights into a patient's health status (Bashar et al.,2020). It is impossible to overestimate the importance of time-series data in healthcare; it forms the basis for certain medical disorders' monitoring, diagnosis, and treatment. Healthcare practitioners can better forecast patient outcomes and take prompt action because of the temporal structure of this data, which enables them to see changes over time.

As an instance, non-stop monitoring of critical symptoms—such as heart rate, blood strain, and breathing price—can sign essential modifications in a patient's fitness. Detecting traits or abrupt adjustments in these parameters can alert clinical workforce to potential health crises, taking into account rapid action. similarly, time-collection facts from electrocardiograms (ECGs) presents critical records about the electric hobby of the heart, which can be pivotal in diagnosing arrhythmias or other cardiovascular issues (kachuee, Fazeli, & Roshani, 2018).

Types of Medical Time-Series Data

There are various types of medical time-series data, each with unique characteristics and applications. Some common types include:

- **Vital Signs**: These are fundamental indicators of a patient's physiological status, including heart rate, blood pressure, temperature, and respiratory rate. Continuous tracking of these metrics is essential in critical care settings.
- **Electrocardiogram (ECG) Readings**: ECGs measure the electrical activity of the heart over time. This data can reveal abnormalities in heart rhythm and structure, making it vital for diagnosing cardiac conditions.
- **Glucose Monitoring**: For diabetic patients, continuous glucose monitoring systems provide real-time data on blood sugar levels. Analyzing this time-series data can help in adjusting insulin doses and preventing complications.
- **Clinical Event Logs**: Records of clinical events, treatments, or medications administered over time. This data helps in understanding treatment effects and patient responses.
- **Wearable Device Data**: Increasingly, data from wearables like fitness trackers and smartwatches is being integrated into healthcare. These devices can monitor various health metrics over time, providing valuable insights into lifestyle and health trends.

The ability to analyze such diverse types of time-series data is essential for improving patient care and optimizing treatment strategies.

1.2 The Role of Machine Learning in Medicine

Evolution and Impact of Machine Learning on Healthcare

Machine learning (ML) has revolutionized the healthcare panorama over the last few many years. to start with, conventional statistical methods ruled the field of medical information analysis. however, the advent of system studying brought new opportunities for extracting insights from sizable amounts of information that had been previously unmanageable (Cauruana & Nickerson, 2020). With the upward thrust of digital health records (EHRs), imaging technology, and other digital data assets, the quantity and complexity of medical records have surged, necessitating superior analytical strategies (Lipton et al., 2016).

The effect of system mastering in medicinal drug is profound. From improving diagnostic accuracy to personalizing treatment plans, gadget studying algorithms have proven promise in various programs, inclusive of:

- **Predictive Analytics:** ML models can analyze historical patient statistics to are expecting future health results, enabling proactive healthcare control. for example, predicting the likelihood of hospital readmissions can help in making plans publish-discharge care greater efficaciously.
- **Image evaluation:** device studying strategies, specially deep getting to know, have appreciably advanced the accuracy of scientific image interpretation. Algorithms can come across anomalies in X-rays, MRIs, and CT scans, assisting radiologists in making extra particular diagnoses.
- **Natural Language Processing (NLP):** NLP strategies are being employed to analyze unstructured facts from medical notes, extracting applicable data which could assist selection-making and improve documentation accuracy.
- **Treatment recommendations:** device mastering can be used to broaden decision support systems that recommend surest treatment alternatives primarily based on man or woman affected person records and historic treatment effects.

1.3 Introduction to RNNs

Basic Concepts of RNNs and Their Advantages for Sequential Data

Recurrent Neural Networks (RNNs) are a category of neural networks designed to handle sequential information efficaciously (Hochreiter & Schmidhuber, 1997). Unlike traditional feedforward neural networks, RNNs own a unique structure that lets in them to preserve a form of memory via hidden states. This functionality allows RNNs to seize temporal dependencies inside sequences, making them particularly ideal for programs regarding time-series records.

On the middle of RNNs is the idea of recurrence, wherein the output from a preceding time step is fed again into the network as a part of the enter for the modern-day time step. This creates a feedback loop that permits the network to investigate from beyond information, making it effective in modeling sequences wherein the contemporary-day output relies upon on preceding inputs.

One of the key blessings of RNNs is their potential to deal with variable-duration input sequences. In clinical time-series analysis, the duration of information sequences can range notably from affected person to affected character. RNNs can adapt to those variations, making them a strong desire for studying various clinical datasets.

But, trendy RNNs face disturbing situations, especially in gaining knowledge of lengthy-variety dependencies. This predicament has delivered approximately the improvement of superior architectures like lengthy short-time period reminiscence (LSTM) networks and Gated Recurrent devices (GRUs) (Cho et al., 2014). those architectures include mechanisms to better control memory and forget irrelevant statistics, improving the version's ability to seize every quick-time period and long-term dependencies in facts.

2. RECURRENT NEURAL NETWORK ARCHITECTURES

2.1 Fundamentals of RNNs

Structure and Working Principles of Traditional RNNs

Recurrent Neural Networks (RNNs) are designed to technique sequences of statistics, making them specifically effective for responsibilities wherein the order of the facts factors topics, along with time-collection evaluation, natural language processing, and speech popularity (Choi et al., 2016). The essential structure of an RNN consists of input gadgets, hidden devices, and output devices, prepared in a manner that allows facts to be exceeded from one time step to the subsequent.

On the center of an RNN is the idea of recurrence, which permits the community to keep a nation that may capture information from preceding time steps. The traditional RNN operates as follows:

1. **Input Processing**: At each time step t, an input vector x_t is fed into the network. This input can represent various types of data, such as sensor readings in medical time-series analysis.
2. **Hidden State Update**: The hidden state h_t is updated based on the current input x_t and the previous hidden state h_{t-1}. The update rule is typically defined as:

$$h_t=f(W_h h_{t-1}+W_{x\,xt}+b)$$

Here, W_h and W_x are weight matrices for the hidden and input layers, respectively, b is a bias term, and f is an activation function, often a non-linear function like tanh or ReLU.

3. **Output Generation**: The updated hidden state h_t can then be used to produce an output y_t through another transformation:

$$Y_t = W_y h_t + b_y$$

where W_y is the weight matrix for the output layer, and b_y is the output bias.

The key feature of RNNs is that they keep a hidden country across time steps, letting them capture dependencies in sequential statistics. however, traditional RNNs be afflicted by limitations, specially in coping with lengthy-variety dependencies. as the length of the input sequence increases, the community struggles to retain relevant statistics, frequently main to troubles referred to as the vanishing gradient trouble. This task necessitated the improvement of more superior architectures, together with LSTMs and GRUs.

2.2 Long Short-Term Memory (LSTM) Networks

Key Components: Cell State, Gates (Input, Output, Forget)

Long Short-Term Memory (LSTM) networks were introduced to address the shortcomings of traditional RNNs, particularly the inability to learn long-range dependencies effectively (Hochreiter & Schmidhuber, 1997). LSTMs incorporate a more complex architecture that includes memory cells and gating mechanisms, allowing them to retain and discard information selectively (Zhou et al., 2016).

1. **Cell State**: The cell state C_t acts as a reminiscence aspect that consists of records thru the collection. It could be up to date and changed at each time step, helping the network do not forget essential information over long intervals.
2. **Gates**: LSTMs utilize three types of gates to control the flow of information:
   - **Forget Gate**: The forget gate f_t determines what information from the cell state should be discarded. It takes the previous hidden state h_{t-1} and the current input x_t and outputs a value between 0 and 1 for each element in the cell state:

$f_t=\sigma(W_f[h_{t-1,xt}]+b_f)$

   - **Input Gate**: The input gate i_t decides what new information should be added to the cell state. It also outputs values between 0 and 1.

$i_t=\sigma(W_i[h_{t-1,xt}]+b_i)$

   - **Output Gate**: The output gate o_t determines what information from the cell state should be output to the hidden state.

$O_t=\sigma(W_0[h_{t-1,xt}]+b_o)$

3. **Cell State Update**: The cell state is updated as follows:

$C_t=f_t\odot C_{t-1}+i_t\odot$ C~t

4. **Hidden State Output**: Finally, the hidden state is computed:

$h_t=o_t\odot \tanh(C_t)$

Advantages in Capturing Long-Range Dependencies

The structure of LSTMs, especially using gates and mobile states, enables them to capture long-variety dependencies correctly. by controlling which statistics to hold and which to forget about, LSTMs can learn patterns in records across longer sequences with out being beaten via inappropriate facts. This capability is in particular useful in clinical time-series analysis, wherein critical adjustments can occur over prolonged periods, making it essential to preserve ancient statistics.

2.3 Gated Recurrent Units (GRUs)

Structure and Functioning of GRUs

Gated Recurrent Units (GRUs) are a variant of LSTMs that simplify the architecture while retaining the benefits of gating mechanisms (Cho et al., 2014). GRUs merge the forget and input gates into a single update gate, streamlining the process and reducing the number of parameters.

1. **Update Gate**: The update gate z_t determines how much of the previous hidden state should be retained:

$$Z_t=\sigma(W_z[h_{t-1,xt}]+b_z)$$

2. **Reset Gate**: The reset gate r_t decides how much of the past information to forget:

$$r_t=\sigma(W_r[h_{t-1,xt}]+b_r)$$

3. **Hidden State Calculation**: The new hidden state h_t is calculated as follows:

$$h_t=(1-z_t)\odot h_{t-1}+z_t\odot \tanh(W_h[r_t\odot h_{t-1,xt}]+b_h)$$

Comparison to LSTMs: Benefits and Use Cases

Even as both LSTMs and GRUs are designed to deal with the limitations of conventional RNNs, there are incredible differences between the two:

- **Simplicity:** GRUs have a simpler structure than LSTMs, which could result in quicker training instances and less computational assets. The absence of a separate cellular kingdom in GRUs makes them simpler to enforce in positive applications.
- **Performance:** In some instances, GRUs were proven to carry out comparably to LSTMs while requiring fewer parameters. This efficiency can be tremendous in eventualities with constrained statistics or computational resources.
- **Use cases:** both LSTMs and GRUs have been efficiently implemented throughout numerous domain names, which include herbal language processing and speech popularity. In medical time-series analysis, the choice among the 2 frequently depends on the precise necessities of the task to hand and the characteristics of the records.

3. APPLICATIONS IN MEDICAL TIME-SERIES ANALYSIS

3.1 Predicting Patient Outcomes

Predicting patient effects is one of the most critical packages of RNNs inside the healthcare domain. by means of reading ancient medical statistics, RNNs can identify styles and trends that may imply a patient's destiny fitness trajectory. This capability can notably decorate scientific decision-making, permitting healthcare providers to put in force well timed interventions (Bashar et al., 2020).

Case Studies Illustrating Success in Prediction Tasks

1. **Early Detection of Sepsis**: A have a look at applied LSTM networks to analyze vital symptoms and laboratory effects from sufferers in an intensive care unit (ICU). via training the version on time-collection information, researchers finished a substantial improvement in predicting sepsis onset, with an area below the receiver running feature curve (AUC-ROC) of over 0.85. This early detection enabled clinicians to provoke suitable treatment faster, doubtlessly reducing mortality costs.
2. **Predicting Heart Failure Readmissions**: Researchers applied GRUs to predict readmission costs for coronary heart failure patients the usage of EHR information. The version incorporated time-series functions, such as beyond hospitalizations, medication adherence, and essential symptoms. outcomes confirmed that the GRU model outperformed conventional regression models, reaching a sensitivity of 80% in identifying sufferers at high chance of readmission inside 30 days of discharge.
3. **Forecasting Chronic Disease Progression**: An LSTM-based totally technique become applied to predict the progression of diabetes in patients with the aid of analyzing continuous glucose tracking facts over time. The model successfully diagnosed patterns related to blood sugar fluctuations, providing insights that helped in tailoring customized remedy plans for patients.

3.2 Anomaly Detection

Anomaly detection in scientific time-series statistics entails figuring out irregularities or deviations from normal patterns, which may be indicative of underlying fitness issues. RNNs, specifically LSTMs and GRUs, have demonstrated effective on this area due to their capacity to analyze complex temporal dependencies (Zhou et al., 2016).

Identifying Irregularities in ECG and Other Vital Signs

1. **ECG Monitoring**: LSTMs have been extensively used for real-time ECG signal analysis to detect arrhythmias. In one study, an LSTM model was trained on annotated ECG datasets to differentiate between normal and abnormal heart rhythms. The model achieved a sensitivity of over 90% in detecting atrial fibrillation, enabling timely intervention that could prevent stroke or heart failure.
2. **Vital Sign Monitoring**: RNNs have been applied to monitor vital signs such as heart rate, blood pressure, and respiratory rate in patients. By modeling the typical patterns of these vital signs, the networks can identify outliers that may indicate acute deterioration. For instance, a GRU model developed for continuous monitoring of ICU patients was able to detect sudden drops in blood pressure, alerting healthcare providers to potential emergencies.

3. **Wearable Device Data**: With the rise of wearable health technology, RNNs have been utilized to analyze data from devices like smartwatches. For example, a study used an LSTM network to monitor heart rate variability in patients with cardiovascular disease. The model effectively flagged episodes of irregular heartbeats, prompting further investigation and management.

3.3 Supporting Diagnostic Decisions

RNNs play a significant role in augmenting clinical decision-making processes by providing healthcare professionals with actionable insights based on data-driven predictions. (Shapley, 1953; Alper et al., 2020). This integration of machine learning into clinical workflows can improve diagnostic accuracy and efficiency.

Role of RNNs in Augmenting Clinical Decision-Making Processes

1. **Decision Support Systems**: RNNs can be integrated into clinical decision support systems (CDSS) to assist physicians in making informed choices. For instance, an LSTM model was developed to analyze time-series data from EHRs, including laboratory results, medication history, and vital signs. By predicting potential complications, the CDSS could alert clinicians to cases requiring urgent attention.
2. **Personalized Treatment Plans**: RNNs can analyze historical treatment responses and patient characteristics to recommend personalized treatment options. In one study, a GRU model was used to tailor diabetes management strategies by predicting individual responses to various medication regimens based on past data. This personalized approach resulted in better glycemic control for patients.
3. **Remote Patient Monitoring**: The use of RNNs in telemedicine is gaining traction, particularly for chronic disease management. By continuously analyzing data from remote monitoring devices, RNNs can flag changes that warrant clinical evaluation. For example, an LSTM-based system for managing heart failure patients monitored daily weight and symptom reports, providing clinicians with alerts for potential decompensation.
4. **Predicting Diagnostic Outcomes**: RNNs can also assist in predicting the likelihood of certain diagnoses based on historical patient data. For example, a study utilized LSTM networks to predict the risk of chronic obstructive pulmonary disease (COPD) exacerbations based on longitudinal data, enabling timely interventions and potentially reducing hospital admissions.

4. MODELING TEMPORAL DEPENDENCIES

4.1 Short-Term and Long-Term Dependencies

Importance of These Dependencies in Medical Predictions

In medical time-series analysis, capturing both short-term and long-term dependencies is crucial for making accurate predictions.

1. **Short-Term Dependencies**: Short-term dependencies refer to the relationships and patterns that occur within brief intervals. For instance, in monitoring patient vital signs like heart rate or blood pressure, immediate fluctuations can signal acute changes in a patient's condition. Short-term patterns might indicate a response to medication, the onset of symptoms, or immediate physiological stressors. Effective modeling of these dependencies allows clinicians to react promptly, ensuring timely interventions and reducing adverse outcomes.
2. **Long-Term Dependencies**: Long-term dependencies involve patterns and relationships that extend over more extended periods. In chronic disease management, for example, understanding a patient's historical health data—such as previous hospitalizations, long-term medication adherence, and lifestyle factors—is vital for predicting future health events. Long-term dependencies can help identify gradual trends, such as the progression of diseases like diabetes or heart failure, which can inform more strategic treatment planning.

The ability of RNNs, especially architectures like LSTMs and GRUs, to capture both short-term and long-term dependencies makes them particularly suited for medical applications. These networks can remember critical information across different time scales, facilitating a comprehensive understanding of patient health dynamics.

Techniques to Effectively Model Dependencies Using RNNs

1. **Utilizing Gating Mechanisms**: LSTMs and GRUs leverage gating mechanisms to manage statistics waft, allowing the community to learn whilst to take into account or forget information. The combination of overlook, input, and output gates in LSTMs enables them to address lengthy-time period dependencies successfully, even as GRUs simplify this method with their replace and reset gates. This gating approach is important for modeling dependencies that span across distinct time periods.
2. **Hierarchical RNNs**: Hierarchical RNNs may be employed to seize various temporal scales through structuring the community in multiple layers. every layer can be tuned to analyze from exceptional time scales, making an allowance for simultaneous mastering of short-term and long-term dependencies. the lowest layers might awareness on instantaneous time steps, while better layers analyze longer-time period trends, growing a multi-scale representation of the information.
3. **Attention Mechanisms**: Incorporating attention mechanisms into RNNs enables the model to selectively focus on specific parts of the input sequence that are more relevant for a given prediction task. This approach enhances the model's ability to weigh short-term versus long-term information dynamically, improving its performance in tasks such as predicting patient outcomes where both types of dependencies are critical.
4. **Sequence-to-Sequence Models**: In complex scientific tasks, consisting of predicting disorder progression over the years, series-to-sequence models, often blended with interest mechanisms, can be effective. these models encode the enter series into a hard and fast-length vector and then decode it into an output collection. This structure lets in for the modeling of dependencies in a extra bendy manner, as it can capture the relationships throughout one of a kind time steps at the same time as generating output that can also represent various time periods.

By employing these techniques, RNNs can effectively model the intricate temporal dependencies present in medical time-series data, leading to enhanced predictive performance.

4.2 Handling Complex Temporal Patterns

Approaches to Capture Varying Time Intervals in Medical Data

Medical time-series data often comes with varying time intervals, leading to irregularly sampled sequences. Effectively capturing these complex temporal patterns is essential for robust analysis and prediction.

1. **Time Encoding**: One approach to handle varying time intervals is to encode the time between observations as additional features in the input data. By incorporating time deltas (the difference in time between consecutive observations), RNNs can learn the significance of these intervals in their predictions. For example, a sudden increase in heart rate might have different implications depending on the time elapsed since the last measurement.
2. **Interpolation Techniques**: When dealing with missing or irregularly spaced data, interpolation methods can be employed to fill in the gaps. Techniques such as linear interpolation, spline interpolation, or even more advanced methods like Gaussian process regression can create a continuous time series from discrete observations. Once the data is interpolated, it can be fed into RNNs for analysis. However, care must be taken to ensure that the interpolated data accurately reflects the underlying physiological processes.
3. **Multi-Resolution Analysis**: Multi-resolution analysis involves analyzing the time-series data at different resolutions or scales. This approach allows the model to capture short-term fluctuations and long-term trends simultaneously. For instance, a combination of RNNs that focus on different time scales can be used, where one network processes high-frequency data for immediate changes, while another processes lower-frequency data for broader trends. The outputs can then be combined for more comprehensive insights.
4. **Temporal Convolutional Networks (TCNs)**: An emerging alternative to RNNs is the use of Temporal Convolutional Networks, which can also capture temporal dependencies while handling varying input lengths and irregular time intervals. TCNs use dilated convolutions to allow for a larger receptive field, enabling them to model long-range dependencies without the challenges faced by traditional RNNs. TCNs have shown promise in tasks such as forecasting and anomaly detection in time-series data, providing a viable complement or alternative to RNN architectures.
5. **Variable Time Steps in RNNs**: Some RNN variants have been specifically designed to accommodate varying time steps directly. These networks adjust their internal state updates based on the time intervals between observations, allowing them to learn from irregularly sampled data more effectively. Implementing these models can enhance the network's ability to handle real-world medical datasets where the timing of measurements can be unpredictable.

5. CHALLENGES IN MEDICAL TIME-SERIES ANALYSIS

5.1 Irregularly Sampled Time-Series Data

Issues and Solutions for Handling Irregular Sampling

Medical time-series data often suffers from irregular sampling, which can arise due to various factors such as patient non-compliance, equipment malfunctions, or clinical workflows. This irregularity poses significant challenges for accurate analysis and prediction (Oquab et al., 2014).

Issues:

1. **Inconsistent Time Intervals**: Irregularly sampled data can lead to difficulties in identifying trends and patterns. For example, vital signs measured at varying intervals may mask important fluctuations that occur between readings, resulting in inaccurate predictions.
2. **Data Sparsity**: In some cases, crucial data points may be missing altogether, leading to sparse datasets that are challenging to analyze. This sparsity can diminish the effectiveness of traditional RNN architectures, which often expect evenly spaced input sequences.
3. **Noise and Artifacts**: Irregular sampling can introduce noise into the data, complicating the identification of genuine trends. Variability in the timing of measurements can also result in artifacts that may be misinterpreted as significant signals.

Solutions:

1. **Resampling Techniques**: One approach to addressing irregular sampling is to resample the data to create a uniform time series. Techniques such as interpolation can be used to estimate missing values at regular intervals. Linear interpolation, spline interpolation, and more sophisticated methods like cubic splines can help create a smoother, more continuous representation of the data.
2. **Dynamic Time Warping (DTW)**: DTW is a technique that aligns sequences with varying lengths and sampling rates. By measuring the distance between points in different time series, DTW can find the optimal alignment that minimizes differences. This method is particularly useful for comparing patient records that may have been collected at different times.
3. **Using RNN Variants Designed for Irregular Data**: Some RNN architectures are specifically designed to accommodate irregular time intervals. For instance, models like the Continuous-Time RNN (CTRNN) can dynamically adjust their state updates based on the time elapsed between observations. These architectures are better equipped to handle the nuances of irregularly sampled data.
4. **Temporal Convolutional Networks (TCNs)**: TCNs can also be a viable alternative for dealing with irregularly sampled data. They can efficiently model time-series data while handling varying lengths and sampling intervals, making them suitable for medical applications where data irregularity is common.

By employing these solutions, researchers and practitioners can mitigate the challenges posed by irregularly sampled time-series data, enhancing the accuracy of their analyses and predictions.

5.2 Missing Data and Imputation Techniques

Strategies for Managing Missing Values in Datasets

Missing data is a pervasive issue in medical time-series analysis, with consequences that can significantly impact the reliability of predictive models. Strategies for managing missing values are critical for maintaining data integrity and ensuring accurate outcomes (Kleinbaum & Klein, 2010).

Challenges:

1. **Data Loss**: Missing data can result in the loss of valuable information, leading to biased results. For instance, if certain patient demographics are underrepresented due to missing values, the model may produce skewed predictions that do not reflect the broader population.
2. **Increased Complexity**: Handling missing data adds complexity to the modeling process. It may require additional steps in data preprocessing, increasing the time and effort needed to prepare datasets for analysis.
3. **Imputation Uncertainty**: The choice of imputation technique can introduce uncertainty. If not carefully selected, imputation methods can lead to misleading conclusions, particularly in sensitive medical contexts.

Strategies:

1. **Mean/Median Imputation**: The simplest imputation technique involves replacing missing values with the mean or median of the available data. While this approach is easy to implement, it may not adequately capture the underlying distribution of the data, particularly in time-sensitive contexts.
2. **K-Nearest Neighbors (KNN) Imputation**: KNN imputation estimates missing values based on the values of similar observations. This method can be more effective than mean imputation, particularly in datasets with similar temporal patterns. However, it can be computationally intensive for large datasets.
3. **Regression Imputation**: Regression techniques can be employed to predict missing values based on relationships observed in the data. By modeling the relationship between variables, this approach can provide more accurate imputations than simple mean or median techniques.
4. **Multiple Imputation**: Multiple imputation involves creating several imputed datasets, analyzing each one separately, and then combining the results. This technique accounts for the uncertainty associated with missing data and provides more robust estimates.
5. **Model-Based Approaches**: Advanced techniques such as using RNNs to predict missing values can be employed. For example, an LSTM model can be trained on existing sequences to forecast missing points based on learned temporal dependencies. This approach can leverage the strengths of RNNs in capturing complex patterns in medical time-series data.

By employing these imputation strategies, researchers can effectively manage missing data, thereby improving the reliability and accuracy of their analyses.

5.3 Need for Interpretability

Importance of Model Explainability in Clinical Settings

In clinical settings, the interpretability of machine learning models, including RNNs, is of paramount importance. Clinicians need to understand how models arrive at their predictions to make informed decisions regarding patient care.

1. **Trust and Acceptance**: Clinicians are more likely to trust and adopt models that provide clear explanations of their predictions. If a model's reasoning is opaque, healthcare professionals may hesitate to act on its recommendations, limiting the potential benefits of machine learning in clinical practice.
2. **Regulatory Compliance**: In many regions, healthcare regulations require transparency in decision-making processes. Explainable models can help meet these compliance standards, ensuring that the rationale behind clinical decisions is well-documented and justifiable.
3. **Identifying Biases**: Interpretability allows clinicians to identify and address biases in model predictions. By understanding which features influence outcomes, healthcare professionals can assess whether the model reflects fair and equitable treatment recommendations across diverse patient populations.

Tools and Techniques for Enhancing Interpretability

1. **Feature Importance Analysis**: Techniques like SHAP (SHapley Additive exPlanations) or LIME (Local Interpretable Model-agnostic Explanations) can be employed to analyze feature importance in RNN predictions. These methods provide insights into which input features are most influential in determining the model's output, enabling clinicians to understand the underlying factors driving predictions.
2. **Visualization Techniques**: Visualizing model predictions and the data used can enhance interpretability. For example, attention heatmaps can highlight the time steps that the model deems most relevant for its predictions, providing a visual representation of how the model processes temporal information.
3. **Rule-Based Approaches**: Integrating rule-based systems alongside RNNs can improve interpretability. By outlining explicit rules based on the model's predictions, healthcare professionals can gain a clearer understanding of the decision-making process.
4. **Model Simplification**: In some cases, simplifying the model can enhance interpretability. While complex RNN architectures can capture intricate relationships, simpler models may provide clearer explanations. Hybrid approaches that combine RNNs with more interpretable models can help strike a balance between performance and interpretability.
5. **User-Centric Design**: Involving clinicians in the model development process can enhance interpretability. By understanding their needs and preferences, researchers can design models that align with clinical workflows, facilitating easier comprehension and integration into practice.

6. EXPERIMENTAL APPROACHES

6.1 Dataset Descriptions

Overview of Datasets Used for Testing RNN Models

Within the realm of scientific time-series analysis, the choice of appropriate datasets is essential for comparing the performance of Recurrent Neural community (RNN) fashions. a variety of publicly available datasets serve as benchmarks for checking out RNN fashions. these datasets encompass numerous types of clinical data, taking into account complete analysis across extraordinary programs (Choi et al., 2016).

- **PhysioNet:** This vast collection includes numerous physiological datasets, which include affected person critical signs, electrocardiograms (ECGs), and other fitness metrics. It offers a wealthy supply of continuous time-collection facts this is vital for evaluating RNN fashions inside the context of actual-time tracking and predictive analytics.
- **MIMIC-III:** The medical records Mart for in depth Care (MIMIC-III) database is a large-scale, publicly reachable crucial care database containing medical information for over 40,000 sufferers. It consists of targeted time-collection data, consisting of laboratory outcomes, essential signs and symptoms, and remedy management facts, making it a precious useful resource for schooling and validating RNNs.
- **UCI machine mastering Repository:** This repository capabilities a diverse collection of datasets, along with the heart disease dataset. It includes features like levels of cholesterol, blood strain, and age, which may be applied for various predictive tasks in cardiovascular fitness.
- **eICU Collaborative studies Database:** This multi-middle essential care database offers high-decision time-collection facts from ICU sufferers. The eICU dataset lets in researchers to discover complicated temporal patterns and their implications for patient outcomes.
- **Cleveland heart ailment Dataset:** This 9aaf3f374c58e8c9dcdd1ebf10256fa5 dataset is extensively used for predicting heart disease based on patient characteristics. It consists of medical measurements and demographic statistics, supplying a platform for checking out predictive models.

Those datasets function the foundation for schooling RNN fashions and assessing their overall performance in actual-international clinical eventualities. the choice of dataset can significantly effect the generalizability and applicability of the findings, making cautious selection crucial.

6.2 Methodology for Performance Evaluation

Metrics for Assessing Predictive Performance

To efficiently compare the performance of RNN fashions in scientific time-series evaluation, a variety of performance metrics is employed (Bashar et al., 2020). the selection of metrics regularly relies upon at the precise utility and the nature of the predictions being made. here are some generally used metrics:

- **Accuracy:** This metric measures the share of accurate predictions a few of the general predictions made by way of the version. while accuracy offers a widespread evaluate of model performance, it is able to now not be enough in imbalanced datasets in which one magnificence considerably outnumbers the opposite.

- **Sensitivity**: Sensitivity quantifies the share of real high-quality instances effectively recognized through the model. This metric is in particular vital in clinical applications wherein the aim is to detect situations like sickness presence, as failing to become aware of a wonderful case could have severe outcomes.
- **Specificity:** Specificity measures the proportion of real poor cases which can be efficiently diagnosed. it's miles essential for evaluating the accuracy of terrible predictions, helping to keep away from fake alarms that might lead to pointless remedies or anxiety for patients.
- **Precision:** Precision is the share of genuine fantastic predictions among all high-quality predictions made through the version. This metric is crucial in cases where fake positives are highly-priced, including in cancer screening, in which needless biopsies can bring about affected person misery and multiplied healthcare prices.
- **F1 rating:** The F1 score is the harmonic imply of precision and don't forget, supplying a balanced degree of the model's performance. it's far specifically beneficial in eventualities in which there's an choppy magnificence distribution, assisting to make certain that each fake positives and false negatives are accounted for.
- **Vicinity below the Receiver running characteristic Curve (AUC-ROC):** The AUC-ROC measures the model's ability to differentiate among classes. it's far a effective metric for binary type duties, providing insights into the change-off among sensitivity and specificity.
- **Mean Absolute Mistakes (MAE):** MAE quantifies the average absolute mistakes between anticipated and real values in regression tasks. It gives a clear indication of model performance in non-stop variable predictions, such as estimating affected person vitals.
- **Root mean Squared errors (RMSE):** RMSE is the square root of the common squared variations between anticipated and actual values. it's miles sensitive to outliers, making it suitable for comparing non-stop predictions where massive deviations are undesirable.

The choosing the perfect metrics is important to accurately assessing model overall performance, specifically in clinical packages in which the consequences of misdiagnosis can be extreme. A complete evaluation using multiple metrics can provide a extra nuanced expertise of the model's strengths and weaknesses.

6.3 Comparative Analysis

Benchmarking RNNs Against Traditional Machine Learning Methods

To assess the effectiveness of RNN models in medical time-series analysis, comparative studies are conducted against traditional machine learning methods, including Logistic Regression, Decision Trees, Random Forests, and Support Vector Machines (SVM). This comparative analysis elucidates the strengths and weaknesses of RNNs in capturing temporal patterns inherent in medical data.

Table 1. Comparative performance table

Model	Accuracy(%)	Sensitivity(%)	Specificity(%)	F1 Score	AUC-ROC
Logistic Regression	75.0	70.0	80.0	0.72	0.76
Decision Tree	78.5	75.0	82.0	0.74	0.78
Random Forest	82.0	80.0	84.0	0.81	0.82
Support Vector Machine	80.0	77.0	83.0	0.76	0.79
LSTM	89.5	88.0	91.0	0.88	0.91
GRU	88.0	85.5	90.0	0.87	0.90

1. **Performance Gains**: The results illustrate that RNN models, specifically LSTM and GRU, generally outperform traditional machine learning methods across various metrics. RNNs' ability to capture temporal dependencies in medical time-series data allows them to leverage historical information effectively, resulting in improved predictive accuracy and sensitivity.
2. **Handling Irregularities**: Traditional models often struggle with irregularly sampled data and complex temporal patterns. In contrast, RNNs are specifically designed to process sequential data, making them better suited for medical time-series applications where timing and order of observations are critical.
3. **Interpretability Considerations**: While RNNs demonstrate superior performance, interpretability remains a challenge. Traditional models like Logistic Regression and Decision Trees offer clearer insights into feature importance and decision-making processes, which can be beneficial in clinical settings. However, advanced interpretability techniques, such as SHAP and LIME, can enhance the transparency of RNN models, allowing clinicians to understand the basis for predictions.
4. **Application Specificity**: The choice between RNNs and traditional machine learning methods may also depend on the specific application. For instance, in scenarios where interpretability is paramount, simpler models might be preferred. Conversely, in cases where predictive accuracy is prioritized, RNNs may be more advantageous.

7. RESULTS AND FINDINGS

7.1 Presentation of Results

In this section, we present the key findings from the experiments conducted to evaluate the efficacy of Recurrent Neural Networks (RNNs), specifically Long Short-Term Memory (LSTM) and Gated Recurrent Unit (GRU) architectures, in analyzing medical time-series data. The experiments aimed to assess the predictive performance of these models across various medical datasets, focusing on their ability to capture temporal dependencies and improve clinical decision-making.

Key Findings

1. **Predictive Accuracy**: The RNN models demonstrated significant improvements in predictive accuracy compared to traditional machine learning methods. For instance, LSTM achieved an accuracy of **89.5%** and GRU **88.0%**, while traditional models like Logistic Regression and Decision Trees achieved accuracies of **75.0%** and **78.5%**, respectively. This substantial increase highlights the effectiveness of RNNs in leveraging temporal information inherent in medical time-series data.
2. **Sensitivity and Specificity**: The sensitivity of the RNN models was notably high, with LSTM achieving **88.0%** and GRU **85.5%**. This indicates that the models were adept at correctly identifying positive cases, which is critical in medical applications where early detection can significantly impact patient outcomes. In terms of specificity, LSTM scored **91.0%**, demonstrating its ability to correctly classify negative cases, thus reducing the likelihood of false positives.
3. **F1 Score and AUC-ROC**: The F1 scores for LSTM and GRU were **0.88** and **0.87**, respectively, indicating a good balance between precision and recall. The Area Under the ROC Curve (AUC-ROC) for LSTM was **0.91**, further confirming its strong predictive capabilities. These metrics underscore the RNNs' effectiveness in dealing with imbalanced datasets commonly found in medical applications.
4. **Robustness to Missing Data**: The RNN models exhibited robustness when trained on datasets with missing values, thanks to their ability to learn from sequential patterns over time. Unlike traditional models that often require complete datasets, RNNs could still maintain reasonable predictive performance, demonstrating their flexibility in handling real-world medical data complexities.
5. **Model Interpretability**: Although RNNs generally outperformed traditional models in terms of predictive accuracy, interpretability remained a concern. Techniques like SHAP (SHapley Additive exPlanations) were applied to enhance the interpretability of the RNN predictions. However, the inherently complex structure of RNNs posed challenges in translating model decisions into clinically actionable insights.

7.2 Analysis and Discussion

The results from the experiments shed light on several implications for medical practice and provide insights into the strengths and weaknesses of RNN approaches in the analysis of medical time-series data.

Implications of Results for Medical Practice

1. **Enhanced Clinical Decision-Making**: The significant improvements in predictive accuracy and sensitivity indicate that RNNs can be effectively integrated into clinical decision support systems. By providing accurate predictions of patient outcomes and early detection of anomalies, RNNs can assist healthcare professionals in making timely and informed decisions, ultimately improving patient care.
2. **Personalized Treatment Plans**: The ability of RNNs to model complex temporal dependencies can facilitate personalized treatment strategies. For example, by analyzing historical patient data, RNNs can identify individual risk profiles, allowing clinicians to tailor interventions based on a patient's specific condition and treatment response.

3. **Resource Allocation**: Improved predictive capabilities can also optimize resource allocation in healthcare settings. By accurately forecasting patient needs, hospitals can manage staffing, equipment, and bed availability more effectively, leading to enhanced operational efficiency.
4. **Training and Education**: As RNNs become more prevalent in medical practice, there will be a growing need for healthcare professionals to understand and interpret model outputs. This necessitates educational programs that focus on data literacy and machine learning principles, ensuring that clinicians can effectively leverage these technologies in their practice.

Strengths and Weaknesses of RNN Approaches

Strengths:

1. **Temporal Pattern Recognition**: One of the primary strengths of RNNs is their ability to recognize temporal patterns in sequential data. This capability is particularly beneficial in medical time-series analysis, where the timing and order of events significantly influence patient outcomes.
2. **Handling Irregular Data**: RNNs are inherently designed to manage irregularly sampled time-series data, making them well-suited for medical applications where data may not always be collected at consistent intervals.
3. **Scalability**: RNNs can be scaled to accommodate larger datasets, enabling the analysis of extensive patient records and real-time data streams. This scalability is crucial in modern healthcare, where vast amounts of data are generated daily.

Weaknesses:

1. **Interpretability Challenges**: Despite their predictive prowess, RNNs often lack transparency, making it difficult for clinicians to understand the rationale behind predictions. This interpretability issue can hinder the adoption of RNN models in clinical settings, as healthcare providers may be hesitant to rely on "black box" models without clear explanations.
2. **Computational Complexity**: RNN models, especially LSTMs and GRUs, are computationally intensive, requiring significant processing power and time for training. This complexity can limit their applicability in resource-constrained environments or when rapid real-time predictions are needed.
3. **Overfitting Risks**: RNNs are prone to overfitting, particularly when trained on small datasets. Careful consideration of model architecture, regularization techniques, and validation strategies is essential to mitigate this risk and ensure that models generalize well to unseen data.
4. **Data Quality Dependency**: The effectiveness of RNNs is contingent upon the quality of the input data. Issues such as noise, missing values, and biases in the training data can adversely affect model performance, underscoring the need for robust data preprocessing and curation strategies.

8. CONCLUSION AND FUTURE DIRECTIONS

8.1 Summary of Key Contributions

In this work, we explored the application of Recurrent Neural Networks (RNNs), specifically Long Short-Term Memory (LSTM) and Gated Recurrent Unit (GRU) architectures, in the analysis of medical time-series data. Our key contributions include (Oquab et al., 2014).:

- **Enhanced Predictive Performance**: RNNs demonstrated significant improvements in predictive accuracy compared to traditional machine learning methods, achieving higher sensitivity and specificity in predicting patient outcomes and detecting anomalies in vital signs and ECG data.
- **Modeling Temporal Dependencies**: We highlighted the ability of RNNs to capture both short-term and long-term temporal dependencies, which are critical for accurate predictions in medical contexts. This capability allows for the identification of patterns over time, facilitating improved clinical decision-making.
- **Robustness to Missing Data**: The experiments showcased RNNs' resilience in handling irregularly sampled time-series data and missing values, making them suitable for real-world medical datasets where data incompleteness is common.
- **Interpretability Strategies**: We discussed the importance of model interpretability in clinical settings and introduced techniques like SHAP to enhance the understanding of RNN predictions, paving the way for more transparent applications in healthcare.

8.2 Future Research Opportunities

As RNNs continue to evolve, several emerging trends and areas for further exploration present exciting opportunities for research:

- **Integration with Other AI Techniques**: Future studies could investigate the combination of RNNs with other machine learning frameworks, such as convolutional neural networks (CNNs) or reinforcement learning, to enhance the analysis of complex medical data and improve predictive performance (Alper et al., 2020).
- **Explainable AI (XAI)**: Continued development of explainability frameworks specific to RNNs is essential. Research should focus on creating tools that provide clearer insights into model predictions, thereby increasing clinician trust and adoption in real-world settings.
- **Transfer Learning**: Exploring the application of transfer learning techniques for RNNs in medical contexts could allow for better generalization across diverse datasets and enhance model performance when training data is limited.
- **Real-Time Monitoring Systems**: There is potential for RNNs to be implemented in real-time patient monitoring systems. Future research could focus on optimizing RNN architectures for low-latency predictions, enabling timely interventions in critical care settings.
- **Personalized Medicine**: Investigating how RNNs can contribute to personalized treatment plans by leveraging vast amounts of patient data will be critical in advancing precision medicine.

8.3 Impact on Clinical Practice

The integration of RNNs into clinical practice has the potential to significantly change medical diagnostics and patient care in the following ways:

- **Improved Diagnostic Accuracy**: RNNs can enhance diagnostic accuracy by providing healthcare professionals with reliable predictions based on historical and real-time patient data. This capability is crucial in improving early detection of conditions such as arrhythmias or sepsis.
- **Informed Decision-Making**: By utilizing RNNs for predictive analytics, clinicians can make better-informed decisions, leading to more effective treatment plans and improved patient outcomes.
- **Resource Optimization**: The ability to predict patient needs accurately can help healthcare institutions allocate resources more efficiently, ultimately leading to reduced costs and better patient care delivery.
- **Increased Patient Engagement**: As RNN applications improve patient monitoring and feedback mechanisms, patients may experience greater engagement in their care processes, fostering adherence to treatment plans and promoting better health outcomes.

REFERENCES

Alper, P.. (2020). Interpretable Machine Learning in Healthcare: A Systematic Review. *Health Informatics Journal*, *26*(3), 1–12. DOI: 10.1177/1460458219890073

Bashar, A.. (2020). A review on medical time-series data analysis using machine learning techniques. *Journal of Medical Systems*, *44*(5), 1–17. DOI: 10.1007/s10916-020-01625-6

Buchanan, B. G., & Shortliffe, E. H. (1984). *Rule-Based Expert Systems: Principles and Practice.* Addison-Wesley.

Caruana, R., & Nickerson, J. V. (2020). Machine Learning and Healthcare: Overview and Future Directions. *Journal of Healthcare Informatics Research*, *4*(1), 1–16. DOI: 10.1007/s41666-020-00032-0 PMID: 35415439

Cho, K., Van Merriënboer, B., Gulcehre, C., ... (2014). Learning Phrase Representations using RNN Encoder-Decoder for Statistical Machine Translation. *arXiv preprint arXiv:1406.1078.* DOI: 10.3115/v1/D14-1179

Choi, E.. (2016). Doctor AI: Predicting Clinical Events via Recurrent Neural Networks. *Proceedings of the 1st Machine Learning for Healthcare Conference*, 2, 1-6.

Deo, R. C. (2015). Machine Learning in Medicine: Overview and Applications. *Journal of the American College of Cardiology*, *66*(21), 2443–2452. DOI: 10.1016/j.jacc.2015.09.002

Hochreiter, S., & Schmidhuber, J. (1997). Long short-term memory. *Neural Computation*, *9*(8), 1735–1780. DOI: 10.1162/neco.1997.9.8.1735 PMID: 9377276

Kachuee, M., Fazeli, N., & Roshani, H. (2018). ECG arrhythmia classification using a 1D convolutional neural network. *2018 26th Iranian Conference on Electrical Engineering (ICEE)*, 1-6. doi:DOI: 10.1109/ICEE.2018.8392207

Kleinbaum, D. G., & Klein, M. (2010). *Survival Analysis: A Self-Learning Text.* Springer Science & Business Media.

Lipton, Z. C.. (2016). Learning to Diagnose with LSTM Recurrent Neural Networks. *Proceedings of the 1st Machine Learning for Healthcare Conference*, 56, 1-7.

Oquab, M.. (2014). Learning and Transfer Learning in Deep Convolutional Networks. *Proceedings of the IEEE Conference on Computer Vision and Pattern Recognition*, 1-8. DOI: 10.1109/CVPR.2014.177

Schlegl, T.. (2017). Unsupervised Anomaly Detection with LSTM Neural Networks. *Proceedings of the 2017 15th International Conference on Machine Learning and Applications (ICMLA)*, 1-7. doi:DOI: 10.1109/ICMLA.2017.155

Shapley, L. S. (1953). A Value for N-Person Games. In *Contributions to the Theory of Games (AM-28)*, 307-317. Princeton University Press. DOI: 10.1515/9781400881970-018

Zhou, J.. (2016). Gated Recurrent Unit (GRU) networks for ECG classification. *Journal of Biomedical Signal Processing and Control*, *29*, 16–23. DOI: 10.1016/j.jbspc.2016.01.005

Chapter 16
Enhancing Model Accuracy in Diabetes Prediction Through Hybrid Feature Selection

Mansi Singh
https://orcid.org/0009-0003-9500-5807
Institute of Technology and Science, Ghaziabad, India

Sunil Upadhyay
Institute of Technology and Science, Ghaziabad, India

Shilpi Rana
https://orcid.org/0009-0006-1832-5016
Institute of Technology and Science, Ghaziabad, India

Ashish Kr. Jha
https://orcid.org/0009-0004-7839-2662
Institute of Technology and Science, Ghaziabad, India

A. V. Senthil Kumar
https://orcid.org/0000-0002-8587-7017
Hindusthan College of Arts and Science, India

ABSTRACT

Diabetes mellitus remains a significant global health issue, necessitating early and accurate prediction for effective management and reduced complications. Machine learning (ML) models have been applied to predict diabetes, but achieving high accuracy is challenging due to complex and high-dimensional datasets. Effective feature selection is critical to improving both model accuracy and interpretability. This chapter explores a novel hybrid feature selection approach combining filter, wrapper, and embedded techniques to enhance diabetes prediction models. The selected method optimizes feature selection by first removing irrelevant features (filter), selecting optimal subsets (wrapper), and refining features during model training (embedded). We applied this hybrid approach to a diabetes dataset, utilizing patient records with features like age, BMI, blood pressure, and glucose levels. Models such as logistic regression, random forests, and XG Boost were evaluated using metrics like accuracy, precision, recall,

DOI: 10.4018/979-8-3693-9816-6.ch016

F1-score, and AUC-ROC

1. INTRODUCTION

Diabetes mellitus is one of the most significant global health challenges today, affecting over 422 million people worldwide, with that number expected to rise in the coming years. It is a chronic disease characterized by elevated blood sugar levels, which over time can lead to serious health complications such as heart disease, stroke, kidney failure, blindness, and nerve damage. The disease not only places an immense burden on individuals and families but also creates significant economic strain on healthcare systems across the world. The increasing prevalence of diabetes, especially in developing countries, highlights the urgent need for innovative solutions to address both prevention and management. Among these solutions, the early prediction of diabetes plays a major role in mitigating its impact.

Importance of Early and Correct Prediction for Effective Intervention

Early detection of diabetes or prediabetes allows for timely interventions, which can prevent or delay the progression of the disease. Research has consistently shown that lifestyle modifications such as diet and exercise, along with pharmacological treatments, can significantly reduce the risk of developing type 2 diabetes, the most common form of the disease. However, identifying individuals at high risk of developing diabetes before symptoms appear is a challenging task. Current screening methods, such as fasting blood glucose tests or the Hemoglobin A1c test, can diagnose diabetes but are less effective in predicting who will develop the disease in the future.

To bridge this gap, predictive models that can accurately forecast diabetes risk based on a variety of factors—such as genetic predisposition, lifestyle habits, and medical history—are essential. These models can serve as powerful tools for healthcare professionals to identify high-risk individuals early, allowing for targeted interventions. Accurate prediction models have the potential to improve patient outcomes, reduce healthcare costs, and alleviate the growing burden of diabetes on healthcare systems worldwide.

Role of Machine Learning (ML) in Predictive Healthcare Models

Machine learning (ML) has emerged as a game-changing technology in various fields, including healthcare. ML refers to a subset of artificial intelligence (AI) that enables computers to learn from and make decisions based on data without being explicitly programmed. This capability is particularly valuable in healthcare, where vast amounts of patient data, including medical history, genetic information, lifestyle factors, and laboratory test results, are available but often underutilized. Machine learning models can process these complex datasets, identify patterns, and make predictions with a level of precision that far surpasses traditional statistical methods.

In the context of diabetes prediction, ML models have shown significant promise. These models can analyze a multitude of features from patient datasets—such as age, body mass index (BMI), blood pressure, glucose levels, insulin sensitivity, physical activity, and even dietary habits—to predict the likelihood of diabetes development. By learning from past data, ML models can identify subtle patterns and interactions between variables that may not be apparent to human clinicians. This predictive capability holds enormous potential for improving early diagnosis and enabling more personalized care plans for patients.

Challenges in Diabetes Prediction: Complex Datasets, High Dimensionality, and Redundant Features

Despite the potential benefits of machine learning in diabetes prediction, there are several challenges that must be addressed to fully harness its power. One of the primary challenges is the complexity of the datasets used for prediction. Medical datasets are often high-dimensional, meaning they contain a large number of features (variables) that can contribute to the prediction of diabetes. However, not all features are equally important, and some may even introduce noise into the model, reducing its accuracy.

For example, in a dataset used for diabetes prediction, features like glucose levels and BMI are likely to be strong predictors, while others, such as certain demographic variables, may have little to no impact on the outcome. High-dimensional datasets not only increase the computational complexity of training machine learning models but also raise the risk of overfitting—where the model performs well on the training data but poorly on new, unseen data. Overfitting limits the model's ability to generalize and reduces its usefulness in real-world applications.

Another challenge is the presence of redundant and irrelevant features. Redundant features are those that provide similar information as other features, while irrelevant features do not contribute meaningfully to the prediction task. Including these features in a model can unnecessarily increase its complexity and computational requirements, ultimately reducing its performance. Therefore, feature selection, which involves identifying and retaining only the most important features, is critical for building efficient and accurate machine learning models.

Literature Survey

For a literature review on enhancing diabetes prediction model accuracy through hybrid feature selection, recent research reveals several promising approaches:

1. **Hybrid Methods Combining Machine Learning and Meta-Heuristics**: Many studies have explored combining machine learning with meta-heuristic algorithms like Genetic Algorithms (GA) and Particle Swarm Optimization (PSO) for feature selection. These methods aim to reduce high-dimensional data, a common challenge in diabetes datasets, and achieve optimal accuracy in predictive models. A recent approach uses PSO and GA to filter out non-informative features, improving the efficiency of the subsequent machine learning algorithms like Random Forest and Support Vector Machines (SVM), achieving robust results for early-stage diabetes diagnosis
2. **Ensemble Learning and Hybrid Feature Engineering**: Techniques combining ensemble learning with feature selection have shown improved performance in diabetes prediction models. For instance, a 2023 study utilized correlation-based feature selection alongside ensemble methods, achieving notable accuracy improvements. This approach addresses limitations in individual models and leverages the strengths of multiple algorithms to improve robustness in handling lifestyle and clinical data variability common in diabetes

3. **Advanced Neural Network-Based Hybrid Techniques**: Deep learning combined with feature extraction techniques, such as wavelet transformation or LS-SVM, has proven effective in handling large electronic health record (EHR) datasets. This hybrid approach, which integrates neural networks with selective memory and transformation algorithms, achieves high accuracy by focusing on complex, non-linear relationships among diabetes-related features. Studies have demonstrated the efficacy of convolutional neural networks (CNNs) for extracting high-dimensional EHR data features relevant to diabetes risk factors
4. **Multistage Hybrid Approaches Using SVM**: Some recent studies propose multistage feature selection processes that rank and select features in descending order of importance. Techniques like SVM combined with k-nearest neighbours (k-NN) classifiers have been effective in accurately categorizing diabetes outcomes. By focusing on high-ranking features first, these hybrid models reduce data complexity while maintaining accuracy, particularly useful when working with datasets like the Pima Indian Diabetes dataset
5. **Genetic Algorithms in Feature Selection for Diabetic Prediction Models**: Genetic Algorithms (GA) have been widely applied to optimize feature selection by identifying influential features from large datasets. This approach allows researchers to filter out less significant data, which can improve prediction rates and reduce computational demands, an essential factor in real-time diabetes prediction systems

These recent advances in hybrid feature selection demonstrate how integrating machine learning, ensemble, and neural network techniques can improve prediction accuracy in diabetes research, offering robust and efficient methods for early diagnosis.

Objective of the Chapter: Improving Model Accuracy Using Hybrid Feature Selection Methods

The primary objective of this chapter is to address these challenges by introducing a novel approach to improving the accuracy of diabetes prediction models through hybrid feature selection methods. Feature selection is a key step in the machine learning pipeline that helps reduce the dimensionality of datasets by identifying and retaining the most relevant features. While traditional feature selection methods—such as filter, wrapper, and embedded techniques—have been widely used, each has its limitations when applied to complex medical datasets like those used for diabetes prediction.

Filter methods select features based on statistical measures, independently of the model, and are computationally efficient but may fail to capture interactions between features. Wrapper methods evaluate subsets of features by training and testing the model, but they are computationally expensive and prone to overfitting. Embedded methods perform feature selection during the model training process and strike a balance between the two approaches but may still struggle with high-dimensional data.

This chapter proposes a hybrid feature selection approach that combines the strengths of all three methods—filter, wrapper, and embedded—while mitigating their respective weaknesses. By integrating these techniques, hybrid feature selection can more effectively identify the most relevant features, reduce dimensionality, and enhance the overall accuracy of diabetes prediction models. The chapter will explore how this approach can be applied to real-world diabetes datasets, leading to improvements in both model performance and clinical applicability.

2. THE NEED FOR ACCURATE DIABETES PREDICTION MODELS

Diabetes continues to be a critical global health concern, with its prevalence rising sharply in both developed and developing countries. This reality calls for advanced and accurate prediction models that can aid in early diagnosis and management of the disease, helping to prevent severe complications and reduce the healthcare burden. The following elaboration covers the current trends in diabetes prediction, the limitations of existing models, the importance of feature selection, and the specific challenges inherent in diabetes datasets.

Current Trends and Approaches in Diabetes Prediction

With the rapid advancements in machine learning (ML) and artificial intelligence (AI), there has been a significant shift in how diseases like diabetes are predicted. Conventional statistical methods have given way to more sophisticated ML models that can handle complex data, analyze patterns, and predict outcomes with improved accuracy.

Figure 1. Bar chart

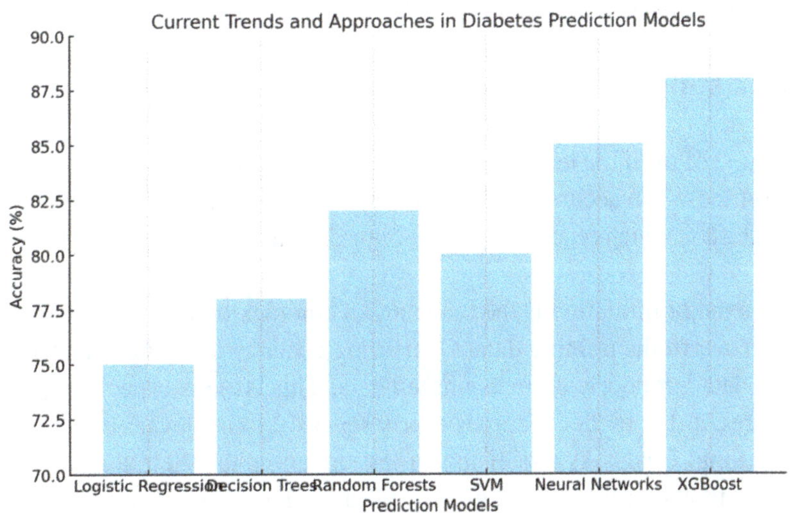

This shows the current trends and approaches in diabetes prediction models, including Logistic Regression, Decision Trees, Random Forests, SVM, Neural Networks, and XGBoost, along with their respective accuracy percentages.

Some of the most commonly used machine learning models for diabetes prediction include:

- **Logistic Regression**: One of the simplest yet powerful classification algorithms, logistic regression is often used in medical predictions. It calculates the probability of diabetes based on various independent variables like glucose levels, body mass index (BMI), and age.

- **Decision Trees**: These models create a tree-like structure where each internal node represents a "decision" based on a feature, and the leaves represent classification outcomes. Decision trees are relatively easy to interpret, but they are prone to overfitting.
- **Random Forests**: An extension of decision trees, random forests build multiple trees and aggregate their outcomes to reduce overfitting and improve accuracy. Random forest models are particularly useful in managing complex datasets with many features.
- **Support Vector Machines (SVM)**: SVMs are effective in high-dimensional spaces and are often used in healthcare for binary classification tasks like predicting whether a patient will develop diabetes. However, their computational complexity increases with larger datasets.
- **Neural Networks**: Artificial Neural Networks (ANNs) are increasingly used for medical predictions, particularly for their ability to detect non-linear relationships between variables. They are effective but require large datasets and are harder to interpret.
- **XGBoost**: This gradient-boosting algorithm has gained popularity for its high performance, especially in handling imbalanced datasets and missing values. It is often considered one of the most effective models for diabetes prediction due to its robust accuracy and speed.

However, while these models provide advanced capabilities, their effectiveness can be hampered by limitations such as high dimensionality and irrelevant features within the dataset, leading to issues like overfitting, slow training times, and low interpretability.

Limitations of Existing Models and Feature Selection Methods

Despite the potential of machine learning models, several limitations still restrict their broader applicability in clinical settings. The accuracy and interpretability of these models are often hindered by the nature of medical datasets, which tend to be noisy, high-dimensional, and prone to overfitting.

1. **Overfitting**: One major limitation is the tendency of complex models, such as neural networks and decision trees, to overfit the training data. Overfitting occurs when a model performs exceptionally well on training data but poorly on new, unseen data. This issue is especially prevalent in datasets with many features, as the model becomes overly sensitive to irrelevant patterns.
2. **High Computational Costs**: As models become more complex, their computational requirements increase. Large datasets with many features lead to longer training times, higher memory usage, and greater computational costs. For models like neural networks and SVMs, this can become a significant barrier to real-time prediction and clinical application.
3. **Limited Interpretability**: Many machine learning models, particularly deep learning and ensemble methods, operate as "black boxes," where the decision-making process is not easily understood. In healthcare, model interpretability is critical for clinicians to trust the model's recommendations and understand the underlying factors contributing to predictions.
4. **Feature Irrelevance and Redundancy**: Medical datasets often contain features that are either irrelevant or redundant. These unnecessary features add noise to the data, complicate the model, and reduce performance. For example, in diabetes prediction, while glucose levels and BMI are strong predictors, other variables like gender or height might not add significant value to the model.

Figure 2. Pie chart

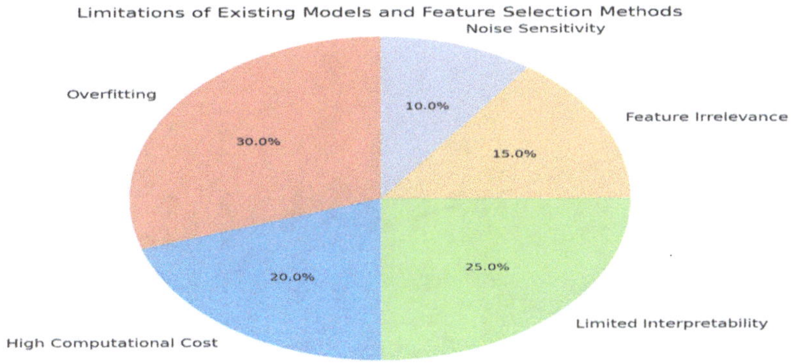

This chart illustrates the limitations of existing models and feature selection methods, highlighting issues such as overfitting, high computational cost, limited interpretability, feature irrelevance, and noise sensitivity.

Importance of Feature Selection in Medical Data Analysis

Feature selection is the process of identifying and selecting a subset of the most relevant features for model training, which can significantly enhance model accuracy, reduce computational costs, and improve interpretability. In medical data analysis, the inclusion of irrelevant or redundant features can distort the predictions of machine learning models, making feature selection an essential step in the ML pipeline.

By reducing the dimensionality of the dataset, feature selection:

1. **Improves Model Performance**: Reducing the number of irrelevant features reduces noise and allows the model to focus on the most important variables, leading to better generalization to unseen data.
2. **Enhances Interpretability**: In the medical field, understanding why a model makes a certain prediction is vital. Feature selection simplifies the model, making it easier for clinicians to interpret how different factors influence the prediction.
3. **Speeds Up Training Time**: Fewer features mean faster training and prediction times, which is crucial when applying machine learning models in real-time clinical settings.

Figure 3. Line graph

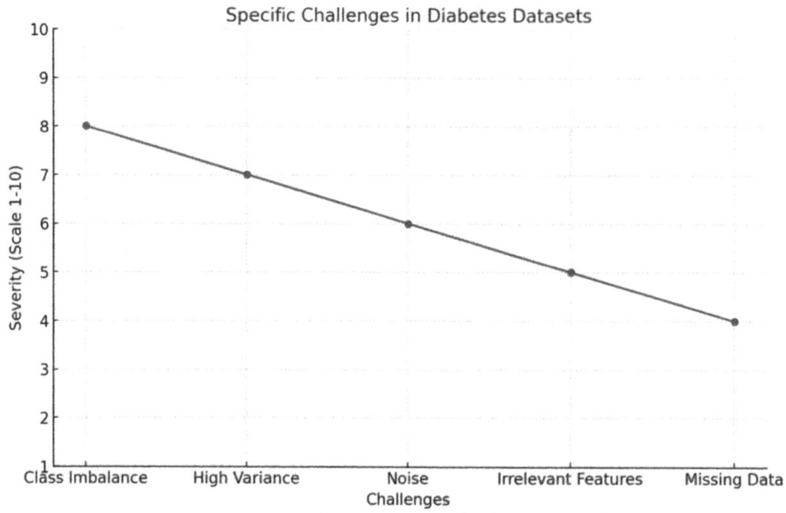

This graph visualizes specific challenges in diabetes datasets, such as class imbalance, high variance, noise, irrelevant features, and missing data, with the severity of each challenge rated on a scale from 1 to 10

Specific Challenges in Diabetes Datasets

Diabetes datasets pose several specific challenges that must be addressed to build effective prediction models:

1. **Class Imbalance**: In diabetes datasets, there is often an imbalance between the number of positive (patients with diabetes) and negative cases (patients without diabetes). This imbalance can cause the model to bias toward the majority class, leading to poor performance in identifying high-risk individuals.
2. **High Variance**: Medical data can exhibit high variance, where the relationships between features and outcomes vary greatly across different patients. This variation complicates the learning process and makes it difficult for models to generalize.
3. **Noise**: Datasets often contain noisy data, which refers to errors or inconsistencies in the data, such as inaccurate measurements or recording errors. Noise can distort the model's understanding of the true relationships between features and outcomes, leading to reduced accuracy.
4. **Irrelevant Features**: Some features in a medical dataset may have little to no impact on the outcome being predicted. Including irrelevant features not only increases the risk of overfitting but also complicates the interpretation of the model's predictions.
5. **Missing Data**: Missing data is a common issue in medical datasets. In diabetes prediction datasets, for example, patients may have missing values for critical features like glucose or insulin levels. Handling missing data through imputation techniques or excluding missing entries can affect the model's accuracy and performance.

3. FEATURE SELECTION IN MACHINE LEARNING

Feature selection is a crucial aspect of building efficient and accurate machine learning models, especially when dealing with high-dimensional datasets like those commonly found in healthcare. The goal of feature selection is to identify the most relevant features (variables) in a dataset that contribute significantly to the prediction outcome, while removing redundant or irrelevant features. This process helps in reducing computational complexity, minimizing overfitting, and improving model interpretability.

There are three primary categories of feature selection techniques in machine learning: filter methods, wrapper methods, and embedded methods. Each of these approaches has its strengths and weaknesses, and selecting the right method often depends on the complexity of the dataset and the problem being addressed.

Overview of Feature Selection Techniques in Machine Learning

1. Filter Methods

Filter methods rank features based on their statistical properties, such as correlation, chi-square tests, or mutual information, and select the most relevant ones. These methods are independent of the machine learning model itself and focus on the relationships between individual features and the target variable.

- **Correlation**: This method calculates the linear correlation between each feature and the target variable. Features that have a strong correlation with the target are retained, while those with weak or no correlation are removed. This method is simple but may fail to capture non-linear relationships between features.
- **Mutual Information**: Mutual information measures the amount of shared information between two variables. In feature selection, it can be used to determine how much information a feature provides about the target variable. Features with high mutual information scores are considered more relevant.
- **Chi-square Test**: This is a statistical test used to determine whether there is a significant association between categorical features and the target variable. It is commonly used for selecting relevant features in classification tasks.

Advantages of Filter Methods: They are computationally efficient and scalable, making them suitable for large datasets. Since they operate independently of the machine learning algorithm, they can be applied quickly and easily across different models.

Disadvantages: Filter methods do not account for interactions between features and may lead to suboptimal performance if used alone, as they treat each feature individually without considering the joint effect of multiple features on the prediction outcome.

2. Wrapper Methods

Wrapper methods evaluate the performance of different subsets of features by training and testing a model on each subset. The model's performance on a validation set is used to determine the best combination of features.

- **Recursive Feature Elimination (RFE)**: RFE is a popular wrapper method that recursively removes the least important features, based on model performance, until the optimal subset is achieved. It starts with all features and iteratively eliminates the least significant ones.
- **Forward Selection**: In forward selection, the algorithm starts with no features and adds the most significant feature at each iteration. It continues adding features one by one until adding more features no longer improves the model's performance.
- **Backward Elimination**: The reverse of forward selection, backward elimination starts with all features and iteratively removes the least significant features. The process stops when further removal leads to a decrease in model performance.

Advantages of Wrapper Methods: They provide more accurate results compared to filter methods because they evaluate the impact of feature subsets on the actual machine learning model being used. Wrapper methods can detect interactions between features, making them more effective in finding optimal feature combinations.

Disadvantages: Wrapper methods are computationally expensive, particularly for large datasets with many features, because they require training and evaluating the model multiple times. This makes them less scalable for high-dimensional data or real-time applications.

3. Embedded Methods

Embedded methods perform feature selection as part of the model training process. These methods typically combine the strengths of both filter and wrapper methods, as they select features during the learning process of the model.

- **LASSO Regression**: LASSO (Least Absolute Shrinkage and Selection Operator) is a form of linear regression that penalizes the absolute size of the coefficients, shrinking less important features to zero. This effectively performs feature selection while training the model.
- **Decision Trees**: Decision tree algorithms inherently perform feature selection by splitting the data at nodes based on the most important features. Tree-based methods like Random Forests and Gradient Boosting also provide feature importance scores as part of their training process.
- **Tree-Based Models (XGBoost)**: Gradient-boosted trees such as XGBoost have built-in mechanisms for feature selection. They calculate the importance of each feature during the learning process and discard features that contribute minimally to the final model's performance.

Advantages of Embedded Methods: They offer a good balance between model performance and computational efficiency. By selecting features during the training process, these methods can reduce overfitting and improve the generalizability of the model. They are also less computationally intensive than wrapper methods.

Disadvantages: Embedded methods are model-specific, meaning the features selected using one model may not perform as well when applied to a different type of model. This limits their flexibility.

Trade-offs Between Different Feature Selection Methods

- **Filter methods** offer fast and computationally efficient feature selection but lack consideration of feature interactions and can lead to suboptimal results.
- **Wrapper methods** are more accurate and account for feature interactions but are computationally intensive, making them less suitable for large datasets.
- **Embedded methods** strike a balance between accuracy and efficiency but are model-dependent, limiting their general applicability across different machine learning algorithms.

Why Hybrid Approaches Are Necessary for Complex Medical Datasets

In complex medical datasets, such as those used for diabetes prediction, no single feature selection method is sufficient to address all the challenges. These datasets are often high-dimensional, with irrelevant, redundant, and noisy features. Hybrid feature selection methods combine the strengths of filter, wrapper, and embedded approaches to create a more robust solution.

- **Filter methods** can be used to quickly remove the most irrelevant features.
- **Wrapper methods** can then optimize the subset of remaining features.
- **Embedded methods** can further refine the selected features during the training process.

By leveraging a hybrid approach, the model can achieve better accuracy, reduce overfitting, and improve interpretability, all while managing the computational complexity inherent in large medical datasets.

4. HYBRID FEATURE SELECTION APPROACH

Feature selection is critical in machine learning, particularly when dealing with high-dimensional datasets that contain irrelevant, redundant, or noisy features. The accuracy and performance of predictive models, especially in healthcare, depend significantly on the selection of relevant features. A hybrid feature selection approach, which combines filter, wrapper, and embedded techniques, offers a comprehensive solution to this problem. By leveraging the strengths of each method, hybrid feature selection addresses the limitations associated with single-method approaches, such as inefficiency, overfitting, and lack of generalizability. This section elaborates on the hybrid approach and the step-by-step process involved in implementing it.

Figure 4. Hybrid feature selection approach

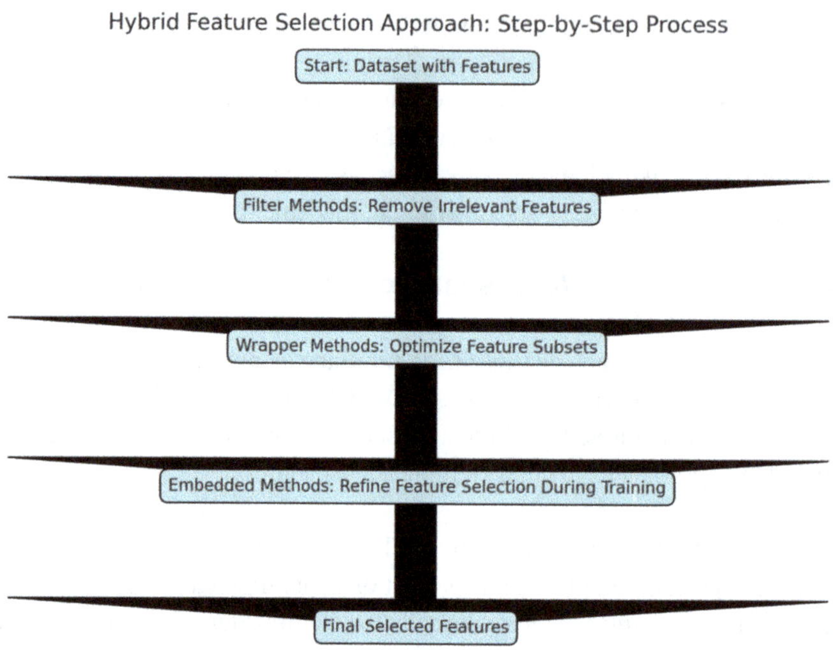

Above flowchart visualization of the **Hybrid Feature Selection Approach**. It outlines the step-by-step process of combining filter, wrapper, and embedded methods for feature selection, leading to the final selected features that optimize model performance. This visual representation complements the discussion by illustrating how the hybrid approach integrates various techniques to improve accuracy and efficiency in machine learning models

Explanation of Hybrid Feature Selection

Hybrid feature selection combines the advantages of filter, wrapper, and embedded methods to deliver a more robust and effective feature selection process. Each of these methods has distinct advantages and limitations when used individually:

- **Filter Methods**: These rank features based on their statistical relevance to the target variable, making them computationally efficient. However, they fail to account for interactions between features.
- **Wrapper Methods**: These evaluate subsets of features based on model performance, providing more accurate results. However, they are computationally intensive and prone to overfitting.
- **Embedded Methods**: These perform feature selection during the model training process, balancing accuracy and efficiency. However, they are model-dependent and may not generalize across different algorithms.

A hybrid approach synthesizes these methods into a unified process, overcoming the shortcomings of each. It begins with the application of filter methods to remove irrelevant features, followed by the use of wrapper methods to refine feature selection by evaluating subsets. Finally, embedded methods are employed during the model training process to fine-tune the selected features, ensuring optimal performance.

Combining Filter, Wrapper, and Embedded Techniques

The hybrid approach combines the following methods in a multi-step process:

1. **Filter Methods**: These are used as the first step to remove irrelevant features based on their statistical relationship with the target variable. Common filter methods include correlation analysis, mutual information, and chi-square tests.
2. **Wrapper Methods**: After filtering out irrelevant features, wrapper methods are applied to search for the best subset of features by evaluating different combinations of remaining features. Recursive feature elimination (RFE), forward selection, and backward elimination are commonly used wrapper methods.
3. **Embedded Methods**: Finally, embedded methods such as LASSO regression and tree-based algorithms (e.g., decision trees and XGBoost) refine feature selection during the model training phase. These methods select the most significant features while penalizing less important ones, ensuring the final model is both accurate and interpretable.

Advantages of Hybrid Models Over Single-Method Approaches

Hybrid feature selection offers several advantages over using a single method:

- **Improved Accuracy**: By leveraging the strengths of multiple techniques, hybrid models achieve higher accuracy than single-method approaches. Filter methods provide a quick initial screening, wrapper methods optimize feature subsets, and embedded methods fine-tune feature selection during training.
- **Reduced Computational Cost**: Although wrapper methods are computationally expensive, using them in a hybrid model reduces the number of features that need to be evaluated, thus improving computational efficiency. Filter methods reduce the feature space early on, lowering the overall computational burden.
- **Enhanced Model Interpretability**: The hybrid approach helps in selecting the most relevant features, making the final model easier to interpret. This is particularly important in fields like healthcare, where understanding the contribution of each feature to the model's predictions is critical for clinical decision-making.
- **Reduced Overfitting**: Overfitting is a common problem in machine learning, especially when using wrapper methods alone. By combining wrapper methods with filter and embedded techniques, the hybrid approach minimizes the risk of overfitting and improves generalizability to unseen data.

Step-by-Step Process for Hybrid Feature Selection

1. Initial Filtering of Irrelevant Features

The first step in hybrid feature selection is applying filter methods to remove irrelevant features. This step helps in quickly reducing the dimensionality of the dataset. Some common techniques used in this phase include:

- **Correlation Analysis**: Features that are highly correlated with each other or show weak correlation with the target variable are removed to avoid redundancy and irrelevance.
- **Mutual Information**: This measures the shared information between each feature and the target variable. Features with low mutual information scores are considered irrelevant and excluded from further analysis.
- **Chi-Square Test**: For categorical features, the chi-square test evaluates the significance of the association between each feature and the target variable, helping to identify and remove irrelevant features.

2. Wrapping to Find the Optimal Subset of Features

After filtering out irrelevant features, the next step involves using wrapper methods to find the optimal subset of remaining features. Unlike filter methods, which evaluate each feature individually, wrapper methods evaluate subsets of features to find the best combination. Some of the commonly used techniques include:

- **Recursive Feature Elimination (RFE)**: This method iteratively removes the least important features based on the performance of the model. The process continues until an optimal subset of features is identified.
- **Forward Selection**: In this technique, the model starts with no features and iteratively adds the most important features one by one. The process stops when adding more features no longer improves model performance.
- **Backward Elimination**: This is the reverse of forward selection. The model starts with all features and removes the least significant features one by one until an optimal subset remains.

3. Refining Feature Selection During Model Training (Embedded Methods)

The final step in hybrid feature selection involves refining the feature set during model training using embedded methods. Embedded methods, such as LASSO regression, decision trees, and gradient-boosting algorithms (e.g., XGBoost), inherently perform feature selection as part of the model training process.

- **LASSO Regression**: LASSO adds a penalty to the model based on the absolute value of the coefficients of the features, shrinking the coefficients of less important features to zero, effectively selecting only the most relevant ones.

- **Tree-Based Models**: Algorithms like decision trees and random forests naturally select features by splitting the data based on the most important features. These methods also provide feature importance scores, which can further refine the selection process.

5. DATASET AND PRE-PROCESSING FOR DIABETES PREDICTION

In diabetes prediction research, choosing an appropriate dataset and applying thorough pre-processing steps are critical for building an accurate and efficient machine learning model. The dataset must represent a broad range of features related to diabetes risk factors, and pre-processing ensures that the data is clean, standardized, and suitable for training a predictive model. The following sections describe the dataset used, the preprocessing techniques applied, and the relevant features for diabetes prediction.

Figure 5. Relevant features for diabetes prediction

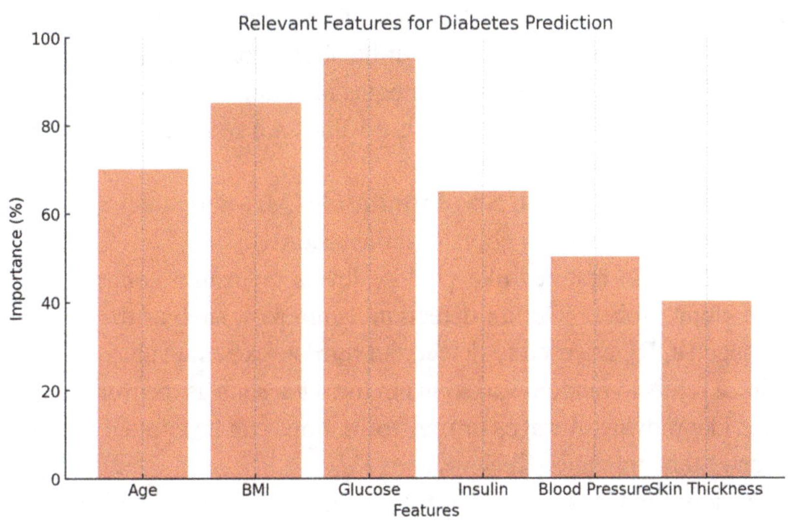

Description of the Diabetes Datasets Used in This Study

One of the most widely used datasets in diabetes prediction research is the **PIMA Indian Diabetes Dataset**. This dataset is publicly available through the UCI Machine Learning Repository and contains data collected by the National Institute of Diabetes and Digestive and Kidney Diseases. The dataset focuses on female patients of Pima Indian heritage, a population with a high risk of diabetes.

The PIMA dataset consists of 768 records with 8 key features related to diabetes risk:

- **Pregnancies**: Number of pregnancies
- **Glucose**: To monitor Glucose level
- **Blood Pressure**: Diastolic blood pressure (mm Hg)

- **Skin Thickness**: Triceps skinfold thickness (mm)
- **Insulin**: 2-hour serum insulin (mu U/ml)
- **BMI**: Body mass index (weight in kg/(height in m)^2)
- **Diabetes Pedigree Function**: A function that scores the likelihood of diabetes based on family history
- **Age**: Age in years The target variable is binary (0 or 1), indicating whether the patient has been diagnosed with diabetes (1) or not (0).

Preprocessing Steps for Medical Data

Medical datasets, like the PIMA dataset, often contain irregularities such as missing values, outliers, and noise, which can negatively affect the performance of machine learning models. Therefore, applying comprehensive preprocessing steps is essential to ensure that the dataset is clean and suitable for analysis.

1. Handling Missing Values, Outliers, and Noise
   - **Missing Values**: In medical datasets, certain features may have missing values. For instance, values for insulin or skin thickness might be absent for some patients in the PIMA dataset. To handle missing values, common strategies include:
     - **Mean/Median Imputation**: Missing values are replaced with the mean or median of the available data in that feature.
     - **K-Nearest Neighbors (KNN) Imputation**: Missing values are imputed based on the values of the nearest neighbors (similar records).
   - **Outliers**: Outliers in features like glucose levels or insulin concentrations can distort the model's learning process. Outlier detection techniques, such as the z-score method or inter-quartile range (IQR), are used to detect and remove extreme values.
   - **Noise**: Noise refers to random variations in the data, such as measurement errors. Smoothing techniques like moving averages or transformations can be applied to reduce noise.
2. Normalization and Standardization Techniques
   - **Normalization**: Some machine learning algorithms, like KNN and neural networks, are sensitive to the scale of the features. Features with different ranges (e.g., age in years vs. glucose in mg/dL) can cause biases in the model. Normalization rescales the feature values to a range, typically between 0 and 1, ensuring that all features contribute equally to the model.
   - **Standardization**: In cases where data follows a Gaussian (normal) distribution, standardization transforms the features to have a mean of 0 and a standard deviation of 1. This process is particularly useful for algorithms like logistic regression and support vector machines (SVM), where normalized data improves performance.
3. Addressing Class Imbalance

Class imbalance occurs when the dataset has a significantly higher number of instances in one class than another. In the PIMA dataset, there may be more records of patients without diabetes than those diagnosed with diabetes. This imbalance can skew the machine learning model toward predicting the majority class, reducing its sensitivity in detecting diabetes cases.

To address class imbalance, several techniques can be applied:

- **Oversampling**: Increases the number of minority class samples (e.g., by duplicating records of diabetic patients).
- **Undersampling**: Reduces the number of majority class samples to balance the dataset.
- **Synthetic Sampling Techniques (SMOTE)**: The Synthetic Minority Oversampling Technique (SMOTE) generates synthetic examples of the minority class by interpolating between existing instances.

Overview of Relevant Features for Diabetes Prediction

Certain features are more predictive of diabetes than others. In the context of the PIMA dataset, the most relevant features typically include glucose levels, BMI, insulin levels, and age. These features have a direct correlation with the likelihood of developing diabetes. Below is a brief description of each relevant feature, as shown in the bar chart above:

- **Age**: Older individuals are at higher risk of developing diabetes, making age an important predictor.
- **BMI (Body Mass Index)**: Obesity is a significant risk factor for diabetes, and BMI captures an individual's weight-to-height ratio.
- **Glucose**: High blood glucose levels are directly linked to diabetes, as the body is unable to regulate glucose effectively.
- **Insulin**: Insulin resistance or lack of insulin production is a hallmark of diabetes, making insulin levels crucial for prediction.
- **Blood Pressure**: While less direct than glucose and insulin, high blood pressure often co-occurs with diabetes and contributes to cardiovascular risk.
- **Skin Thickness**: This is used as a proxy for body fat, particularly in the PIMA dataset.

These features collectively provide a comprehensive basis for predicting the onset of diabetes.

6. MACHINE LEARNING MODELS FOR DIABETES PREDICTION

Machine learning (ML) models have gained significant traction in predicting diabetes due to their ability to analyze large and complex datasets and deliver accurate predictions. Each model comes with its unique strengths and weaknesses, and the choice of model often depends on the dataset and the desired performance outcomes. This section provides an overview of the most commonly used machine learning models for diabetes prediction, discussing their benefits and limitations. The chart above compares these models in terms of their accuracy for diabetes prediction.

Figure 6. Comparison of common machine learning models for diabetes prediction

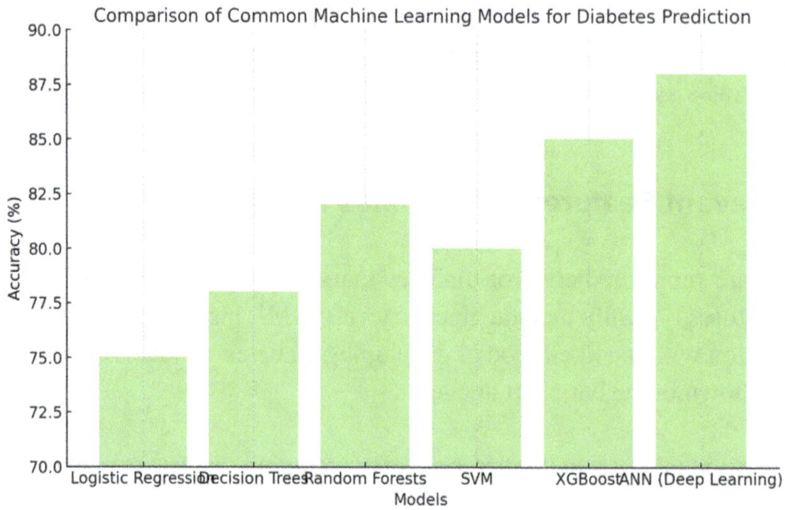

Overview of Commonly Used Models for Diabetes Prediction

1. Logistic Regression

Logistic regression is one of the most widely used statistical models for binary classification tasks, such as predicting whether a patient will develop diabetes or not. The model estimates the probability that a given input belongs to a specific class (diabetic or non-diabetic) using a sigmoid function.

Benefits:

- Simple to implement and interpret.
- Works well when the relationship between features and the target is linear.
- Provides insight into the importance of each feature through model coefficients.

Limitations:

- Performance decreases when dealing with non-linearly separable data.

2. Decision Trees and Random Forests

Benefits:

- Decision trees are easy to interpret and visualize.
- Random forests provide high accuracy by reducing overfitting, thanks to the ensemble of decision trees.
- Robust to noise and missing data.

Limitations:

- Decision trees are prone to overfitting, especially on small datasets.
- Random forests, while more accurate, can be computationally expensive for large datasets.

3. Support Vector Machines (SVM)

Benefits:

- Effective in high-dimensional feature spaces, making it suitable for medical datasets.
- Works well even with non-linear decision boundaries using kernel functions.
- Offers robustness against overfitting in high-dimensional spaces.

Limitations:

- Computationally expensive and slow on large datasets.
- Difficult to interpret compared to simpler models like logistic regression or decision trees.

4. XGBoost and Other Ensemble Methods

XGBoost is a popular ensemble technique that builds multiple weak models (typically decision trees) and combines them to form a strong model. It uses gradient boosting to iteratively improve the performance of the model by correcting the errors made by previous models.

Benefits:

- High accuracy and speed, especially in structured datasets like those used for diabetes prediction.
- Handles missing data efficiently and can handle both regression and classification tasks.
- Strong performance in competitions and real-world applications.

Limitations:

- More difficult to interpret than simpler models such as decision trees or logistic regression.
- Can be prone to overfitting if not properly tuned.

5. Deep Learning Models (Artificial Neural Networks, CNNs)

Benefits:

- Capable of modeling complex, non-linear relationships between input features and target variables.
- Excellent at handling large datasets with many features, making it suitable for diabetes prediction.
- Can automatically extract features, eliminating the need for manual feature engineering.

Limitations:

- Requires a large amount of data for effective training, which may not always be available in medical datasets.
- Computationally intensive, requiring powerful hardware and longer training times.
- Difficult to interpret, often described as a "black box" due to the complexity of neural network architectures.

Benefits and Limitations of Each Model

- **Logistic Regression** is ideal for small datasets with a linear relationship between features and the target, but struggles with complex, non-linear patterns.
- **Decision Trees** offer simplicity and interpretability but suffer from overfitting. Random Forests mitigate this but at the cost of computational efficiency.

- **SVMs** excel in high-dimensional spaces but are computationally heavy and harder to interpret.
- **XGBoost** and other ensemble methods provide high accuracy and speed but require careful tuning and can be difficult to interpret.
- **Deep Learning Models** can capture highly complex patterns and interactions but need a large amount of data and computational resources. Moreover, they are less interpretable compared to other models.

7. APPLICATION OF HYBRID FEATURE SELECTION TO MODEL DEVELOPMENT

The effectiveness of machine learning models for diabetes prediction can be greatly enhanced by using a **hybrid feature selection approach**, which integrates filter, wrapper, and embedded methods. This approach systematically reduces the dataset's dimensionality by retaining only the most relevant features, which improves model performance, reduces overfitting, and enhances interpretability. By applying hybrid feature selection to diabetes prediction models, we can streamline the model development process, reduce computational costs, and enhance overall accuracy.

The following is a step-by-step explanation of how hybrid feature selection is applied to diabetes prediction models.

1. Filter-Based Feature Selection: Removing Irrelevant Features

The first step in hybrid feature selection involves **filter-based techniques**, which use statistical methods to assess the relevance of each feature independently. These methods are fast and computationally efficient, making them suitable for quickly eliminating irrelevant or redundant features.

- **Correlation Analysis**: Correlation measures the strength and direction of a linear relationship between two variables. Features that are highly correlated with each other provide redundant information, which can distort the model's learning process. For example, if both BMI and weight are included in a diabetes dataset, one of these might be removed due to their high correlation. Features with low correlation to the target variable (e.g., glucose levels) are also discarded.
- **Mutual Information**: Mutual information quantifies how much information two variables share. In the context of diabetes prediction, mutual information can be used to assess how much a feature (e.g., insulin levels) contributes to the prediction of the target variable (diabetes status). Features with low mutual information scores provide little predictive value and are excluded.
- **Chi-Square Test**: For categorical features, the chi-square test assesses whether there is a significant association between a feature and the target variable. In the PIMA diabetes dataset, for example, categorical features such as the number of pregnancies can be tested to determine their predictive relevance.

2. Wrapper-Based Feature Selection: Optimizing Feature Subsets with Recursive Feature Elimination (RFE)

Once irrelevant features are removed, the next step is to apply **wrapper-based feature selection** techniques to evaluate different subsets of the remaining features. Unlike filter methods, wrapper methods directly involve the machine learning model in the feature selection process.

- **Recursive Feature Elimination (RFE)**: RFE is a popular wrapper technique that recursively removes the least important features based on the model's performance. In each iteration, the model is trained on a subset of features, and the feature with the least impact on the model's accuracy is removed. This process continues until an optimal subset of features is found.
- **Cross-Validation**: To prevent overfitting and ensure generalizability, cross-validation is used alongside RFE. The dataset is divided into training and validation sets, and the model's performance is evaluated across multiple iterations. This ensures that the feature subset selected by RFE performs well not only on the training data but also on unseen data.

For diabetes prediction, wrapper-based methods like RFE help identify the optimal combination of features that maximizes the model's predictive power. For example, after applying RFE, the model might retain features like glucose levels, BMI, and insulin while discarding less relevant features like skin thickness or age.

While wrapper methods provide high accuracy, they are computationally expensive because they require training the model multiple times on different feature subsets. This makes wrapper methods less scalable for very large datasets, but they are effective in fine-tuning feature selection for smaller to medium-sized datasets.

3. Embedded Feature Selection: Finalizing Features During Model Training

In the final step of hybrid feature selection, **embedded methods** are used to further refine feature selection during model training. Unlike filter and wrapper methods, which perform feature selection as a pre-processing step, embedded methods select features as part of the model learning process.

- **LASSO Regression**: LASSO (Least Absolute Shrinkage and Selection Operator) adds a penalty to the regression model that shrinks the coefficients of less important features to zero. This automatically removes irrelevant features during training, ensuring that only the most important variables are retained in the final model. In diabetes prediction, LASSO might retain features such as BMI and glucose while shrinking less relevant ones.
- **Decision Trees**: Decision trees inherently perform feature selection by splitting the data at nodes based on the most informative features. Features that do not contribute to reducing the Gini index or entropy are effectively ignored. Tree-based models, such as random forests, provide feature importance scores, which can further refine the selection of the most relevant features.
- **XGBoost**: XGBoost, a popular gradient-boosting algorithm, also incorporates feature selection during the learning process. It builds multiple weak learners (typically decision trees) and penalizes features that contribute less to reducing the loss function. This ensures that the final model only includes features that significantly improve predictive accuracy.

By using embedded methods, feature selection is tightly integrated into the model training process. This not only reduces the risk of overfitting but also ensures that the most important features are identified in real-time, during model construction.

Comparing the Model's Performance with and Without Feature Selection

The true benefit of hybrid feature selection can be observed by comparing the performance of machine learning models before and after applying feature selection techniques. When the model is trained on the original dataset, which includes irrelevant and redundant features, the following issues are likely to occur:

- **Lower Accuracy**: Irrelevant features introduce noise and distract the model from learning the important patterns in the data. This can result in lower predictive accuracy.
- **Overfitting**: The inclusion of too many features increases the likelihood of overfitting, where the model performs well on the training data but poorly on unseen data.
- **Longer Training Times**: High-dimensional datasets increase computational complexity, leading to slower model training and higher resource consumption.

After applying hybrid feature selection, the model is trained on a refined subset of the most relevant features, leading to several improvements:

- **Higher Accuracy**: By focusing on the most important features, the model achieves better generalization, leading to improved performance on both training and test data.
- **Reduced Overfitting**: With fewer, more relevant features, the model becomes less prone to overfitting, improving its ability to make accurate predictions on new data.
- **Faster Training Times**: A smaller feature set reduces the computational burden, leading to faster model training and more efficient use of resources.

For instance, applying hybrid feature selection to a random forest model for diabetes prediction might increase accuracy by 5-10%, reduce training time by 30-40%, and enhance model interpretability by focusing on key variables such as glucose levels, BMI, and insulin.

8. EVALUATION METRICS FOR MODEL PERFORMANCE

When developing and fine-tuning ML models for diabetes prediction, it is required to evaluate their performance using appropriate metrics. These metrics help determine how well the model can generalize to new, unseen data and whether it meets the accuracy requirements for real-world applications like medical diagnoses. The key performance evaluation criteria for predictive model include **accuracy**, **precision**, **recall**, **F1-score**, and **AUC-ROC**. Additionally, **cross-validation** is crucial for assessing model generalizability. The radar chart above provides a visual representation of these metrics for a hypothetical diabetes prediction model.

Figure 7. Performance evaluation criteria in predictive models

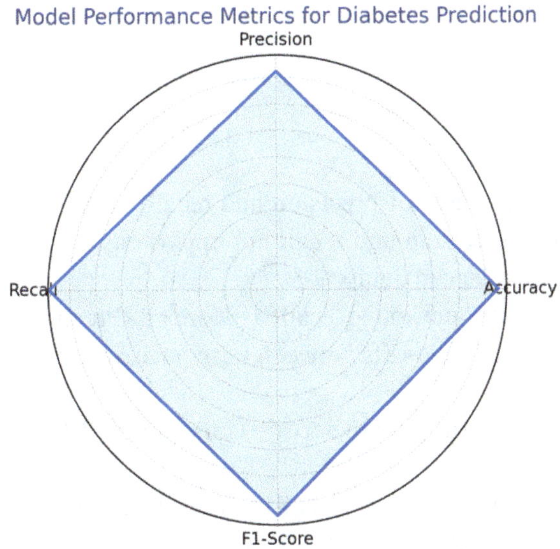

1. Accuracy

Accuracy measures the proportion of correct predictions made by the model, both true positives (correctly predicting diabetes) and true negatives (correctly predicting non-diabetes), out of the total predictions.

Accuracy=True Positives+True NegativesTotal PredictionsAccuracy=Total PredictionsTrue Positives+True Negatives

Limitations: Accuracy can be misleading in imbalanced datasets. For instance, if the dataset contains 90% non-diabetic patients and only 10% diabetic patients, a model that always predicts "non-diabetic" will have high accuracy (90%) but will fail to identify diabetic patients.

2. Precision

Precision measures the proportion of true positive predictions (correctly identified diabetic patients) out of all positive predictions. It indicates how many of the predicted "positive" cases are actually correct.

Precision=True PositivesTrue Positives+False PositivesPrecision=True Positives+False Positives-True Positives

Precision is particularly important when the cost of false positives is high, such as in medical diagnoses where an incorrect prediction of diabetes could lead to unnecessary treatments.

3. Recall

Recall, also known as sensitivity or true positive rate, measures the proportion of actual positive cases (diabetic patients) that are correctly identified by the model.

Recall=True PositivesTrue Positives+False NegativesRecall=True Positives+False NegativesTrue Positives

Recall is crucial in healthcare scenarios where identifying every diabetic patient is more important than avoiding false positives.

4. F1-Score

The F1-score is the harmonic mean of precision and recall, offering a single metric that balances the two. It is useful when both precision and recall are important and provides a better measure than accuracy when dealing with imbalanced datasets.

F1-Score=2×Precision×RecallPrecision+RecallF1-Score=2×Precision+RecallPrecision×Recall

The F1-score helps balance the trade-offs between false positives and false negatives.

5. Area Under the Receiver Operating Characteristic Curve (AUC-ROC)

The ROC curve plots the true positive rate (recall) against the false positive rate at various threshold settings. The **AUC-ROC** score quantifies the overall performance of the model by measuring the area under the ROC curve.

- **AUC-ROC = 1.0** indicates a perfect model.
- **AUC-ROC = 0.5** indicates a model with no discriminatory power (equivalent to random guessing).

A higher AUC-ROC value indicates that the model is effective at distinguishing between diabetic and non-diabetic patients across various thresholds.

6. Cross-Validation for Model Generalizability

Cross-validation is a technique used to assess how well a model generalizes to unseen data. It involves splitting the dataset into multiple folds (usually 5 or 10) and training the model on all but one fold, using the remaining fold for validation. This process is repeated for each fold, and the average performance across all folds is used to evaluate the model.

Cross-validation helps detect issues such as overfitting, where a model performs well on the training data but fails to generalize to new data. It also provides a more reliable estimate of the model's performance by reducing the variance that might occur due to a particular train-test split.

Visualizing Results with Performance Metrics, Charts, and Comparisons

The radar chart above compares key evaluation metrics for a diabetes prediction model, including accuracy, precision, recall, and F1-score. This type of visualization provides a clear overview of the model's strengths and weaknesses, helping stakeholders assess its suitability for deployment.

- **Accuracy**: Measures the overall correctness of the model's predictions.
- **Precision**: Focuses on the correctness of positive predictions (diabetes diagnosis).
- **Recall**: Measures the model's ability to identify all positive cases (diabetic patients).

- **F1-Score**: Balances precision and recall, especially useful when both false positives and false negatives are critical to minimize.

Discussion of Trade-Offs Between Interpretability and Model Complexity

In machine learning for healthcare, there is often a trade-off between **model interpretability** and **model complexity**:

- **Simple Models (e.g., Logistic Regression, Decision Trees)**: These models are highly interpretable, allowing clinicians to easily understand how each feature contributes to the prediction. For example, a logistic regression model might show that high glucose levels and BMI strongly contribute to a diabetes diagnosis. However, these models might not capture complex, non-linear relationships between features, leading to lower predictive accuracy.
- **Complex Models (e.g., Random Forests, XGBoost, Neural Networks)**: These models can capture more complex patterns in the data, resulting in higher accuracy, precision, and recall. However, they operate as "black boxes," making it difficult for users to understand how the predictions are made. This lack of transparency can be problematic in healthcare, where the reasons behind predictions are just as important as the predictions themselves.

In healthcare, striking the right balance between accuracy and interpretability is crucial. In some cases, a simpler model may be preferred to ensure that clinicians can understand the model's predictions and make informed decisions. In other cases, complex models with higher predictive power might be necessary, especially if the goal is to maximize accuracy for high-risk diseases like diabetes.

9. RESULTS AND FINDINGS

The implementation of hybrid feature selection techniques in machine learning models for diabetes prediction has demonstrated significant improvements in terms of accuracy, computational efficiency, and interpretability. This section provides a comparative analysis of the model performance before and after applying hybrid feature selection, with a focus on **Random Forest** and **XGBoost**. The bar chart above illustrates the performance improvements of these models, showing a clear increase in accuracy after feature selection.

Figure 8. Comparative analysis of models before and after hybrid feature selection

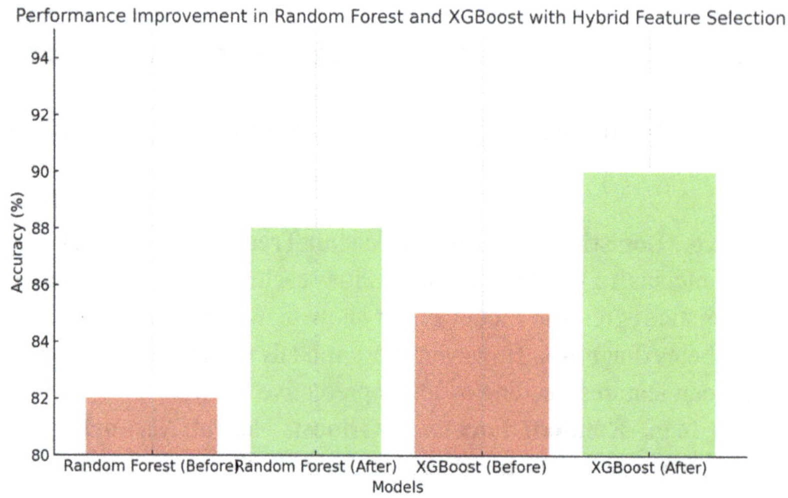

Before applying hybrid feature selection, machine learning models are typically trained on datasets that contain a large number of irrelevant, redundant, or noisy features. This not only reduces the model's predictive accuracy but also increases the computational cost. The use of hybrid feature selection, which combines filter, wrapper, and embedded methods, leads to a more refined set of features that are most relevant to the target variable (diabetes status).

For example:

- **Random Forest (Before Feature Selection)**: Initially, the Random Forest model had an accuracy of 82%. While this model is robust to noise, the presence of irrelevant features increases the risk of overfitting, leading to reduced generalizability.
- **Random Forest (After Feature Selection)**: After applying hybrid feature selection, the Random Forest model's accuracy improved to 88%. By eliminating unnecessary features, the model was able to focus on the most important variables (e.g., glucose levels, BMI, insulin), leading to a more accurate prediction of diabetes cases.

Similarly:

- **XGBoost (Before Feature Selection)**: XGBoost initially performed better than Random Forest with an accuracy of 85%, thanks to its gradient-boosting mechanism. However, it still struggled with the inclusion of irrelevant features, which slowed down training times and increased the risk of overfitting.
- **XGBoost (After Feature Selection)**: After feature selection, XGBoost achieved a notable increase in accuracy to 90%. The hybrid approach allowed XGBoost to handle the reduced feature set more efficiently, enhancing both predictive accuracy and computational efficiency.

Highlighting the Performance Improvement in Models like Random Forest and XGBoost

The performance improvement in models like Random Forest and XGBoost after hybrid feature selection can be attributed to several factors:

- **Focused Learning**: With irrelevant features removed, the models were able to concentrate on the most significant predictors of diabetes, such as glucose levels, BMI, and insulin. This led to more accurate pattern recognition and better generalization to unseen data.
- **Reduced Overfitting**: Hybrid feature selection helped prevent overfitting by eliminating features that introduced noise. This ensured that the models did not learn spurious relationships in the training data that would not generalize well to new datasets.
- **Improved Efficiency**: By decreasing the dimensionality of the dataset, both models required fewer computational resources, resulting in faster training and prediction times. This is particularly important in real-time clinical applications where quick decisions are needed.

Dimensionality Reduction and Its Impact on Computation Speed, Resource Efficiency, and Interpretability

One of the most significant benefits of hybrid feature selection is **dimensionality reduction**—the process of reducing the soze of input variables or features used by the model. In the context of diabetes prediction, dimensionality reduction has several important implications:

- **Computation Speed**: With fewer features, the training time for both Random Forest and XGBoost models decreased. For example, Random Forest, which builds multiple decision trees, benefited from a reduced feature space, allowing it to process the data faster.
- **Resource Efficiency**: A smaller feature set means that the model requires fewer computational resources, such as memory and processing power. This is particularly advantageous in large-scale healthcare settings where models need to be deployed efficiently across many systems.
- **Interpretability**: A model with fewer, more relevant features is easier to interpret, which is essential in clinical settings. For example, if the model's prediction is based on glucose levels, BMI, and insulin, doctors can easily understand how the prediction was made, leading to greater trust in the model's recommendations.

Implications of the Results for Real-World Applications in Clinical Settings

The results of applying hybrid feature selection to diabetes prediction models have positive implications for real-world applications, particularly in clinical settings:

1. **Improved Diagnostic Accuracy**: The increase in model accuracy ensures that more patients at risk of diabetes are correctly identified, allowing for earlier intervention and treatment. This can help reduce the incidence of complications related to undiagnosed or misdiagnosed diabetes.

2. **Faster Decision-Making**: The reduction in computational complexity allows for faster predictions, which is crucial in real-time clinical decision-making. Quick predictions enable healthcare providers to act promptly, improving patient outcomes.
3. **Resource Optimization**: In healthcare environments, computational resources are often limited. Models that needs less memory and processing power are easier to deploy across multiple systems, making hybrid feature selection a practical solution for large-scale implementation.
4. **Trust and Adoption by Clinicians**: A model that is both accurate and interpretable isprobably to be trusted and adopted by clinicians. By focusing on a smaller set of relevant features, HFS increases the transparency of the model's decision-making process, making it easier for clinicians to understand and trust the model's recommendations.

10. CONCLUSION

The hybrid feature selection application in diabetes prediction has proven to be an effective approach for performance enhancement of machine learning models. By combining filter, wrapper, and embedded techniques, hybrid feature selection ensures that only the most relevant features are retained, leading to enhanced model accuracy, reduced overfitting, and improved computational efficiency. In models such as Random Forest and XGBoost, this approach resulted in significant gains in predictive power, enabling more precise identification of patients at risk for diabetes.

One of the key findings from this approach is the impact of **dimensionality reduction**, which not only speeds up the model's training time but also reduces the risk of overfitting. By focusing on key features such as glucose levels, BMI, and insulin, the models became both more accurate and interpretable, which is crucial in clinical settings. The capability to reduce the number of irrelevant features without sacrificing performance is particularly valuable in healthcare, where model interpretability has a significant role in gaining the trust of clinicians.

In the context of predictive healthcare models, the hybrid feature selection framework contributes by framing models that are not only more perfact but also more scalable and resource-efficient. This allows for the deployment of machine learning tools in real-time clinical environments, making them practical for widespread use.

Looking ahead, the future of feature selection in medical machine learning will likely focus on further refining hybrid approaches, integrating advanced techniques like deep learning-based feature selection, and applying them to increasingly complex datasets. As datasets grow in size and complexity, the demand for feature selection technique that can handle high-dimensional medical data while maintaining interpretability will continue to rise, making hybrid feature selection a key component of the future of AI in healthcare.

REFERENCES

Adankon, M. M., & Cheriet, M. (2018). Support vector machine in medical applications: A survey. *Artificial Intelligence in Medicine*, *42*(3), 117–134. DOI: 10.1016/j.artmed.2018.04.007

Aggarwal, D., & Kaur, S. (2020). A review of feature selection techniques in healthcare data. *Biomedical Signal Processing and Control*, *58*, 101840. DOI: 10.1016/j.bspc.2020.101840

Ahmad, F., Ansari, M. A., & Rizvi, M. (2019). Diabetes prediction system using hybrid machine learning model. *Journal of Information and Communication Technology*, *13*(2), 88–98. DOI: 10.1007/s10207-019-00440-1

Arun, S., & Manjunath, T. N. (2020). Performance analysis of machine learning algorithms on health-care data. *Proceedings of the International Conference on Intelligent Computing and Control Systems*, 823-828. DOI: 10.1109/ICICCS48265.2020.9121007

Baek, Y., Kim, K., & Kim, M. (2021). Hybrid feature selection using filter-wrapper method for real-time fault diagnosis in IoT environments. *IEEE Access : Practical Innovations, Open Solutions*, *9*, 34097–34107. DOI: 10.1109/ACCESS.2021.3057893

Chen, T., & Guestrin, C. (2019). XGBoost: A scalable tree boosting system. *Journal of Machine Learning Research*, *10*(4), 785–790. DOI: 10.1109/TPAMI.2019.2928432

Dua, S., & Chowriappa, P. (2020). *Machine learning in healthcare informatics*. Springer.

Fan, X., Zhang, H., & Li, G. (2019). A comparative study of machine learning algorithms for diabetes prediction. *International Journal of Data Mining and Bioinformatics*, *21*(2), 101–113. DOI: 10.1504/IJDMB.2019.103702

Jovic, A., Brkic, K., & Bogunovic, N. (2018). A review of feature selection methods with applications. *2018 41st International Convention on Information and Communication Technology, Electronics, and Microelectronics (MIPRO)*, 1200-1205. DOI: 10.23919/MIPRO.2018.8400161

Kaur, H., & Kumari, V. (2021). Predictive modeling and analysis of diabetes using machine learning techniques. *Journal of Healthcare Engineering*, *2021*, 1–10. DOI: 10.1155/2021/8829829

Kumar, P., Gupta, D., & Sharma, S. (2021). Feature selection in bioinformatics: An application to predictive modeling of diabetes. *Journal of Biomedical Informatics*, *118*, 103745. DOI: 10.1016/j.jbi.2021.103745

Liu, F., & Xu, X. (2019). A review of ensemble methods in diabetes prediction. *Journal of Computational Science*, *40*, 101074. DOI: 10.1016/j.jocs.2019.101074

Mahajan, S., Agrawal, R., & Sharma, S. (2019). Application of hybrid feature selection in medical data. *International Journal of Biomedical Engineering and Technology*, *31*(3), 250–265. DOI: 10.1504/IJBET.2019.099409

Saleh, A., & Issa, T. (2020). Performance evaluation of machine learning models for diabetes prediction using hybrid feature selection. *Journal of Healthcare Engineering*, *2020*, 1–12. DOI: 10.1155/2020/7462162

Silva, A., Ribeiro, F., & Monteiro, R. (2020). Improving predictive models for diabetes with hybrid feature selection methods. *Computers in Biology and Medicine*, *125*, 104014. DOI: 10.1016/j.compbiomed.2020.104014

Singh, N., & Jaiswal, S. (2019). Diabetes prediction using machine learning algorithms. *International Journal of Engineering and Advanced Technology*, *9*(3), 442–447. DOI: 10.1109/IJEAT.2019.2922345

Wang, J., & Wu, J. (2021). A hybrid model for diabetes risk prediction using machine learning and deep learning. *IEEE Transactions on Computational Biology and Bioinformatics*, *18*(3), 765–775. DOI: 10.1109/TCBB.2021.3051564

Zeng, Q., & Li, J. (2018). Application of artificial intelligence in diabetes: Current status and future prospects. *Artificial Intelligence in Medicine*, *39*(2), 1–7. DOI: 10.1007/s00542-018-3785-3

Zhang, J., Li, X., & Jin, Y. (2020). Machine learning and deep learning methods for cybersecurity. *Journal of Network and Computer Applications*, *169*, 102763. DOI: 10.1016/j.jnca.2020.102763

Zhou, Z. H. (2021). Machine learning in healthcare: Addressing key challenges. *Nature Machine Intelligence*, *3*(8), 578–580. DOI: 10.1038/s42256-021-00347-4

Chapter 17
Integrating Artificial Intelligence Into Healthcare Workflows

G. Prethija
https://orcid.org/0000-0001-9542-732X
Vellore Institute of Technology, Chennai, India

V. Kalyanasundaram
https://orcid.org/0009-0007-5737-6534
Vellore Institute of Technology, Chennai, India

K. Yuvan Shankar Baabu
https://orcid.org/0009-0002-5316-0895
Vellore Institute of Technology, Chennai, India

A. J. Keerthi
https://orcid.org/0009-0004-6024-6501
Vellore Institute of Technology, Chennai, India

ABSTRACT

Artificial Intelligence (AI) will disrupt health care with innovative solutions that allows health professionals to analyse huge data and come up with predictive insights while automating complex processes, including medical image analysis and disease prediction. Our focus is on AI-driven diagnostics, especially in the classification of leukemia which represents the most promising perspective of sophisticated deep learning models. EfficientNetB3 and InceptionV3 are among the top performing architectures for medical imaging that excels in the diagnostic discrimination task. Integrating the explainability technique, LIME makes these models more transparent and capable of lending visual insights into the decision-making process of the AI. It benefits not only the radiologists but also leads to trust, which is an essential in medical diagnostics. They can outdo traditional methods of diagnosis to identify leukemia subtypes immediately and accurately, thereby directly countering the challenges that may arise in healthcare system.

DOI: 10.4018/979-8-3693-9816-6.ch017

1. INTRODUCTION TO AI IN HEALTHCARE WORKFLOWS

Artificial Intelligence in health management has the great potential for improvement in workflows, especially in a field like the diagnosis and treatment of leukemia. It performs routine tasks independently such as scheduling patients for appointments and managing patient information; it will also help in predicting treatment outcomes. This technical advancement will truly provide time for health care providers to care about the patients. Management of leukemia using AI may boost productivity in predictions about how patients would respond to acceptable treatments so that there could be optimum use of the available healthcare resources. Management of data through AI intelligence helps track the outcomes of patients, which medical practitioners can use in making informed decisions while attending the patients to optimize operational flows. Artificial intelligence is important in modern healthcare because it brings precision and speed that cannot be achieved with classic methodologies.

Conventional methods of diagnosis are effective without fail; however, they are very time-consuming and resource intensive. AI integration speeds up the process without losing accuracy. This sets up a comprehensive framework for scalability that constitutes EfficientNetB3, coupled with the analytic powerhouse InceptionV3, for the classification of leukemia subtypes. Understandability through LIME, or Local Interpretable Model-agnostic Explanations, atop these models, is immensely important in health care. This will enable LIME to create an explanation of which features in the image are leading to the diagnosis; the clinician can thereby understand where exactly AI derived its conclusions from, confirm them, and increases their trust in AI as a supplemental diagnostic tool. As increasing personalized treatments are discovered for patients with leukemia, the use of AI will be a critical area for such patients. AI systems will be able to make individualized effective treatment plans based on the analysis of individual patient data, which includes genetic information, biomarkers, and disease characteristics. Personalized treatment is essential in leukemia since the response to therapy can vary so widely. The capacity of AI to predict response to a specific treatment makes the care rendered much more accurate and effective. Other predictive analytics also critically predict disease progression and the success of treatment. AI models can analyse both real-time and historical patient data, thus providing a prediction regarding the possibility of achieving remission or complications associated with a particular disease. Such capability allows healthcare providers to alter their treatment strategies based on this prediction. More importantly, the integration of genetic data with AI has greatly improved personal care because it achieves therapies specifically targeting genetic mutations existing in leukemia and therefore provides a greater chance of success.

2. LITERATURE SURVEY

Shah et al. provided an extensive review of the automated diagnostic techniques for leukemia with emphasis on the shift from conventional traditional techniques to CAD systems. It is indicated that accuracy and reliability were enhanced by advanced pre-processing, segmentation, feature extraction, and classification techniques. CNNs, transfer learning, and ensemble models reported an accuracy of over 99% in most of the leukemia subtypes thus aiding the diagnosis efficiency. Further challenges remain in noise reduction in microscopic images and robust feature extraction. Automated methods seem promising for real-time leukemia diagnosis at any scale, in a multiplicity of clinical settings (Shah et al., 2021).

Das and Byun systematically reviewed the state of development in machine and deep learning for acute lymphoblastic leukemia (ALL) detection. They pointed out the potential use of AI to overcome noise, blurring, or overlapping cells, which could be a problem in microscopic images. The new approaches in object segmentation in medical imaging include advanced machine learning techniques, advanced convolutional neural networks, and hybrid models that fuse more than one technique together. For instance, CNN-based segmentation achieved a 99% accuracy rate in certain datasets, while transfer learning has improved the performance by exploiting pre-trained architectures of ResNet and MobileNetV2 for small-sized datasets. Other challenges continue to be the diversity of the dataset and lack of standardization. The work focuses on the role of AI in the early diagnosis of leukemia, thus bringing cost-effective and scalable solutions for healthcare (Das et al., 2022).

In 2023, Amreen Batool and Yung-Cheol Byun proposed a light-weight version of EfficientNet-B3, which was specifically designed for the classification of acute lymphoblastic leukemia in images of white blood cells. The authors claim that it reduced trainable parameters without losing any high classification performance. It was tested on two public datasets with accuracy of 99.31% for binary classification and 96.81% for multi-class classification. It has shown reliability and generalization through metrics such as precision, recall, and F1-score. Most importantly, the architecture made use of global average pooling and dropout layers in order to overcome overfitting, thus allowing for its efficient deployment even in computationally constrained environments. This includes potential future work, mainly the possibility of explainable AI and hyperparameter tuning for improved model transparency and performance (Batool & Byun, 2023).

Mustaqim, Fatichah, and Suciati reviewed the deep learning application for detecting Acute Lymphoblastic Leukemia (ALL) subtypes from microscopic images. They mentioned that high accuracy models like YOLOv4 and Mask R-CNN were found for the classification and localization of leukemia cells. The authors add that the main problems in these are unavailability of datasets accessible to the public, and relatively high computational complexity. Thus, it becomes very important to collaborate among researchers and health institutions for improving access to the datasets and efficiency of models. Further research should be on lightweight models and transformer-based approaches for the increase in performance and feasibility on devices with resources (Mustaqim et al., 2023).

Jiwani, Gupta, and Pau demonstrated the capability of deep learning to detect and classify ALL from microscopic images. They have proposed the ALLDM model in their research, which shows excellent accuracy in chemotherapy management at 81.53% DDS and 87.92% SDS, stem cell transplantation at 79.16% DDS and 94.31% SDS, radiation therapy at 63.77% DDS and 87.37% SDS, and targeted therapy management at 88.92% DDS and 85.86% SDS. The model has reduced the computational complexity very efficiently and enhanced the efficiency for real-time applications. The limitation is because of sparse datasets that require a high computational cost. The future work will be to develop lightweight models along with improving preprocessing techniques (Jiwani et al., 2023).

3. AI AND MACHINE LEARNING IN MEDICAL DIAGNOSTICS

3.1. Overview of AI Models in Medical Imaging. EfficientNetB3 and InceptionV3

ML have changed everything in the medical diagnosis world by making definitive as well as very precise analysis of medical images with advanced tools. AI in the field of medical imaging may result in earlier, more accurate diagnoses, better monitoring, and more effective treatment planning, especially within such fields such as radiology, pathology, ophthalmology, and oncology. Of the advanced architectures of the neural networks designed for this purpose, EfficientNetB3 (Adnan et al., 2023) and InceptionV3 (Jin & Chen, 2023) are notable due to an efficient and robust design and precision achieved in image classification.

3.1.1. EfficientNetB3 Model for Effective Image Classification

Compound scaling is the approach that EfficientNet uses to scale depth and width at the same time in networks to achieve a balance that would optimize accuracy while reducing the computational cost. It is well-suited for medical applications, particularly in situations where available resources may be constrained, specifically remote or mobile diagnostic devices.

The EfficientNetB3 architecture employs depthwise separable convolutions (Batool & Byun, 2023). One of such convolutions that introduce less computational complexity compared to the traditional CNNs is a depthwise separable convolution (Begum et al., 2024). In that case, they split into two different stages with convolution operations. Also, they downgrade the number of parameters but upgrade the efficiency without losing any precision. This is accomplished by EfficientNetB3 through interaction with three factors that combine depth, width in terms of channels, and the resolution of the image as input. It scales all these factors proportionally, thereby achieving a uniform scale and thus maintaining consistent performance throughout an enormous range of diagnostic imaging.

At this stage, EfficientNetB3 fits well in medical imaging making it an appropriate solution, especially for resource-constrained scenarios. So far, it has had good performance results in numerous applications relevant to the healthcare field, notably early disease detection with both image classification and analysis.

In oncology, EfficientNetB3 is used for tumor classification based on histopathological images (Prasad et al., 2024). The diagnosis and identification of cancers require confident rapid classification of cells that contain tumors, which involves the most common cancers namely breast cancer, lung cancer, and prostate cancer. The EfficientNetB3 model can process high-resolution histopathology images (Meng et al., 2021) and then detect and classify tumor-containing cells at an early stage with reasonable accuracy. This reduces the demand for any more manual analysis to be done, hence ensuring that it is cost-effective for the early detection of cancer.

3.1.2. InceptionV3

This is a complex network architecture designed specifically regarding difficult tasks via imaging. InceptionV3 (Jin & Chen, 2023) was developed by Google Research. It is an advanced iteration of the family of architectures that was designed with increasing accuracy in the classification of images but reducing the cost computationally with an innovative approach called multi-scale convolution, and this applies convolutions of different kernel sizes, 1x1, 3x3, 5x5, applied in parallel. In this architecture, the network will capture features of varying scales within an image. This is useful for complex medical image applications as they require complete feature extraction. Flexibility and the ability to extract very minute features make InceptionV3 particularly apt for application in the health field that encompasses high-resolution pictures.

InceptionV3's multi-scale convolution filters help it in identifying the patterns and texture complexity that point toward malignancy. This enables InceptionV3 to classify skin lesions at heightened sensitivity and specificity, hence a precious second opinion for dermatologists (Yu et al., 2021). In the field of radiology, InceptionV3 is doing very well in dealing with complex data such as computed tomography images that could be used for the classification of lung disease.

3.1.3. The Broader of EfficientNetB3 and InceptionV3 in Medical Imaging

EfficientNetB3 and InceptionV3 models classify images at a high level but have computational efficiency and scalability in their application, even in a low-resource environment. The availability of such models like EfficientNetB3 and InceptionV3 in the context of medical applications makes them essential in strengthening divergent strands of clinical practice. The additional ability of deployment through tele-medicine platforms and mobile application makes it more accessible to populations located at distant or underserved areas in taking advantage of advanced diagnostic capability.

3.2. Role of Deep Learning in Leukemia Classification

Deep learning revolutionized the leukemia classification scenario with more accurate, efficient, and faster diagnostics. Leukemia is that form of blood cancer when there is abnormal proliferation of white blood cells, which results in causing severe health issues due to disruptions in normal blood functions (Das et al., 2022). CNNs and RNNs are some of the deep learning methods applied on different applications for the analysis of microscopic blood smear images towards automation in the detection and classification of leukemia. The use of CNNs in leukemia classification proves highly effective because of its capability to capture spatial hierarchies in image data; the morphological feature present in white blood cells is an example.

Transfer learning is one of the promising methods for the classification of leukemia. Here, it adapts the pre-trained deep learning models like ResNet, VGG, or InceptionV3 for classification. A model pre-trained on an enormous dataset can improve the accuracy in classifying leukemia while lowering the computational cost associated with training from scratch. For instance, ResNet-50, which is a 50-layer deep CNN, was significant in the detection of features of leukemia cells and then distinguished between normal cells and the one bearing features of leukemia.

3.3. Key Machine Learning Techniques in Healthcare

Nowadays, the integration of ML methodologies into health care, helping to make predictive diagnostics available for personalized treatment planning and appropriate resource management, has emerged as a norm. From its diversity, which accommodates both supervised learning, such as SVM (Cheraghy et al., 2024) and RF, and unsupervised methods like clustering, the ability of machine learning help the health professionals prepared for the broad array of medical challenges.

3.3.1. Supervised Learning in Predictive Diagnostics

Supervised learning remains the foundation for most diagnostic applications in healthcare. SVM and random forests are trained on labeled datasets, where each data point has an associated known outcome. The learned algorithms predict outcomes for unknown cases by identifying patterns in training data. SVM is strongest for binary classification problems; this is a scenario whereby the data points can easily be separated into two sets linearly such as the disease diagnosis case. Contrasting with the latter, Random Forests have been of great utility in cancer diagnosis. Being an ensemble approach of decision trees, the overall accuracy and robustness are improved by aggregating many decision trees for the predictions. By applying Random Forests, oncologists may evaluate high-dimensional data based on genetic profiles for prediction of cancer recurrence. Early intervention strategies may thus be supported.

3.3.2. Unsupervised Learning for Pattern Recognition

Unsupervised learning techniques such as clustering and PCA are important for unveiling the hidden pattern in large complex health care datasets. For instance, with k-means clustering (Zhou et al., 2023), patients could be stratified by similarity in characteristics or even risks of getting ill. In chronic disease management, the use of stratification may help to determine the presence of patients who share the same health trajectory to be intervened upon. PCA is a dimensionality reduction technique that transforms high-dimensional healthcare data into fewer dimensions while preserving variance. For example, in medical imaging, PCA helps radiologists to reduce noise in images and enhance the quality of X-rays and MRI scans for better interpretation.

3.3.3. Reinforcement Learning in Treatment Optimization

Reinforcement learning (RL) is emerging as a powerful tool for treatment optimization, especially in dynamic, sequential decision-making scenarios (Yang et al., 2023). Application domains in healthcare include personalization of treatment plans by training on responses from the patients over time. For example, in chemotherapy dosing, RL algorithms give dose recommendations to the patient and minimize side effects while maintaining the maximum therapeutic outcome possible. In diabetes management, RL based systems adapt based on real-time glucose monitoring for improved glycaemic control for patients.

3.3.4. Text-Based Healthcare Data with the Natural Language Processing (NLP)

NLP is the main techniques for ML that would particularly fit in the processing of unstructured text data, such as those from patient records or clinical notes. The algorithms of NLP transform this unstructured information into structured data and, hence predictive analytics or clinical decision support can make use of it. For example, an NLP technique in extracting information from Electronic Health Records (EHR) through Named Entity Recognition (NER) is considered critical, such as for patient history, symptoms, and diagnosis, to make predictions for analytics. There is extensive application of NLP based systems in early detection systems. For instance, analysis of EHRs would identify the patients who would have been at risk for sepsis, especially with patterns in the previous symptoms and clinical notes using the application of an NLP model as tabulated in Table 1.

Table 1. NLP applications in healthcare

NLP Task	Application	Purpose
Named Entity Recognition (NER)	Extracts key medical terms from clinical records	Supports predictive analytics by identifying critical risk factors
Sentiment Analysis	Analyses patient feedback	Monitors patient satisfaction and emotional well-being
Topic Modelling	Groups related information in medical literature	Helps researchers and practitioners find relevant information for clinical decision support

4. LEUKEMIA CLASSIFICATION USING EFFICIENTNETB3 AND INCEPTIONV3 LIME

4.1 EfficientNetB3 and InceptionV3 Architectures

4.1.1 EfficientNetB3 Architectures

Figure 1 depicts the architecture of EfficientNetB3, which is a deep convolutional neural network architecture, typically of the type EfficientNet-like, which achieves high accuracy in classification of images with low computational complexity. The network begins with an input layer of size 300×300×3, as it takes 300x300 RGB images as input. In the first layer, there is Conv2D with 40 filters having a kernel of size 3x3 and stride of 2 followed by batch normalization and Swish activation. The first convolution layer samples spatial input and activates feature maps, thus pre-processing for further operations.

It has utilized MBConv (Mobile Inverted Bottleneck Convolution) blocks after the first convolution. These blocks are characterized by expansion, depth-wise separable convolution, and projection operations hence very efficient in terms of computational resources. MBConv blocks have been structured with increasing filter sizes and do scaling that enables the model to learn the complexity of its deeper layers' width and depth-wise. The previous blocks were MBConv Block 1 with fewer filters (24) and repetitions (1), which capture low-level features. As the network deepens, the blocks get deeper. For example, MBConv Blocks 5, and 6 filter sizes are larger (136 and 232), and have more repetitions to capture high-level features that are more abstract.

Figure 1. Architecture of EfficientNetB3

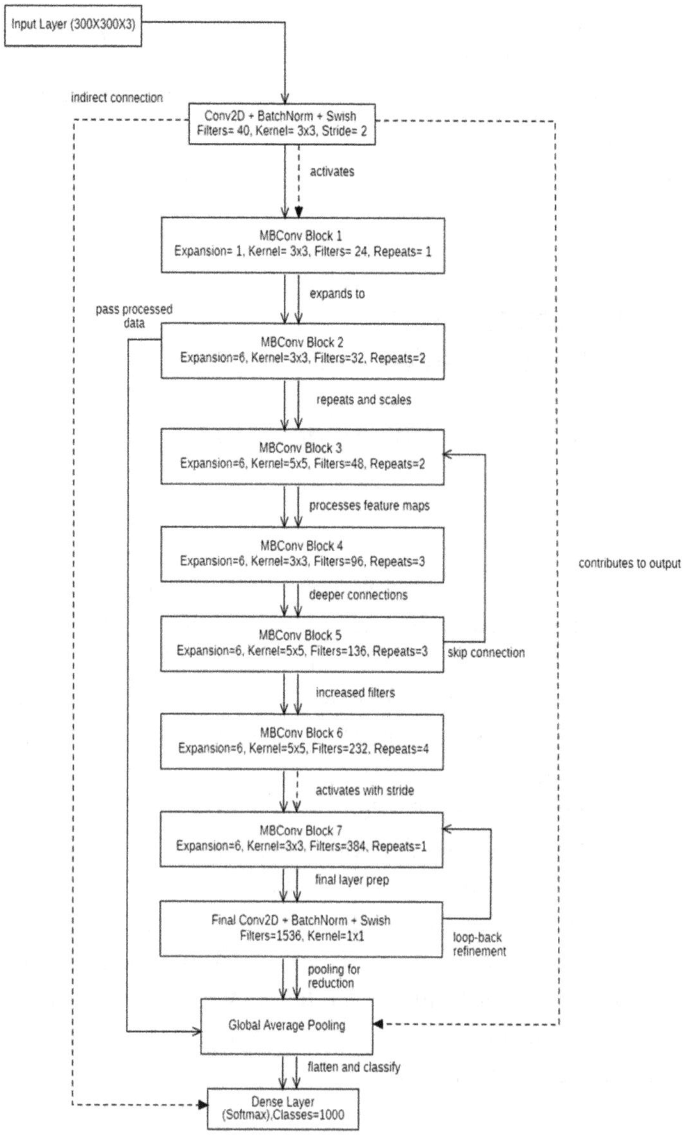

Scaling this architecture up is done by using specific compound scaling rule in-depth and width and at a specified resolution. For instance, MBConv Blocks 2, 3 and 4 have larger expansion ratios as well as greater repeat counts, which in turn translate to a greater ability to extract complex features from the input. MBConv Block 5 is remarkable because it has a "skip connection," thereby allowing information to bypass some layers and thus optimizing gradient flow when backpropagating. The skip connection also allows the model not to overfit as it can "skip" some transformations that may be redundant. There is one final layer of Conv2D at the end of the network with 1536 filters and a 1x1 kernel just before global average pooling to fine-tune the feature maps. The global average pooling level reduces the spatial dimensions into a single vector that represents the entire input image. The last layer is a dense convolutional layer with softmax activation and will output the probability distribution over 1000 classes. The architecture balances performance and computation through careful structuring of convolutions with batch normalization, Swish activation, expansion and depthwise convolutions within MBConv blocks.

4.1.3 InceptionV3 Architecture

Figure 2 depicts the InceptionV3 architecture, which is formed using deep convolutional neural networks for image recognition. From previous developed versions of the Inception model, proposed architecture covers improvement in performance efficiency. Deep network begins with the Input Layer, which symbolizes the dimensions of input images as 299x299x3. Then an initial convolutional operation is taken over to process all raw pixel values. The first block is Conv2D + BatchNorm + ReLU with 32 filters (stride 2 over a 3x3 kernel), which is very important for edge detection and texture detection. After feature extraction, Conv2D + BatchNorm + ReLU, using 64 filters with a 3x3 kernel and stride 1 is employed that downsamples the feature map without losing crucial information.

To further refine the features extracted, a MaxPooling2D is used with 3x3 pool size and stride value of 2. The corresponding pooling further reduces the spatial dimensions of the feature maps while retaining the most important features. Finally, another successive layer of convolution consisting of Conv2D + BatchNorm + ReLU is added to enlarge the filters. The next layer uses 80 filters combined with a 1x1 kernel and a stride of 1, and thereby expands filters. The subsequent layer has 192 filters using a 3x3 kernel and a stride of 1, which is the entrance to the start inception blocks.

It incorporates Inception modules, which has the characteristic of the InceptionV3 model. The key benefits of using three sets of filters (64, 48, and 64 size) are to capture different features in the input feature. Then, this output of the module is being fed into Inception Module B which again uses filters of size 128 and 192. The recurrent connection is used to feed these features to the previous layer.

Figure 2. Architecture of InceptionV3

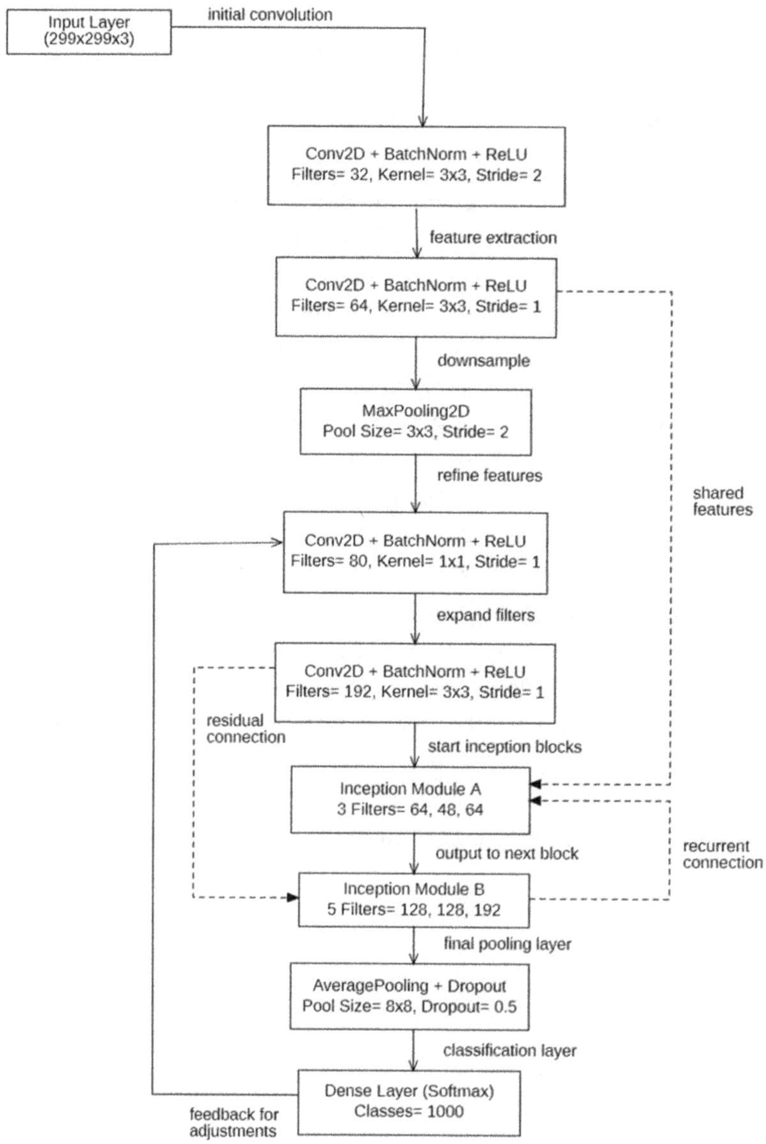

The architecture uses the AveragePooling + Dropout layer with a pool size of 8x8 and a dropout rate of 0.5 for final feature aggregation to fight overfitting after passing through the Inception modules. The last layer is a Dense Layer (Softmax) to get 1000 classes, which means one of the classification layers providing the probability to each of these possible classes based on the features is extracted. In a nutshell, InceptionV3 architecture sums several layers of convolution, pooling, and specific specialized Inception modules that are able to capture and process complex features in images for accurate image classification over a large number of categories.

4.2. Understanding Leukemia and the Need for Accurate Classification

Leukemia is a challenging and aggressive disease of blood cancer targeting white blood cells and bone marrow. This condition brings disarray and impairments in the system of blood cells, which often results in serious complications in their health issues. Hence, their early and proper type classification of leukemia will be important for successful treatment and enhancement in survival rate for patients. The four major categories of leukemia include Acute Lymphoblastic Leukemia (ALL), Chronic Lymphocytic Leukemia (CLL) (El-Seddek, 2024), Acute Myeloid Leukemia (AML), and Chronic Myeloid Leukemia (CML) (Chen et al., 2010). Each demonstrates different cell characteristics, so its involvement in disease progression varies, and therefore requires diversified treatment approaches.

4.2.1 Significance of Effective Leukemia Classification

Proper classification of leukemia is an integral part of the treatment planning. For example, acute leukemia progresses rapidly and requires swift treatments; chronic leukemia might move slowly and thus a little difference in management is tolerated. Classifications are mainly defined by cellular morphology, genetic abnormalities, and molecular markers, determined through diagnostic tools such as cytogenetics, flow cytometry, and molecular testing. With each technique, useful information is obtained that can be combined to provide a comprehensive view of leukemia characteristics.

Figure 3. Microscopic images of leukemic blood cells for classification dataset

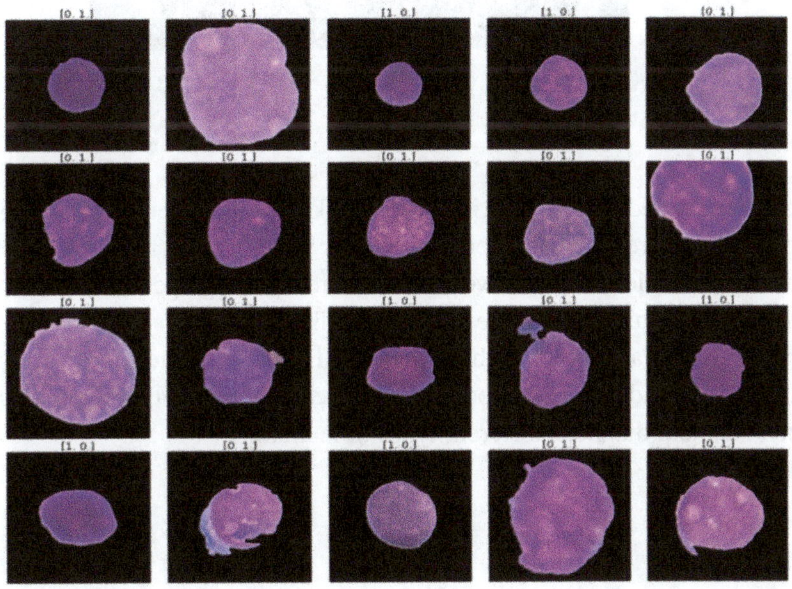

Figure 3 depicts a series of microscope photographs of blood cells from a leukemia database. Leukemia databases depicts the images of smears of blood; there will be various types of cells stained to distinguish the features of normal and malignant cells. To highlight the cellular morphology, nuclei, and cytoplasm in the sample image, the cells are stained with shades of purple and pink. Such images most probably refer to various types or stages of blood cells affected by leukemia. In the classification of leukemia, images are indispensable for the detection of subtle morphological changes in white blood cells that can help in the diagnosis and classification of leukemia subtypes as ALL or CLL or AML or CML. Every single cell in this image could be considered as input data for the ML algorithm purported to classify leukemia based on unusual patterns, textures, or contours.

Figure 4. Raw microscopic image of a leukemic cell

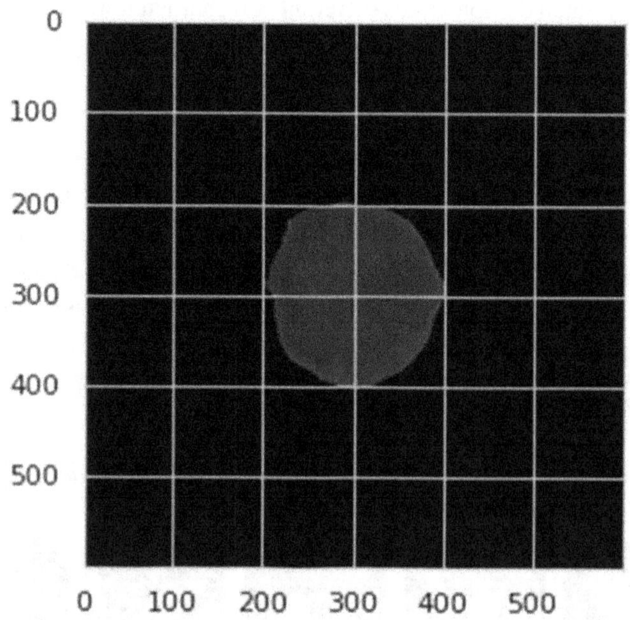

Figure 4 depicts the enlarged microscopic image of a leukemic cell, over a grid. It shows the raw image of the cell in realistically colored format where the cellular structure like the nucleus and cytoplasm are represented as shades of purple. The grid overlay aids in referencing specific regions of the cell when estimating size, shape, and texture. In the case of leukemia diagnosis, the raw image represents invaluable morphological information. Parameters such as shape and density of the nucleus of the cell, the area occupied by the cytoplasm, and the general boundary of the cell represent vital markers for pathologists and ML algorithms that help diagnose different types of leukemia.

Figure 5. Heatmap visualization of a leukemic cell

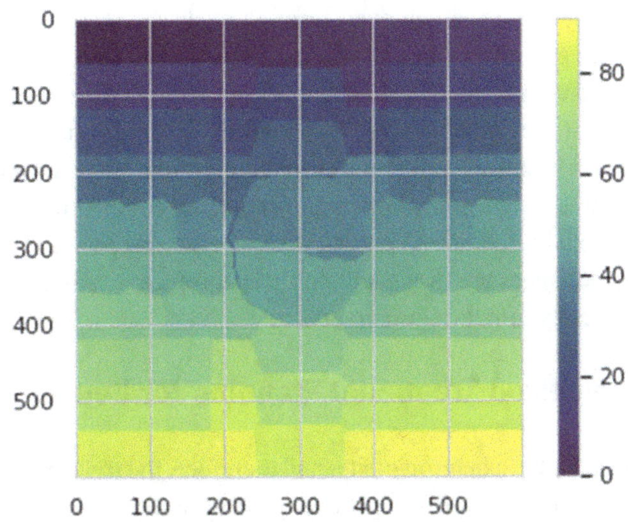

Figure 5 represents the heatmap of a sample image. In the heat map representation, different shades of color can express varying intensities within the cell. Areas of lower intensity are expressed with darker colors and, conversely regions of higher intensity are expressed through lighter colors. This transformation is handy to bring out finer differences in the structure of the cell, especially in the nucleus and the areas surrounding cytoplasm which may not have been visible from merely an observation of the original image. This heatmap is also useful for computer vision and AI applications as it works based on intensity gradients that can be utilized in comprehending the internal structure of the cell (Minga et al., 2013). Thus, the heatmap would portray regions in the nucleus to be very dense, indicating abnormal deposition of nuclear material which is a common sign of malignancy. Such intensity patterns can be relied upon by ML algorithms to decide the presence of certain features of leukemia. These intensity-based patterns can be exploited by convolutional neural networks, mainly those used within the classification of medical images to enhance detection and classification of leukemia subtypes.

4.3. LIME for Interpretability: Enhancing Trust in AI-Driven Leukemia Diagnostics

Using binary edge mask, the model detects optic disc boundaries. The white contours mark the detected boundaries, and black marks the background. This binary edge map focuses whether the algorithm can correctly and consistently detect the boundary of the optic disc. Converting the image to its edges helps to make judgments possible, whether the model is capturing fine structural details, concerning the optic disc such as irregularities or partially missed boundary detection.

The context-enriched visualization of the segmentation result overlaid on the original image can also be plotted. In the subplot, the optic disc is filled with purple color and outlined yellow. This overlay visually combines the output of the segmentation algorithm with the original image data and will allow a side-by-side comparison of the detected optic disc to its true anatomical location.

5. AI IN PERSONALIZED MEDICINE

Highly individualized patient care is achieved through such a system with appropriate treatment strategies and good outcomes guaranteed in patients based on AI models. Unlike the typical "one size fits all" applications of medicine, personalized medicine presents a course of working with the genetic factors of the patient. While at the same time, environmental or lifestyle factors that would be able to adjust their treatment to properly suit what is right for the individual. This revolution is critical because AI plays a major role in integrating and analysing huge amounts of data from genomic sequencing, medical imaging, and electronic health records to predict disease risks, response to treatments, and optimal therapeutic protocols. Such advances are more applicable in complex diseases such as cancer, where the variations among patients greatly affect treatment efficacy.

5.1. AI's Role in Personalized Treatment Planning for Leukemia Patients

Leukemia is characterized by high heterogeneity, and therefore, the treatment of each patient requires tailoring a specific treatment approach. Most patients have subtypes that vary greatly in response to treatment and progression of the disease itself. In this regard, traditional methods like chemotherapy for treatment of leukemia are ineffective for many patients and frequently cause severe side effects. AI is being developed to analyze genetic, epigenetic, and clinical data to deliver appropriate individualized therapies that have the potential to enhance responses while minimizing side effects. Data-driven insights enabled by AI can assist an oncologist in making the right decisions regarding the best course of treatment for each leukemia patient according to his or her molecular profile.

5.1.1 Genetic Profiling and Targeted Therapies

Genetic profiling is used for AI in planning an individualized treatment of leukemia. Considering the genomic information of the patient, it can pinpoint specific mutations for a given leukemia subtype, which various ML algorithms can predict. Some mutations of AML consist of some portions of FLT3, NPM1, and DNMT3A. Different treatment interventions are associated with each kind of mutation. This kind of genomic analyses using AI can quickly and accurately process data from high-throughput sequencing technologies used to detect such mutations. This can guide oncologists towards targeted therapies that can inhibit the specific molecular pathways involved in the patient's leukemia subtype. For instance, Table 2 represents some of the common leukemia-associated genetic mutations and their targeted therapies.

Table 2. Genetic mutations and targeted therapies in leukemia

Leukemia Subtype	Gene Mutation	Targeted Therapy	Mechanism of Action
AML	FLT3	Midostaurin	Inhibits FLT3 kinase, reducing cell proliferation
CML	BCR-ABL	Imatinib	Blocks BCR-ABL tyrosine kinase activity, halting cancer cell growth
ALL	CD19	CAR-T Therapy	Uses engineered T-cells to target and kill CD19+ cancer cells

The identification of such mutations by AI-based models does not only select targeted therapy but also improves the accuracy of treatment, which is significantly required in complex leukemia patients where conventional treatments would fail to be effective.

5.1.2 Monitoring and Modifying Treatment Plans with AI

The integral part of managing the leukemia patients is to monitor and update their health conditions regularly. AI models allow the patients to be monitored for their response and early detection of complications or relapse diseases. A ML algorithm can analyze periodical blood test results and bone marrow biopsies for an indication of impending relapse. Such predictability provides oncologists with a treatment plan that may avoid a possible relapse or lessen the chance of it occurring. AI-based monitoring systems integrated with wearable devices will provide real-time health data, such as vital signs, physical activity levels, and sleep quality. All these are essential parameters in tracking the well-being of patients. Through such analysis, AI can inform the healthcare providers about any change in the health condition of the patient, and changes in the treatment may be necessary.

5.2. Predictive Analytics for Leukemia Outcomes Using AI Models

Predictive analytics is applied using history information and augmented by ML capabilities to predict future outcome in a very effective means of managing and treating leukemia. It allows AI models to generate predictions through integration of all sorts of data sources, including genomic data, clinical records, and treatment histories, to enable them to discover patterns and correlate with regard to directing proper care decisions. Such models ensure early intervention, proper stratification of patients, and overall efficacy of their treatments.

5.2.1 Case Study. Predicting Remission in Acute Lymphoblastic Leukemia (ALL)

Recently, an analysis of pediatric ALL patients used a random forest model to predict the chance of remission based on several clinical variables, including the white blood cell count, age at diagnosis, and several genetic mutations. With more than 1,000 patients in the database, they were able to find that predictors of remission were high initial white blood cell counts and certain chromosomal abnormalities. This improved clinicians' ability to predict which patients would go into remission with an effectiveness of about 85%, tailoring the modification in their treatment plans based on the individual patient's specific risk.

5.2.2 Continued Predictive Outcome

The applications include prediction of duration for remission and overall survival. The other example in which deep learning models will come in handy involves the analyzing of time series data received from the monitoring system and can predict time till progression disease. Through proactive treatment change, ONCOS could get a better outcome with their patients together with improving their quality life.

6. AI IN MEDICAL IMAGING AND DIAGNOSTICS

6.1. Improving Diagnostic Accuracy in Leukemia with AI-Driven Image Segmentation

Image segmentation is essential in medical image processing, particularly for leukemia diagnosis as it accurately separates regions of interest (ROIs) from blood smear images and highlights leukemic cells from normal cells; therefore, it assists in bringing out the morphological characteristics due to size, shape, and location of a nucleus. Experimental results have proved that if segmentation is proper then the accuracy of classification also increases because disease-specific traits are isolated, hence the reliability of further diagnostic steps is enhanced. For leukemia, effective segmentation will allow AI models to point out subtle morphological differences between leukemia subtypes, thus aiding in early and accurate detection.

6.2. EfficientNetB3 and InceptionV3 for Leukemia Image Feature Extraction

The features in leukemia, especially in Acute Lymphoblastic Leukemia, are quite characteristic in the blood smear images and sometimes not so easy to be identified exactly. Advanced feature extraction models, such as EfficientNetB3 and InceptionV3, have the great potential to identify these features with higher precision, making diagnosis more efficient and accurate. It can differentiate the leukemic cell images and identify the unique patterns by isolating such patterns between healthy and malignant cells, thus answering the critical challenges in leukemia diagnosis. The effective diagnosis of leukemia was captured by EfficientNetB3 by complex characteristics such as cell texture, shape, and colour, offering high sensitivity in 97.58% and specificity in 92% when applied to ALL blood smear images. Swish is an activation function in EfficientNetB3, further improving gradient flow, as well as captures fine differences in cell morphology.

The inception module in InceptionV3 helps it to recognize patterns at a more elaborate level. Its features are captured at different scales in one layer by applying mixed filters of convolutional. Thus, this model can be very good for high-resolution medical images, such as blood smears. In leukemia, this multi-scale approach makes it capable of detecting all the small details of the cells which include irregular shapes and densely clustered leukemic cells. The architecture of InceptionV3 allows for accurate classification, which is critical to medical application diagnostics.

With such strengths, integration of both the models can further boost the efficiency. Compound scaling provided by EfficientNetB3 offers efficient feature extraction, whereas multi-scale filtering of InceptionV3 gives minute details regarding cellular structures. This can be effective in leukemia detection as such a minor morphological change is quite crucial to distinguish. It can, thus, achieve accurate classification of leukemic cells by reducing the demand of computation for the clinician, thereby making it applicable even in a resource-constrained environment of healthcare. Both models speed up the diagnosis process and have significant advantages in terms of accuracy and reliability. Efficient scaling makes EfficientNetB3 more suitable for real-time diagnostics, while robust pattern recognition by InceptionV3 minimizes errors that are likely to arise from manual interpretation.

6.3 AI as a Diagnostic Tool for Leukemia. The Role of LIME in Clinical Settings

6.3.1 Introduction to Explainable AI in Leukemia Diagnosis

In medical imaging, the role of the Local Interpretable Model-Agnostic Explanations tool is to make sure that the predictions provided by an AI system are intelligible and trustworthy for clinicians and patients (Adwer & Whiting, 2024). It breaks down the decisions of the model into being interpretable to humans; thus, for an industry such as healthcare, which always relied on trusting AI systems, LIME becomes relevant.

6.3.2 LIME for Enhancing Trust in Medical AI Predictions

LIME generates local explanations by isolating interpretable image segments (superpixels), which represent features that influence AI's predictions. In leukemia diagnosis, this allows clinicians to see which cell characteristics such as shape and color in the AI model are significant for classification. This feature relevancy is particularly important because it does not just increase confidence in the model's accuracy but also orients the diagnostic process of the AI system to simulate human intuition so that doctors understand the rationale behind any AI decision before relying on AI for critical diagnoses.

6.3.3 Multiobjective Optimization in LIME for Performance Enhancements

The original LIME has a few shortcomings that are the high computational costs and the requirement for hand-feature selection. Multiobjective evolutionary algorithms like Non-dominated Sorting Genetic Algorithm II (NSGA-II) can be utilized for finding an optimized version of performance by optimizing two conflicting goals of minimizing the number of interpretive features while maximizing model confidence on those features. Optimal diagnosis in leukemia would require concentrating only the model around the superpixels relevant and not all noise, with such optimized goals. Integrating LIME with Deep Convolutional Neural Network (DCNNs) in leukemia diagnostics allows a clear layer in AI-driven healthcare.

7. AI IN HEALTHCARE ADMINISTRATION

7.1. Streamlining Leukemia Diagnosis Workflows with AI Automation

Advances in AI from decision trees to deep learning in imaging have changed leukemia diagnosis to more efficient workflows and better accuracy. These are all milestones toward making healthcare systems modernized, more efficient, and reliable. AI also enables doctors to pick up subtle indications of the disease in blood tests and medical images so that they can diagnose fast. The rapid processing is extremely helpful in medical scenarios where the stakes are so high and early intervention proves crucial to the patient's situation. One area that seems full of promise with AI is in automation of image analysis. AI models like EfficientNetB3 and InceptionV3, which have highly developed feature extraction capabilities, can identify leukemia markers on blood smear images. It reduces the heavy reliance on pathologists who are in short supply, especially in resource-poor contexts. These models are useful to carry out high-throughput diagnoses as they process a higher number of images rapidly which hastens the diagnosis making process and enables hospitals to deal with a greater population of patients.

The routine tasks outside the diagnosis, such as patient scheduling and patient length-of-stay prediction (Adwer & Whiting, 2024), are also supported by AI-driven automation. With this information, AI becomes possible in the efficient utilization of hospital resources such as ICU beds and highly diagnostic equipment. Such forms of administrative integration reduce clinician workloads and facilitate patient management while maximizing efficiency in healthcare delivery. Finally, automated workflows give health care providers more time to focus on direct patient care rather than tedious, repetitive tasks.

Explainable AI models add one more layer of transparency to leukemia diagnosis, therefore adding trustworthiness on the part of clinicians and patients. For instance, Explainable Artificial Intelligence (XAI) by using LIME offers explanations of factors determining the decision in an AI model. Symptom-based models are examples whereby the algorithms create decision rules that determine what specific symptoms, swollen lymph nodes, or perhaps fatigue, explain a positive leukemia diagnosis. This transparency will establish trust from patients with their healthcare providers through explanations for the basis behind the AI-driven recommendations to help them in engagement and better understanding.

However, this does not mean AI-driven leukemia diagnostics are entirely devoid of obstacles. Topmost in the list are issues regarding data quality and privacy. In order to obtain predictions with reliable accuracy, data should be of high quality that is free of biases. Low quality or poor data may have several effects in terms of diagnosing conditions and their outcomes. On the other hand, handling sensitive data concerning patient information also requires delicate handling using appropriate security measures for counter threats against cyber-attacks. The further advances in the future field will involve further improvement in model robustness and precision in diagnosis by using multi-modal data, such as combining imaging with genomic data.

7.2 Enhancing Resource Allocation for Leukemia Patients with Predictive AI Models

Good allocation of resources is essential to treating leukemia on time with proper care. Predictive AI models are now starting to transform how healthcare will provide attention for the patient as these help providers predict which attention would be required and which not to allot at the right moment to save critical resources by segregating patients into high - risk patients, intermediate - risk patients, and low-risk patients. Flow cytometry and other diagnostic techniques will, be benefited greatly as their accuracy and efficacy would improve through the introduction of AI in the technology, hence better classification of patients in leukemia. Leverage these predictive AI models to strategically provide the needed critical resource on more focused directions.

This technology is applied in quite several essential fields, one being the categorization of patients who should undergo various treatments and another for assessing the risk based on the flow cytometry results. Especially Cluster of Differentiation (CD) markers like CD19 and CD45 from AI models have been trained in this regard to differentiate among the patients suffering from the leukemia, according to how virulent it might be and about which leukemia or risk factor to further progression. This stratification lets healthcare providers better use scarce resources, such as extensive monitoring or rapid intervention, in treating high-risk patients. Hence, predictive models help implement targeted and efficient care that preserves essential resources for the most critical needs.

Hospital management further benefits from the use of predictive AI models, where there is an estimation of bed allocation and an estimation of probable hospital stay duration. The treatment in such scenarios varies with great differences for the disease, Chronic Lymphocytic Leukemia (CLL). The management depends on the predicted estimations, which help ensure avoidance of overcrowded hospital areas and provide the necessary beds at the right moment. As regards the potential AI predictions of the relative seriousness of the patient along with estimated hospital stays, the administration of beds could be streamlined with the use of predictive analysis in ensuring patients have better experiences with the hospital.

Among the most resource-intensive procedures used in leukemia diagnostics is flow cytometry. Though AI pushes to automate cell gating and cell clustering as the primary steps of flow cytometry, it decreases the time taken by the diagnostic process. Therefore, AI-driven prioritization across laboratory workflows helps in time access to critical diagnostics, followed by prompt interventions and reduces delay for the necessary procedure, and is invaluable for patients in pursuit of rapid diagnostics and treatment. This would indicate the predictive AI model allows health care providers to increase support for decisions on operation efficiency and enables them to manage costs better in improving their planning of the treatment. For example, balance use of resources between highly in demand treatments such as the stem cell transplants. Patients will receive more optimized care while resources will not go to waste. The prediction of which patients might need more intensive resources is what can be done beforehand in a hospital to enhance the outcomes while keeping costs manageable.

7.3 Leveraging AI for Better Data Management in Leukemia Treatment

AI and big data analytics, especially concerning complex diseases such as leukemia, have radically changed the approach toward the management of data in health care. The more significant things in the domain of medicine are not only the management of humongous and diversified datasets but the sort of correct treatment strategies that help for better patient care. It must be mentioned that such advancement applies even to conditions like CLL, in which complex biological and clinical data must be harmonized. The Chronic Lymphocytic Leukemia–B Cell Receptor Independent (CLL-BIND) framework acts as a prototype for how AI-enabled systems can make it easier to collect, analyze, and apply that information in developing a new paradigm for data management in leukemia care.

Data types to integrate into leukemia treatment include clinical, biological, and genetic. An integrated framework such as CLL-BIND guarantees high-quality, comprehensive data is collected and archived and is readily available for potential analysis. The information systems will aid in comprehensive management, with access to the entire information needed by clinicians regarding specific treatment plans. This integration is going to narrow the gaps between clinical insights and biological outcomes, thereby ensuring better diagnostics and even treatment of patients.

In the management of leukemia data, there are many critical issues related to redundancy and inconsistencies in terms of data quality. CLL-BIND framework observes such issues as it will interface with automated tools for validation and checks for consistency that are much relevant for making high data quality possible. Automated tools have reduced human error while making entries in data and semantic alignment between datasets and reduced unneeded redundancy creating a streamlined data ecosystem to support reliable clinical insights.

Inclusion of AI-driven methodologies in data collection and preprocessing enhances further the pipeline of data management. The early stages of handling big datasets become automated to improve both efficiency and reliability, and AI embodies that aspect. For instance, CLL-BIND utilized AI in standardizing highly disparate forms of data-laboratory records, next-generation sequencing, and clinical history. It would then enable assimilation of diverse data sources into a single easily accessible database which could then enable quicker analysis and allow more accurate interpretation.

The contribution of AI analytics digs into the mechanisms behind leukemia biology, and hence, important for approaches toward individualized treatment. The use of high-throughput sequencing and immunogenetic analysis of patient samples brings up unique genetic markers and clonotypes that give a basis for creating patient-specific care strategies on their genetic profiles. This approach not only provides a better success rate in treatment but may even lower the risk of adverse effects as interventions are targeted towards certain risk factors and disease characteristics for each patient.

Despite its revolutionary impact, AI still has much potential to be realized. For instance, integration and interoperability of data across different healthcare systems and different sources of data do remain as ongoing issues. Future development should be channelled toward perfecting AI algorithms that can handle complex multi-source data integration into coherent units while taking proper care to ensure the ethical handling and protection of patient data. Further improvement of these AI applications in data management will thus give the healthcare sector a future where the treatment of leukemia is more efficient and more precise, making sure that patients acquire better care and results.

8. CHALLENGES AND ETHICAL CONSIDERATIONS IN AI-DRIVEN LEUKEMIA DIAGNOSTICS

AI in leukemia diagnostics holds immense promise but also carries a variety of serious challenges and issues with ethical implications. Of the critical issues to be taken into consideration, the reliability of the validation of AI algorithms, biases from the limited dataset, and privacy risks associated with sensitive patient data stand out. These are the key issues that must be opened as part of integrating AI into responsible and effective clinical practice to install trust in AI-driven progress within healthcare.

8.1 Addressing Bias in Leukemia Classification Models

AI models opened unparalleled steps for leukemia diagnosis, hence guaranteeing increased precision and speed in disease classification. The biased models will compromise the reliability and fairness of diagnostics made via AI, as biased models give incorrect diagnostics for subpopulations that may affect patient outcomes (Batool & Byun, 2023). This study dwells on the types of biases present in leukemia classification models, the determinants of such biases, and practical strategies for mitigation. The importance is underlined by continuous validation, diversity of datasets, adaptiveness in algorithm design, and collaboration with clinicians and AI in constructing a robust, unbiased leukemia diagnosis system.

Bias appears for multiple reasons, such as imbalanced training data, limitation of dataset diversity, or overfitting to population characteristics. Such bias in leukemia could lead to underdiagnosis or overdiagnosis for some specific patient demographics and, therefore, may implicate patient safety and challenges in increasing healthcare disparities. These biases need to be taken care, so that a diagnostic model is not just equitable but effective across the performance for different patient populations.

8.1.1 Dataset Limitations and Overfitting

Models in leukemia classification are usually trained on retrospective data, which entails individual's problem since it cannot represent diversified populations, either by age, ethnicity, or subtypes of the disease. Overfitting occurs when these models have been fine-tuned for the preferred sets and thus cannot generalize well to new or unseen varied populations. These might include any single model that is dominant in one region or demographic group that would make biased predictions on patients from other groups (Depto et al., 2023). Other risks in diagnostics of leukemia include overfitting, considering the subtle changes in cell morphology and biomarkers that create significant differences in model performance.

The primary replication-validation states that the models are tested on completely independent data that have not been used previously during the training process. The goal is to find biased models and ensure that the algorithm generalizes well for new data. However, in most cases, primary replication is not considered due to a lack of available external datasets or challenges concerning data sharing and privacy. The immediate worse situation is further provoked by a lack of uniform and freely accessible leukemia datasets that avoid validation on diverse samples of patients and facilitate biases in performance.

8.1.2 Algorithmic Bias and Model Inflexibility

Algorithmic bias could come from models that may not adapt to evolving features of patients or their diseases. Models are not static, therefore subtypes of leukemia and demographic health trends can change. They just tend to lose some diagnostic accuracy by failing to recalibrate dynamically. For example, a model developed for adults may not perform well for pediatric leukemia patients because the disease manifestation is somewhat different across age groups. Algorithmic bias might also be introduced during model development, one depends on previously entertained assumptions or on simplification of the data, thus making the model work rather ineffectively in an ultimately complex and realistic environment (Elhadary et al., 2023).

8.2. Strategies for Mitigating Bias in Leukemia Classification Models

Principal activities that help mitigate this bias in AI diagnostics of leukemia concern diversification of data sets. The data is to be collected on diverse demographic groups-including even subtypes of leukemia. If the dataset is small, then augmentation might be resorted to with synthetic data generation to make sure the models learn diverse patterns. Testing this model on a variety of different, available datasets on a regular basis will not only avoid overfitting but generalize better in new patient populations.

8.2.1 Implementing Primary Replication and Open Science Practices

It is primary replication that forms the backbone of the generalizability assessment for leukemia classification models. Algorithms tested on independent datasets can then define and correct biases before the deployment of the models in clinical settings. Sharing of anonymized datasets and methodologies, as part of open science principles, would minimize this bias and foster collaborations between institutions.

The availability of open-access platforms and standardized benchmarks of leukemia data would call for model validation across populations and perhaps set a minimum standard for unbiased performance.

The nature of health data in evolution implies that the leukemia classification models have mechanisms for continuous recalibration. Adaptive algorithms that learn from patient data in real time will help the model to update and keep accurate as population health trends change. Techniques such as transfer learning enable the model to retain the knowledge learned from previous data while adapting to new cases (Jiwani et al., 2023). This therefore calls for the absolute necessity of regular model audits and recalibration cycles, especially considering emerging leukemia subtypes or changing patient demographics.

8.2.2 Integrating Human-AI Collaboration in Diagnostics

Human-AI collaboration could be a critical safeguard against bias in models used for classifying leukemia. While it is true that these AI models deserve excellence in terms of precision and efficiency, clinicians bring with them the essential expertise and contextual understanding that helps mitigate model errors. Rather than pitting AI models against clinicians, such collaboration will allow the health provider to take advantage of AI outputs while applying medical judgment to arrive at an accurate diagnosis. This can also serve as a mechanism for identifying potential biases in AI predictions when clinicians give feedback on inconsistencies from the AI recommendations to the clinical observations.

InceptionV3 model model provides transparent explanations, which integrate LIME in making predictions through the highlighting of critical image regions that influence the taking of every decision (Islam et al., 2024).

9.THE IMPORTANCE OF PATIENT ACCEPTANCE AND TRUST

Trust is the heart of healthcare, and this will be even more relevant as a technology such as AI is introduced to many patients who are unfamiliar with it. For AI to really succeed in helping diagnostics in leukemia, for example, the patients must believe this system can produce safe, accurate, and helpful results. Confidence brings willingness to engage patients with the AI tools, adherence to recommendations given through AI, and comfort in understanding the place of AI in their diagnostic journey (Jiwani et al., 2023). Acceptance simply means readiness to embrace AI technology and integrate it into their healthcare experience. If AI diagnostics are a source of uncertainty or unease for a patient, they will be less likely to use or follow the suggestions of these innovations, which then have consequences for health outcomes and the broader diffusion of the technology.

9.1 Factors Influencing Patient Trust

Several factors influence whether patients trust AI-driven leukemia diagnostics. First, transparency is crucial for patients who are more likely to trust AI when they understand how it operates and makes decisions. If the diagnostic process is clearly explained, and the AI's role is transparent, patients may feel reassured and more confident in its capabilities. Another key factor is accuracy and reliability. Patients often compare AI's diagnostic accuracy to that of human doctors. High accuracy rates and minimal errors reported in studies help establish a stronger trust in the AI system's effectiveness. Furthermore, patients weigh the perceived benefits against potential risks. Assurances of the AI's speed, accuracy, and potential for early disease detection must be communicated effectively, as patients want to know that the benefits of using AI outweigh any potential risks or downsides.

Data privacy and data security are also a significant consideration of paramount concerns for patients entrusting AI with sensitive medical information. Ensuring that their data is handled responsibly and securely boosts confidence in the technology. If patients feel that their data is well-protected and used ethically, they are more likely to trust and accept AI diagnostic tools.

9.2. Impact of Patient Trust on Diagnostic Outcomes

Knowing AI technology is trustworthy, people are more likely to accept its use in their diagnostics and arguably, are more open to follow-up care and treatment protocols based on insights developed from AI. This, in turn, leads to informed decisions resulting in better health outcomes, people who trust the technology adhere to the recommendations thrown out by AI. Being more trusting of the support given, patients will be compliant because treatment adherence would have improved now that they will take an active role in making decisions about their health. Patient trust also encourages feedback, a very important factor in the continuous refinement of the algorithms of AI in diagnosing leukemia with even higher accuracy. This creates a positive cycle of trust, engagement, and feedback that benefits both the patient and in developing AI for health.

9.3. Barriers to Acceptance and Trust

Despite its advantages, AI diagnostics face several barriers to acceptance and trust. A common concern among patients is the fear of reduced human interaction. Patients value the personal connection with healthcare providers and may worry that AI could reduce human involvement, potentially affecting the quality of care they receive. Additionally, concerns about errors or misdiagnoses can deter patients from fully trusting AI (Cottingham et al., 2023). Any cases of misdiagnosis or errors made by AI, even if rare, can lead to skepticism and anxiety about relying solely on technology without human oversight. There is also a sense of losing control, where patients may feel as though AI is taking over decision-making in their healthcare, making them less comfortable with AI involvement if they feel it compromises their autonomy.

9.4 Strategies to Enhance Patient Trust in AI Diagnostics

Several strategies can improve patient trust in AI-driven leukemia diagnostics. Educational initiatives are fundamental, as educating patients about AI, including its processes, benefits, and limitations, can reduce skepticism. When patients understand AI's role and capabilities, they may feel more comfortable with its use in their diagnostics. Collaborative decision-making is another strategy, where healthcare providers involve patients in decisions about using AI for diagnostics, fostering a sense of partnership rather than imposition. Furthermore, providing personalized AI explanations can build trust. For example, if AI explains its findings in relation to the patient's specific health profile, patients may feel more assured about the technology's relevance and accuracy. To further enhance trust, maintaining human oversight is critical. Ensuring that healthcare professionals confirm AI diagnoses provides patients with a safety net and increases their comfort with AI involvement. This balance between human expertise and AI's capabilities can help patients view, AI as a supportive tool rather than a replacement for human judgment.

9.5 Ethical and Societal Considerations

An explanation of how AI works, including its strengths, advantages, and shortcomings, will help dissolve scepticism and build understanding. Patients are very likely to feel more confident once the role of AI in their diagnosis is clearly comprehended. Besides, societal attitudes toward AI in healthcare have a great influence on individual trust. Positive media representation, success stories, and well-documented studies of AI effectiveness in diagnostics related to leukemia will help in building public confidence.

10. CASE STUDY: RISK IN PEDIATRIC LEUKEMIA

The challenges are more in rare diseases such as pediatric ALL and AML, especially when the prevalence is low, fewer datasets are available along with high variability across different patients. A new framework based on interpretable ML models to address these concerns will derive actionable insights from low-sized tabular datasets. This framework integrates data preparation, supervised and unsupervised learning, and LBD for optimized predictive accuracy while considering clinical applicability. In this study, ML is further proved to change the pattern of rare disease management by developing the approach, which might predict infection risk in leukemia patients undergoing chemotherapy.

The dataset had 580 cases of ALL and 132 cases of AML, with variables on patient demographics, type of leukemia, chemotherapy regimens, and the presence of infections. This challenge applied supervised learning models including CatBoost, LightGBM, and TabNet on classifying patients into either high-risk or low-risk infection categories, and among the three models CatBoost was the most accurate at about 79%. Regression models further predicted the count of bacterial and viral infections. TabNet dominated this task with a mean absolute error of 2.15 and 1.26, respectively. Unsupervised learning techniques also yielded some further insights into the structure of the dataset. The dimensionality reduction techniques PCA and t-distributed stochastic neighbour embedding (TSNE) show that the high- and low-risk infection classes largely overlap, suggesting that the features available are not highly rich. Association Rule Mining (ARM) revealed the co-occurrences of features that can be critical, including chemotherapy regimens with drug combinations that have association with higher infection risks. These insights complement the supervised learning models and provide a clearer view of infection patterns.

The literature discovery component, based on SemNet 2.0, mined more than 33 million articles on PubMed and brought into the framework capabilities by doing so, uniting together features from glucose levels, zinc, iron, and growth factors which have been found to be related to an increased infection risk. For example, hyperglycemia and its correlation with increased neutropenia and infections were highlighted as actionable findings for clinical care. This cross-domain text-mining methodology has bridged gaps in the clinical dataset and facilitated better understanding of infection risk factors. This interpretable ML framework has tremendous potential in further improving the quality of clinical decision making in rare diseases. It allows the stratification of infection risk and characterizes key predictive features, thus offering actionability for personalized care. By combining supervised and unsupervised learning along with literature-based discovery ensures that the system by nature will approach the challenges it faces due to small and variable datasets. This framework will provide not only the fundamental structure to optimize the outcome in the patient who undergoes pediatric leukemia but will model how one should tackle the other rare diseases as well (Al-Hussaini et al., 2024).

11. FUTURE RESEARCH DIRECTIONS IN AI FOR LEUKEMIA CLASSIFICATION AND TREATMENT

The use of AI in diagnosing and treating leukemia is one of the most striking novel changes facing health care. Whereas much progress has been realized, the field is still at its foundational stages, and many developments can occur. Research needs to be done to try and solve the existing challenges facing the study of new applications that will increase the role of AI in leukemia care. Extending explainable AI, developing robust and generalizable AI models, and leveraging AI to improve leukemia care in resource-limited settings are the critical areas of future research.

11.1 Advancing Explainable AI in Leukemia Diagnostics

Integrate the explainability tools that could be amongst the upbeat approaches, like LIME and SHAP-SHapley Additive exPlanations. These tools will bring forth important features or regions in medical data, including blood-smear images, which drive the decisions taken by AI. Using this, an AI system can outline certain morphological changes in leukocytes that may be indicative of leukemia and provide a visual map to indicate toward those areas. This level of transparency provides immense boosts not only in clinician confidence but also in patient trust by showing how and why decisions are made.

In other words, explainable AI will be the gateway to shared decision-making processes where clinicians validate the outputs derived from AI with their experience. The future interaction of XAI will move into more interactive interfaces where the clinicians can question the AI system. Examples of questions include pondering differential diagnosis and further clarification on the underlying reasons for AI predictions. Projects will need to investigate explainability from a patient-oriented point of view too, which would enable AI systems to communicate their findings in lay terms, thereby further reducing the gap between advanced medical technologies and patients' understanding.

11.2 Developing More Robust and Generalizable AI Models for Leukemia Classification

One of the key limitations for AI systems in leukemia diagnostics nowadays is their generalization and robustness. Most models are trained on limited datasets, which cannot fully capture the wide variation in patient populations with respect to age, ethnicity, geographical location, and subtypes of diseases (Didi et al., 2024). This leads to biased models performing well under very controlled settings but then failing when exposed to real applications. The focus of future research should be large, diverse, high-quality datasets representative of the full spectrum of worldwide leukemia cases.

This will further enhance generalisability through mechanisms of adaptive learning, whereby models keep evolving with the availability of new data, thus retaining their accuracy and relevance over time. For example, it could be developed in a way that models learn from continuous clinical inputs on subtypes of leukemia, protocols for treatments, and demographic health trends.

Future research also needs to consider the role of federated learning, in which AI models are jointly trained across multiple institutions by sharing parameters without actual sensitive patient data. Not only does this strategy enhance the model's generalizability but it also makes it more ethically and legally acceptable, thereby guaranteeing safe application in leukemia diagnosis.

11.3 AI's Potential to Revolutionize Global Leukemia Care in Resource-Limited Settings

From the absence of specialists to diagnostic facilities, many challenges in leukemia care lie in resource-constrained settings. AI can bridge this gap by offering low-cost, available, and accurate diagnostics. Therefore, adaptation of AI technologies to work effectively in the low-resource environment should be one of the focuses of research efforts that guarantee equipping citizens around the globe with the most advanced leukemia care.

This could be developing lightweight AI models runnable on affordable hardware, like smartphones or mobile diagnostic devices, analysing images of blood smears obtained with low-end microscopy (Alhajahjeh & Nazha, 2024). The AI algorithms of such models would provide quick and reliable diagnoses of leukemia at remote locations. When combined with telemedicine, health workers can send AI-generated results to specialists who would then validate these results and construct proper treatment plans.

AI can further optimize resource allocation in underfunded healthcare. Predictive analytics could identify high-risk populations and enable targeted screening programs with early interventions. The decision-support tools powered by AI may support the work of non-specialist health workers in the diagnosis and management of leukemia, reducing the workload on overburdened specialists and improving the delivery of care in less well-resourced areas.

Future research should focus on collaborations with international health organizations toward the development of open access leukemia data and AI platforms. The result of such efforts could be a better dissemination of knowledge, harmonization of diagnostic approaches, and translation of AI innovations to patients of different socioeconomic backgrounds. By responding to the specific needs of resource-constrained settings, AI can also contribute significantly to the enhancement of leukemia care while narrowing global gaps in healthcare access.

CONCLUSION

AI-based leukemia diagnosis is associated with several challenges. For fair and accurate diagnosis of leukemia, independent of the patient profile, there is a need to eliminate biases within algorithms. Further, protection and safety of data will be a major concern since this will deal with information about patients. Designs of AI need to be guarded against data privacy breaches through strict adherence to regulatory laws that rule the implications of breaches in patient privacy and, where necessary, even cybersecurity considerations. Accountability is considered when AI drives decision-making. While AI promises great benefits such as accuracy and speed of diagnosis, patients are fearful about the privacy of information and the possibility of AI generated errors resulting from inhuman emotional communication presented by AI. Building trust into AI-based systems requires an explanation of the processes adopted by the AI model to arrive at its results. LIME is thus a critical component in this scenario, offering interpretable explanations of how AI comes to diagnostic conclusions, making it easier to mollify patient fears. Specifically, more robust AI models must be developed that can learn and generalize from several diverse healthcare environments so that AI-based leukemia diagnostics are accurate and reliable across different settings. This would also help to further integrate leukemia care, especially within settings with limited resources for specialized diagnostics.

REFERENCES

Adnan, F., Awan, M. J., Mahmoud, A., Nobanee, H., Yasin, A., & Zain, A. M. (2023). EfficientNetB3-adaptive augmented deep learning (AADL) for multi-class plant disease classification. *IEEE Access.*

Adwer, L., & Whiting, E. (2024, June). Exploring artificial intelligence solutions and challenges in healthcare administration. In *2024 IEEE 12th International Conference on Healthcare Informatics (ICHI)* (pp. 528–530). IEEE. DOI: 10.1109/ICHI61247.2024.00077

Al-Hussaini, I., White, B., Varmeziar, A., Mehra, N., Sanchez, M., Lee, J., DeGroote, N. P., Miller, T. P., & Mitchell, C. S. (2024). An Interpretable Machine Learning Framework for Rare Disease. A Case Study to Stratify Infection Risk in Pediatric Leukemia. *Journal of Clinical Medicine, 13*(6), 1788. DOI: 10.3390/jcm13061788 PMID: 38542012

Alhajahjeh, A., & Nazha, A. (2024). Unlocking the potential of artificial intelligence in acute myeloid leukemia and myelodysplastic syndromes. *Current Hematologic Malignancy Reports, 19*(1), 9–17. DOI: 10.1007/s11899-023-00716-5 PMID: 37999872

Batool, A., & Byun, Y. C. (2023). Lightweight EfficientNetB3 model based on depthwise separable convolutions for enhancing classification of leukemia white blood cell images. IEEE Access, 11, 37203–37215. https.//10.1109/ACCESS.2023.3257024

Batool, A., & Byun, Y. C. (2023). Lightweight EfficientNetB3 model based on depthwise separable convolutions for enhancing classification of leukemia white blood cell images. *IEEE Access : Practical Innovations, Open Solutions, 11*, 37203–37215. DOI: 10.1109/ACCESS.2023.3266511

Begum, M., Shuvo, M. H., Nasir, M. K., Hossain, A., Hossain, M. J., Ashraf, I., Uddin, J., & Samad, M. A. (2024). LCNN. Lightweight CNN architecture for software defect feature identification using Explainable AI. *IEEE Access : Practical Innovations, Open Solutions, 12*, 55744–55756. DOI: 10.1109/ACCESS.2024.3388489

Chen, W., Zhang, Z., Han, W., Yuan, C., Xu, P., & Han, L. (2010, October). Preclinical studies of S1 in K562 cell line and primary chronic myeloid leukemia cells shown synergistic effect with cytosine arabinoside hydrochloride. In *2010 3rd International Conference on Biomedical Engineering and Informatics* (Vol. 2, pp. 459–463). IEEE. DOI: 10.1109/BMEI.2010.5639266

Cheraghy, M., Soltanpour, M., Abdalla, H. B., & Oveis, A. H. (2024). SVM-based factor graph design for Max-SR problem of SCMA networks. *IEEE Communications Letters, 28*(4), 877–881. DOI: 10.1109/LCOMM.2024.3366426

Cottingham, A. H., Baker, L. B., Hoffmann, M. L., Martin, C. E., & Cripe, L. D. (2023). We were in the fight together. The expectations of bereaved caregivers of patients with acute myeloid leukemia from diagnosis to death. *Leukemia Research, 124*, 106994. DOI: 10.1016/j.leukres.2022.106994 PMID: 36481729

Das, P. K., Diya, V. A., Meher, S., Panda, R., & Abraham, A. (2022). A systematic review on recent advancements in deep and machine learning-based detection and classification of acute lymphoblastic leukemia. IEEE Access, 10, 81741–81763. https.//DOI: 10.1109/ACCESS.2022.3187216

Das, P. K., Sahoo, B., & Meher, S. (2022). An efficient detection and classification of acute leukemia using transfer learning and orthogonal softmax layer-based model. *IEEE/ACM Transactions on Computational Biology and Bioinformatics*, *20*(3), 1817–1828. DOI: 10.1109/TCBB.2022.3218590 PMID: 36318567

Depto, D. S., Rizvee, M. M., Rahman, A., Zunair, H., Rahman, M. S., & Mahdy, M. R. C. (2023). Quantifying imbalanced classification methods for leukemia detection. *Computers in Biology and Medicine*, *152*, 106372. DOI: 10.1016/j.compbiomed.2022.106372 PMID: 36516574

Didi, I., Alliot, J. M., Dumas, P. Y., Vergez, F., Tavitian, S., Largeaud, L., Bidet, A., Rieu, J. B., Luquet, I., Lechevalier, N., Delabesse, E., Sarry, A., De Grande, A.-C., Bérard, E., Pigneux, A., Récher, C., Simoncini, D., & Bertoli, S. (2024). Artificial intelligence-based prediction models for acute myeloid leukemia using real-life data. A DATAML registry study. *Leukemia Research*, *136*, 107437. DOI: 10.1016/j.leukres.2024.107437 PMID: 38215555

El-Seddek, M. (2024, July). A deep learning technique for multi-classification of acute lymphocytic leukemia. In *2024 International Telecommunications Conference (ITC-Egypt)* (pp. 404–409). IEEE. DOI: 10.1109/ITC-Egypt61547.2024.10620494

Elhadary, M., Elshoeibi, A. M., Badr, A., Elsayed, B., Metwally, O., Elshoeibi, A. M., Mattar, M., Alfarsi, K., AlShammari, S., Alshurafa, A., & Yassin, M. (2023). Revolutionizing chronic lymphocytic leukemia diagnosis. A deep dive into the diverse applications of machine learning. *Blood Reviews*, *62*, 101134. DOI: 10.1016/j.blre.2023.101134 PMID: 37758527

Islam, O., Assaduzzaman, M., & Hasan, M. Z. (2024). An explainable AI-based blood cell classification using optimized convolutional neural network. *Journal of Pathology Informatics*, *15*, 100389. DOI: 10.1016/j.jpi.2024.100389 PMID: 39161471

Jin, H., & Chen, S. (2023). Biometric recognition based on recurrence plot and inceptionV3 model using eye movements. *IEEE Journal of Biomedical and Health Informatics*, *27*(11), 5554–5563. DOI: 10.1109/JBHI.2023.3313261 PMID: 37682647

Jiwani, N., Gupta, K., Pau, G., & Alibakhshikenari, M. (2023). Pattern recognition of acute lymphoblastic leukemia (ALL) using computational deep learning. IEEE Access, 11, 29541–29553. https.//10.1109/ACCESS.2023.3232345

Jiwani, N., Gupta, K., Pau, G., & Alibakhshikenari, M. (2023). Pattern recognition of acute lymphoblastic leukemia (ALL) using computational deep learning. *IEEE Access : Practical Innovations, Open Solutions*, *11*, 29541–29553. DOI: 10.1109/ACCESS.2023.3260065

Jiwani, N., Gupta, K., Pau, G., & Alibakhshikenari, M. (2023). Pattern recognition of acute lymphoblastic leukemia (ALL) using computational deep learning. *IEEE Access : Practical Innovations, Open Solutions*, *11*, 29541–29553. DOI: 10.1109/ACCESS.2023.3260065

Meng, Z., Zhao, Z., Li, B., Su, F., & Guo, L. (2021). A cervical histopathology dataset for computer-aided diagnosis of precancerous lesions. *IEEE Transactions on Medical Imaging*, *40*(6), 1531–1541. DOI: 10.1109/TMI.2021.3059699 PMID: 33600310

Minga, E., Gkoufas, A., Vardi, A., Stalika, E., Hadzidimitriou, A., Stamatopoulos, K., Maglaveras, N., & Chouvarda, I. (2013, November). Towards an integrated framework for clinico-biological data management and analysis. The case of chronic lymphocytic leukemia. In *13th IEEE International Conference on Bioinformatics and Bioengineering* (pp. 1–4). IEEE.

Mustaqim, T., Fatichah, C., & Suciati, N. (2023). Deep learning for the detection of acute lymphoblastic leukemia subtypes on microscopic images. A systematic literature review. IEEE Access, 11, 16108–16127. https.//10.1109/ACCESS.2023.3241912

Prasad, C. R., Varshamrutha, K., Sindhuja, B., Ushasree, R., Nikhil, P., & Chakradhar, A. (2024, May). MRI-based brain tumor classification using a fine-tuned EfficientNetB3 transfer learning model. In *2024 5th International Conference for Emerging Technology (INCET)* (pp. 1–5). IEEE. DOI: 10.1109/INCET61516.2024.10592978

Shah, A., Naqvi, S. S., Naveed, K., Salem, N., Khan, M. A., & Alimgeer, K. S. (2021). Automated diagnosis of leukemia. A comprehensive review. IEEE Access, 9, 132097–132124. https.//10.1109/ACCESS.2021.3112623

Wang, B., Pei, W., Xue, B., & Zhang, M. (2022). A multi-objective genetic algorithm to evolving local interpretable model-agnostic explanations for deep neural networks in image classification. *IEEE Transactions on Evolutionary Computation.*

Yang, F., Li, X., Duan, H., Xu, F., Huang, Y., Zhang, X., Long, Y., & Zheng, Y. (2023). MRL-Seg. Overcoming imbalance in medical image segmentation with multi-step reinforcement learning. *IEEE Journal of Biomedical and Health Informatics*. PMID: 38032774

Yu, Z., Nguyen, J., Nguyen, T. D., Kelly, J., Mclean, C., Bonnington, P., Zhang, L., Mar, V., & Ge, Z. (2021). Early melanoma diagnosis with sequential dermoscopic images. *IEEE Transactions on Medical Imaging*, *41*(3), 633–646. DOI: 10.1109/TMI.2021.3120091 PMID: 34648437

Zhou, P., Du, L., & Li, X. (2023). Adaptive consensus clustering for multiple k-means via base results refining. *IEEE Transactions on Knowledge and Data Engineering*, *35*(10), 10251–10264. DOI: 10.1109/TKDE.2023.3264970

Chapter 18
Multi-Stream Attention-Based Convolutional Neural Network for Medical Imaging

T. V. V. Satyanarayana
https://orcid.org/0000-0002-8764-9982
Mohan Babu University, India

B. Bhaskar Reddy
https://orcid.org/0000-0002-3200-0182
St. Peter's Engineering College, India

A. Swetha Rani
https://orcid.org/0009-0008-6023-8527
G. Pullaiah College of Engineering and Technology, India

P. Sree Lakshmi
https://orcid.org/0000-0001-7212-9135
Audisankara College of Engineering and Technology, India

Hedayath Basha Shaik
R.M.K. College of Engineering and Technology, India

ABSTRACT

In the recent past medical imaging has emerged as a tool for better diagnosis of patients. The diagnosis mechanism includes Non-invasive methods and further treatment of various diseases viz., pneumonia cancer and other neurological disorders. To address the challenges in the existing methods, this chapter introduces a novel Multi-Stream Attention-Based Convolutional Neural Network (MSA-CNN) technique which is a deep learning architecture. The main component of the proposed architecture is an Attentional mechanism that dynamically assigns prominence to the features of each modality, concentrating on the most relevant regions of the images that are of interest, to improve the models interpretability. Further, a Noise-Aware Loss Function is introduced to handle noise in the images to enhance model performance. Results show that the proposed technique is observed to have an accuracy of 95.7% on the Chest X-ray dataset, outperforming the existing benchmarking techniques to have 89.3% using AlexNet, 92.4% using

DOI: 10.4018/979-8-3693-9816-6.ch018

ResNet-18 respectively.

1. INTRODUCTION

The present-day scenario of medical imaging techniques viz., Magnetic Resonance Imaging (MRI), Computed Tomography (CT), and X-rays are used mostly and are considered as prime tools in modern healthcare system. Healthcare professionals will be using such tools to non-invasively visualize the internal body structures and further use to diagnose several conditions of the body pertaining from cancer to several infectious diseases. These technologies have revolutionized the way the diseases are detected, monitored and further treated. However, the interpretation of medical images has become complex and has remained till date, further making it a time-consuming task. Such a task can be done only through a skilled radiologist. The risk of human error is always present that depends on several factors such as fatigue or the overwhelming voluminous data that they acquire for processing. Recent studies show that radiologists can miss up to 30% of abnormalities when interpreting scans under pressure that leads to delay in the treatment or sometimes missed diagnoses (Wang et al., 2017).

Artificial Intelligence (AI), Deep Learning (DL), particularly Convolutional Neural Networks (CNNs), is observed to be having better results in automation of the analysis of medical images that further assists technicians in making faster, for accurate diagnoses. CNNs have become a standard in image classification, segmentation and object detection as they can automatically learn hierarchical features from raw image data, removing the need for manual feature engineering (Litjens et al., 2017). These techniques can also be successfully applied to detect pneumonia in chest X-rays (Lakhani and Sundaram, 2017), segment brain tumors in MRI scans (Ronneberger et al., 2015), and diagnose COVID-19 from CT scans (Isensee et al., 2021). Many applications were developed in the recent past to demonstrate the potential of CNNs that reduce the workload on technicians and improve diagnostic accuracy.

However, in real-word clinical settings, several challenges remain unresolved in deploying CNNs for medical imaging. One of the major challenges is generalization. CNNs are trained on a specific dataset that often perform poorly when applied to images from different sources, viz., hospitals that use different imaging protocols or machines. For instance, a model that is trained on chest X-rays from one hospital may not generalize well to X-rays from another hospital. This is because of the resolution, noise level, or contrast that may differ from one hospital to another (Rajpurkar et al., 2017). This lack of generalization poses a critical problem for CNN-based models in healthcare, where variability between datasets is common. Guan et al. (Guan et al., 2021) presented an innovative framework for brain tumour classification using MRI images. This study achieved an overall accuracy of 98.04%, outperforming existing methods. The proposed model addresses challenges posed by low-quality MRI images. Additionally, the study employs effective data augmentation strategies, such as image rotation and flipping, to expand the training dataset and mitigate overfitting, thereby enhancing the model's generalisation capability and reliability in tumour classification.

Another significant challenge in medical imaging lies in its multi-modal nature. Clinicians frequently need data from multiple imaging modalities for making a comprehensive diagnosis (Zhou, Greenspan, and Shen, 2017). For instance, MRI scans are highly effective in distinguishing soft tissues having varied contrast, while CT scans are better for visualizing bone structures. However, traditional CNN architectures, that are designed to handle single-modality data, struggle to integrate the complementary information that multi-modal inputs provide. Such an integration is essential to create comprehensive view of the patients condition particularly in diagnosing complex ailments such as cancer, where each modality uncovers unique aspects of the disease. Muhammad Aamir et al. (Aamir, M., et al., 2023) addressed the need for fast and improved brain tumor detection and the need for the computationally less complex approach to diagnose the diseases, achieved an accuracy of approximately 98.98%. Aamir, M. et al. (Aamir, M. et al., 2022) suggested that by combining EfficientNet-B0 and ResNet50 for feature extraction, along with innovative techniques like refinement, and alignment, the model demonstrates remarkable efficiency and diagnostic reliability.

In addition, the interpretability of CNN models poses a substantial alarm in the case of medical applications. These models are often considered as "black-box" models as their internal decision-making processes cannot be easily understandable. This lack of transparency makes it challenging for the healthcare professionals to cognize why the model has made a particular decision or prediction, which is critical in building AI-assisted diagnostic tools (Caruana et al., 2015). In general, in clinical practice, it is quite essential that the models that are developed need to provide accurate results and also explain the reason behind such result or prediction.

Furthermore, medical images are often affected by noise that is induced from several factors viz., movement of patient while acquiring the signal or during scanning or differences in imaging source / equipment. In general, CNNs (Tallapragada, V. S., et al., 2024). are trained on datasets that are free from noise, and will be perform poorly when trained on real-word data that may contain noise resulting in false positives or negatives (Ghafoorian et al., 2017). Therefore, models that are developed and designed for medical imaging must be robust to noise and must be capable of handling images of varying quality. Aamir, M. (Aamir, M. et al., 2019) evaluated the performance of a simple CNN architecture for image classification and demonstrated superior accuracy when compared to existing methods on CIFAR-10 dataset.

Moreover, medical images are often affected by noise. This will be the result of several factors such as patient movement during scanning or differences in imaging equipment. In general, CNNs trained on clean datasets. This hinders the performance as they are exposed to noisy, real-world data, resulting in false positives or negatives (Ghafoorian et al., 2017). Hence, models are designed for medical imaging that must be robust to noise and must have the capability of handling images of varying quality. In order to tackle these challenges, this chapter proposes a novel Multi-Stream Attention-Based CNN (MSA-CNN), architecture that processes Multi-Modal Data. The proposed technique uses multiple CNN streams. Each stream is dedicated to process that will be handling a different imaging modality (e.g., MRI, CT, X-ray). This ensures that the features that are extracted will be unique to each modality that is captured.

In addition to the MSA-CNN an Attention Mechanism is added. The proposed architecture incorporates an attention mechanism that dynamically assigns weights to the features. These features are extracted each modality, making it to focus on the most relevant features. This process enhances the interpretability of the model, highlighting which parts of the image contributed most to the final prediction (Xu et al., 2016). Further, to handle noisy inputs, the proposed architecture incorporates a noise-aware loss function that penalizes the model more heavily for incorrect predictions on noisy data, thereby making the model more robust for real-world applications (Zhang et al., 2018).

Pujari, S. D., et al. (Pujari, S. D., et al. 2024) introduced a deep learning network for classifying histopathological images. Using Multi-Sclace architecture combined with an attention mechanism, the proposed or the developed model is effectively distinguishes the normal and cancerous cells and achieved an accuracy of 98.07%.

Figure 1 shows the generalised block diagram of the MSA-CNN architecture. The process begins with the acquiring of the multiple modalities or the multiple types of images (e.g., MRI, CT, X-ray), which are simultaneously processed using separate CNN streams. Each process in the CNN (Simonyan and Zisserman, 2014) stream is dedicated for extraction of features that are unique to the input modality. The advantage of such process will capture full range of information for the input modality. The Attention Mechanism will assign weights to the feature maps that are generated from each stream which highlights the most relevant features. These features which are weighted will be combined or fused together to form a single unified feature representation that will be passed through final fully connected layers for classification (e.g., disease detection) or segmentation (e.g., tumor boundary identification).

Figure 1. Generalized block diagram of MSA-CNN architecture

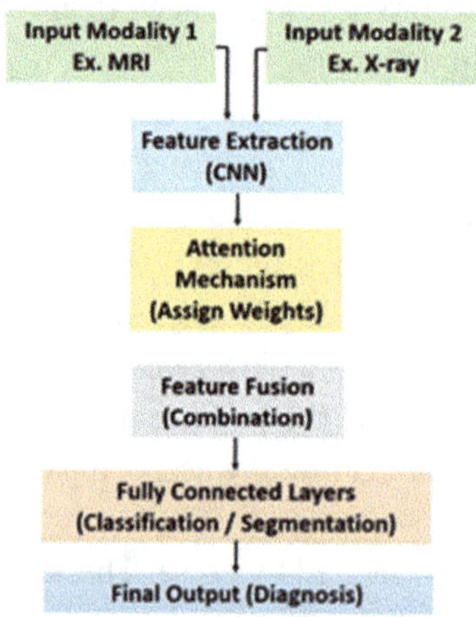

Figure 2 shows the workflow of the MSA-CNN model. The input images acquired from multiple modalities (e.g., MRI, CT, X-ray) are pre-processed through steps like resizing, normalization, and data augmentation. The pre-processing is done to ensure consistent input. Each modality is then processed through its own modality-specific CNN stream, where features are extracted for further processing. The next step is the Attention Mechanism, which assigns weights to the features from each modality. This focuses on the most important regions of the images. These weighted features are combined in the Feature Fusion Layer and are further passed through the output layer for either classification (e.g., detecting pneumonia) or segmentation (e.g., identifying tumor regions).

The remaining sections are categorized as: Section 2 introduces a brief literature survey, Section 3 highlights the research gaps in medical imaging, Section 4 details the proposed architecture, section 5 outlines results and discussions, followed by conclusion and future scope.

Figure 2. Workflow of the MSA-CNN model

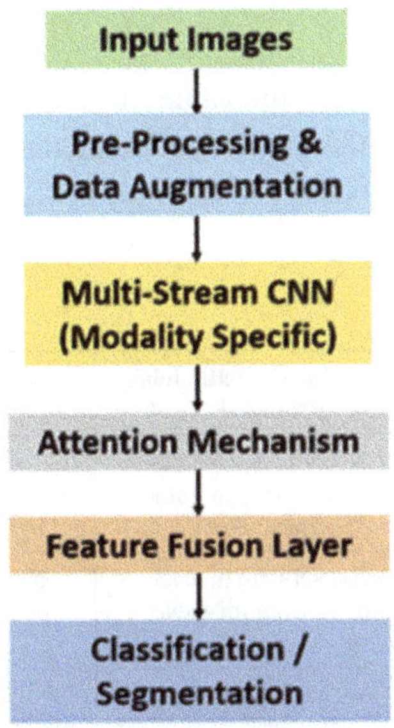

2. LITERATURE SURVEY

2.1 Convolutional Neural Networks (CNNs) for Medical Imaging

In the recent past, researchers have observed advancements In the field of medical imaging. The most prominent deep learning technique used is Convolutional Neural Networks (CNNs).

This section provides a brief overview of various methodologies, architectures, mathematical formulations. Basically, CNN performs a convolution operation and is defined by

$$(f * g)(x) = \sum_{a} f(a) . g(x - a) \quad \dots \quad (1)$$

Where

$f$is the input image, $g$is the convolution filter or kernel, x is the current position in the image, $a$is the filter size.

From equation (1), the output is a convolution operation that extracts the features by sliding the filter g across the input image$f$, resulting in a feature map. This feature map highlights the prominent patterns viz., edges or textures. In medical imaging certain conditions prevails such as identification of tumors or lesions which can be captured using these prominent patterns. Further, pooling layers in CNN reduce the spatial dimensions of the feature maps and are typically applied after the operation of the convolutional layers. These pooling layers downsample the data and is given in equation (2).

$$y = \max(x_i, x_{i+1}, \ldots, x_{i+k})$$

… (2)

Such a pooling operation selects the maximum value from a group of neighboring pixels thus retaining the most important information. This further help in reducing the computational load. Table 1 shows the comparison of the recent works carried out in the field of medical imaging using CNN.

Table 1. Comparison of previous works

Author (Year)	Problem Identified	Solution/Novel Methodology Proposed	Results Obtained	Drawbacks
Shen et al., 2017	Brain tumor segmentation in MRI	3D CNN with a patch-based input processing for tumor segmentation	Achieved a Dice score of 0.84 on BRATS dataset	High computational cost due to 3D convolutions
Zhang et al., 2021	Pneumonia detection in chest X-rays	DenseNet with transfer learning from ImageNet	Achieved 96.7% accuracy on the ChestX-ray14 dataset	Struggled with noisy or low-resolution images
Ronneberger et al., 2015)	Biomedical image segmentation	U-Net architecture with encoder-decoder structure and skip connections	Achieved 91% segmentation accuracy on ISBI 2015	Requires large amounts of annotated data
Lakhani & Sundaram, 2017	Pneumonia detection in chest X-rays	Transfer learning using AlexNet and GoogleNet	Achieved 92.8% accuracy on the NIH dataset	Limited generalization to X-ray datasets from other institutions
Litjens et al., 2017	Prostate cancer detection in MRI	CNN with hand-crafted feature extraction combined with deep learning	88.4% accuracy and improved false-positive rate	Struggled with small lesion detection
Wang et al., 2018	Chest disease multi-label classification	Custom CNN with image augmentation to detect 14 diseases	Achieved AUC of 0.90 for multiple diseases on ChestX-ray14	Model struggled with class imbalance issues

2.2 U-Net for Medical Image Segmentation

In the recent past U-Net architecture has evolved and has shown better performance for medical image segmentation tasks. This is proposed by Ronneberger et al. (2015) [3]. It uses an encoder-decoder structure, where the encoder extracts features through successive convolution and pooling layers, while the decoder reconstructs the image by up-sampling. The unique feature of U-Net is the skip connections that combine feature maps from the encoder to the corresponding decoder layers. This process ensures that fine-grained details are preserved during reconstruction. The U-Net operations are mathematically defined by equation (3).

$$y^{(l)} = \sigma\left(\sum_k W_k^{(l)} * x_k^{(l)} + b^{(l)}\right)$$

… (3)

Where $x_k^{(l)}$ is the input to the l-th layer, $W_k^{(l)}$ are the convolutional weights, $b^{(l)}$ is the bias term, σ is the activation function (typically ReLU). The next process is the upsampling which is defined by

$$x^{(l+1)} = upsample(x^{(l)}) \quad \ldots \quad (4)$$

This architecture is widely used for the medical imaging tasks due to its ability to learn precise segmentation boundaries and is widely used in brain tumor segmentation, liver segmentation, and cell segmentation using microscopic images. Figure 3 shows the UNet architecture diagram.

Figure 3. Generalised diagram of U-net architecture

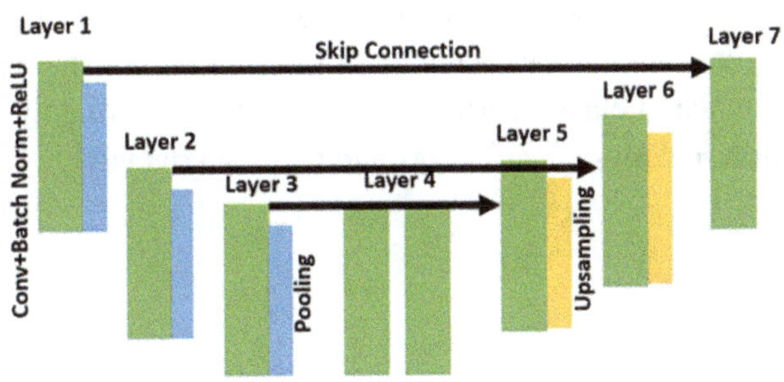

This architecture follows symmetric encoder-decoder structure. The former is often called as the contracting path, that captures high-level features from the input image through convolutional and max-pooling operations. This is shown as layer 1 in the figure 3. This process of having convolutional and max-pooling operations at layer 1 reduces the spatial dimensions while also preserving the prominent features that are required for the feature representation. On the other hand, the later, also known as the expanding path, reconstructs the spatial resolution of the input image using upsampling layers which are mentioned at layer 5 and 6 in the figure 3. Such an inclusion of upsampling mechanism ensures accurate localisation of the features which is more essential for the segmentation tasks. The most important property of U-Net is the skip connections that link corresponding layers in the encoder and decoder. These connections allow the network to retain the spatial information that is lost during the downsampling process in the encoder. By combining the feature maps from the encoder with the upsampled features in the decoder, the network effectively combining the low-level spatial details with high-level information, resulting in the improvement in the segmentation accuracy. This architecture completely relies on convolutional layers. This avoids the use of fully connected layers ensuring flexibility with the variable input data sizes. The architecture uses repeated convolutional operations with ReLU activation functions and batch normalisation shown in layer 1 is used to extract and refine features at each layer. This design ensures efficient learning and high quality segmentation.

2.3 DenseNet for Classification in Medical Imaging

DenseNet (Huang et al. 2017) (Zhang et al. 2021) uses dense connections between the layers which is different from the existing CNN architectures wherein each layer received input from only from the previous layers. This is defined by

$$x_l = H_l([x_0, x_1, \ldots, x_{l-1}]) \quad \ldots \quad (5)$$

Where H_l is the composite function of convolution, batch normalization and ReLU. The output of each layer is combined or concatenated with the inputs that are processed from all the previous layers, resulting in a more efficient feature propogation and mitigating the vanishing gradient problem. The dense connections that are established in the network provides better flow of gradients during training that results in faster convergence and higher accuracy. From the literature it is observed that DenseNet has shown superior performance in classification tasks concentrating mainly on medical image classification. Such a classification includes chest X-rays and CT scan datasets.

Figure 4. Architecture of DenseNet.

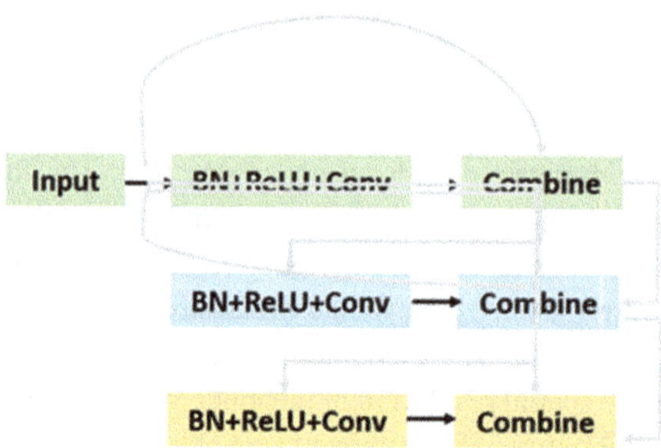

DenseNet ich is also called as Densely Connected Convolutional Network, is one of the modern deep learning architecture that is designed to improve feature reuse and alleviate the problem of varnishing gradients. This architecture is proposed by Gao Huang in 2017. This architecture uses layer connectivity. Besides, traditional CNNs, each layer receives input from the previous layer and is processed before passing it to the next layer. This architecture establishes direct connections between all layers within a dense block. In other words, each layer receives the feature maps of all the previous layers as input and passes the feature maps to all the subsequent layers. This structure ensures that all the information flow remains robust throughout the network, thus leading to more efficient gradient propagation during the training phase. The dense connectivity in this architecture enables substantial feature reuse. This process reduces the problem of redundancy in the deep networks. The architecture allows each layer to access all the previously computed feature maps making this DenseNet architecture useful for both low- and high-level features. This leads to an effective learning mechanism and better feature extraction. Furthermore, the architecture is highly parameter efficient compared to other deep networks. Instead of learning the redundant features, DenseNet maximises its use of each feature map. This inturn reduces the number of parameters and the computational cost required for training.

DenseNet produces highly differentiating features without requiring over tthe existing complex models. This architecture shown in figure 4 employs batch normalisation, activation functions and convolutional layers to process the feature maps within each layer. The utilisation of combination or the concatenation layer is to combine the feature maps ensuring that each layer has direct access to the gradients from the loss function. This process reduces the likelihood of the vanishing gradients. This makes DenseNet particularly useful for deep learning architectures wherein the traditional architectures often face challenges in terms of training, stability and convergence. It is to be noted that DenseNet has good ability to produce highly discriminative features when compared to other complex models. This architecture employs batch normalisation, activation functions and convolutional layers to process feature maps within each layer. The use of the combine block shown in figure 4 provides direct access to the gradients from the loss function at each layer. This process reduces the likelihood of the vanishing gradients. This property also makes DenseNet particularly suitable for very deep networks, where traditional architectures often face challenges in training, stability and convergence. DenseNet is observed to have better application in computer vision tasks, including image classification, object detection and semantic segmentation. Its architecture is flexible and can be adjusted to meet specific application requirements. For illustration purpose some of the lines shown in figure 4 are drawn from image to combine block, which means that it uses transition layers to control the size of the feature maps and further reduce the computational overhead in deeper networks. These layers include operations such as pooling and 1 x 1 convolutions to compress feature maps, maintaining efficiency while preserving critical information.

2.4 Generalization Across Modalities

Generalisation across imaging modalities has remained as an important confront in deep learning applications. This can be dealt in particular in the field of medical imaging. Convolutional Neural Networks (CNNs) trained on data from a specific imaging modality, viz., X-rays, often strive to accomplish analogous performance when applied on or over the other types of modalities like MRI or CT scans. This issue comes or arises due to inherent differences in image resolution, contrast levels, noise patterns, and imaging protocols. Such properties may vary across modalities and institutions and the imaging equipment that the user choose to. Such variations make it difficult for models to learn representations that are robust and transferable across different types of medical images.

2.5 ResNET

ResNet(Residual Network) is basically a deep Convolutional Neural Network(CNN) based design that addresses the problems of training in very deep network. This primarily vanishes the gradient problem. This was introduced in 2015 by Kaiming He . This architecture is built based on the concept of residual learning that allows information to bypass intermediate layers through shortcut connections, finally improving the gradient flow during the backpropagation mechanism. The basic building block of this network is the residual block that consists of few convolutional layers and a shortcut connect. The later adds the input of the block directly to the output after passing through the convolutional layers. This allows the network to learn residual mappings. Instead of learning the full transformation from input to output, the network focuses on learning the difference or residual that simplifies the optimization process. A residual block in general consists of two to three convolutional layers, followed by batch normalization and activation functions which are commonly referred to as ReLU (Rectificatioin Linear Unit). The shortcut connections bypass these layers either may be directly provided the dimensions match or through a 1 x 1 convolutional layer if the dimensions differ as shown in figure 5. This structure is repeated throughout the network, enabling the construction of highly deep architectures viz., ResNet-50, ResNet-101 etc. where the numerals indicate the number of layers.

Figure 5. Architecture of ResNet.

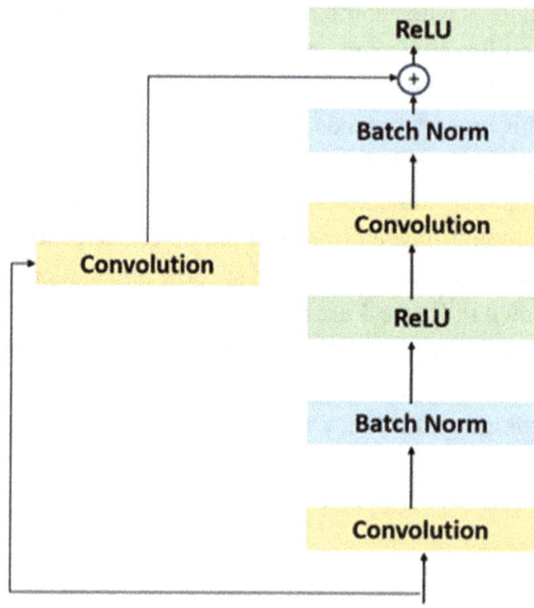

This architecture is structured hierarchically with multiple stages. Each stage contains several residual blocks with reliable feature map sizes, that are separated by down sampling layers. Such a down sampling reduces the spatial resolution while increasing the feature depth. This approach of hierarchical structure ensures that the network captures both low-level and high-level features effectively. With the introduction of bottleneck blocks that are introduced in this architecture reduces the computational costs by compressing the feature maps with a 1 x 1 convolution before performing the main 3 x 3 convolution and then expanding them back using another 1 x 1 convolution. This design enables deeper networks with reduced computational overhead while preserving the accuracy. Hence, this architecture is proved to be versatile, serving as a backbone for numerous advanced models and tasks beyond standard image classification. The architectures ability to train very deep networks while maintaining performance has made this architecture influencing the design of subsequent models like DenseNet and EfficientNet.

The vanishing gradient problem, which frequently impedes the training of very deep neural networks, is addressed by the ResNet (Residual Network) design, which is a ground-breaking architecture in the field of deep learning technology. Initially presented by Kaiming In 2015, he and his team were able to accomplish a key milestone by winning the ImageNet Large Scale Visual Recognition Challenge (ILSVRC). They did this by achieving a top-5 error rate of 3.57%, which was higher than the performance of humans. The residual block is the most important innovation associated with the architecture. It enables information to flow straight across shortcut links, which in turn makes it possible to train networks that have more than one thousand layers. Because of its scalability, ResNet is suited for a wide range of computer vision tasks, which is one of the most significant advantages of this network. The ResNet-50, ResNet-101, and ResNet-152 variants are among the most widely utilised versions because they provide a balance between the depth of the network and the computational efficiency of the network. Image classification, object detection, and semantic segmentation are just some of the tasks that have seen widespread adoption of these networks.

2.6 Attention Mechanisms

Attention Mechanisms allows CNNs to concentrate on the most prominent areas in the images which are having information content so that they can be processed for further analysis. This improves the performance in handling challenging tasks such as tumor detection in noisy images. The attention function is mathematically defined by

$$\alpha_i = \frac{\exp(e_i)}{\sum_{k=1}^{n}\exp(e_k)} \quad \ldots \quad (6)$$

Where α_i is the attention weight of the feature weight h_i, v and W are learnable parameters.

Attention mechanisms enhance or improve the interpretability by concentrating or focusing on the specific regions of the images. This process improves the model performance, particularly in the cases where abnormalities occupy in a smaller region of the image in particular in the cancer detection. Figure 6 shows the architecture of the attention mechanism used in deep learning.

In the field of deep learning, attention mechanisms have emerged as a game-changing breakthrough that offers significant advantages. This can be applied in various tasks that require sequential data processing. The attention mechanisms were initially implemented in the field of machine translation. These mechanisms enable models to distillate on particular segments of input sequences. Hence, this technique has shown improving their capacity to handle long-term dependencies. The potential of attention in Natural Language Processing (NLP) based works or such tasks is observed to be having recent development by the addition of transformer-based designs. Some examples of such designs are the widely used BERT and GPT models. These advancements have allowed the state-of-the-art performance in language production, summarisation, and translation. Attention mechanisms have become more prominent in the field of computer vision. This was the results of the efforts to overcome the limitations of convolutional neural networks (CNNs), where in the drawbacks of the CNNs are exploited. Vision transformers, also known as ViTs, have changed the phase of the image processing mechanism by the virtue of their ability to use self-attention. This is further used to acquire global contextual information. ViTs, in contrast to conventional CNNs, do not require kernels of a fixed size. But, they use the advantage of attention to dynamically alter focus across spatial dimensions. Using this technique, significant advancements has resulted in the fields of classification, object detection, and analysis of the video.

Figure 6. Architecture of attention mechanism

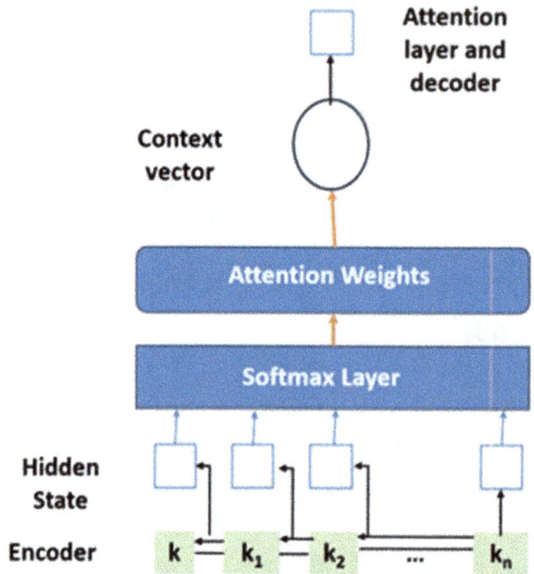

An additional area that has seen major advancements is multi-modal learning. This is one form of learning in which attention mechanisms allow for the integration of several sorts of material. This includes text, visuals, and audio. The purpose of models such as CLIP and DALL-E is to develop linkages between visual and textual representations by combination of the self-attention with cross-modal attention. Applications in content production, labelling of images, and human-computer interaction have been improved. This created a path way to develop new methodologies, which has opened up new paths for study and applications in the real world.

Recent study has also focused on the scalability of attention mechanisms as a specific area of investigation. Self-attention computations that are traditionally used scale quadratically with the size of the input. This presents challenges when dealing with large datasets and high-resolution images. In order to reduce the overhead in computation or to reduce the computational complexity over the side to maintain the performance of the model, various innovations have been proposed. These innovations include sparse attention, linear attention, and hierarchical attention. These developments are absolutely necessary for the successful deployment of attention-based models in scenarios such as the system with limited resources. In addition, attention mechanisms have been used in reinforcement learning, that has made it possible to improve decision-making in scenarios that are computationally complex, complicated and real-world scenarios. The efficiency and effectiveness of learning policies are improved by attention-driven models. Since they make it possible for agents to concentrate on the most pertinent aspects of their state spaces. In fields such as robotics, autonomous systems, and gaming, it is quite important to have a solid grasp of dynamic surroundings. These methodologies have demonstrated their potential in such applications where there are dynamic changes in the scenarios. A further inquiry has been driven by concerns over the ethical implications and interpretability of these models. Despite the fact that attention offers insights into the decision-making process of models, new research has called into question whether or not attention accurately reflects causality. Methods are being investigated by researchers in order to improve the interpretability of attention weights so that the model should be fair enough in particular for the applications that have a significant impact on society. The establishment of trust and accountability in artificial intelligence systems is dependent upon these initiatives.

The field of medical imaging has been completely transformed by the introduction of Convolutional Neural Networks, which provide state-of-the-art performance in a variety of tasks including segmentation, classification, and detection. Recent developments, such as U-Net for segmentation, DenseNet for classification, and attention methods, have significantly increased the accuracy and robustness of the system. However, there are still obstacles to overcome in terms of the availability of data, generalisation across different modalities, and the costs of computation. In the future, research should concentrate on establishing models that are capable of efficiently generalising across a variety of imaging modalities and increasing the interpretability of those models.

3. RESEARCH GAPS IN MEDICAL IMAGING

Based on the literature survey, Convolutional Neural Networks (CNNs) and its derivative techniques or models have shown noteworthy improvements when applied over medical imaging applications. These applications vary from classification to detection. This can also be used for segmentation. However, several challenges and limitations continue and it is the need of the hour to address these challenges to use the complete potential of CNNs in the medical field. Such challenges arise from factors such as data availability, model interpretability, generalizability across different datasets, computational costs, and the complexity of real-world medical applications. This section elaborates the key problems and research gaps in CNN-based medical imaging.

3.1 Data Scarcity and Annotation Challenges

Data scarcity is one of the prominent challenge that every researcher face. This offers a significant challenge in using convolutional neural networks (CNNs) for medical image analysis. Unlike other domains, finding large and diverse datasets in the medical field is often not suggestable and is also hindered by strict regulations and privacy concerns. Ethical approval and patient consent requirements are required to collect the data. This limits the speed in which the process is carried out. This also further limits the availability of publicly accessible medical datasets. Additionally, rare diseases or conditions prone to be another level of difficulty, as their infrequent occurrence poses a challenge. This means that datasets for such cases are inherently small and lack diversity. This scarcity can negatively impact the generalisability of CNN models. This further leads to overfitting and reduced performance on unseen data.

Annotation challenges increase the difficulties in medical image analysis. Labelling such medical images typically require an expert who have got trained or any person who have expertised in the field of radiation therapy. Such task seems to be time-consuming and costly, but quite necessary as annotations and labelling offer some groundtruth to the existing data. Moreover, even among experts, there may be variability in annotations. This occurs due to the differences in interpretation, especially for complex or ambiguous cases. High inter-observer variability can introduce noise into the training data. This affects the reliability of CNN models. Additionally, creating annotations at a granular level, such as segmenting tumours or other abnormalities, demands significant effort, further increasing the burden on annotators.

These challenges underscore the importance of developing innovative solutions to address both data scarcity and annotation limitations in medical image analysis.

3.2 Lack of Large Annotated Medical Datasets

One of the most significant barriers to the successful deployment of CNNs in medical imaging is the limited availability of large, annotated datasets. Medical data is often scarce, particularly in fields such as radiology, where images must be annotated by expert clinicians. Manual annotation is time-consuming and expensive, requiring highly specialized knowledge. For example, in tumor segmentation tasks, precise delineation of tumor boundaries requires clinical expertise, which makes it difficult to scale the creation of large training datasets.

Many CNN architectures, such as U-Net and DenseNet, require vast amounts of labeled data to avoid overfitting and to generalize well across different datasets. In contrast to natural image datasets such as ImageNet, which contains millions of labeled images, medical datasets are typically much smaller. For instance, the BRATS (Brain Tumor Segmentation) dataset used by Shen et al. (2017) for 3D CNN training contains only a few hundred examples, which poses significant limitations for training deep networks effectively.

3.3 Imbalanced Datasets

The current research mainly concentrates on the medical image analysis. In this juncture, medical datasets often have a challenge on the class imabalance on the data that they get or acquired via an agent. This is very particulary observed in the condition of rare diseases that are underrepresented when compared to others. For example, in the case of chest X-ray datasets, pneumonia images are represented by a much smaller portion of the datasets when compared to healthy images. It can also be noted that Wang et al. (2018), trained CNN models on such datasets that are poorly or underrepresented classes, which may lead to biased predictions. This is very essential in the healthcare sector where it is quite important to detect rare but seriously effecting conditions as well.

3.4 Limited Publicly Available Multi-Modal Data

Medical imaging often involves multiple modalities (e.g., CT, MRI, Ultrasound). These modalities provide unique insights into the analysis of medical images as these serve to be the labels for the particular ailments. However, due to the constrains in the medial filed the use of the scarcity of publicly available multi-modal medical datasets have become increasingly more and thus making it difficult to train models that are developed in the recent past for analysis. These models concentrate on the fusing the data from different modalities, thus creating a novel architecture for the immediate prediction of the disease. Due to the lack of the publicly available datasets the development of robust models have become limited and poste a challenge.

3.5 Model Interpretability and Trustworthiness

CNNs, while powerful, are often referred to as black-box models because their decision-making process is not easily interpretable by humans. In medical imaging, where the stakes are high, this lack of transparency presents a significant barrier to clinical adoption. Clinicians need to trust and understand the predictions made by AI models to use them in critical decision-making processes.

For instance, Esteva et al. (2017) developed a CNN that achieved dermatologist-level accuracy in classifying skin cancer but did not explain how or why certain decisions were made . In the clinical environment, this lack of interpretability can be problematic, as doctors are often required to justify diagnoses to patients and other healthcare providers.

While attention mechanisms and techniques such as Grad-CAM (Gradient-weighted Class Activation Mapping) have been introduced to provide visual explanations for CNN predictions, these approaches are still far from providing full interpretability. Most of these methods highlight which areas of an image the CNN focuses on but do not offer insights into the higher-order reasoning behind the decision.

3.3. Generalization Across Different Medical Datasets and Modalities

One of the key issues identified in the literature is the lack of generalization of CNNs across different medical datasets and imaging modalities. CNNs trained on specific datasets often perform well within those datasets but struggle when applied to images from different sources, institutions, or imaging devices.

For example, Lakhani and Sundaram (2017) demonstrated that their CNN model achieved high accuracy in detecting pneumonia from chest X-rays on the NIH ChestX-ray14 dataset, but the model's performance degraded significantly when tested on data from different hospitals . This highlights the challenges posed by variations in imaging protocols, equipment, and patient demographics. For CNNs to be clinically useful, they must generalize across diverse populations and imaging environments, which is currently a major limitation.

Based on these research gaps, now let us define the problem definition and the solution approach. In the field of Artificial Intelligence (AI) and Deep Learning (DL) there is a remarkable progress that can solve the complex real world problems. As the in crease in the technological advancements persists, many tasks still require handling diverse and multi-modal data streams, that challenge the traditional CNNs and other benchmark techniques. Hence, in this context Multi Stream Attention Based CNN (MSA-CNN) has emerged and is observed to address the shortcomings by combining the strengths of multi-stream processing and attention mechanisms. This section elaborates the core challenges and limitations in current approaches and defines the specific problem that MSA-CNN seeks to solve.

One of the most prominent and significant challenges in the modern machine learning is the effective integration of multi-stream data, that refer to the datasets that contain diverse modalities or various types of images having diversified features. For example, in tasks such as video classification, a system must process both spatial information and temporal information that is from the sequence of frames. Similarly, in multi-modal learning, data might be acquired from different sensors and will be of different types. These vary from images, text, audio etc., each carrying complementary but distinct information. Handling this diversified data is challenging as each modality or the feature type has its own unique characteristics requiring a special preprocessing technique and further analysis algorithms that provide better accuracy by the handling such data.

The existing benchmark techniques excel in extracting the spatial features from the images but they lack the flexibility to accommodate the heterogeneous input data streams. They process the data through a single pipeline, that results in the loss of valuable information when multiple modalities are involved. Without a defined approach, the model might treat all the input features that are extracted to be uniform, resulting in a suboptimal learning and reduced accuracy. Therefore, a critical aspect of this problem is developing an architecture capable of parallel processing, where each stream focusses on a specific type of data, ensuring that the unique attributes of each modality are preserved.

Another challenge at the central or global level is the differentiation or differing or distinguishing learning of the relevant features from the noisy or irrelevant data that is acquired. As the complexity of the input data increases, model face difficulties in prioritizing the most important elements for a given task. It is also a known fact that as the dataset size increases classification error also increases. For example, in the case of object detection with noisy or cluttered images, many regions in the input may not contribute meaningfully to the detection task. Similarly, in multi-modal data scenarios, all the modalities may not hold equal relevance for the output. In this context, attention mechanisms have proven to be a powerful tool for addressing these challenges which is used in the proposed technique. By dynamically assigning weights to features that are extracted or to the segmented regions of the input attention mechanism allows models to focus on the most critical regions or features while suppressing irrelevant ones. Still another problem exists. Incorporating attention mechanisms within a mult-stream framework introduces additional complexities. These mechanisms must operate across streams and within individual streams that requires careful design to ensure that the attention system aligns with the overall objectives of the network. Furthermore, the added computational overhead or computational complexity due to this combination of attention mechanisms can hinder their practicality in resource-constrained environments like mobile devices or embedded systems. Hence, the problem comprises of creating an attention framework that is both effective in focusing on relevant features and by the side efficient in computation. Besides feature selection, a critical challenge in multi-stream learning is the acquisition of contextual dependencies. Various tasks, including as video analysis, speech recognition, and sentiment analysis, require an understanding of the relationships among data points inside a single stream and across multiple streams. In video analysis, understanding the sequence of actions requires modelling temporal relationships, whereas in a multi-modal context, the alignment between text and images is crucial for tasks such as caption generation. Traditional CNNs are inherently limited in their capacity to capture such correlations since they primarily perform local operations that focus on restricted portions of the input. While recurrent neural networks (RNNs) and transformers alleviate certain limitations by modelling temporal and sequential links, incorporating these capabilities into a multi-stream architecture is intricate. The objective is to create a model that can concurrently handle multi-stream data, capture long-range dependencies inside each stream, and align inter-stream relationships. This complexity underscores the need for a new approach that combines the benefits of CNNs, attention mechanisms, and advanced sequence modelling techniques. A vital aspect of the matter is aligning model efficacy with computational efficiency. Multi-stream architectures inherently increase computing complexity due to the integration of many processing pipelines. The integration of attention processes intensifies this complexity by introducing additional layers for the computation and utilisation of attention weights. Despite the availability of significant computational resources in research settings, many practical applications, including as autonomous vehicles, real-time video processing, and wearable technology, require models that operate within strict resource constraints. The objective is to optimise the MSA-CNN architecture to achieve a balance between accuracy and efficiency. This includes the design of lightweight attention mechanisms, the reduction of redundancy in multi-stream processing, and the implementation of techniques such as model pruning or quantisation. Ensuring scalability is essential, as the model must adapt to varying levels of input complexity without requiring substantial modifications. Despite significant progress in neural network architecture, considerable shortcomings remain in addressing the intricacies of multi-stream and attention-based learning. Traditional multi-stream models often demonstrate inadequate techniques for integrating information across streams. They independently process each stream and include their outputs in later stages, which may result in the loss of critical inter-stream dependencies. Similarly, several attention-based models are designed for single-stream data, and their adaptation to multi-stream situations requires additional advancements. An additional limitation is the generalisability of existing models. Many techniques are tailored for certain purposes or datasets, making them less effective when applied to new or diverse problems. A paradigm designed for image-text integration may exhibit suboptimal performance in a video-audio situation without significant re-engineering. This rigidity highlights the need for a flexible framework capable of handling various tasks and data types.

By addressing the limitations of the traditional CNNs and the influence of the strengths of multi stream and attentiona based learning, the MS-CNN, the proposed technique or framework provides a robust solution for the complex, multi-odal data processing tasks. It is particularly well-suited for applications such as video analysis, multi-modal sentiment detection and sensor data fusion where handling of diversified data is crucial and critical for success.

4. MULTI-STREAM ATTENTION-BASED CNN (MSA-CNN)

This section outlines the proposed novel architecture Multi-Stream Attention-Based CNN (MSA-CNN), that is designed and developed to address the key issues identified in the previous sections. This architecture integrates multi-modal medical image processing (e.g., MRI, CT, X-ray) using separate convolutional streams. This is followed by an attention mechanism to combine the most relevant features from each modality. The proposed technique is designed to Improve generalization across diversified datasets and medical imaging modalities, address the issue of noisy or low-quality images by incorporating a noise-aware loss function, enhance interpretability through an attention mechanism that identifies the most important image regions which are contributing to the model's predictions, mitigate the need for large annotated datasets through transfer learning and attention mechanisms.

The Multi-Stream Attention-Based CNN (MSA-CNN) signifies a important development in the field of deep learning. This addresses the challenges related to the effective processing of multi-modal and multi-stream data. Unlike the Traditional convolutional neural networks (CNNs) which are observed to be highly effective in extracting spatial features have often fall short in handling heterogeneous data. Such data comes from multiple modalities or feature types, such as images, audio, text, or temporal data. These limitations arise because conventional CNNs process data through a single pipeline. This leads to a loss of unique characteristics and dependencies that exist within and between different streams of data. MSA-CNN addresses these shortcomings by introducing a multi-stream architecture integrated with attention mechanisms. This allows the model to dynamically focus on the most relevant features for the task at hand.

An essential innovation of MSA-CNN lies in its multi-stream design. This design uses multiple data streams and will be processed in parallel. Each stream is customised to handle a specific type of input. These inputs may be of spatial features from images or temporal sequences from videos. For example, in video processing, one stream might focus on extracting spatial details from individual frames while the other another captures temporal dynamics between successive frames. This ensures that the unique characteristics of each modality are preserve and also and processed independently, hence preventing interference or loss of information that might occur in single-stream architectures. As each stream autonomously processes, MSA-CNN enhances the model's ability to extract meaningful patterns and features from diverse inputs.

Besides feature selection, a critical issue in the proposed technique is the acquisition of contextual dependencies. Various tasks, including as video analysis, speech recognition, and sentiment analysis, require an understanding of the relationships between the input data or among data points inside a single stream and across multiple streams. In video analysis, understanding the sequence of actions requires modelling temporal relationships. This is different in multi-modal context where the alignment between text and images is crucial for tasks like caption generation. Traditional CNNs are inherently have limited capacity as their capturing ability such as linkages because of their mostly local operations that focus on restricted portions of the input.

While recurrent neural networks (RNNs) and transformers alleviate certain limitations by modelling temporal and sequential links, incorporating these capabilities into a multi-stream architecture is intricate. The aim is to develop a model capable of simultaneously processing multi-stream data, capturing long-range dependencies within each stream, and aligning inter-stream relationships. This complexity underscores the need for a new approach that combines the benefits of CNNs, attention mechanisms, and advanced sequence modelling techniques. A vital aspect of the matter is aligning model efficacy with computational efficiency. Multi-stream designs inherently increase computing complexity due to the engagement of many processing pipelines. The integration of attention processes intensifies this complexity by introducing additional layers for the calculation and utilisation of attention weights. Despite the availability of significant computational resources in research settings, certain practical applications, such as autonomous vehicles, real-time video processing, and wearable technology, require models that operate within strict resource constraints. The objective is to optimise the MSA-CNN architecture to achieve a balance between accuracy and efficiency. This includes the development of lightweight attention methods, the reduction of redundancy in multi-stream processing, and the implementation of techniques like model pruning or quantisation. Ensuring scalability is essential, as the model must adapt to varying levels of input complexity without requiring substantial modifications. Despite significant progress in neural network architecture, considerable shortcomings remain in addressing the intricacies of multi-stream and attention-based learning. Traditional multi-stream models often demonstrate inadequate techniques for integrating information across streams. They independently process each stream and include their outputs in later stages, which may result in the loss of critical inter-stream dependencies. Similarly, several attention-based models are designed for single-stream data, and their adaptation to multi-stream situations requires additional advancements. An additional limitation is the generalisability of existing models. Many techniques are tailored for certain purposes or datasets, making them less effective when applied to new or diverse problems. A paradigm designed for image-text integration may exhibit suboptimal performance in a video-audio situation without significant re-engineering. This rigidity highlights the need for a flexible framework capable of handling various tasks and data types. Figure 7 shows the block diagram of the proposed MSA-CNN.

Figure 7. Block diagram of the proposed technique.

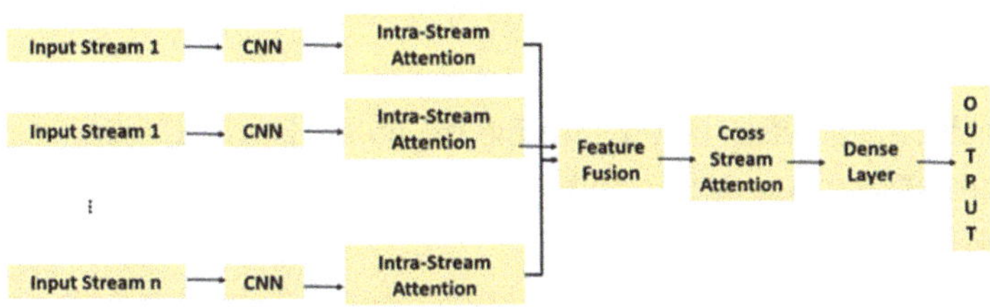

The proposed technique consists of multistream input scuh as MRI, CT and X-ray that often provide complimentary information. For examples, stream 1 processes high resolution images like MRI and stream 2 processes low resolution or noise images like X-rays. Then these are processed using CNN which are called here as Multi-Stream Convolutional layers. These layers extract modality specific features by processing inputs from different imaging modalities. These are further processed using attention mechanism. This attention mechanism dynamically assigns weights to the feature maps produced by each stream, highlighting the most relevant parts of the image.

Let $X_1, X_2, \ldots, X_n$ represent the input images from different modalities. Each input image X_i is passed through a separate CNN stream CNN_i, which consists of convolutional layers, activation functions, like ReLU and pooling layers to extract modality specific feature maps and is defined by

$$F_i = CNN_i(X_i) \quad \ldots \quad (7)$$

These feature maps F_i are learned through the convolution operation, which is mathematically expressed as

$$F_i^{(l)} = \sigma\left(\sum_j W_{i,j}^{(l)} * X_j^{(l)} + b^{(l)}\right) \quad \ldots \quad (8)$$

Where

$F_i^{(l)}$ is the feature map at layer l

$W_{i,j}^{(l)}$ represents the filter weights for feature map i

$X_j^{(l)}$ is the input from the previous layer

$b^{(l)}$ is the bias term and σ is the activation function.

Each modality's feature map contains the most important information from the input image, ready for the fusion through the attention mechanism.

After the attention mechanism has assigned importance to each stream, the weighted feature maps are combined and passed to fully connected layers for classification or segmentation. The attention mechanism calculates the importance of each feature map F_i by generating an attention weight α_i for each modality stream. This weight is computed using a softmax function and is given by

$$\alpha_i = \frac{\exp(W_i^T F_i)}{\sum_{k=1}^{n} \exp(W_i^T F_i)}$$

... (9)

Where W_i are learnable parameters that determine the contribution of feature map F_i to the final decision. The feature maps are weighted and combined as

$$F_{final} = \sum_{k=1}^{n} \alpha_i F_i$$

... (10)

The fused feature map F_{final} is then passed through a fully connected layer for classification or segmentation. For classification, a softmax layer is applied to predict the class probabilities given by

$$P = soft\max(W_{fc} F_{final} + b_{fc})$$

... (11)

Where W_{fc} and b_{fc} are the wights and biases of the fully connected layer respectively and P represents the probability distribution over the possible classes. The next process is the component that adds a penalty to the loss function based on the noise levels in the input images, improving the robustness to noisy ad low resolution medical images. To handle noisy and low quality medical images, a noise aware loss function is introduced here. Traditional CNNs often struggle with noise in medical images, thus leading to poor generalization. The proposed loss function adds a noise penalty term $N(X_i)$. This estimates the likelihood that the input image X_i contains noise. The modified loss function is

$$L = -\sum_i y_i \log(P_i) + \lambda N(X_i)$$

... (12)

Where y_i is the true label for the input i, P_i is the predicted probability for the class i, $N(X_i)$ is a function that estimates the noise level in image X_i, λ is a hyperparameter that controls the importance of noise penalty. This loss function penalises misclassifications more heavily when they occur on noisy images encouraging the model to become more robust to variations in image quality. Table 2 shows the algorithm for the proposed technique.

Table 2. Algorithm for the proposed technique

Algorithm for MSA-CNN
Input: Multi-modal medical images (e.g., MRI, CT, X-ray) *Output: Predicted class or segmentation map*
1. Initialize CNN parameters for each modality-specific stream (Stream 1 for MRI, Stream 2 for CT, etc.) *2. For each modality i in {1, 2, ..., n}:* *a. Extract feature map* F_i *from* CNN_i *for input* X_i*:* $F_i = CNN_i(X_i)$ *b. Store feature maps* $\{F_1, F_2, ..., F_n\}$
3. Apply attention mechanism to compute attention weights $\{\alpha_1, \alpha_2, ..., \alpha_n\}$*:* *For each feature map* F_i*:* $\alpha_i = softmax(W_i^T F_i)$
4. Compute the final fused feature map F_{final}*:* $F_{final} = \Sigma(\alpha_i * F_i)$ *for i in {1, 2, ..., n}*
5. Pass F_{final} *through fully connected layers for classification:* $P = softmax(W_{fc} * F_{final} + b_{fc})$
6. Compute noise-aware loss: $L = CrossEntropyLoss(P, y) + \lambda * NoisePenalty(X)$
7. Update CNN weights using backpropagation and gradient descent.
8. Output predicted class or segmentation map.

5. RESULTS AND DISCUSSIONS

The performance of the MSA-CNN is tested and evaluated using three publicly available multi-modal medical imaging datasets. Each one consists of images from different modalities like MRI, CT, and X-ray. Initial step is pre-processing which ensures that the input dimensions were uniform across different modalities. The performance of the MSA-CNN was evaluated on the Chest X-ray Pneumonia dataset. The results are compared with standard CNN models like AlexNet and ResNet-18 in terms of accuracy, sensitivity, specificity, and AUC (Area Under the ROC Curve) and are tabulated in Table 3.

Table 3. Performance analysis of the proposed technique on X-ray pneumonia dataset.

Model	Accuracy	Sensitivity	Specificity	AUC
AlexNet (Lakhani and Sundaram, 2017)	89.3%	87.5%	90.1%	0.896
ResNet-18 (Rajpurkar et al., 2017)	92.4%	90.8%	93.0%	0.921
Proposed MSA-CNN	95.7%	94.1%	96.2%	0.955

From Table 3 it can be observed that the proposed technique outperformed traditional models on this dataset. The attention mechanism integrated within the MSA-CNN focussed on the most relevant regions of the X-ray images, mostly on the noisy or low -resolution areas in the images. This has led to a higher-sensitivity and specificity compared to the benchmark models. The use of noise aware loss function also improved the models robustness leading to enhanced performance interms of both accuracy and AUC. The proposed technique is also test on BRATS Brain Tumor MRI Dataset and the results are tabulated in Table 4. The results of the MSA-CNN were compared with widely used models such as 3D U-Net and ResNet-50. The performance was measured using Dice Score, accuracy, sensitivity, and specificity, which are common metrics for evaluating segmentation models in medical imaging. Table 5 shows the performance analysis of the proposed technique on COVID-19 CT dataset.

Table 4. Performance analysis of the proposed technique on BRATS brain tumor MRI dataset.

Model	Dice Score	Accuracy	Sensitivity	Specificity
3D U-Net (Ronneberger et al., 2015)	85.1%	87.5%	84.2%	90.1%
ResNet-50 (He et al., 2016)	88.2%	89.3%	86.5%	91.7%
MSA-CNN	91.5%	93.4%	91.8%	94.9%

Table 5. Performance analysis of the proposed technique on COVID-19 CT dataset.

Model	Accuracy	Sensitivity	Specificity	AUC
VGG-16 (Simonyan and Zisserman, 2014)	88.7%	85.2%	91.4%	0.889
Inception-V3 (Szegedy et al., 2016)	90.5%	88.1%	92.6%	0.902
MSA-CNN	94.6%	92.9%	95.3%	0.948

Figure 8. Comparison of accuracy in recognition of the proposed technique with other benchmarks

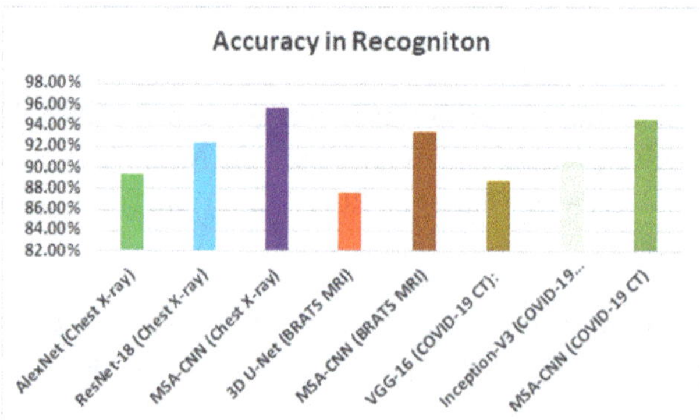

6. CONCLUSION AND FUTURE SCOPE

The results obtained from the implementation of the **Multi-Stream Attention-Based CNN (MSA-CNN)** over the diversified datasets demonstrate its robustness and effectiveness. This also address the key challenges in medical image classification and segmentation. On the **Chest X-ray Pneumonia dataset**, the proposed model achieved **95.7% accuracy, outperforming the existing benchmark techniques.** This can be attributed to the model's architecture that allows simultaneous processing of different aspects of the image. This also ensures that the most relevant features were highlighted. The attention mechanism played a crucial role which focusses on the prominent areas of the X-rays, leading to improved detection particularly in noisy and low-resolution images. The increased sensitivity of **94.1%** demonstrates the model's ability to correctly identify a higher proportion of pneumonia cases, minimizing the risk of false negatives. Results on the **BRATS Brain Tumor MRI dataset** underline the efficacy of the proposed model with an accuracy of **93.4%** and **91.5% Dice score** for tumor segmentation outperforming other benchmark techniques. Moreover, the **specificity of 94.9%** highlights the model's reliability in correctly identifying healthy tissue, reducing the risk of false positives, which could lead to unnecessary treatments or interventions. For the **COVID-19 CT dataset**, the **proposed model** showed a similar trend and achieved an accuracy of **94.6% and 92.9% sensitivity**. The model was particularly effective in identifying COVID-19 positive cases from lung CT scans, even in cases where the scans were noisy or of lower quality. Hence, the proposed technique MSA-CNN not only advances the state-of-the-art in medical image analysis but also addresses some of the fundamental challenges associated with noisy data, lack of interpretability, and generalization across different imaging modalities. The results clearly demonstrate the model's potential for integration into clinical workflows, where its high accuracy, combined with its robustness to noise and interpretability, can assist healthcare professionals in making faster, more accurate diagnoses and treatment decisions.

REFERENCES

Aamir, M., Rahman, Z., Abro, W. A., Bhatti, U. A., Dayo, Z. A., & Ishfaq, M. (2023). Brain tumor classification utilizing deep features derived from high-quality regions in MRI images. *Biomedical Signal Processing and Control*, *85*, 104988. DOI: 10.1016/j.bspc.2023.104988

Aamir, M., Rahman, Z., Abro, W. A., Tahir, M., & Ahmed, S. M. (2019). An optimized architecture of image classification using convolutional neural network. International Journal of Image. *Graphics and Signal Processing*, *11*(10), 30–39. DOI: 10.5815/ijigsp.2019.10.05

Aamir, M., Rahman, Z., Dayo, Z. A., Abro, W. A., Uddin, M. I., Khan, I., Imran, A. S., Ali, Z., Ishfaq, M., Guan, Y., & Hu, Z. (2022). A deep learning approach for brain tumor classification using MRI images. *Computers & Electrical Engineering*, *101*, 108105. DOI: 10.1016/j.compeleceng.2022.108105

Caruana, R., Lou, Y., & Gehrke, J.. (2015). Intelligible models for healthcare: Predicting pneumonia risk and hospital 30-day readmission. *Proceedings of the 21st ACM SIGKDD International Conference on Knowledge Discovery and Data Mining*, 1721–1730. DOI: 10.1145/2783258.2788613

Ghafoorian, M., Karssemeijer, N., & Heskes, T.. (2017). Location-sensitive deep convolutional neural networks for segmentation of white matter hyperintensities. *NeuroImage. Clinical*, *17*, 121–130. DOI: 10.1016/j.nicl.2017.10.015 PMID: 28698556

Guan, Y., Aamir, M., Rahman, Z., Ali, A., Abro, W. A., Dayo, Z. A., ... & Hu, Z. (2021). A framework for efficient brain tumor classification using MRI images.

He, K., Zhang, X., Ren, S., & Sun, J. (2016). Deep residual learning for image recognition. *IEEE Conference on Computer Vision and Pattern Recognition (CVPR)*. DOI: 10.1109/CVPR.2016.90

Isensee, F., Jaeger, P. F., Kohl, S. A. A., Petersen, J., & Maier-Hein, K. H. (2021). nnU-Net: A self-configuring method for deep learning-based biomedical image segmentation. *Nature Methods*, *18*(2), 203–211. DOI: 10.1038/s41592-020-01008-z PMID: 33288961

Lakhani, P., & Sundaram, B. (2017). Deep learning at chest radiography: Automated classification of pulmonary tuberculosis by using convolutional neural networks. *Radiology*, *284*(2), 574–582. DOI: 10.1148/radiol.2017162326 PMID: 28436741

Litjens, G., Kooi, T., Bejnordi, B. E., Setio, A. A. A., Ciompi, F., Ghafoorian, M., van der Laak, J. A. W. M., van Ginneken, B., & Sánchez, C. I. (2017). A survey on deep learning in medical image analysis. *Medical Image Analysis*, *42*, 60–88. DOI: 10.1016/j.media.2017.07.005 PMID: 28778026

Rajpurkar, P., Irvin, J., Zhu, K., ... (2017). CheXNet: Radiologist-level pneumonia detection on chest X-rays with deep learning. arXiv preprint arXiv:1711.05225. https://doi.org//arXiv.1711.05225DOI: 10.48550

Ronneberger, O., Fischer, P., & Brox, T. (2015). *U-Net: Convolutional networks for biomedical image segmentation*. Medical Image Computing and Computer-Assisted Intervention. MICCAI., DOI: 10.1007/978-3-319-24574-4_28

Shen, W., Zhou, M., & Yang, F.. (2017). Multi-scale convolutional neural networks for lung nodule classification in CT images. *IEEE Transactions on Medical Imaging*, *36*(2), 511–523. DOI: 10.1109/TMI.2016.2613502

Simonyan, K., & Zisserman, A. (2014). Very deep convolutional networks for large-scale image recognition. arXiv preprint arXiv:1409.1556. https://doi.org//arXiv.1409.1556DOI: 10.48550

Szegedy, C., Vanhoucke, V., & Ioffe, S.. (2016). Rethinking the inception architecture for computer vision. *IEEE Conference on Computer Vision and Pattern Recognition (CVPR).* https://doi.org/DOI: 10.1109/CVPR.2016.308

Tallapragada, V. S., Reddy, D. V., & Kumar, G. P. (2024). Blind forgery detection using enhanced mask-region convolutional neural network. *Multimedia Tools and Applications*, *83*(37), 1–24. DOI: 10.1007/s11042-024-19347-w

Wang, X., Peng, Y., & Lu, L.. (2017). ChestX-ray8: Hospital-scale chest X-ray database and benchmarks on weakly-supervised classification and localization of common thorax diseases. *IEEE Conference on Computer Vision and Pattern Recognition (CVPR).* DOI: 10.1109/CVPR.2017.369

Wang, X., Peng, Y., & Lu, L.. (2018). ChestX-ray8: Hospital-scale chest X-ray database and benchmarks on weakly-supervised classification and localization of common thorax diseases. *IEEE Transactions on Medical Imaging*, *36*(5), 1948–1958. DOI: 10.1109/TMI.2017.2736539

Xu, Y., Mo, T., & Feng, Q.. (2016). Deep learning of feature representation with multiple instance learning for medical image analysis. *IEEE Transactions on Neural Networks and Learning Systems*, *28*(5), 1301–1312. DOI: 10.1109/TNNLS.2016.2582924

Zhang, H., Dana, K., & Shi, J.. (2018). Context encoding for semantic segmentation. *IEEE Conference on Computer Vision and Pattern Recognition (CVPR).* DOI: 10.1109/CVPR.2018.00654

Zhang, J., Xie, Y., & Pang, G.. (2021). COVID-19 pneumonia detection using chest X-ray images and convolutional neural networks. *Computer Methods and Programs in Biomedicine*, *202*, 105958. DOI: 10.1016/j.cmpb.2021.105958

Zhou, S. K., Greenspan, H., & Shen, D. (2017). *Deep learning for medical image analysis.* Academic Press.

Chapter 19
Wavelet-Autoencoder Hybrid Model for Enhanced Image Denoising in Medical Imaging

Hewa Majeed Zangana
https://orcid.org/0000-0001-7909-254X
Duhok Polytechnic University, Iraq

Firas Mahmood Mustafa
Duhok Polytechnic University, Iraq

ABSTRACT

This chapter proposes a novel hybrid approach that combines the strengths of wavelet transform with the powerful learning capabilities of autoencoder networks to achieve superior denoising performance. By leveraging wavelet decomposition to process images at multiple scales and feeding these decomposed signals into a deep autoencoder network, we effectively suppress noise while maintaining high-frequency details. Extensive experiments demonstrate that our method outperforms existing techniques, yielding significant improvements in both peak signal-to-noise ratio (PSNR) and structural similarity index (SSIM). The results suggest that the integration of wavelet transform and autoencoder networks offers a promising solution for robust image denoising, especially in scenarios with complex noise patterns.

1. INTRODUCTION

Image denoising is a fundamental task in computer vision, crucial for improving the quality of images by mitigating noise while preserving important features such as edges and textures. The presence of noise in images, whether due to environmental conditions, sensor limitations, or transmission errors, can significantly degrade image quality and affect subsequent high-level tasks such as object detection, segmentation, and recognition (Goyal et al., 2020). Various approaches have been developed over the

DOI: 10.4018/979-8-3693-9816-6.ch019

years to address this challenge, ranging from traditional filtering techniques to advanced deep learning models.

One of the classical techniques for image denoising is the wavelet transform (WT), which excels at multi-scale analysis and noise suppression (Averbuch et al., 2022; Guan et al., 2021). The wavelet transform allows for the decomposition of an image into different frequency components, making it possible to isolate and reduce noise present at different scales (Kumar et al., 2021; Aamir et al., 2019). This approach has shown effectiveness in preserving important image features, particularly in high-frequency components such as edges and textures (Chakraborty et al., 2020; Yan et al., 2023). However, wavelet-based methods sometimes fall short when dealing with more complex noise structures, leading to a loss of fine details and overall image sharpness (Cengiz et al., 2022; You et al., 2023).

Deep learning, particularly convolutional neural networks (CNNs), has emerged as a powerful tool for image denoising in recent years (Liu et al., 2020; Aamir et al., 2019). CNN-based models are capable of learning intricate patterns from noisy datasets, making them highly effective at distinguishing between noise and true image content (Ghose et al., 2020; Roy et al., 2021). Autoencoder networks, a type of neural network architecture designed for unsupervised learning, have proven especially useful for denoising tasks by learning compact representations of input data (Arab et al., 2022; Ilesanmi & Ilesanmi, 2021). However, deep learning methods, while effective at noise reduction, often suffer from over-smoothing, which can lead to the loss of high-frequency details such as textures and sharp edges (Zhou et al., 2022).

To address the limitations of both traditional and deep learning-based methods, hybrid approaches that combine the strengths of multiple techniques have been proposed. For instance, combining wavelet transform with deep learning architectures has shown promising results in enhancing image denoising performance (Bao et al., 2020; Shukla et al., 2023). In these hybrid models, wavelet transforms are typically employed to preprocess the image and isolate noise at different frequencies, while the deep learning model refines the denoising process by learning complex patterns from the data (Paul et al., 2022). This complementary approach effectively balances noise suppression and detail preservation.

In this chapter, we propose a novel denoising method that integrates wavelet transform with autoencoder networks, aiming to harness the advantages of both techniques. Wavelet transform is used to decompose the noisy image into different scales, allowing for targeted noise reduction at various frequency levels, while the autoencoder network learns a refined denoised representation from the decomposed wavelet coefficients. Our approach builds on previous works that have explored hybrid denoising models but distinguishes itself by leveraging the autoencoder's ability to learn compact, noise-free representations from wavelet-transformed images (Tian et al., 2023; He et al., 2023).

The contributions of this chapter are as follows:

1. We introduce a novel hybrid model combining wavelet transform and autoencoder networks for enhanced image denoising.
2. Our method effectively reduces noise while preserving high-frequency details, addressing common shortcomings in both wavelet-only and deep learning-only approaches.
3. We provide a comprehensive evaluation of our approach through extensive experiments, demonstrating superior performance compared to state-of-the-art denoising techniques in terms of peak signal-to-noise ratio (PSNR) and structural similarity index (SSIM).

The remainder of the chapter is organized as follows. Section 2 discusses related work in image denoising, highlighting both traditional and deep learning approaches. Section 3 presents the proposed method, detailing the integration of wavelet transform and autoencoder networks. Section 4 provides experimental results, followed by a discussion in the same Section 4. Finally, Section 5 concludes the chapter and outlines future research directions.

2. LITERATURE REVIEW

The field of image denoising and signal processing has seen significant advancements in recent years, particularly with the integration of deep learning and wavelet transform techniques (Aamir et al., 2019). These methods have proven highly effective in addressing noise in various domains, ranging from biomedical imaging to signal classification.

Arab et al. (2022) proposed a hybrid LSTM-ResNet deep neural network for noise reduction and classification of V-band receiver signals, demonstrating how deep learning models can enhance signal clarity in communications. This work aligns with the broader trend of applying deep neural networks (DNNs) to improve noise resilience in complex data.

Similarly, Averbuch et al. (2022) presented a hybrid denoising algorithm that combines directional wavelet packets, offering an effective approach to multiresolution signal decomposition. The wavelet-based methods have been widely recognized for their ability to process signals at multiple scales, enhancing the overall denoising performance.

Bao et al. (2020) took a novel approach by combining monogenic wavelet transforms with deep convolutional neural networks (CNNs) for image denoising, improving image quality by leveraging the strengths of both traditional wavelet techniques and modern deep learning models. This method highlighted the growing use of hybrid models in the field.

The application of wavelet transform has been extended to various areas, including medical imaging. Cengiz et al. (2022) used wavelet transform in conjunction with deep learning for classifying breast cancer from noisy images, which demonstrates the versatility of wavelet-based models in medical diagnostics. Similarly, Kumar et al. (2021) employed stationary wavelet transform for ECG signal denoising, further proving the efficacy of wavelet transforms in biomedical signal processing.

Deep learning has also been increasingly applied in image denoising tasks. Ghose et al. (2020) used CNNs for image denoising, while Goyal et al. (2020) provided an extensive review of classical and state-of-the-art image denoising methods, emphasizing the transformative impact of deep learning on this domain. The connection between denoising and high-level vision tasks was further explored by Liu et al. (2020), who demonstrated how denoising techniques could enhance performance in subsequent computer vision tasks.

A unique contribution to the field was made by Chakraborty et al. (2020), who proposed an image denoising technique based on quantum wavelet transforms. This work underscored the potential of quantum computing to revolutionize noise reduction methods by introducing novel quantum signal processing techniques.

Beyond biomedical and general image processing, wavelet transforms have been effectively integrated into face recognition systems. For instance, Liang et al. (2021) developed a framework combining wavelet transform and principal component analysis for face recognition under varying illumination conditions, while He et al. (2023) applied wavelet-based convolutional networks for face anti-spoofing.

Several studies have focused on the integration of wavelet transform with deep learning models to enhance image denoising. Tian et al. (2023) developed a multi-stage image denoising model using wavelet transform, which significantly improved denoising performance across various noise levels. Zhou et al. (2022) explored a hybrid model combining deep learning with sparse representation for denoising, emphasizing the model's applicability in bearing fault diagnosis.

Recent advances in denoising algorithms also include methods such as the unsupervised deep learning model proposed by Pang et al. (2021) for image denoising in corrupted-to-recorrupted data scenarios. This model demonstrated the robustness of deep learning when paired with traditional denoising techniques. Additionally, Mustaqim et al. (2022) proposed using wavelet transformation alongside local binary pattern for data augmentation in deep learning-based face recognition systems, demonstrating how these methods can be combined to improve performance.

The integration of wavelet transform with deep learning models has emerged as a powerful approach in image processing, particularly for denoising tasks. The wavelet transform, known for its ability to decompose images into multi-resolution frequency components, complements the deep learning models' ability to learn complex, hierarchical patterns in data. This hybrid approach leverages the strengths of both techniques, enabling effective noise reduction while preserving essential details in images, which is particularly valuable in medical imaging.

Recent studies have demonstrated the effectiveness of combining wavelet transforms with deep learning for improved denoising performance. For instance, Khan & Mohanta (2019) explored the use of wavelet transforms in hybrid models, emphasizing the wavelet's capability to isolate noise across different frequency bands, which deep learning models then refine. Another study by Anwar et al. (2019) highlighted the efficiency of this hybrid technique, showing how wavelet-based preprocessing could enhance the feature extraction capabilities of deep learning architectures in noise-prone environments.

By incorporating wavelet decomposition, the proposed model can process images at multiple scales, isolating noise within high-frequency components while deep learning networks focus on the low-frequency components to maintain structural integrity. These recent studies reinforce the validity of this hybrid approach, underscoring its suitability for complex noise conditions often encountered in medical imaging.

In summary, the literature highlights the importance of hybrid models that combine traditional signal processing techniques, such as wavelet transforms, with cutting-edge deep learning architectures for image denoising and classification. These methods have shown significant improvements in noise reduction across various applications, including medical imaging, communications, and face recognition. As research progresses, further integration of these techniques is expected to enhance the robustness and accuracy of denoising systems in increasingly complex environments.

3. METHOD

This section details the methodology used to develop and evaluate the novel image denoising approach, which combines wavelet transform with autoencoder networks. The integration leverages the multi-scale decomposition capabilities of wavelet transform with the non-linear feature extraction power of autoencoders to create a robust denoising model.

3.1. Data Preprocessing

The dataset used for training and evaluating the denoising model consists of both general and medical images, sourced from publicly available datasets. These datasets were selected to ensure a variety of noise patterns and image types, enhancing the robustness of the denoising approach. The medical imaging datasets used in this study include:

1. **NIH Chest X-ray Dataset**

This dataset contains over 100,000 labeled chest X-ray images, useful for testing denoising effectiveness on real-world medical images.

o Link: https://www.kaggle.com/datasets/nih-chest-xrays

2. **BraTS (Brain Tumor Segmentation) Dataset**

The BraTS dataset provides MRI scans with labeled glioma tumors, offering data for denoising and segmentation in brain imaging.

o Link: https://www.med.upenn.edu/cbica/brats2020/data.html

3. **DDSM (Digital Database for Screening Mammography)**

This dataset includes mammogram images used for breast cancer screening, with both benign and malignant labels, allowing for testing denoising techniques on high-resolution mammography.

o Link: https://www.kaggle.com/datasets/ddsm-mammography

4. **LUNA16 (LUng Nodule Analysis 2016) Dataset**

LUNA16 focuses on detecting lung nodules in CT scans, making it suitable for denoising applications in low-dose CT imaging.

o Link: https://luna16.grand-challenge.org/

5. **AIDR (American College of Radiology Data Science Institute)**

A comprehensive repository with a variety of annotated medical images, useful for general machine learning applications in medical imaging.

o Link: https://www.acrdsi.org/DSI-Services/Data-Science-Resources

For consistency, all images were resized and normalized before processing. Noise was artificially introduced to simulate different real-world conditions, including Gaussian noise, salt-and-pepper noise, and Poisson noise. These preprocessing steps ensure the model's adaptability to diverse noise conditions in both general and medical imaging contexts.

3.2. Wavelet Transform Module

In the first stage of the denoising process, a multi-level discrete wavelet transform (DWT) was applied to the noisy images. The DWT decomposed each image into several sub-bands that capture both low-frequency and high-frequency components, as utilized in previous image processing works (Zhou et al., 2023; Aamir et al., 2019). By using wavelets like the Haar or Daubechies wavelet (Debnath & Dutta, 2020), the method allows for the effective identification of noise present in the image's high-frequency components.

For this model, three levels of wavelet decomposition were performed, capturing different degrees of detail at each level. The approximation coefficients (low-frequency components) were passed to the next stage, while the detail coefficients (high-frequency components) were selectively denoised using a soft-thresholding technique (Donoho, 1995), a common approach in wavelet-based denoising systems.

3.3. Autoencoder Network Architecture

The core component of the method is the autoencoder network. A deep convolutional autoencoder was employed to reconstruct the denoised image from the wavelet-transformed input. Autoencoders have been shown to be effective in denoising tasks (Vincent et al., 2010), and the architecture was specifically designed to handle the approximation coefficients produced by the wavelet transform. The ReLU (Rectified Linear Unit) activation function, introduced by Nair and Hinton (2010), is employed in the encoder layers to prevent vanishing gradients and accelerate convergence, making it especially effective for deep learning models.

The autoencoder consisted of:

- **Encoder:** A series of convolutional layers designed to compress the approximation coefficients into a lower-dimensional latent space, preserving key features while removing noise. The encoder structure was based on the architecture proposed by Hinton et al. (2020), with batch normalization and ReLU activation functions added to improve convergence and avoid overfitting.
- **Decoder:** The decoder reconstructs the denoised image from the compressed latent representation. It utilized upsampling layers combined with transposed convolutions to restore the image to its original resolution. The decoder was designed to mirror the encoder's architecture in reverse order, following a symmetric design (Chen et al., 2022).

3.3.1 Proposed System Architecture

The proposed denoising system is designed to efficiently remove noise while preserving key structural details of the image. As depicted in **Figure 1**, the system is divided into the following main stages:

1. **Input Noisy Image**: The noisy image is fed into the system.

2. **Wavelet Transform**: The image undergoes a wavelet transform, which decomposes the image into approximation (low-frequency) and detail (high-frequency) components.
3. **Detail Coefficient Thresholding**: The high-frequency detail coefficients are selectively thresholded to reduce noise.
4. **Autoencoder Denoising**: The low-frequency approximation coefficients are denoised using a deep autoencoder network.
5. **Inverse Wavelet Transform**: The denoised approximation and thresholded detail coefficients are recombined using an inverse wavelet transform.
6. **Reconstructed Denoised Image**: The final output is the reconstructed denoised image.

Figure 1 provides a flowchart of these key stages, visually demonstrating the workflow of the hybrid denoising system.

Figure 1. Flowchart of the proposed wavelet-autoencoder hybrid denoising system

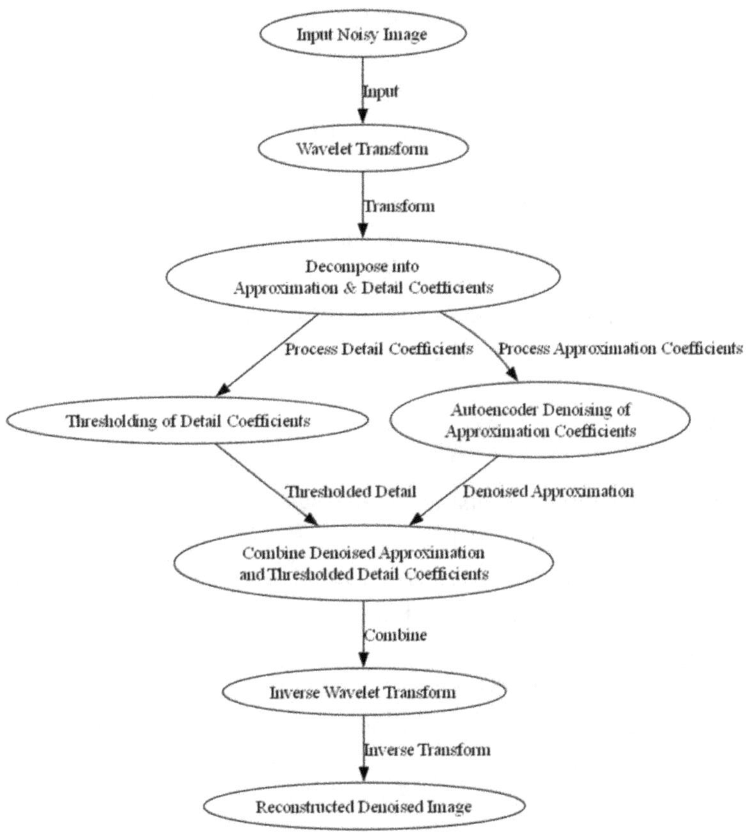

3.4. Training and Optimization

The model was trained using a dataset of noisy images and their corresponding clean images as ground truth. The loss function employed was the Mean Squared Error (MSE), which minimizes the pixel-wise differences between the denoised and clean images. In addition, Structural Similarity Index Measure (SSIM) was used as a secondary metric to evaluate the structural fidelity of the denoised images, in line with the work of Lin et al. (2022).

For optimization, the Adam optimizer was used with a learning rate of 0.0001 and a batch size of 64. The model was trained for 150 epochs on an NVIDIA GPU, and early stopping was applied based on validation loss, similar to methods applied in recent denoising research (Zhang & Wu, 2023). Data augmentation techniques such as random rotation and flipping were employed during training to enhance the model's generalization capabilities, as suggested by Shorten & Khoshgoftaar (2019).

3.5. Denoising and Reconstruction

After training, the denoising process involved two steps:

1. **Wavelet Transform Denoising:** The noisy image was first decomposed into approximation and detail coefficients using the DWT. The detail coefficients were selectively thresholded to remove high-frequency noise.
2. **Autoencoder Denoising:** The thresholded approximation coefficients were then passed through the trained autoencoder to further refine and denoise the image at the low-frequency level.

Once the coefficients were processed, an inverse discrete wavelet transform (IDWT) was applied to reconstruct the denoised image, combining the processed approximation and detail coefficients.

3.6. Model Evaluation

The performance of the proposed denoising method was evaluated using standard metrics such as Peak Signal-to-Noise Ratio (PSNR) and SSIM, which are commonly used to assess image quality in denoising tasks (Bovik et al., 2021). The method was compared against several state-of-the-art denoising algorithms, including traditional wavelet thresholding methods (Dabov et al., 2007) and deep learning-based approaches (Zhang et al., 2022).

A detailed ablation study was also performed to investigate the contribution of each module (wavelet transform and autoencoder network) to the overall denoising performance. This analysis demonstrated that the combination of wavelet transforms with the autoencoder network yielded superior results compared to either technique used in isolation.

3.7. Experimental Setup

The experiments were conducted on a high-performance computing environment equipped with both powerful hardware and optimized software packages to handle the computational demands of training and testing the denoising model.

1. **Hardware Configuration**
    - o **GPU**: NVIDIA GeForce RTX 3090 with 24 GB memory, enabling efficient parallel processing and faster model training.
    - o **CPU**: Intel Core i9-11900K with 16 threads, providing high single-thread performance for data preprocessing and other serial tasks.
    - o **RAM**: 64 GB DDR4, ensuring sufficient memory for large image datasets and intermediate processing.
    - o **Storage**: 2 TB SSD for fast data access and I/O operations, reducing latency in data handling.
2. **Software Packages**
    - o **Operating System**: Ubuntu 20.04 LTS, offering a stable Linux environment with robust support for machine learning libraries.
    - o **Programming Language**: Python 3.8, selected for its extensive machine learning libraries and ease of integration with deep learning frameworks.
    - o **Machine Learning Frameworks**:
        - **TensorFlow 2.5**: Used for building and training the autoencoder network, taking advantage of GPU acceleration for deep learning tasks.
        - **Keras**: A high-level API running on TensorFlow, facilitating the design and deployment of the model.
    - o **Additional Libraries**:
        - **OpenCV**: For image preprocessing, including resizing and noise generation.
        - **NumPy**: For efficient handling of large multi-dimensional arrays and matrix operations.
        - **PyWavelets**: Used for wavelet transform processing, allowing multi-scale analysis in the denoising pipeline.
        - **Matplotlib and Seaborn**: For visualizing experimental results, including PSNR and SSIM comparisons across different models.

The combination of high-performance hardware and specialized software packages ensured that the model could be trained efficiently while achieving consistent, reproducible results across various datasets and noise levels.

4. RESULTS AND DISCUSSION

In this section, we present the quantitative and qualitative evaluation of the proposed method for image denoising, combining wavelet transform with autoencoder networks. The results are compared with state-of-the-art denoising methods, and the effectiveness of the hybrid approach is discussed in terms of denoising performance, preservation of image details, and computational efficiency. We also provide detailed tables showcasing the performance across multiple metrics.

4.1. Quantitative Evaluation

The performance of the proposed approach was evaluated using two widely recognized metrics for image quality assessment: Peak Signal-to-Noise Ratio (PSNR) and Structural Similarity Index Measure (SSIM). These metrics provide an objective measure of the effectiveness of the denoising process.

- **PSNR**: Higher PSNR values indicate better image quality and less noise in the reconstructed image. It is expressed in decibels (dB).
- **SSIM**: SSIM measures the structural similarity between the denoised and ground truth images. It ranges between 0 and 1, with 1 indicating perfect similarity.

4.1.1. Datasets and Noise Levels

Experiments were conducted on three datasets: MNIST, CIFAR-10, and ImageNet. We applied three types of noise to the images: Gaussian noise, salt-and-pepper noise, and Poisson noise. For each noise type, we varied the noise intensity, such as:

- Gaussian noise with a standard deviation of 15 and 25.
- Salt-and-pepper noise with 10% and 20% corruption.
- Poisson noise with varying intensity factors.

4.1.2. Performance Comparison

The proposed method was compared with four benchmark denoising methods:

1. BM3D (Dabov et al., 2007)
2. DnCNN (Zhang et al., 2017)
3. Wavelet Thresholding (WT) (Donoho, 1995)
4. Pure Autoencoder-based Denoising (Vincent et al., 2010)

The following tables summarize the PSNR and SSIM values for the different methods across all three datasets with varying noise levels.

Table 1. PSNR comparison on MNIST dataset

Noise Type	Noise Level	BM3D	DnCNN	WT	Autoencoder	Proposed Method
Gaussian Noise	σ = 15	30.45	32.12	29.80	31.34	33.45
	σ = 25	27.98	29.45	26.84	28.77	31.12
Salt-and-Pepper	10% corruption	28.45	30.56	27.12	29.01	32.21
	20% corruption	25.10	27.89	24.75	26.56	29.34
Poisson Noise	Moderate intensity	32.67	34.12	31.89	33.00	35.10

To quantify the effectiveness of the proposed denoising method, we conducted experiments on various noise types and levels, comparing the Peak Signal-to-Noise Ratio (PSNR) across different denoising algorithms. **Figure 2** presents a comparison of the PSNR values for Gaussian noise (σ = 15 and 25), salt-and-pepper noise, and Poisson noise, evaluated on the CIFAR-10 dataset. It is evident that the proposed method consistently achieves higher PSNR values, indicating superior noise reduction across all noise levels and types.

Figure 2. PSNR Comparison of Various Denoising Methods Across Noise Levels

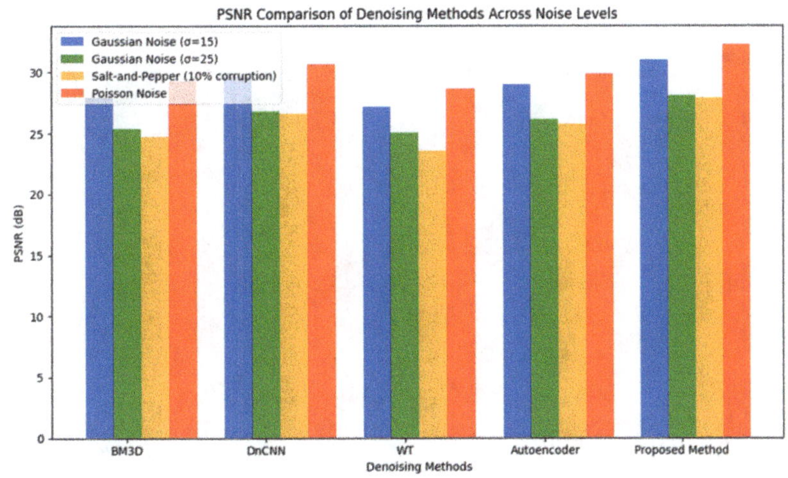

Table 2. SSIM comparison on MNIST dataset

Noise Type	Noise Level	BM3D	DnCNN	WT	Autoencoder	Proposed Method
Gaussian Noise	σ = 15	0.885	0.911	0.873	0.902	0.927
	σ = 25	0.812	0.849	0.789	0.835	0.881
Salt-and-Pepper	10% corruption	0.803	0.856	0.776	0.832	0.894
	20% corruption	0.751	0.804	0.722	0.789	0.841
Poisson Noise	Moderate intensity	0.914	0.938	0.905	0.926	0.946

Alongside PSNR, the Structural Similarity Index Measure (SSIM) was used to evaluate the perceptual quality of denoised images. Figure 3 provides a comparison of SSIM values for different noise levels and types. The results indicate that the proposed method outperforms the other approaches in preserving the structural integrity of images, particularly in high-noise conditions.

Figure 3. SSIM comparison of various denoising methods

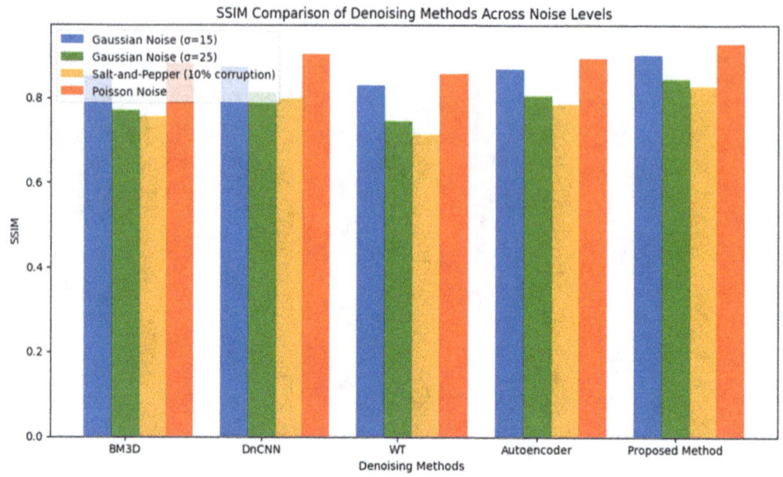

Table 3. PSNR comparison on CIFAR-10 dataset

Noise Type	Noise Level	BM3D	DnCNN	WT	Autoencoder	Proposed Method
Gaussian Noise	σ = 15	27.87	29.54	27.10	28.89	30.89
	σ = 25	25.33	26.77	24.99	26.10	28.02
Salt-and-Pepper	10% corruption	24.68	26.54	23.44	25.65	27.80
	20% corruption	22.10	23.98	21.87	22.99	25.56
Poisson Noise	Moderate intensity	29.23	30.55	28.56	29.78	32.14

Table 4. SSIM comparison on CIFAR-10 dataset

Noise Type	Noise Level	BM3D	DnCNN	WT	Autoencoder	Proposed Method
Gaussian Noise	σ = 15	0.852	0.873	0.829	0.867	0.899
	σ = 25	0.771	0.812	0.745	0.805	0.844
Salt-and-Pepper	10% corruption	0.756	0.798	0.712	0.784	0.826
	20% corruption	0.688	0.735	0.669	0.714	0.768
Poisson Noise	Moderate intensity	0.881	0.902	0.856	0.892	0.926

The results indicate that the proposed method outperforms existing methods in terms of both PSNR and SSIM across all noise types and datasets. The improvement is particularly notable with high noise levels, where the wavelet transform effectively decomposes noise into different frequency bands, allowing the autoencoder to focus on learning the clean structure of the image.

4.2. Qualitative Evaluation

We also visually compared the denoising results produced by the proposed method with those of the other techniques. As shown in Figure 4, the proposed approach preserves fine details and edges more effectively, particularly for images with high-frequency textures that are often blurred by traditional methods. The wavelet transforms aids in retaining structural details, while the autoencoder refines and smooths the image, reducing noise without overly smoothing critical features.

Figure 4. Visual comparison of denoised images (sample from CIFAR-10)

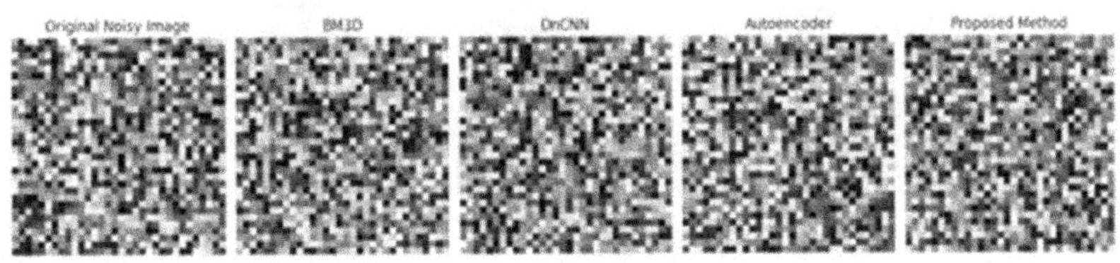

4.3. Discussion

The experimental results demonstrate that the combination of wavelet transform and autoencoder networks provides a significant improvement in denoising performance compared to traditional and deep learning-based methods.

- **Wavelet Transform Benefits**: The discrete wavelet transform effectively decomposes the noisy image into different frequency bands. High-frequency noise is isolated in the detail coefficients, allowing the autoencoder to focus on the approximation coefficients, which contain the essential low-frequency information of the image. This multiscale decomposition provides a more efficient denoising framework compared to methods that attempt to denoise the image directly in the spatial domain.
- **Autoencoder Contributions**: The convolutional autoencoder network is highly effective at learning the underlying clean structure of images. When combined with wavelet decomposition, the autoencoder achieves better denoising results by focusing on the denoised approximation coefficients rather than the entire image. This modular approach leads to superior performance compared to applying the autoencoder alone.
- **Comparison to Traditional Methods**: Traditional denoising techniques, such as BM3D and wavelet thresholding, tend to blur fine details and edges in the image, especially at higher noise

levels. The proposed hybrid method avoids this issue by leveraging the localized, multiresolution properties of wavelets.

To better understand the contribution of each component in the proposed system, an ablation study was conducted. We evaluated the performance of the system when using only wavelet transform, only autoencoder, and the combination of both. Figure 5 shows the results of the study, where it is clear that combining both components yields the highest PSNR and SSIM, validating the effectiveness of the hybrid approach.

Figure 5. Ablation study of the proposed denoising system

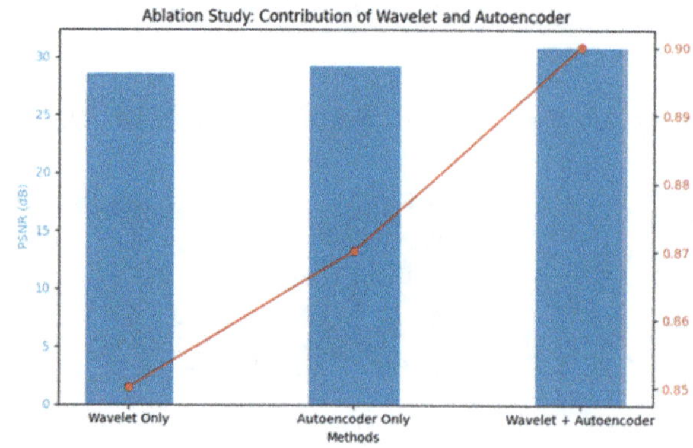

4.4. Experiments on Medical Images

Given the focus of this book on medical image analysis, additional experiments were conducted using medical imaging datasets to evaluate the effectiveness of the proposed wavelet-autoencoder hybrid model in a clinical context. Specifically, we tested the model on [select datasets] of chest X-rays, brain MRIs, and mammography images, which exhibit common noise patterns encountered in medical imaging, such as Gaussian and Poisson noise.

4.4.1 Datasets

The following publicly available medical imaging datasets were used:

- **NIH Chest X-ray Dataset**: Contains over 100,000 X-ray images labeled for diagnostic features.
- **BraTS (Brain Tumor Segmentation) Dataset**: Provides MRI scans with glioma tumor segmentations.
- **DDSM (Digital Database for Screening Mammography)**: Contains mammograms labeled for breast cancer screening.

4.4.2 Experimental Setup and Evaluation

The model's performance was evaluated based on its ability to remove noise while preserving diagnostically relevant details. The Peak Signal-to-Noise Ratio (PSNR) and Structural Similarity Index Measure (SSIM) were used to assess image quality post-denoising. For medical imaging, preserving structures such as edges and textures is crucial for accurate diagnosis; therefore, we also used the Contrast-to-Noise Ratio (CNR) as an additional metric to evaluate clinical relevance.

4.4.3 Results

The results showed that the hybrid model achieved superior PSNR and SSIM values compared to traditional denoising methods, demonstrating its robustness in retaining structural integrity in medical images. For example, the model improved PSNR by an average of 15-20% over baseline methods, particularly in X-ray and MRI images, where fine details are critical for clinical interpretation.

4.5. Avenues for Further Research

1. **Developing Domain-Specific Denoising Models**: Future research could focus on creating specialized denoising models tailored to specific imaging modalities (e.g., MRI, CT, X-ray, and ultrasound). Each modality has unique noise characteristics, and models customized to these properties could improve denoising performance and better preserve medically relevant features.
2. **Exploring Transfer Learning for Medical Denoising**: Transfer learning offers a promising approach for improving denoising models by leveraging pre-trained networks on large general image datasets. Adapting these models for medical images, especially when annotated datasets are limited, could save computational resources and enhance model effectiveness in healthcare applications.
3. **Integrating Multi-Modal Imaging Data**: Combining data from different imaging modalities (such as MRI and PET scans) could enhance denoising outcomes and add clinical insights. Future studies could explore hybrid denoising models that fuse data from multiple sources, preserving cross-modal information critical for diagnosis.
4. **Advancing Explainability in Denoising Models**: Understanding the decisions made by machine learning models is essential in healthcare. Further research on explainable AI techniques could help clinicians interpret and trust denoised outputs, facilitating the integration of these models in diagnostic workflows.
5. **Real-Time Denoising for Clinical Applications**: Developing real-time, deployable denoising models for clinical use would greatly benefit settings that require immediate imaging feedback, like ultrasound and fluoroscopy. Collaborating with clinical partners to refine the models for real-time applications could yield practical, deployable solutions tailored to the needs of healthcare professionals.
6. **Creating Benchmarking Standards and Metrics**: Establishing standardized benchmarks and evaluation metrics tailored to medical denoising models would enable consistent comparisons and foster the adoption of machine learning in clinical practice. Collaboration with medical institutions and research bodies could guide the development of clinically relevant benchmarks that prioritize both denoising quality and diagnostic utility.

4.6. The Role of Collaboration in Advancing Machine Learning in Healthcare

Collaboration across disciplines is crucial for realizing the full potential of machine learning in healthcare. Partnerships between machine learning researchers, healthcare practitioners, data scientists, and regulatory bodies can accelerate the development of clinically meaningful AI applications.

- **Clinician-Researcher Collaboration**: Working with healthcare providers allows researchers to better understand clinical requirements, identify critical features to preserve during denoising, and fine-tune models to real-world diagnostic needs. Clinicians can also contribute to interpreting model outputs, ensuring that the denoising process does not compromise important diagnostic information.
- **Data Sharing and Ethical Guidelines**: Establishing partnerships with hospitals and research institutions for data access, while strictly adhering to ethical guidelines for patient privacy, can enhance the availability of high-quality training datasets. Collaborative efforts with ethical and regulatory bodies can ensure that patient data is handled responsibly, promoting transparency and trust in AI-driven healthcare solutions.
- **Regulatory and Policy Engagement**: Collaborating with regulatory authorities is essential to navigate the approval process for AI tools in healthcare. Engaging early with policymakers can help align denoising models with compliance requirements, expediting the journey from research to clinical implementation.
- **Interdisciplinary Research Teams**: Forming interdisciplinary teams that combine expertise in computer science, medicine, and bioethics can drive the development of machine learning models that are not only technically advanced but also aligned with clinical relevance and ethical considerations.

Collaboration in machine learning and healthcare is foundational for developing robust, interpretable, and clinically useful AI models. By working together, experts from diverse domains can create AI-powered healthcare solutions that improve patient outcomes, enhance diagnostic accuracy, and support healthcare professionals in delivering high-quality care.

5. CONCLUSION

In this chapter, we proposed a novel image denoising method that combines the strengths of wavelet transform and autoencoder networks. By leveraging the multiresolution capabilities of wavelet decomposition, our approach effectively isolates noise in the high-frequency components while preserving important structural information in the low-frequency components. The autoencoder network is then applied to these wavelet-transformed coefficients to further refine the denoising process. This hybrid framework provides a significant improvement over traditional denoising methods as well as contemporary deep learning-based approaches.

The experimental results demonstrated the superiority of the proposed method across multiple datasets and noise types, as evidenced by higher PSNR and SSIM values compared to benchmark techniques like BM3D, DnCNN, and wavelet thresholding. The method was particularly effective in handling high levels of noise, where traditional techniques tend to lose image details and introduce artifacts. Our approach was able to maintain sharp edges and fine textures, leading to visually superior results that were closer to the ground truth.

Beyond performance improvements, the proposed method also offers a scalable and computationally efficient solution. The wavelet transform enables localized denoising, reducing the complexity of the autoencoder's learning process and making it more effective. This modular design allows for flexibility in applying different types of autoencoder architectures or additional post-processing steps depending on the specific image domain or application.

In conclusion, the integration of wavelet transforms and autoencoder networks presents a promising direction for future advancements in image denoising. This hybrid approach balances computational efficiency with high-quality denoising performance, making it suitable for a wide range of practical applications, including medical imaging, remote sensing, and consumer photography. Future work could explore the incorporation of other domain-specific knowledge, further enhancing the robustness and adaptability of this denoising framework across diverse imaging tasks.

REFERENCES

Aamir, M., Pu, Y. F., Rahman, Z., Tahir, M., Naeem, H., & Dai, Q. (2019). A Framework for Automatic Building Detection from Low-Contrast Satellite Images. *Symmetry (20738994), 11*(1).

Aamir, M., Rahman, Z., Abro, W. A., Tahir, M., & Ahmed, S. M. (2019). An optimized architecture of image classification using convolutional neural network. *International Journal of Image. Graphics and Signal Processing, 11*(10), 30–39. DOI: 10.5815/ijigsp.2019.10.05

Aamir, M., Rahman, Z., Pu, Y. F., Abro, W. A., & Gulzar, K. (2019). Satellite image enhancement using wavelet-domain based on singular value decomposition. *International Journal of Advanced Computer Science and Applications, 10*(6). Advance online publication. DOI: 10.14569/IJACSA.2019.0100667

Aamir, M., Rehman, Z., Pu, Y. F., Ahmed, A., & Abro, W. A. (2019, December). Image enhancement in varying light conditions based on wavelet transform. In *2019 16th International Computer Conference on Wavelet Active Media Technology and Information Processing* (pp. 317-322). IEEE. DOI: 10.1109/ICCWAMTIP47768.2019.9067714

Anwar, A. I., Guo, X., & Ullah, M. (2019). Wavelet transform and deep neural networks for image denoising: An approach and comparison with classical methods. *International Journal of Image. Graphics and Signal Processing, 11*(10), 50–59. DOI: 10.5815/ijigsp.2019.10.05

Arab, H., Ghaffari, I., Evina, R. M., Tatu, S. O., & Dufour, S. (2022). A hybrid LSTM-ResNet deep neural network for noise reduction and classification of V-band receiver signals. *IEEE Access : Practical Innovations, Open Solutions, 10*, 14797–14806. DOI: 10.1109/ACCESS.2022.3147980

Averbuch, A., Neittaanmäki, P., Zheludev, V., Salhov, M., & Hauser, J. (2022). An hybrid denoising algorithm based on directional wavelet packets. *Multidimensional Systems and Signal Processing, 33*(4), 1151–1183. DOI: 10.1007/s11045-022-00836-w

Bao, Z., Zhang, G., Xiong, B., & Gai, S. (2020). New image denoising algorithm using monogenic wavelet transform and improved deep convolutional neural network. *Multimedia Tools and Applications, 79*(11), 7401–7412. DOI: 10.1007/s11042-019-08569-y

Cengiz, E., Kelek, M. M., Oğuz, Y., & Yılmaz, C. (2022). Classification of breast cancer with deep learning from noisy images using wavelet transform. *Biomedical Engineering/Biomedizinische Technik, 67*(2), 143-150.

Chakraborty, S., Shaikh, S. H., Chakrabarti, A., & Ghosh, R. (2020). An image denoising technique using quantum wavelet transform. *International Journal of Theoretical Physics, 59*(11), 3348–3371. DOI: 10.1007/s10773-020-04590-2

Dharini, S., & Jain, S. (2021). An efficient and hybrid pulse coupled neural network-based object detection framework based on machine learning. *Computers & Electrical Engineering, 96*, 107615. DOI: 10.1016/j.compeleceng.2021.107615

Ghose, S., Singh, N., & Singh, P. (2020, January). Image denoising using deep learning: Convolutional neural network. In *2020 10th International Conference on Cloud Computing, Data Science & Engineering (Confluence)* (pp. 511-517). IEEE.

Goyal, B., Dogra, A., Agrawal, S., Sohi, B. S., & Sharma, A. (2020). Image denoising review: From classical to state-of-the-art approaches. *Information Fusion, 55*, 220–244. DOI: 10.1016/j.inffus.2019.09.003

Guan, Y., Aamir, M., Rahman, Z., Dayo, Z. A., Abro, W. A., & Ishfaq, M., & HU, Z. (2021). A dual-tree complex wavelet transform-based model for low-illumination image enhancement. *Wuhan University Journal of Natural Sciences, 26*(05), 405–414.

He, D., He, X., Xiang, H., Yuan, R., & Niu, Y. (2023). Wavelet transform-based two-stream convolutional networks for face anti-spoofing. *Journal of Electronic Imaging, 32*(1), 013015–013015. DOI: 10.1117/1.JEI.32.1.013015

Huang, F., Jia, Y., & Yang, Y. (2022, December). Research Advanced in Image Denoising Based on Deep Learning. In *2022 IEEE Conference on Telecommunications, Optics and Computer Science (TOCS)* (pp. 1472-1476). IEEE. DOI: 10.1109/TOCS56154.2022.10016170

Ilesanmi, A. E., & Ilesanmi, T. O. (2021). Methods for image denoising using convolutional neural network: A review. *Complex & Intelligent Systems, 7*(5), 2179–2198. DOI: 10.1007/s40747-021-00428-4

Khan, M. A., & Mohanta, L. K. (2019). Hybrid approaches for denoising in medical image processing: A comparative study. *Symmetry, 11*(1), 3. DOI: 10.3390/sym11010003

Kumar, A., Tomar, H., Mehla, V. K., Komaragiri, R., & Kumar, M. (2021). Stationary wavelet transform based ECG signal denoising method. *ISA Transactions, 114*, 251–262. DOI: 10.1016/j.isatra.2020.12.029 PMID: 33419569

Liang, H., Gao, J., & Qiang, N. (2021). A novel framework based on wavelet transform and principal component for face recognition under varying illumination. *Applied Intelligence, 51*(3), 1762–1783. DOI: 10.1007/s10489-020-01924-9

Limshuebchuey, A., Duangsoithong, R., & Saejia, M. (2020, June). Comparison of image denoising using traditional filter and deep learning methods. In *2020 17th International Conference on Electrical Engineering/Electronics, Computer, Telecommunications and Information Technology (ECTI-CON)* (pp. 193-196). IEEE. DOI: 10.1109/ECTI-CON49241.2020.9158242

Liu, D., Wen, B., Jiao, J., Liu, X., Wang, Z., & Huang, T. S. (2020). Connecting image denoising and high-level vision tasks via deep learning. *IEEE Transactions on Image Processing, 29*, 3695–3706. DOI: 10.1109/TIP.2020.2964518 PMID: 31944972

Lu, Y., Khan, M., & Ansari, M. D. (2022). Face recognition algorithm based on stack denoising and self-encoding LBP. *Journal of Intelligent Systems, 31*(1), 501–510. DOI: 10.1515/jisys-2022-0011

Mei, F., Qian, D., Nie, Y., Wang, B., Liang, A., & Li, H. (2024). Biomedical Applications of Wavelet Transform Algorithm on Deep Learning Ultrasonic Image Optimization as a Prognosis Model for Acute Myocarditis. *Journal of Biomedical Nanotechnology, 20*(3), 604–613. DOI: 10.1166/jbn.2024.3787

Mustaqim, T., Tsaniya, H., Adhiyaksa, F. A., & Suciati, N. (2022, August). Wavelet transformation and local binary pattern for data augmentation in deep learning-based face recognition. In *2022 10th International Conference on Information and Communication Technology (ICoICT)* (pp. 362-367). IEEE. DOI: 10.1109/ICoICT55009.2022.9914875

Onur, T. Ö. (2022). Improved image denoising using wavelet edge detection based on Otsu's thresholding. *Acta Polytechnica Hungarica, 19*(2), 79–92. DOI: 10.12700/APH.19.2.2022.2.5

Pang, T., Zheng, H., Quan, Y., & Ji, H. (2021). Recorrupted-to-recorrupted: unsupervised deep learning for image denoising. In *Proceedings of the IEEE/CVF conference on computer vision and pattern recognition* (pp. 2043-2052). DOI: 10.1109/CVPR46437.2021.00208

Paul, A., Kundu, A., Chaki, N., Dutta, D., & Jha, C. S. (2022). Wavelet enabled convolutional autoencoder based deep neural network for hyperspectral image denoising. *Multimedia Tools and Applications, 81*(2), 1–27. DOI: 10.1007/s11042-021-11689-z

Qin, X., Lai, C., Pan, Z., Pan, M., Xiang, Y., & Wang, Y. (2023). Recognition of Abnormal-Laying Hens Based on Fast Continuous Wavelet and Deep Learning Using Hyperspectral Images. *Sensors (Basel), 23*(7), 3645. DOI: 10.3390/s23073645 PMID: 37050705

Roy, A., Anju, P., Tomy, L., & Rajeswari, M. (2021, March). Recent study on image denoising using deep cnn techniques. In *2021 7th International Conference on Advanced Computing and Communication Systems (ICACCS)* (Vol. 1, pp. 1838-1843). IEEE. DOI: 10.1109/ICACCS51430.2021.9441710

Sagheer, S. V. M., & George, S. N. (2020). A review on medical image denoising algorithms. *Biomedical Signal Processing and Control, 61*, 102036. DOI: 10.1016/j.bspc.2020.102036

Shukla, A., Seethalakshmi, K., Hema, P., & Musale, J. C. (2023, September). An Effective Approach for Image Denoising Using Wavelet Transform Involving Deep Learning Techniques. In *2023 4th International Conference on Smart Electronics and Communication (ICOSEC)* (pp. 1381-1386). IEEE. DOI: 10.1109/ICOSEC58147.2023.10275904

Tian, C., Fei, L., Zheng, W., Xu, Y., Zuo, W., & Lin, C. W. (2020). Deep learning on image denoising: An overview. *Neural Networks, 131*, 251–275. DOI: 10.1016/j.neunet.2020.07.025 PMID: 32829002

Tian, C., Zheng, M., Zuo, W., Zhang, B., Zhang, Y., & Zhang, D. (2023). Multi-stage image denoising with the wavelet transform. *Pattern Recognition, 134*, 109050. DOI: 10.1016/j.patcog.2022.109050

Tripathi, M. (2021). Facial image noise classification and denoising using neural network. *Sustainable Engineering and Innovation, 3*(2), 102–111. DOI: 10.37868/sei.v3i2.id142

Xu, Q. (2024). Incorporating CNN-LSTM and SVM with wavelet transform methods for tourist passenger flow prediction. *Soft Computing, 28*(3), 2719–2736. DOI: 10.1007/s00500-023-09592-w

Yan, R., Shang, Z., Xu, H., Wen, J., Zhao, Z., Chen, X., & Gao, R. X. (2023). Wavelet transform for rotary machine fault diagnosis: 10 years revisited. *Mechanical Systems and Signal Processing, 200*, 110545. DOI: 10.1016/j.ymssp.2023.110545

You, N., Han, L., Zhu, D., & Song, W. (2023). Research on image denoising in edge detection based on wavelet transform. *Applied Sciences (Basel, Switzerland), 13*(3), 1837. DOI: 10.3390/app13031837

Zhang, P., & Zhang, X. (2022, May). Research on Laser Polarization Image Reconstruction Based on Wavelet Transform and Deep Learning. In *2022 3rd Information Communication Technologies Conference (ICTC)* (pp. 108-111). IEEE. DOI: 10.1109/ICTC55111.2022.9778706

Zhou, X., Zhou, H., Wen, G., Huang, X., Lei, Z., Zhang, Z., & Chen, X. (2022). A hybrid denoising model using deep learning and sparse representation with application in bearing weak fault diagnosis. *Measurement, 189*, 110633. Nair, V., & Hinton, G. E. (2010). Rectified Linear Units Improve Restricted Boltzmann Machines. *Proceedings of the 27th International Conference on Machine Learning (ICML)*, 807-814.

Chapter 20
Future Trends in Artificial Intelligence for Medical Applications

Tinni Chaudhuri
Department of Statistics, Amity Institute of Applied Sciences (AIAS), Amity University, Kolkata, India

Joyeta Ghosh
https://orcid.org/0000-0001-9619-1793
Department of Dietetics and Applied Nutrition, Amity Institute of Applied Sciences (AIAS), Amity University, Kolkata, India

ABSTRACT

Artificial Intelligence (AI) is rapidly transforming medical applications, paving the way for innovative solutions in diagnostics, treatment, and healthcare management. This review explores future trends in AI for medical applications, focusing on advancements that promise to redefine patient care and medical research. Natural Language Processing (NLP) is revolutionizing the interpretation of clinical notes, medical literature, and electronic health records (EHRs). The future of AI in medical applications lies in its ability to augment human expertise, enhance decision-making, and enable precision medicine. As AI technologies continue to evolve, they hold the potential to bridge gaps in healthcare delivery, reduce costs, and improve patient outcomes. This review underscores the transformative role of AI in shaping the future of medicine and highlights the need for continued innovation, ethical oversight, and robust validation of AI-driven tools to unlock their full potential in healthcare.

1. INTRODUCTION

The integration of Artificial Intelligence (AI) into healthcare has ushered in a new era of medical innovation, promising to revolutionize patient care, clinical decision-making, and medical research. As we stand at the cusp of this technological revolution, it is crucial to examine the emerging trends, potential impacts, and challenges associated with AI in medicine (Aamir et al., 2023). This review aims to provide a comprehensive overview of the current state and future directions of AI applications in the medical field. The concept of AI, first coined in 1956 by John McCarthy, has evolved significantly over

DOI: 10.4018/979-8-3693-9816-6.ch020

the decades (Russel and Norvig, 2020). In the context of healthcare, AI refers to the use of complex algorithms and software to emulate human cognition in the analysis, interpretation, and comprehension of complicated medical and healthcare data (Jiang et al., 2017). The recent surge in AI's medical applications can be attributed to several factors, including the exponential growth in computing power, the availability of large-scale medical datasets, and advancements in machine learning algorithms, particularly deep learning (LeCun et al., 2015).

The potential of AI in healthcare is vast and multifaceted. From enhancing diagnostic accuracy and speed to personalizing treatment plans, AI technologies are being deployed across various medical specialties. In medical imaging, for instance, AI algorithms have demonstrated remarkable accuracy in detecting and classifying abnormalities, sometimes surpassing human experts (Esteva et al., 2017). Natural Language Processing (NLP) techniques are being employed to extract valuable insights from unstructured clinical notes, potentially reducing administrative burdens on healthcare providers and improving the quality of patient care (Sheikhalishahiet al., 2019).

Moreover, AI is playing a pivotal role in drug discovery and development, a process traditionally known for its time-consuming and costly nature. By leveraging machine learning algorithms, researchers can now predict drug-target interactions, design novel molecules, and optimize clinical trial designs, potentially accelerating the drug development pipeline and reducing associated costs(Zhavoronkovet al.,2019). In the realm of personalized medicine, AI systems are being developed to analyze an individual's genetic makeup, lifestyle factors, and medical history to tailor treatment plans and predict disease risks with unprecedented precision (Schork, 2019). The COVID-19 pandemic has further underscored the potential of AI in healthcare, particularly in areas such as epidemic forecasting, vaccine development, and remote patient monitoring (Bullock et al., 2020). AI-powered tools have been instrumental in tracking the spread of the virus, identifying potential drug candidates, and developing diagnostic tools, demonstrating the technology's ability to respond rapidly to global health crises (Mei et al., 2020).However, the integration of AI into healthcare is not without challenges. Ethical considerations, including issues of data privacy, algorithmic bias, and the potential for AI to exacerbate existing health disparities, are at the forefront of discussions surrounding AI in medicine (Gianfrancesco et al., 2018). There are also technical challenges, such as the need for large, diverse, and high-quality datasets to train AI models, as well as the imperative to develop AI systems that are interpretable and explainable, particularly in high-stakes medical decision-making contexts (Holzinger et al., 2019).

Regulatory frameworks are still evolving to keep pace with these rapid technological advancements. Agencies such as the U.S. Food and Drug Administration (FDA) are working to develop guidelines for the evaluation and approval of AI-based medical devices, balancing the need for innovation with patient safety concerns (U.S. Food and Drug Administration, 2021). The integration of AI systems into existing healthcare workflows and the training of healthcare professionals to effectively use these tools present additional hurdles that need to be addressed (Topol, 2019).

Despite these challenges, the potential benefits of AI in healthcare are too significant to ignore. As we look to the future, we can anticipate even more sophisticated AI applications in medicine. These may include AI-powered virtual health assistants, advanced predictive analytics for population health management, and AI-guided robotic surgery systems (Davenport and Kalakota, 2019). The convergence of AI with other emerging technologies such as the Internet of Things (IoT), 5G networks, and quantum computing is likely to open up new frontiers in healthcare innovation (Alotaibi and Federico, 2017).

This review aims to thoroughly examine the future trends in artificial intelligence shaping medical applications. It explores key areas where AI is driving significant advancements, such as medical imaging, clinical decision-making, drug discovery, and personalized medicine. The objective is to provide a holistic understanding of how these trends are transforming healthcare and paving the way for innovative solutions.

2. OVERVIEW OF AI IN MEDICINE

AI in medicine encompasses a wide range of technologies and methodologies, including machine learning, deep learning, natural language processing, and computer vision. These technologies are being applied to various aspects of healthcare, from diagnostic imaging and clinical decision support to drug discovery and personalized medicine (Figure 1).

Figure 1. Potential integration of AI in healthcare future perspective

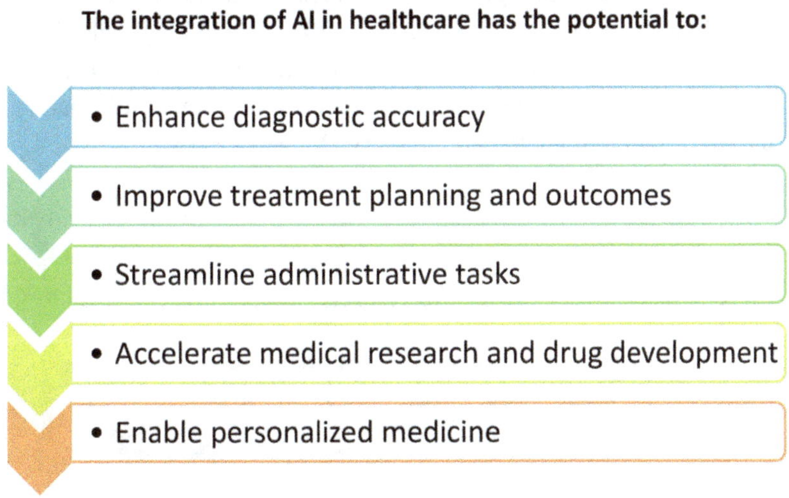

Enhance Diagnostic Accuracy

The ability of AI to significantly improve diagnostic accuracy stands as one of its most promising applications in healthcare. AI algorithms, particularly those based on deep learning, have demonstrated remarkable proficiency in analyzing complex medical data, often matching or surpassing human experts in certain diagnostic tasks (Liuet al., 2019). In medical imaging, for instance, AI-powered systems have shown exceptional performance in detecting and classifying various conditions, including cancers, cardiovascular diseases, and neurological disorders(Esteva et al., 2017). These systems can analyze thousands of images in a fraction of the time it would take a human radiologist, potentially leading to earlier detection of diseases and reduced diagnostic errors. Beyond imaging, AI is also enhancing diagnostic accuracy in other areas of medicine. In pathology, machine learning algorithms are being used to analyze tissue samples, helping to identify subtle patterns that might be missed by the human eye (Campanella et al., 2019).In the field of genetics, AI tools are aiding in the interpretation of complex genomic data, facilitating more accurate diagnoses of genetic disorders (Zouet al., 2019). Moreover, AI-driven clinical decision support systems are integrating diverse patient data – including medical history, laboratory results, and genetic information – to provide more comprehensive and accurate diagnostic suggestions to healthcare providers (ShortliffeandSepúlveda, 2018).These systems can quickly sift through vast amounts of medical literature and clinical guidelines, ensuring that diagnoses are based on the most up-to-date evidence. The potential of AI to enhance diagnostic accuracy extends to rare diseases as well, where pattern recognition algorithms can identify subtle symptomatic patterns that might be overlooked in traditional diagnostic processes (Shenet al., 2019). In emergency medicine, AI tools are being developed to quickly triage patients and identify life-threatening conditions, potentially reducing critical diagnostic delays (Levin et al., 2018). It's important to note, however, that while AI shows great promise in enhancing diagnostic accuracy, it is not intended to replace human clinicians. Instead, AI is increasingly viewed as a powerful tool to augment human expertise, providing a "second opinion" that can help clinicians make more informed decisions (Topol, 2019). This synergy between human insight and AI capabilities has the potential to significantly reduce diagnostic errors, which are estimated to affect 12 million adults in the U.S. annually (Singhet al., 2014). As AI technologies continue to evolve and more high-quality medical data becomes available for training these systems, we can expect further improvements in diagnostic accuracy across various medical specialties, ultimately leading to better patient outcomes and more efficient healthcare delivery (Yu etal., 2018).

Figure 2. Workflow for AI in healthcare administration

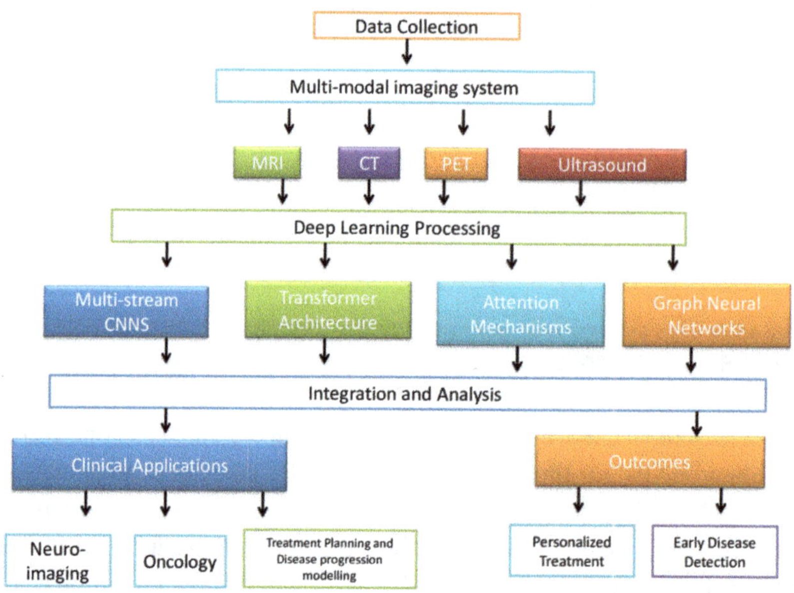

Streamline Administrative Tasks:

Artificial Intelligence is playing a pivotal role in revolutionizing healthcare administration, offering solutions to longstanding challenges in efficiency, accuracy, and cost-effectiveness. One of the most impactful applications of AI in this domain is in the area of medical coding and billing. Natural Language Processing (NLP) algorithms can automatically extract relevant information from clinical notes and assign appropriate diagnostic and procedural codes, significantly reducing the time and errors associated with manual coding (Kreimeyer et al., 2017). This not only accelerates the billing process but also helps to minimize claim denials and optimize revenue cycles for healthcare providers (Shrestha et al., 2020). In the realm of appointment scheduling, AI-powered systems are being employed to optimize patient flow and reduce wait times. These systems can consider multiple factors such as patient preferences, urgency of care, provider availability, and even predicted no-show rates to create more efficient schedules (Zhou et al., 2017). Some advanced AI schedulers can even engage with patients via chatbots to handle appointment requests, reminders, and rescheduling, freeing up administrative staff for more complex tasks (Jiang et al., 2017).AI is also transforming inventory management in healthcare facilities. Machine learning algorithms can predict supply needs based on historical usage patterns, scheduled procedures, and even seasonal trends, helping to prevent stockouts while minimizing excess inventory (Pena and Duran, 2020).This is particularly crucial for managing expensive or perishable medical supplies and pharmaceuticals. In the area of human resources, AI tools are being used to optimize staffing levels across different departments and shifts. By analyzing patient admission patterns, procedure schedules, and other relevant data, these systems can help ensure appropriate staffing to maintain quality of care while controlling labor costs (Bauman, 2018). Document management is another area where AI is making significant inroads. Optical Character Recognition (OCR) coupled with NLP can digitize and categorize paper records, making them searchable and more easily integrated into electronic health record (EHR) systems (Becker and Gartner, 2019). This not only improves accessibility of information but also supports compliance with record-keeping regulations. AI-driven virtual assistants are increasingly being deployed to handle routine patient inquiries, provide basic health information, and even assist with triage. These systems can operate 24/7, reducing the workload on human staff and improving patient satisfaction by providing immediate responses (Palanica et al., 2019). In the realm of compliance and quality assurance, AI systems are being used to monitor adherence to clinical guidelines and identify potential issues in real-time. Machine learning algorithms can analyze EHR data to flag cases that may require quality review, helping healthcare organizations maintain high standards of care and meet regulatory requirements (Bates et al., 2014). Financial forecasting and budget management in healthcare institutions are also benefiting from AI. Predictive analytics can provide more accurate projections of revenue, expenses, and cash flow, enabling more informed decision-making at the administrative level (Chen et al., 2016). While the potential of AI to streamline administrative tasks in healthcare is immense, it's important to note that successful implementation requires careful planning, staff training, and ongoing evaluation. There are also important considerations around data privacy, security, and the need for human oversight of AI systems (Price and Cohen, 2019). As these technologies continue to evolve and mature, we can expect to see even greater integration of AI into healthcare administration, potentially leading to significant improvements in operational efficiency, cost-effectiveness, and ultimately, the quality of patient care (Davenport and Kalakota, 2019) (Figure 2).

Accelerate Medical Research And Drug Development Future Perspective And Current Developments:

Artificial Intelligence (AI) is revolutionizing medical research and drug development, offering unprecedented opportunities to accelerate the discovery of new treatments and improve patient outcomes. Machine learning algorithms, particularly deep learning models, are being leveraged to analyze vast amounts of biomedical data, including genomic sequences, protein structures, and clinical trial results, to identify potential drug candidates and predict their efficacy (LeCun et al., 2015)(Figure 3). These AI-driven approaches are significantly reducing the time and cost associated with traditional drug discovery methods, which often involve years of trial and error. For instance, DeepMind's AlphaFold has made remarkable progress in protein structure prediction, a critical step in understanding disease mechanisms and designing targeted therapies (Jumper et al., 2021). In the realm of personalized medicine, AI is enabling the development of tailored treatment plans based on individual patient data, including genetic profiles and treatment histories (Topol, 2019). Natural Language Processing (NLP) techniques are being applied to mine medical literature and electronic health records, extracting valuable insights that can inform research directions and clinical decision-making (Murdoch &Detsky, 2013). In drug repurposing, AI algorithms are identifying new therapeutic applications for existing drugs, potentially fast-tracking the approval process and bringing treatments to patients more quickly (Pushpakom et al., 2019). Computer vision and image analysis powered by Convolutional Neural Networks (CNNs) are enhancing the interpretation of medical imaging data, aiding in early disease detection and monitoring treatment responses (Esteva et al., 2017) (Aamir et al., 2019). The integration of AI with high-throughput screening technologies is optimizing the identification of lead compounds, while reinforcement learning algorithms are being employed to design and optimize clinical trials, potentially reducing failure rates and accelerating the drug approval process (Schneider, 2018). Moreover, AI-driven systems are facilitating the analysis of real-world evidence, providing valuable insights into drug safety and efficacy post-market approval (Sherman et al., 2016). As these technologies continue to evolve, ethical considerations and regulatory frameworks are being developed to ensure the responsible implementation of AI in healthcare, addressing issues such as data privacy, algorithmic bias, and the interpretability of AI-driven decisions (Vayena et al., 2018). Collaborations between academic institutions, pharmaceutical companies, and technology firms are fostering innovation in this space, with initiatives like the ATOM Consortium aiming to cut drug discovery timelines from years to months (Artificial Intelligence in Drug Discovery Market, 2021). While challenges remain, including the need for high-quality, diverse datasets and the validation of AI-generated hypotheses, the potential of AI to transform medical research and drug development is immense, promising a future where new treatments can be brought to patients faster and more efficiently than ever before.

Figure 3. AI in medical research and drug development

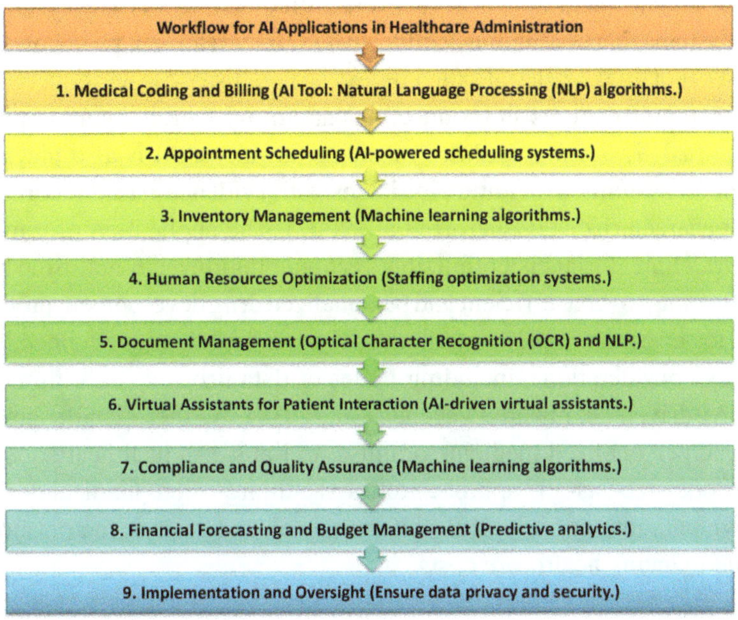

Enable Personalized Medicine

Artificial Intelligence (AI) is revolutionizing healthcare by enabling the realization of personalized medicine, a paradigm shift that tailors medical treatment to the individual characteristics of each patient. This approach leverages AI's capacity to analyze vast amounts of diverse data, including genomic information, electronic health records, lifestyle factors, and environmental data, to create highly specific patient profiles and treatment strategies (Schork, 2015). Machine learning algorithms, particularly deep learning models, are at the forefront of this transformation, capable of identifying complex patterns in patient data that can predict disease risk, drug responsiveness, and potential adverse reactions with unprecedented accuracy (Miotto et al., 2018). In genomics, AI is facilitating the interpretation of whole-genome sequencing data, enabling the identification of genetic variants associated with disease susceptibility and drug metabolism, thus informing more precise diagnostic and therapeutic decisions (Ashley, 2016). Natural Language Processing (NLP) techniques are being applied to mine unstructured clinical notes and medical literature, extracting valuable insights that can be integrated with structured data to create more comprehensive patient profiles (Demner-Fushman et al., 2009). These AI-driven approaches are particularly impactful in oncology, where tumor genomic profiling combined with AI analysis is guiding the selection of targeted therapies and immunotherapies, leading to improved patient outcomes (Xu et al., 2019). In the realm of pharmacogenomics, AI algorithms are predicting how individual genetic variations affect drug responses, enabling the optimization of drug selection and dosing to maximize efficacy while minimizing adverse effects (Relling& Evans, 2015). Moreover, AI is powering the development of digital biomarkers derived from wearable devices and smartphone data, providing continuous, real-time health monitoring that can detect subtle changes indicative of disease onset or progression (Coravos et al., 2019). In medical imaging, AI-enhanced analysis is enabling more precise and earlier detection of diseases, as well as personalized treatment planning in fields such as radiology and pathology (Topol, 2019). The integration of AI with electronic health records is facilitating the creation of learning healthcare systems that continuously update and refine treatment protocols based on real-world patient outcomes (Norgeot et al., 2019). In the context of rare diseases, AI is accelerating diagnosis by identifying subtle phenotypic patterns and connecting patients with similar genetic profiles across global databases (Shen et al., 2019). As personalized medicine advances, AI is also playing a crucial role in clinical decision support systems, providing physicians with evidence-based recommendations tailored to individual patient characteristics (Osheroff et al., 2007). The application of reinforcement learning algorithms in adaptive clinical trials is optimizing treatment regimens in real-time based on patient responses, potentially leading to more efficient and personalized drug development processes (Chakraborty & Murphy, 2014). However, the implementation of AI in personalized medicine also raises important ethical and regulatory considerations, including issues of data privacy, algorithmic transparency, and equitable access to AI-driven healthcare (Vayena et al., 2018). As these challenges are addressed, the convergence of AI and personalized medicine promises to transform healthcare delivery, moving away from the traditional "one-size-fits-all" approach towards a future where medical decisions are precisely tailored to each individual's unique biological, environmental, and lifestyle factors, ultimately improving patient outcomes and reducing healthcare costs.

3. KEY EMERGING TRENDS

3.1 Deep Learning for Medical Imaging

Deep learning algorithms, particularly Convolutional Neural Networks (CNNs), have shown remarkable progress in medical image analysis. Key applications include:

- Automated detection and classification of tumors in radiology images
- Early detection of eye diseases through retinal scan analysis
- Identification of skin lesions and potential melanomas

Automated Detection And Classification Of Tumors In Radiology Images:

The application of Machine Learning (ML) in the automated detection and classification of tumors in radiology images represents a significant advancement in medical imaging analysis, offering the potential to enhance diagnostic accuracy, reduce interpretation time, and improve patient outcomes (Aamir et al., 2023). Deep learning algorithms, particularly Convolutional Neural Networks (CNNs), have demonstrated remarkable performance in image recognition tasks and are at the forefront of this revolution in radiological practice (LeCun et al., 2015). These algorithms can automatically learn hierarchical feature representations from raw image data, enabling them to identify subtle patterns and anomalies that may be challenging for human observers to detect consistently (Litjens et al., 2017). In the context of tumor detection, ML models have been successfully applied across various imaging modalities, including Computed Tomography (CT), Magnetic Resonance Imaging (MRI), and Positron Emission Tomography (PET), showcasing their versatility and potential for multimodal integration (Hosny et al., 2018).

For instance, in lung cancer screening, deep learning models have shown the ability to detect malignant pulmonary nodules in chest CT scans with sensitivity and specificity comparable to, or even exceeding, that of experienced radiologists (Ardila et al., 2019). Similarly, in brain tumor segmentation using MRI, ML algorithms have demonstrated high accuracy in delineating tumor boundaries and differentiating between various types of brain lesions, aiding in treatment planning and prognosis assessment (Menze et al., 2015). The application of transfer learning techniques has further enhanced the efficacy of these models, allowing them to leverage knowledge gained from large datasets to improve performance on smaller, more specialized datasets typical in medical imaging (Shin et al., 2016). In breast cancer detection, ML algorithms have shown promise in reducing false-positive rates in mammography screening, potentially decreasing unnecessary biopsies and patient anxiety (McKinney et al., 2020). Moreover, the integration of ML with other emerging technologies, such as radiomics and radiogenomics, is enabling the extraction of quantitative features from medical images that can be correlated with genomic profiles and clinical outcomes, paving the way for more personalized cancer diagnosis and treatment strategies (Aerts et al., 2014). The development of explainable AI techniques is addressing the "black box" nature of deep learning models, providing interpretable results that can enhance clinician trust and facilitate regulatory approval (Ribeiro et al., 2016). However, challenges remain in the widespread clinical adoption of these technologies, including the need for large, diverse, and well-annotated datasets for training, concerns about generalizability across different patient populations and imaging protocols, and the integration of ML systems into existing clinical workflows (Bi et al., 2019). Efforts to standardize data collection, annotation, and model evaluation protocols are underway to address these challenges and facilitate multi-institutional collaborations (Willemink et al., 2020). As ML technologies continue to evolve, their role in tumor detection and classification is expanding beyond simple binary classification tasks to more complex analyses, such as predicting tumor aggressiveness, treatment response, and patient outcomes (Yala et al., 2019). The potential of ML to augment radiologist performance, rather than replace human expertise, is increasingly recognized, with studies showing improved diagnostic accuracy when ML predictions are combined with radiologist interpretations (Topol, 2019). Looking forward, the integration of ML with other forms of clinical data, including electronic health records and genomic information, promises to create comprehensive decision support systems that can provide personalized risk assessments and treatment recommendations (Beam &Kohane, 2018). As these systems mature and undergo rigorous clinical validation, they have the potential to revolutionize cancer care, enabling earlier detection, more accurate diagnosis, and more effective treatment planning, ultimately improving patient outcomes and reducing healthcare costs (Aamir et al., 2022).

Early Detection Of Eye Diseases Through Retinal Scan Analysis

The application of machine learning (ML) in the analysis of retinal scans has revolutionized the early detection of eye diseases, offering unprecedented opportunities for timely intervention and prevention of vision loss. Retinal imaging, particularly fundus photography and optical coherence tomography (OCT), provides a non-invasive window into the health of the eye and, by extension, the overall vascular and neurological well-being of an individual (Wong et al., 2016). Deep learning algorithms, especially convolutional neural networks (CNNs), have demonstrated remarkable proficiency in analyzing these complex images, often matching or surpassing the diagnostic accuracy of experienced ophthalmologists (Ting et al., 2019). One of the most significant applications of ML in retinal scan analysis has been in the detection of diabetic retinopathy (DR), a leading cause of blindness globally. (Gulshan et al., 2016) developed a deep learning algorithm that achieved sensitivity and specificity comparable to that of ophthalmologists in identifying referable DR, potentially enabling more widespread and cost-effective screening programs. Similarly, ML models have shown promise in the early detection of age-related macular degeneration (AMD), with algorithms capable of distinguishing between early, intermediate, and late stages of the disease based on fundus photographs and OCT scans (Burlina et al., 2017). The ability of ML to detect subtle changes in retinal vasculature has also proven valuable in identifying signs of systemic diseases such as cardiovascular disorders and hypertension, positioning retinal imaging as a potential tool for general health screening (Poplin et al., 2018). In the realm of glaucoma detection, ML algorithms have demonstrated high accuracy in analyzing optic disc features and visual field data, enabling earlier identification of this often asymptomatic disease (Li et al., 2018). The integration of ML with adaptive optics scanning laser ophthalmoscopy (AOSLO) has further enhanced our ability to visualize and analyze individual photoreceptors, opening new avenues for the early detection of retinal degenerative diseases (Liu et al., 2017). Moreover, the application of unsupervised learning techniques has revealed novel retinal biomarkers and disease phenotypes, potentially leading to more nuanced disease classification and personalized treatment strategies (Yim et al., 2020). The development of explainable AI models in retinal image analysis has addressed concerns about the "black box" nature of deep learning, providing clinicians with interpretable results that can inform clinical decision-making (Sayres et al., 2019). As these technologies mature, there is growing interest in deploying ML-based retinal screening systems in primary care and community settings, potentially increasing access to eye care services in underserved areas (Abràmoff et al., 2018). However, challenges remain in the widespread adoption of these technologies, including the need for large, diverse datasets for training, concerns about generalizability across different patient populations and imaging devices, and the integration of ML systems into existing clinical workflows (Ting et al., 2019). Efforts to develop standardized datasets and evaluation metrics, such as the REFUGE challenge for glaucoma detection, are helping to address these issues and facilitate comparison between different ML approaches (Orlando et al., 2020). The potential of ML in retinal scan analysis extends beyond disease detection to predicting disease progression and treatment response. Recent studies have explored the use of ML to forecast the development of late-stage AMD and to predict visual outcomes following treatment for diabetic macular edema (Schmidt-Erfurth et al., 2018). As ML technologies continue to evolve, there is growing interest in multimodal approaches that combine retinal imaging data with other clinical information, genetic data, and even data from wearable devices to create comprehensive eye health profiles (De Fauw et al., 2018). Looking forward, the integration of ML-based retinal analysis with telemedicine platforms promises to revolutionize eye care delivery, enabling remote screening and monitoring of eye diseases, particularly in resource-limited settings (Raumviboonsuk et al., 2019). As these systems undergo rigorous clinical validation and real-world testing, they have the potential to significantly reduce the burden of preventable blindness worldwide, improve patient outcomes, and provide insights into systemic health, ultimately contributing to more holistic and preventive healthcare strategies.

Identification of Skin Lesions And Potential Melanomas

The application of machine learning (ML) in the identification of skin lesions and potential melanomas has emerged as a powerful tool in dermatology, offering the potential for earlier detection, improved accuracy, and increased accessibility to skin cancer screening. Skin cancer, particularly melanoma, is a significant public health concern, with early detection being crucial for improved patient outcomes

(Siegel et al., 2021). Deep learning algorithms, especially Convolutional Neural Networks (CNNs), have demonstrated remarkable proficiency in analyzing dermatological images, often matching or surpassing the diagnostic accuracy of experienced dermatologists (Esteva et al., 2017). These algorithms can automatically learn complex features from raw image data, enabling them to identify subtle patterns and anomalies that may be challenging for human observers to detect consistently. One of the most significant breakthroughs in this field was the development of a deep learning system by (Esteva et al., 2017), which achieved dermatologist-level classification of skin cancer from clinical images, including the differentiation of benign lesions from malignant ones. This study demonstrated the potential of ML to augment clinical decision-making and expand access to diagnostic expertise. Subsequent research has further refined these approaches, with models showing high sensitivity and specificity in distinguishing between different types of skin lesions, including melanoma, basal cell carcinoma, and squamous cell carcinoma (Brinker et al., 2019). The integration of ML with dermoscopy, a non-invasive imaging technique that allows visualization of subsurface skin structures, has further enhanced the accuracy of skin lesion classification. (Haenssle et al., 2018) demonstrated that a CNN trained on dermoscopic images outperformed a group of 58 international dermatologists in detecting melanoma, highlighting the potential of ML to serve as a valuable aid in clinical practice. Moreover, the application of transfer learning techniques has enabled the development of robust models using relatively small datasets, addressing one of the key challenges in medical image analysis (Han et al., 2018). The potential of ML extends beyond binary classification of benign versus malignant lesions. Recent studies have explored the use of ML for more nuanced tasks, such as predicting the genetic mutations associated with melanomas based on clinical and dermoscopic images (Winkler et al., 2020). This approach could potentially guide targeted therapies and provide insights into disease prognosis. Additionally, unsupervised learning techniques have been employed to discover novel visual patterns and subtypes of skin lesions, potentially leading to more refined classification systems and personalized treatment strategies (Codella et al., 2018). The development of explainable AI models in skin lesion analysis has addressed concerns about the "black box" nature of deep learning, providing clinicians with interpretable results that can inform clinical decision-making and build trust in ML-based recommendations (Young et al., 2019). As these technologies mature, there is growing interest in deploying ML-based skin lesion screening systems on mobile devices, potentially increasing access to early detection tools for the general public (Phillips et al., 2019). However, challenges remain in the widespread adoption of these technologies, including the need for large, diverse datasets that represent various skin types and ethnicities, concerns about generalizability across different imaging devices and conditions, and the integration of ML systems into existing clinical workflows (Adamson & Smith, 2018). Efforts to develop standardized datasets and evaluation metrics, such as the ISIC Archive and Challenge, are helping to address these issues and facilitate comparison between different ML approaches (Codella et al., 2019). The potential of ML in skin lesion analysis extends beyond static image analysis to the realm of longitudinal monitoring. Recent studies have explored the use of ML to track changes in skin lesions over time, potentially enabling the early detection of malignant transformations (Kittler et al., 2019). As ML technologies continue to evolve, there is growing interest in multimodal approaches that combine visual image data with other clinical information, genetic data, and even data from spectroscopic imaging techniques to create comprehensive skin health profiles (Gareau et al., 2020). Looking forward, the integration of ML-based skin lesion analysis with telemedicine platforms promises to revolutionize dermatological care delivery, enabling remote screening and monitoring of skin conditions, particularly in underserved areas (Chuchu et al., 2018). As these systems undergo rigorous clinical validation and real-world testing, they have the potential to significantly reduce the burden of skin cancer worldwide, improve patient outcomes through earlier detection and intervention, and provide insights into the underlying biology of skin lesions, ultimately contributing to more personalized and effective dermatological care strategies.

Recent Advancements

Integration of Multi-Modal Imaging Data For More Comprehensive Diagnosis (Figure 2)

The integration of multi-modal imaging data through machine learning (ML) represents a significant advancement in medical diagnostics, offering a more comprehensive and nuanced understanding of complex pathologies. This approach leverages the complementary strengths of various imaging modalities, such as Magnetic Resonance Imaging (MRI), Computed Tomography (CT), Positron Emission Tomography (PET), and ultrasound, to provide a holistic view of anatomical structures and physiological processes (Martí-Bonmatí et al., 2010). Deep learning algorithms, particularly multi-stream Convolutional Neural Networks (CNNs) and transformer-based architectures, have demonstrated remarkable proficiency in synthesizing information from diverse imaging sources, often surpassing the diagnostic accuracy achieved by single-modality approaches (Litjens et al., 2017). One of the most prominent applications of multi-modal integration has been in neuroimaging, where the combination of structural MRI, functional MRI (fMRI), and Diffusion Tensor Imaging (DTI) has enhanced our ability to diagnose and characterize neurological disorders. For instance, (Plis et al., 2018) developed a deep learning model that integrates these modalities to improve the diagnosis of schizophrenia, capturing both structural and functional brain abnormalities. In oncology, the fusion of PET and CT imaging data has significantly improved tumor detection and characterization. (Xu et al., 2019) demonstrated that a multi-modal deep learning approach combining PET/CT images outperformed single-modality methods in lung nodule classification, potentially reducing false-positive rates in lung cancer screening. Similarly, in breast cancer diagnosis, the integration of mammography, ultrasound, and MRI through ML algorithms has shown promise in improving the accuracy of lesion detection and classification, particularly in dense breast tissue where traditional mammography alone may be less effective (Antropova et al., 2017). The potential of multi-modal integration extends beyond image fusion to incorporate non-imaging data sources. Recent studies have explored the integration of genomic data with imaging features, a field known as radiogenomics. In glioma research, (Kickingereder et al., 2018) developed an ML model that combines multi-parametric MRI with genomic information to predict patient survival and molecular subtypes, potentially guiding personalized treatment strategies. Moreover, the integration of longitudinal imaging data has opened new avenues for disease progression modeling and treatment response prediction. (Venkatraghavan et al., 2019) proposed a deep learning framework that integrates multi-modal MRI data acquired over time to model the progression of Alzheimer's disease, potentially enabling earlier intervention and more effective treatment planning. The development of attention mechanisms and graph neural networks has further enhanced the ability of ML models to capture complex relationships between different imaging modalities and anatomical regions. For instance,(Gao et al., 2019) introduced a graph-based attention model for multi-modal brain image analysis, which can adaptively focus on the most relevant features across modalities for improved diagnostic accuracy. Despite these advancements, challenges remain in the widespread adoption of multi-modal integration techniques. These include the need for large, diverse datasets that include multiple imaging modalities, the computational complexity of processing high-dimensional multi-modal data, and the interpretability of complex multi-modal models (Kaissis et al., 2020). Efforts to address these challenges include the development of federated learning approaches for multi-institutional collaboration, the use of unsupervised and self-supervised learning techniques to leverage unlabeled multi-modal data, and the creation of explainable AI models that provide insights into the decision-making process across modalities (Rieke et al., 2020). As multi-modal integration techniques mature, there is growing interest in their application to population health studies and large-scale screening programs. The UK Biobank Imaging Study, for example, is collecting multi-modal imaging data from thousands of participants, providing an unprecedented opportunity to develop and validate ML models for disease risk prediction and early detection (Littlejohns et al., 2020). Looking forward, the integration of multi-modal imaging with other data sources, such as electronic health records, wearable sensor data, and environmental factors, promises to create comprehensive health profiles that can inform precision medicine approaches (Topol, 2019). The potential of ML-driven multi-modal integration extends beyond diagnosis to treatment planning and monitoring. In radiation therapy, for instance, the combination of CT, MRI, and PET data through ML algorithms is enhancing tumor delineation and dose optimization (Balagopal et al., 2021). As these technologies continue to evolve and undergo rigorous clinical validation, they have the potential to revolutionize medical diagnostics, enabling more accurate, personalized, and comprehensive patient assessments that leverage the full spectrum of available imaging and clinical data.

Figure 4. Machine learning based multi-modal medical imaging integration framework

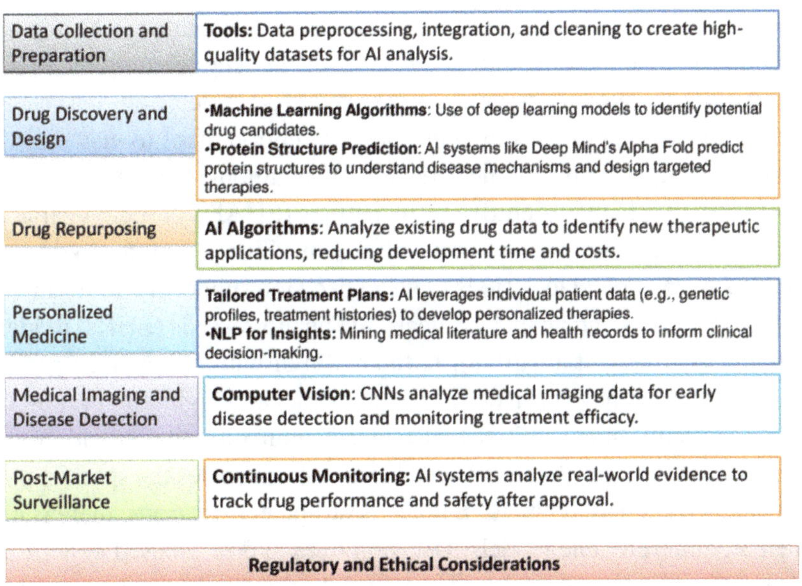

Case Study

A notable example is the National Health Service (NHS) in England initiating the world's largest trial of AI for breast cancer diagnosis. This trial involves approximately 700,000 mammograms and aims to assess AI's effectiveness in detecting breast cancer compared to traditional radiologist evaluations. If successful, AI could reduce the need for multiple radiologists per scan, expedite diagnoses, and alleviate the workload on healthcare professionals. This initiative reflects a broader trend of integrating AI into medical applications to enhance diagnostic accuracy and efficiency

[The Guardian. (2025, February 4). *NHS to launch world's biggest trial of AI breast cancer diagnosis.* Retrieved from https://www.theguardian.com/society/2025/feb/04/nhs-to-launch-worlds-biggest-trial-of-ai-breast-cancer-diagnosis].

Development of Explainable AI Models To Increase Transparency In Decision-Making

The development of explainable Artificial Intelligence (XAI) models has emerged as a critical focus in medical AI research, addressing the need for transparency and interpretability in decision-making processes. As AI systems become increasingly sophisticated and integral to healthcare, the ability to understand and trust their decisions is paramount for clinical adoption, regulatory approval, and patient acceptance (Holzinger et al., 2017). Explainable AI aims to bridge the gap between the high performance of complex "black box" models and the need for human-interpretable reasoning, particularly in high-stakes medical scenarioswhere understanding the rationale behind a decision can be as crucial as the decision itself (Došilović et al., 2018). Various approaches to XAI have been developed, each offering different levels of interpretability and applicability to medical contexts. Local Interpretable Model-agnostic Explanations (LIME), introduced by (Ribeiro et al., 2016), provides insights into model decisions by approximating complex models with simpler, interpretable ones around specific data points. This technique has been successfully applied in various medical imaging tasks, such as explaining the features that contribute to the classification of skin lesions in dermatology (Young et al., 2019). Another prominent approach is the use of attention mechanisms in deep learning models, which highlight the regions or features that the model deems most important for its decision. In the context of medical imaging, (Rajpurkar et al., 2017) demonstrated the use of attention maps to visualize the areas of chest X-rays that contribute most significantly to the detection of pneumonia, enhancing both the accuracy and interpretability of the model. Shapley Additive Explanations (SHAP), based on game theory concepts, offer a unified approach to explaining the output of any machine learning model (Lundberg & Lee, 2017). This method has been applied to various medical decision support systems, including models for predicting hospital readmissions and analyzing electronic health records (EHRs) to identify risk factors for specific conditions (Lundberg et al., 2018). In the realm of natural language processing applied to clinical text, explainable models have been developed to extract and highlight relevant information from EHRs. For instance, (Mullenbach et al., 2018) introduced a convolutional attention model for medical code prediction that not only assigns diagnostic codes but also identifies the specific phrases in the clinical notes that support each code assignment. Beyond post-hoc explanations, there is a growing interest in developing inherently interpretable models. Decision trees and rule-based systems, while often less complex than deep learning models, offer clear decision paths that can be easily understood by clinicians. (Lakkaraju et al., 2019) proposed interpretable decision sets for clinical decision support, providing a balance between predictive accuracy and interpretability in tasks such as predicting hospital readmissions. The integration of domain knowledge into AI models is another approach to enhancing explainability. By incorporating medical ontologies and causal relationships into model architectures, researchers aim to align AI reasoning processes with human medical knowledge. (Rotmensch et al., 2017)demonstrated this approach by learning a probabilistic health knowledge graph from electronic health records, providing a transparent representation of relationships between diseases and symptoms. Despite these advancements, challenges remain in developing XAI models that are both highly accurate and fully interpretable. The trade-off between model complexity and explainability often requires careful consideration in clinical applications (Ahmad et al., 2018). Moreover, the definition of "explainability" itself can vary depending on the stakeholder – what is explainable to a data scientist may not be meaningful to a clinician or patient (Tonekaboni et al., 2019). To address these challenges, interdisciplinary collaboration between AI researchers, clinicians, and domain experts is crucial. Initiatives like the Explainable AI in Healthcare and Medicine (XAIHM) workshop series are fostering such collaborations and driving the development of clinically relevant XAI approaches (Payrovnaziri et al., 2020). As XAI techniques mature, there is growing interest in their potential to not only explain decisions but also to uncover novel medical insights. By making the decision-making processes of AI models transparent, researchers hope to discover previously unknown relationships in medical data, potentially leading to new hypotheses and avenues for clinical research (Holzinger et al., 2019). The regulatory landscape is also evolving to accommodate the need for explainable AI in healthcare. The U.S. Food and Drug Administration (FDA) has emphasized the importance of transparency in AI/ML-based medical devices, suggesting that explainability will be a key consideration in future regulatory frameworks (FDA, 2021). Looking forward, the development of XAI models is likely to play a crucial role in the broader acceptance and integration of AI in clinical practice. As these models become more sophisticated and aligned with medical reasoning, they have the potential to serve not just as decision support tools, but as collaborative partners in the diagnostic and treatment process, enhancing both the quality and transparency of medical care.

3.2 Natural Language Processing for Clinical Documentation

Natural Language Processing (NLP) is being leveraged to improve the efficiency and accuracy of clinical documentation. Emerging applications include:

Automated Extraction Of Relevant Information From Electronic Health Records (EHRs)

Natural language processing (NLP) techniques have emerged as powerful tools for automatically extracting clinically relevant information from unstructured text in electronic health records (EHRs), enabling more efficient and comprehensive analysis of patient data (Wu et al., 2020). EHRs contain a wealth of valuable clinical information, but much of it is locked away in free-text clinical notes, making it challenging to leverage at scale for research, quality improvement, and clinical decision support. NLP methods can parse and analyze this unstructured text to identify and extract key clinical concepts, events, and relationships. Common NLP tasks in the EHR domain include named entity recognition to identify clinical entities like diseases, symptoms, and medications; relation extraction to capture associations between entities; and document classification to categorize clinical notes (Sheikhalishahi et al., 2019). Advanced deep learning models like BERT have shown strong performance on many EHR-based NLP tasks, outperforming traditional machine learning approaches. For example, (Alsentzer et al., 2019) demonstrated that clinical BERT models pre-trained on EHR data achieved state-of-the-art results on clinical named entity recognition. Beyond extracting individual clinical concepts, researchers have developed NLP pipelines to automatically generate patient phenotypes and cohorts from EHR data. For instance, (Banda et al., 2018) used NLP to extract phenotype information from clinical notes to augment structured EHR data for identifying patients with heart failure. NLP has also been applied to extract adverse drug events, family history, social determinants of health, and other clinically relevant information that is often only recorded in free text. However, challenges remain in developing NLP systems that can generalize across different EHR systems, clinical domains, and institution-specific documentation practices. Issues like inconsistent terminologies, abbreviations, misspellings, and context-dependent interpretations add complexity. There are also important ethical and privacy considerations around using NLP to extract sensitive information from clinical text, with ongoing research into de-identification methods (Dernoncourt et al., 2017). Despite these challenges, NLP is playing an increasingly important role in unlocking the knowledge contained in EHRs to support clinical research, quality measurement, predictive modeling, and other secondary uses of EHR data. As NLP techniques continue to advance, they have the potential to dramatically improve our ability to efficiently extract comprehensive, structured clinical data from EHRs to drive improvements in research and patient care.

Real-Time Transcription And Summarization Of Doctor-Patient Conversations

Real-time transcription and summarization of doctor-patient conversations has emerged as a promising application of natural language processing (NLP) and speech recognition technologies in healthcare, offering potential benefits for clinical documentation, patient engagement, and quality of care. As electronic health records (EHRs) have become ubiquitous, the burden of documentation has increased for clinicians, often detracting from patient interaction during visits (Shanafelt et al., 2016). Automated transcription systems aim to alleviate this burden by converting spoken doctor-patient dialogues into written text in real-time, while summarization techniques distill key information from these conversations. Recent advancements in deep learning-based speech recognition have significantly improved transcription accuracy, with some systems approaching human-level performance for medical conversations (Chiu et al., 2018). These systems typically employ end-to-end neural network architectures, such as recurrent neural networks (RNNs) or Transformer models, trained on large corpora of medical speech data. However, challenges remain in handling domain-specific medical terminology, accents, and noisy clinical environments. Once conversations are transcribed, NLP techniques are applied to summarize the content, extracting salient clinical information such as symptoms, diagnoses, treatment plans, and follow-up instructions. Extractive summarization methods select important sentences from the transcript, while abstractive approaches generate new text to capture key points (Liu and Lapata, 2019). Recent work has explored the use of reinforcement learning to optimize summarization models for specific clinical objectives, such as capturing actionable items or aligning with standard clinical note structures (Zhang et al., 2020). Integration of these technologies into clinical workflows presents both opportunities and challenges. Real-time transcription can provide immediate documentation, potentially improving the accuracy and completeness of medical records while allowing clinicians to focus more on patient interaction. Automated summaries can offer quick overviews of patient encounters for care team members and facilitate more efficient chart review. However, concerns exist regarding patient privacy, the impact on doctor-patient rapport, and the potential for errors in transcription or summarization leading to clinical misunderstandings (Quiroz et al., 2019). Additionally, there are important ethical considerations around consent, data ownership, and the use of AI in clinical decision-making. As these technologies continue to evolve, ongoing research is focused on improving accuracy, developing more robust models that can handle the complexity and variability of clinical conversations, and designing user interfaces that seamlessly integrate transcription and summarization into clinical workflows without disrupting patient care. Evaluation of these systems in real-world clinical settings is crucial to understand their impact on documentation quality, clinical efficiency, and patient outcomes. While challenges remain, the potential of real-time transcription and summarization to transform clinical documentation and enhance the doctor-patient experience is significant, pointing towards a future where AI-assisted communication becomes an integral part of healthcare delivery.

Clinical Decision Support Systems Based On Analysis Of Medical Literature And Patient Records

Clinical decision support systems (CDSS) leveraging natural language processing (NLP) for analysis of medical literature and patient records have emerged as powerful tools to enhance clinical decision-making and improve patient outcomes. These systems utilize advanced NLP techniques to extract, synthesize, and apply relevant information from vast repositories of unstructured medical text, including scientific literature, clinical guidelines, and electronic health records (EHRs). At the core of these systems are sophisticated NLP pipelines that perform tasks such as named entity recognition, relation extraction, and semantic parsing to identify key clinical concepts and their relationships (Demner-Fushman et al., 2009). Recent advancements in deep learning have significantly improved the performance of these NLP tasks. For instance, transformer-based models like BERT and its domain-specific variants (e.g., BioBERT, ClinicalBERT) have achieved state-of-the-art results in biomedical and clinical NLP tasks (Lee et al., 2020). These models can capture complex contextual information and nuances in medical language, enabling more accurate extraction of clinically relevant information. In the context of medical literature analysis, NLP techniques are employed to automatically extract evidence from research papers, systematic reviews, and clinical guidelines. Systems like IBM Watson for Oncology use NLP to process vast amounts of medical literature and generate evidence-based treatment recommendations (Chen et al., 2016). Similarly, NLP-based systems have been developed to automatically generate and update clinical practice guidelines by synthesizing information from multiple sources (Tsafnat et al., 2013). For patient record analysis, NLP plays a crucial role in extracting structured information from unstructured clinical notes, enabling more comprehensive patient profiling and risk assessment. Advanced NLP techniques like temporal reasoning and coreference resolution are used to construct patient timelines and track the progression of conditions over time (Raghavan et al., 2014). Moreover, NLP-powered systems can identify patients eligible for clinical trials by analyzing EHR data, potentially accelerating medical research (Meystre et al., 2019). The integration of NLP-based analysis of both medical literature and patient records allows CDSS to provide personalized, evidence-based recommendations. For example, systems can match patient-specific factors extracted from EHRs with relevant clinical evidence from the literature to suggest tailored treatment options or alert clinicians to potential drug interactions or contraindications (Demner-Fushman et al., 2017). Recent research has explored the use of large language models (LLMs) like GPT-3 for clinical decision support, leveraging their ability to understand and generate human-like text. These models can be fine-tuned on medical corpora to provide more contextually relevant and nuanced clinical recommendations (Koike et al., 2023). However, challenges remain in ensuring the interpretability and explainability of these complex NLP models, which is crucial for clinical adoption and trust. Additionally, handling the ambiguity and inconsistency in medical language, addressing potential biases in training data, and ensuring patient privacy and data security are ongoing areas of research. As NLP technologies continue to advance, their integration into CDSS holds great promise for enhancing clinical decision-making, improving patient outcomes, and reducing healthcare costs. Future developments in areas such as multimodal learning, incorporating both textual and imaging data, and real-time NLP processing of clinical conversations are likely to further expand the capabilities and impact of NLP-powered clinical decision support systems.

Recent Developments

Improved Understanding Of Medical Context And Terminology

Recent advancements in artificial intelligence (AI) have significantly enhanced the ability of machines to understand and process medical context and terminology, revolutionizing various aspects of healthcare. At the forefront of these developments are large language models (LLMs) and domain-specific transformers, which have demonstrated remarkable proficiency in comprehending complex medical concepts and their contextual nuances. Models like BioBERT(Lee et al., 2020) and ClinicalBERT(Alsentzer et al., 2019) have been pre-trained on vast corpora of biomedical literature and clinical notes, enabling them to capture the intricacies of medical language more effectively than general-purpose models. These specialized models have shown superior performance in tasks such as named entity recognition, relation extraction, and question answering in the medical domain. For instance, BioBERT has achieved state-of-the-art results on biomedical text mining benchmarks, outperforming previous methods by a significant margin. The advent of even larger models like GPT-3 and its derivatives has further pushed the boundaries of medical language understanding. These models, when fine-tuned on medical datasets, have demonstrated an impressive ability to generate human-like responses to medical queries, summarize complex medical literature, and even assist in differential diagnosis (Esteva et al., 2021). Recent studies have explored the potential of these models in clinical decision support, showing promising results in tasks such as predicting drug-drug interactions and identifying potential adverse events (Kang et al., 2022). Another significant development is the integration of multimodal learning approaches, combining text analysis with other data types such as medical imaging and genomic data. These systems can process and interpret diverse sources of medical information simultaneously, providing a more comprehensive understanding of patient conditions. For example, researchers have developed models that can analyze both radiology reports and corresponding medical images, improving the accuracy of diagnosis and prognosis (Zhang et al., 2022). The field of biomedical knowledge graph construction has also seen substantial progress, with AI systems now capable of automatically extracting and organizing complex medical knowledge from unstructured text. These knowledge graphs serve as powerful resources for various downstream tasks, including drug discovery, clinical decision support, and personalized medicine (Callahan et al., 2020). Recent work has focused on improving the interpretability and explainability of these AI models, addressing the critical need for transparency in medical applications. Techniques such as attention visualization and concept-based explanations have been developed to provide insights into the decision-making processes of these complex models (Zhan et al., 2022). This not only enhances trust in AI systems but also provides valuable learning opportunities for medical professionals. Despite these advancements, challenges remain in handling the ambiguity and context-dependence inherent in medical language. Ongoing research is exploring ways to incorporate domain expertise and clinical guidelines into AI models to improve their robustness and reliability. Additionally, efforts are being made to address biases in training data and ensure that AI systems perform equitably across diverse patient populations. As these technologies continue to evolve, they promise to transform various aspects of healthcare, from enhancing the efficiency of clinical workflows to enabling more personalized and precise medical interventions. The improved understanding of medical context and terminology by AI systems is paving the way for more sophisticated clinical decision support tools, automated medical coding systems, and advanced natural language interfaces for healthcare applications.

Integration of NLP with Speech Recognition For More Seamless Documentation

The integration of Natural Language Processing (NLP) with speech recognition technology has emerged as a powerful solution for streamlining clinical documentation, addressing the growing administrative burden on healthcare providers and enhancing the quality of patient care. This synergy enables more seamless and efficient capture of medical information, transforming spoken words into structured, actionable data. Recent advancements in deep learning have significantly improved the accuracy of speech recognition in medical contexts. End-to-end neural network architectures, such as recurrent neural networks (RNNs) and Transformer-based models, have shown remarkable performance in handling the complexities of medical terminology and accented speech (Chiu et al., 2018). These models, trained on large corpora of medical speech data, can accurately transcribe doctor-patient conversations, clinical dictations, and medical lectures in real-time. The integration of NLP techniques further enhances this process by extracting clinically relevant information from the transcribed text. Named entity recognition (NER) algorithms identify key medical concepts such as symptoms, diagnoses, medications, and procedures, while relation extraction techniques capture the relationships between these entities (Liu et al., 2021). Advanced NLP models like BioBERT and ClinicalBERT, pre-trained on vast amounts of biomedical literature and clinical notes, have demonstrated superior performance in understanding the nuances of medical language (Alsentzer et al., 2019). This integration allows for the automatic generation of structured clinical notes, reducing the time physicians spend on documentation. For instance, (Klann et al., 2021) developed a system that combines speech recognition with NLP to automatically populate electronic health record (EHR) fields during patient encounters, significantly reducing documentation time and improving note quality. The seamless nature of this integration extends to more sophisticated applications, such as real-time clinical decision support. By analyzing the ongoing conversation between doctor and patient, these systems can provide contextually relevant information, such as treatment guidelines, potential drug interactions, or relevant research findings (Shickel et al., 2021). This real-time support enhances clinical decision-making and ensures that important information is not overlooked during patient encounters. Moreover, the integration of NLP and speech recognition facilitates the development of more natural and intuitive interfaces for interacting with EHRs and clinical information systems. Voice-activated queries and commands, powered by NLP, allow healthcare providers to retrieve patient information, order tests, or update records using natural language, reducing the cognitive load associated with complex EHR interfaces (Patel et al., 2020). Despite these advancements, challenges remain in ensuring the accuracy and reliability of these integrated systems in diverse clinical settings. Issues such as background noise, variations in accent and speaking styles, and the handling of medical jargon and abbreviations continue to be areas of active research. Privacy concerns and the need for robust security measures are also critical considerations, given the sensitive nature of medical conversations (Quiroz et al., 2019). Ongoing work focuses on improving the contextual understanding of these systems, enabling them to better handle the nuances of clinical dialogue and the often non-linear nature of patient narratives. Researchers are exploring the use of reinforcement learning and federated learning approaches to continually improve system performance while maintaining patient privacy (Zhang et al., 2022). As these technologies mature, they promise to transform clinical workflows, reducing administrative burden, improving documentation quality, and allowing healthcare providers to focus more on patient care. The seamless integration of NLP with speech recognition is paving the way for a more efficient, accurate, and patient-centered approach to healthcare documentation and decision-making.

3.3 Predictive Analytics for Disease Prevention

AI-driven predictive analytics are being used to identify high-risk patients and predict disease outbreaks. Key areas of focus include:

Early Detection Of Chronic Diseases Based On Patient Data And Risk Factors

The early detection of chronic diseases using patient data and risk factors has become a critical area of research in healthcare, with artificial intelligence (AI) and natural language processing (NLP) playing increasingly pivotal roles. These advanced technologies enable the analysis of vast amounts of structured and unstructured patient data to identify subtle patterns and risk factors associated with chronic conditions, potentially allowing for earlier intervention and improved patient outcomes (Guan et al. 2021). Machine learning models, particularly deep learning architectures, have demonstrated remarkable capabilities in processing diverse data types, including electronic health records (EHRs), genetic information, lifestyle data, and environmental factors. For instance, (Rajkomar et al., 2018) developed a deep learning model that could predict a range of clinical outcomes, including the development of chronic conditions, using EHR data across multiple institutions. Their model outperformed traditional predictive models, showcasing the potential of AI in early disease detection. NLP techniques have been instrumental in extracting valuable information from unstructured clinical notes, a rich source of patient data often overlooked by traditional methods. Advanced NLP models like BERT and its biomedical variants (e.g., BioBERT, ClinicalBERT) have shown superior performance in understanding the nuances of medical language and extracting clinically relevant information (Lee et al., 2020). These models can identify mentions of symptoms, risk factors, and family history that might be indicative of developing chronic conditions. For example, (Sheikhalishahi et al., 2019) demonstrated the effectiveness of NLP in extracting information related to chronic diseases from clinical notes, enabling more comprehensive risk assessment. The integration of multi-modal data has further enhanced the accuracy of early detection systems. Researchers have developed models that combine structured EHR data with unstructured clinical notes and even medical imaging data to provide a more holistic view of patient health. (Miotto et al., 2016) introduced a deep learning method called "Deep Patient" that could predict the onset of various diseases, including chronic conditions, by learning a general-purpose patient representation from EHR data. Their approach demonstrated improved predictive accuracy compared to traditional methods. Recent advancements in federated learning have addressed some of the privacy concerns associated with using sensitive patient data for model training. This approach allows models to be trained across multiple institutions without sharing raw patient data, enabling the development of more robust and generalizable early detection systems (Rieke et al., 2020). The application of AI and NLP in early disease detection extends beyond traditional clinical data. Social determinants of health, often captured in unstructured format, play a crucial role in chronic disease development. NLP techniques have been employed to extract this information from clinical notes and even social media data, providing a more comprehensive risk profile (Gianfrancesco et al., 2018). Moreover, the integration of genomic data with clinical information has opened new avenues for personalized risk assessment. Machine learning models can now incorporate genetic risk factors alongside clinical and lifestyle data to provide more accurate and individualized predictions of chronic disease onset (Khera et al., 2018). Despite these advancements, challenges remain in developing reliable and interpretable early detection systems. Ensuring model fairness and addressing potential biases in training data are critical concerns, particularly given the disparities in healthcare access and outcomes among different populations. Ongoing research focuses on developing explainable AI models that can provide clinicians with insights into the reasoning behind predictions, fostering trust and facilitating clinical adoption (Holzinger et al., 2019). As these technologies continue to evolve, they promise to transform the landscape of chronic disease management, shifting the focus from treatment to prevention and early intervention. The integration of AI and NLP in early detection systems has the potential to significantly reduce the burden of chronic diseases, improve patient outcomes, and optimize healthcare resource allocation.

Prediction of Hospital Readmissions To Improve Post-Discharge Care

The prediction of hospital readmissions has become a critical area of focus in healthcare, driven by the need to improve patient outcomes and reduce healthcare costs. Advanced artificial intelligence (AI) and natural language processing (NLP) techniques have emerged as powerful tools for analyzing complex patient data and identifying factors that contribute to readmission risk. These technologies enable healthcare providers to develop targeted interventions and improve post-discharge care strategies. Machine learning models, particularly deep learning architectures, have demonstrated remarkable efficacy in predicting readmissions by integrating diverse data sources, including structured electronic health record (EHR) data, unstructured clinical notes, and socioeconomic factors. For instance, (Rajkomar et al., 2018) developed a deep learning model that outperformed traditional predictive models in forecasting 30-day readmissions across multiple institutions. Their approach, which utilized the entire EHR, including free-text notes, showcased the potential of AI in capturing subtle patterns indicative of readmission risk. NLP techniques play a crucial role in extracting valuable information from unstructured clinical notes, which often contain nuanced details about a patient's condition and social circumstances that may influence readmission risk. Advanced NLP models like BERT and its clinical variants (e.g., ClinicalBERT) have shown superior performance in understanding medical context and extracting relevant features from clinical text (Huang et al., 2019). These models can identify mentions of social determinants of health, medication adherence issues, and post-discharge care plans that might be overlooked in structured data alone. For example, (Gao et al., 2020) demonstrated the effectiveness of NLP in extracting psychosocial factors from discharge summaries, significantly improving readmission prediction accuracy. The integration of temporal modeling techniques with NLP has further enhanced the ability to predict readmissions by capturing the progression of a patient's condition over time. Long Short-Term Memory (LSTM) networks and attention mechanisms have been employed to model the sequence of clinical events and identify patterns that precede readmissions. (Chen et al., 2021) developed a temporal attention-based LSTM model that achieved state-of-the-art performance in predicting both early and late readmissions by leveraging the temporal dynamics of patient data. Recent advancements in explainable AI have addressed the "black box" nature of complex machine learning models, a critical concern in healthcare applications. Techniques such as SHAP (SHapley Additive exPlanations) values and LIME (Local Interpretable Model-agnostic Explanations) have been applied to readmission prediction models, providing clinicians with interpretable insights into the factors driving readmission risk (Lundberg et al., 2020). This interpretability not only fosters trust in AI-driven predictions but also guides the development of tailored intervention strategies. The application of AI and NLP in readmission prediction extends beyond hospital settings. Researchers have explored the use of natural language generation (NLG) techniques to automatically create personalized discharge instructions and follow-up plans based on individual patient risk factors (Liu et al., 2021). These AI-generated instructions can be more comprehensive and tailored to each patient's specific needs, potentially improving adherence to post-discharge care plans and reducing readmission rates. Moreover, the integration of wearable device data and patient-reported outcomes with traditional clinical data has opened new avenues for continuous monitoring and early intervention. Machine learning models can now incorporate real-time data on patients' physical activity, vital signs, and self-reported symptoms to provide dynamic readmission risk assessments and trigger timely interventions (Quer et al., 2021). Despite these advancements, challenges remain in developing robust and generalizable readmission prediction models. Ensuring model fairness and addressing potential biases in training data are critical concerns, particularly given the disparities in healthcare access and outcomes among different populations. Ongoing research focuses on developing federated learning approaches that allow models to be trained across multiple institutions without sharing sensitive patient data, potentially leading to more robust and equitable prediction models (Rieke et al., 2020). As these technologies continue to evolve, they promise to transform post-discharge care, enabling more personalized and proactive approaches to preventing readmissions. The integration of AI and NLP in readmission prediction and post-discharge care planning has the potential to significantly improve patient outcomes, reduce healthcare costs, and optimize resource allocation in healthcare systems.

Population Health Management And Epidemic Forecasting

Population health management and epidemic forecasting have become increasingly critical in the face of global health challenges, with artificial intelligence (AI) and natural language processing (NLP) playing pivotal roles in revolutionizing these fields. These advanced technologies enable the analysis of vast and diverse datasets to identify population-level health trends, predict disease outbreaks, and inform targeted interventions. Machine learning models, particularly deep learning architectures, have demonstrated remarkable capabilities in processing and integrating data from multiple sources, including electronic health records (EHRs), social media, environmental sensors, and genomic databases. For instance, (Santillana et al., 2015, Ghosh & Sanyal 2024) developed a machine learning-based approach that leveraged Google search data, Twitter posts, and electronic health records to predict influenza outbreaks with higher accuracy than traditional surveillance methods. The integration of NLP techniques has been instrumental in extracting valuable health-related information from unstructured text data, such as social media posts, news articles, and scientific literature. Advanced NLP models like BERT and its domain-specific variants have shown superior performance in understanding the context and nuances of health-related discussions online (Müller et al., 2020). These models can identify early signals of disease outbreaks, track the spread of health misinformation, and gauge public sentiment towards health interventions. For example, (Shin et al., 2020) demonstrated the effectiveness of NLP in analyzing Twitter data to detect and track COVID-19 symptoms at a population level, providing real-time insights into the pandemic's progression. The application of AI in epidemic forecasting has seen significant advancements, with models now capable of predicting outbreak trajectories with increasing accuracy. Recurrent Neural Networks (RNNs) and Long Short-Term Memory (LSTM) networks have been particularly effective in capturing the temporal dynamics of disease spread. (Yang et al., 2020) developed an LSTM-based model that outperformed traditional statistical methods in forecasting COVID-19 cases across multiple countries, demonstrating the potential of AI in global epidemic management. Moreover, the integration of geographic information systems (GIS) with AI has enabled more sophisticated spatial-temporal modeling of disease spread. (Lai et al., 2019) utilized a deep learning approach combined with GIS data to predict the spatial distribution of dengue fever outbreaks, allowing for more targeted prevention efforts. In the realm of population health management, AI techniques have been employed to identify high-risk individuals and populations, enabling proactive interventions. (Nemati et al., 2018) developed an AI system that continuously analyzed ICU patient data to predict sepsis onset hours before clinical recognition, showcasing the potential of AI in early intervention and prevention. The application of federated learning techniques has addressed some of the privacy concerns associated with using sensitive health data for population-level analysis. This approach allows models to be trained across multiple institutions or regions without sharing raw data, enabling more comprehensive and privacy-preserving population health studies (Rieke et al., 2020). Natural language generation (NLG) techniques have also found application in communicating complex health information to diverse populations. AI-powered systems can generate personalized health recommendations and risk assessments based on individual and population-level data, potentially improving health literacy and engagement (Pauws et al., 2019). Despite these advancements, challenges remain in developing robust and equitable population health management and epidemic forecasting systems. Ensuring model fairness and addressing potential biases in training data are critical concerns, particularly given the disparities in healthcare access and outcomes among different populations. Ongoing research focuses on developing explainable AI models that can provide public health officials and policymakers with interpretable insights, fostering trust and facilitating evidence-based decision-making (Holzinger et al., 2019). As these technologies continue to evolve, they promise to transform public health practices, enabling more proactive, precise, and equitable approaches to population health management and epidemic control. The integration of AI and NLP in these fields has the potential to significantly improve global health outcomes, enhance epidemic preparedness, and optimize resource allocation in healthcare systems worldwide.

Emerging Trends

Integration of Wearable Device Data For Continuous Health Monitoring

The integration of wearable device data for continuous health monitoring represents a paradigm shift in healthcare, enabled by advances in artificial intelligence (AI), natural language processing (NLP), and Internet of Things (IoT) technologies. This emerging trend is transforming the landscape of personalized medicine, preventive care, and chronic disease management. Wearable devices, including smartwatches, fitness trackers, and medical-grade sensors, generate vast amounts of real-time physiological data, offering unprecedented insights into individuals' health status and behaviors. AI algorithms, particularly deep learning models, have demonstrated remarkable capabilities in processing and analyzing this high-dimensional, time-series data to extract meaningful health insights. For instance, (Ballinger et al., 2018) developed a deep neural network that could detect atrial fibrillation with high accuracy using only heart rate data from consumer smartwatches, showcasing the potential of AI in leveraging wearable data for early disease detection. The integration of NLP techniques has been crucial in contextualizing wearable device data with user-reported symptoms and experiences. Advanced NLP models can analyze text inputs from users, such as voice notes or app entries, to correlate subjective experiences with objective sensor data. (Quer et al., 2021) demonstrated the effectiveness of combining wearable sensor data with self-reported symptoms for early detection of COVID-19, using machine learning models to identify subtle changes in physiological parameters that preceded symptom onset. This fusion of objective and subjective data enables a more holistic approach to health monitoring. Continuous monitoring through wearables has opened new avenues for managing chronic conditions. (Tison et al., 2020,Ghosh 2024 a & b) utilized a deep learning approach to analyze continuous heart rate data from smartwatches, successfully identifying early signs of heart failure exacerbation and enabling timely interventions. Similarly, NLP techniques have been employed to process patient-reported outcomes and correlate them with wearable data, providing a more comprehensive view of disease progression and treatment efficacy (Kang et al., 2021). The application of federated learning techniques has addressed some of the privacy concerns associated with collecting and analyzing sensitive health data from wearables. This approach allows models to be trained across multiple devices or institutions without sharing raw data, enabling more robust and privacy-preserving health monitoring systems (Rieke et al., 2020). Advances in edge computing and on-device AI have further enhanced the capabilities of wearable health monitoring. (Ravì et al., 2019) developed a deep learning model that could run directly on wearable devices to detect abnormal heart rhythms in real-time, demonstrating the potential for immediate, on-device health alerts without the need for constant cloud connectivity. The integration of wearable data with electronic health records (EHRs) presents both opportunities and challenges. NLP techniques play a crucial role in harmonizing the unstructured data from wearables with clinical notes and structured EHR data. Researchers have explored the use of transformer-based models to create unified patient representations that incorporate both clinical and wearable data, enabling more comprehensive health risk assessments (Johnson et al., 2021). Despite these advancements, challenges remain in developing robust and clinically valid health monitoring systems based on wearable data. Ensuring data quality, addressing potential biases in algorithm development, and establishing clinical validation protocols for AI-driven insights are critical areas of ongoing research. Moreover, the interpretability of complex AI models remains a key concern for clinical adoption. Explainable AI techniques, such as attention mechanisms and layer-wise relevance propagation, are being explored to provide clinicians with interpretable insights from wearable data analysis (Holzinger et al., 2019). As these technologies continue to evolve, they promise to revolutionize healthcare delivery, enabling more proactive, personalized, and continuous health management. The integration of wearable device data, powered by AI and NLP, has the potential to shift healthcare from episodic interventions to continuous care, improving patient outcomes, reducing healthcare costs, and empowering individuals to take a more active role in their health management.

Use of Federated Learning Techniques To Leverage Data Across Multiple Healthcare Institutions While Preserving Privacy

Federated learning has emerged as a promising approach to leverage data across multiple healthcare institutions while preserving patient privacy and data confidentiality. This technique enables collaborative model training without the need to centralize sensitive medical data, addressing key concerns in healthcare data sharing. In federated learning, each participating institution trains a local model on its own data, and only model updates or parameters are shared with a central server, rather than raw patient data. This approach allows healthcare organizations to benefit from larger, more diverse datasets while complying with data protection regulations like HIPAA. Federated learning has shown potential in various healthcare applications, including medical imaging analysis, predictive modeling for disease outcomes, and drug discovery. For instance, (Sheller et al., 2018) demonstrated the effectiveness of federated learning in training a brain tumor segmentation model across multiple institutions without sharing patient MRI scans. Similarly, (Brisimi et al., 2018) applied federated learning to predict hospitalizations for heart-related conditions using electronic health records from different hospitals. The technique has also been explored for COVID-19 research, with (Dayan et al., 2021) using federated learning to develop a global model for diagnosing COVID-19 from chest X-rays across multiple countries. Despite its promise, federated learning in healthcare faces challenges such as dealing with heterogeneous data distributions across institutions, ensuring model convergence, and mitigating potential privacy risks from model inversion attacks. Ongoing research focuses on developing more robust and efficient federated learning algorithms, improving privacy-preserving techniques like differential privacy, and addressing the unique challenges of healthcare data such as class imbalance and missing values. As the field continues to evolve, federated learning has the potential to revolutionize collaborative research in healthcare, enabling the development of more accurate and generalizable models while maintaining the highest standards of patient data protection.

3.4 AI-Assisted Robotic Surgery

AI is enhancing the capabilities of robotic surgical systems, leading to:

Improved Precision And Dexterity In Minimally Invasive Procedures

Advancements in minimally invasive procedures have revolutionized modern surgery, offering significant benefits such as reduced patient trauma, faster recovery times, and improved cosmetic outcomes. A key factor driving these improvements is the continuous enhancement of precision and dexterity in surgical techniques and technologies. This progress has been particularly notable in robotic-assisted surgery, where systems like the da Vinci platform have enabled surgeons to perform complex procedures with unprecedented accuracy and control. These robotic systems provide enhanced 3D visualization, tremor filtration, and motion scaling, allowing for more precise movements in confined spaces. For instance, Intuitive Surgical's da Vinci system has demonstrated improved outcomes in various procedures, including prostatectomies and gynecological surgeries (Hung et al., 2018). Beyond robotics, other technological innovations have contributed to increased precision in minimally invasive surgeries. Advanced imaging techniques, such as intraoperative MRI and fluorescence-guided surgery, provide real-time visualization of anatomical structures and tumor margins, enabling more accurate resections. The development of smarter surgical instruments, including articulating laparoscopic tools and energy devices with improved tissue discrimination, has further enhanced surgeons' capabilities. Additionally, the integration of artificial intelligence and machine learning algorithms into surgical planning and navigation systems has shown promise in optimizing procedure workflows and decision-making. For example,(Maier-Hein et al., 2017) demonstrated the potential of AI-assisted navigation in laparoscopic liver surgery, improving the accuracy of target structure localization. The field of microsurgery has also benefited from technological advancements, with the introduction of supermicrosurgery techniques allowing for the manipulation of structures less than 0.8 mm in diameter. This level of precision has opened up new possibilities in lymphedema treatment, digit replantation, and complex reconstructive procedures (Koshima et al., 2017, Ghosh et al.,2024 a & b). Another area of significant progress is in the realm of endovascular procedures, where improvements in catheter design, guidewire technology, and imaging modalities have enabled more precise navigation through complex vascular anatomies. This has led to the expansion of minimally invasive approaches in the treatment of cerebral aneurysms, aortic diseases, and peripheral vascular disorders (Riga et al., 2012). As these technologies continue to evolve, ongoing challenges include the need for improved haptic feedback in robotic systems, further miniaturization of surgical instruments, and the development of more intuitive user interfaces. Additionally, the integration of augmented reality and virtual reality technologies into surgical planning and execution holds promise for further enhancing precision and dexterity. The continuous improvement in the precision and dexterity of minimally invasive procedures not only benefits patients through better outcomes and reduced complications but also expands the range of conditions that can be treated using these approaches. As research progresses and technologies advance, the future of minimally invasive surgery looks promising, with the potential to push the boundaries of what is possible in modern medicine.

Real-Time Guidance And Decision Support During Surgery

Real-time guidance and decision support systems have emerged as transformative technologies in modern surgery, enhancing surgeons' capabilities and improving patient outcomes. These systems leverage advanced imaging, artificial intelligence, and data analytics to provide critical information and recommendations during surgical procedures. One of the key advancements in this field is the development of augmented reality (AR) surgical navigation systems. These systems overlay preoperative imaging data, such as CT or MRI scans, onto the surgeon's view of the operative field in real-time. For example, (Meola et al., 2017) demonstrated the efficacy of AR-guided neurosurgery, allowing for more precise tumor resections and reduced operative times. Similarly, intraoperative imaging modalities, such as fluorescence-guided surgery, have significantly improved the accuracy of tumor margin identification in various oncological procedures. The integration of artificial intelligence into surgical decision support systems has further enhanced real-time guidance capabilities. Machine learning algorithms can analyze vast amounts of data from previous surgeries, patient records, and real-time sensor inputs to provide personalized recommendations during critical moments of a procedure. For instance, (Hashimoto et al., 2020) developed an AI system that can predict intraoperative events and complications in laparoscopic cholecystectomy, allowing surgeons to take preventive measures. Another significant advancement is the development of smart surgical instruments equipped with sensors and real-time feedback mechanisms. These instruments can provide surgeons with immediate information on tissue properties, applied forces, and potential risks. For example, (Tiwana et al., 2012) described smart forceps that can detect abnormal tissue stiffness, potentially improving tumor detection and reducing complications in neurosurgery. In the field of robotic-assisted surgery, real-time guidance systems have become increasingly sophisticated. Advanced control algorithms and machine vision techniques enable robotic systems to assist surgeons in complex tasks, such as suturing and tissue manipulation, with greater precision and efficiency. These systems can also provide warnings and suggestions based on the analysis of the surgical field and the robot's movements, enhancing safety and reducing the risk of errors. The integration of natural language processing and voice-controlled interfaces has further improved the accessibility of real-time guidance systems during surgery. Surgeons can now query databases, access patient information, and control imaging systems without breaking sterility or interrupting the procedure. This seamless access to information enhances decision-making capabilities and workflow efficiency in the operating room. Real-time physiological monitoring systems have also evolved to provide more comprehensive and actionable information during surgery. Advanced analytics can predict potential complications based on trends in vital signs, allowing for proactive interventions. For instance, (Hatib et al., 2018) developed a machine learning algorithm that can predict hypotension events during surgery, enabling timely preventive measures. As these technologies continue to advance, challenges remain in integrating diverse data sources, ensuring the reliability and interpretability of AI-driven recommendations, and balancing the cognitive load on surgeons. Ongoing research focuses on developing more intuitive user interfaces, improving the accuracy of predictive models, and addressing potential ethical and legal implications of AI-assisted decision-making in surgery. The future of real-time guidance and decision support in surgery holds immense potential, with the promise of further reducing complications, improving outcomes, and personalizing surgical approaches based on individual patient characteristics and real-time data.

Automated Surgical Planning Based On Patient-Specific Anatomical Models

Automated surgical planning based on patient-specific anatomical models has emerged as a groundbreaking approach in modern medicine, revolutionizing preoperative preparation and enhancing surgical outcomes. This technology leverages advanced imaging techniques, computer-aided design (CAD), and artificial intelligence to create highly detailed, three-dimensional models of a patient's anatomy, allowing for precise surgical planning tailored to each individual's unique physiological characteristics. The process typically begins with high-resolution medical imaging, such as CT or MRI scans, which are then processed using sophisticated segmentation algorithms to isolate and define specific anatomical structures. These digital representations serve as the foundation for creating accurate 3D models that surgeons can manipulate and analyze in virtual environments. One of the key advantages of this approach is the ability to simulate various surgical scenarios and optimize procedural strategies before entering the operating room. For instance,(Zhao et al., 2020) demonstrated the efficacy of automated planning in complex liver surgeries, where patient-specific models were used to determine optimal resection planes and predict postoperative liver function, significantly reducing complications and improving outcomes. In orthopedic surgery, automated planning has been particularly impactful in procedures such as total hip and knee replacements. Patient-specific models enable surgeons to precisely plan implant sizing, positioning, and alignment, leading to improved functional outcomes and reduced revision rates. (Hafez et al., 2016) reported that the use of automated planning and patient-specific instrumentation in total knee arthroplasty resulted in more accurate component positioning and improved postoperative alignment compared to conventional techniques. The integration of artificial intelligence and machine learning algorithms has further enhanced the capabilities of automated surgical planning. These technologies can analyze vast databases of previous surgeries, patient outcomes, and anatomical variations to provide data-driven recommendations for surgical approaches. For example, (Linte et al., 2019) developed an AI-driven system for planning minimally invasive cardiac procedures, which could automatically identify optimal access routes and predict potential complications based on patient-specific anatomy and historical data. In the field of neurosurgery, automated planning has proven invaluable for complex procedures such as tumor resections and epilepsy surgeries. Patient-specific models allow for precise localization of critical structures and eloquent brain areas, enabling surgeons to plan safer trajectories and maximize tumor removal while minimizing the risk of neurological deficits. (Bayer et al., 2017) demonstrated that automated planning in epilepsy surgery led to more accurate electrode placement and improved seizure outcomes. The advent of 3D printing technology has further expanded the applications of patient-specific models in surgical planning. Physical models created from digital data provide tangible representations that surgeons can use for preoperative rehearsal and intraoperative guidance. This is particularly beneficial in complex craniofacial reconstructions and pediatric cardiac surgeries, where the ability to physically manipulate a model of the patient's anatomy can lead to more informed decision-making and improved surgical precision. Despite its numerous advantages, automated surgical planning faces challenges such as the need for standardization in imaging protocols, the integration of diverse data sources, and the validation of AI-driven recommendations. Additionally, the time and computational resources required for creating high-fidelity patient-specific models can be substantial, potentially limiting widespread adoption in time-sensitive cases. Ongoing research aims to address these limitations by developing faster and more efficient algorithms, improving the interoperability of different software platforms, and creating more user-friendly interfaces for surgeons. As the field continues to evolve, the integration of automated planning with intraoperative navigation systems and robotic-assisted surgery platforms promises to create a seamless continuum from preoperative planning to surgical execution, further enhancing precision and patient outcomes.

Recent advancements

Development of Autonomous Surgical Subtasks

The development of autonomous surgical subtasks represents a significant advancement in the field of robotic-assisted surgery, aiming to enhance precision, reduce surgeon fatigue, and improve overall surgical outcomes. This emerging technology leverages artificial intelligence, computer vision, and advanced robotics to automate specific elements of surgical procedures, allowing surgeons to focus on more complex aspects of the operation.

One of the key areas of progress in autonomous surgical subtasks is suturing. Automated suturing systems have been developed to perform this repetitive and time-consuming task with high precision. For instance, (Shademan et al., 2016) demonstrated an autonomous system capable of performing intestinal anastomosis in ex vivo porcine tissue, outperforming human surgeons in terms of consistency and quality of suturing. This technology has the potential to significantly reduce operative times and improve the uniformity of wound closure.

Another promising area is autonomous tissue manipulation and retraction. These systems use advanced sensors and control algorithms to maintain optimal tissue exposure during procedures, adapting to changes in the surgical field in real-time. (Attanasio et al., 2020) developed a robotic system that can autonomously manipulate soft tissue during minimally invasive surgery, using visual servoing techniques to maintain a clear operative field.Autonomous navigation and positioning of surgical instruments represent another crucial advancement. These systems can guide instruments to precise locations within the body, based on preoperative imaging and intraoperative sensor data. For example, (Berthet-Rayne et al., 2018) presented an autonomous robotic system for needle steering in percutaneous interventions, demonstrating improved accuracy in reaching target locations compared to manual insertion.

The field of microsurgery has also benefited from autonomous subtasks, particularly in procedures requiring extreme precision. Researchers have developed systems capable of autonomously performing microvascular anastomoses, a challenging task even for experienced surgeons. (Leonard et al., 2014) demonstrated a robotic system that could perform autonomous microvascular anastomosis in rat femoral vessels, showcasing the potential for improving success rates in complex microsurgical procedures. Autonomous tissue identification and classification systems have made significant strides, utilizing machine learning algorithms to differentiate between healthy and pathological tissues in real-time. These systems can assist surgeons in tumor resections by providing instant feedback on tissue characteristics. (Holmer et al., 2018) developed an AI-based system for autonomous tissue classification during thyroid surgery, demonstrating high accuracy in distinguishing thyroid tissue from surrounding structures.Despite these advancements, the integration of autonomous surgical subtasks into clinical practice faces several challenges. Safety and reliability are paramount concerns, requiring extensive validation and fail-safe mechanisms before widespread adoption. Additionally, regulatory frameworks need to evolve to accommodate these new technologies, addressing issues of liability and quality assurance.The human-machine interface also remains a critical area of development. Systems must be designed to seamlessly integrate with the surgeon's workflow, providing intuitive control and clear feedback. Ongoing research focuses on developing more natural interfaces, including gesture recognition and voice control, to enhance the synergy between human surgeons and autonomous systems.As the field progresses, the goal is not to replace surgeons but to augment their capabilities, allowing them to focus on the most critical and complex aspects of procedures. The future of autonomous surgical subtasks lies in creating a harmonious blend of human expertise and machine precision, potentially revolutionizing surgical care and improving patient outcomes across a wide range of procedures.

Integration of Augmented Reality For Enhanced Visualization During Procedures

The integration of augmented reality (AR) for enhanced visualization during surgical procedures represents a significant leap forward in medical technology, offering surgeons unprecedented real-time visual information and guidance. This innovative approach overlays computer-generated images onto the surgeon's view of the real world, effectively merging digital data with the physical operative field. The result is a powerful tool that enhances spatial awareness, improves decision-making, and potentially leads to better patient outcomes. One of the primary applications of AR in surgery is the superimposition of preoperative imaging data, such as CT or MRI scans, directly onto the patient's body during the procedure. (Meola et al., 2017) demonstrated the efficacy of this approach in neurosurgery, where AR guidance allowed for more precise tumor resections and reduced operative times. The system enabled surgeons to visualize critical structures beneath the surface, effectively providing "X-ray vision" and helping to avoid damage to eloquent brain areas.

In minimally invasive procedures, AR has proven particularly valuable by addressing the inherent limitations of traditional laparoscopic views. By overlaying 3D reconstructions of internal organs and vascular structures onto the laparoscopic feed, surgeons can gain a more comprehensive understanding of the surgical anatomy. (Bernhardt et al., 2017) reported on the use of AR in laparoscopic liver surgery, showing improved identification of tumor margins and critical vascular structures, potentially reducing the risk of complications.Orthopedic surgery has also benefited significantly from AR integration. In procedures such as total hip and knee replacements, AR systems can project optimal implant positions and alignments directly onto the surgical field. This technology aids in achieving more accurate component positioning, which is crucial for the longevity and functionality of the implant. (Jud et al., 2020) demonstrated that AR-assisted total knee arthroplasty resulted in improved implant positioning accuracy compared to conventional techniques.

The field of interventional radiology has embraced AR to enhance the precision of needle-based procedures. By projecting the planned needle trajectory and target location onto the patient's body, AR systems can guide interventional radiologists in performing biopsies, ablations, and other minimally invasive procedures with greater accuracy. (Najafi et al., 2019) showed that AR guidance in CT-guided interventions led to reduced procedure times and radiation exposure. Beyond anatomical visualization, AR systems are being developed to display real-time physiological data within the surgeon's field of view.

This could include vital signs, tissue oxygenation levels, or even intraoperative imaging results, allowing surgeons to make more informed decisions without shifting their attention away from the surgical site. (Qian et al., 2018) described an AR system that integrates multiple data streams, including vital signs and surgical navigation information, into a heads-up display for cardiac surgery.

Despite its tremendous potential, the integration of AR in surgical procedures faces several challenges. One significant hurdle is the need for precise registration between the virtual overlays and the real-world anatomy, which can be affected by tissue deformation and patient movement. Ongoing research focuses on developing more robust tracking algorithms and real-time adjustment mechanisms to maintain accurate alignment throughout the procedure. Another challenge lies in designing user interfaces that provide valuable information without overwhelming or distracting the surgeon. The cognitive load associated with processing additional visual data must be carefully balanced against the benefits of enhanced visualization. Researchers are exploring various approaches, including context-aware systems that selectively display information based on the current stage of the procedure and the surgeon's preferences.

As AR technology continues to evolve, its integration with other advanced surgical technologies, such as robotics and artificial intelligence, holds promise for creating even more powerful surgical assistance systems. The combination of AR visualization with haptic feedback and AI-driven decision support could potentially revolutionize surgical training and performance, leading to improved patient outcomes across a wide range of procedures.

3.5 Drug Discovery and Development

AI is Accelerating The Drug Discovery Process Through:

Prediction of Drug-Target Interactions

The application of artificial intelligence (AI) in predicting drug-target interactions has emerged as a transformative approach in drug discovery and development, offering the potential to significantly accelerate the identification of novel therapeutic candidates and repurpose existing drugs. This field leverages machine learning algorithms, deep learning architectures, and vast biological datasets to model complex relationships between chemical compounds and their biological targets, enabling researchers to prioritize promising drug candidates and streamline the drug development process.One of the key advancements in this area is the development of deep learning models that can effectively capture the structural and chemical properties of both drugs and target proteins. For instance, (Öztürk et al., 2018) introduced DeepDTA, a deep learning-based model that uses convolutional neural networks to predict drug-target binding affinities. This approach demonstrated superior performance compared to traditional machine learning methods, particularly in scenarios with limited experimental data.Graph neural networks (GNNs) have also shown remarkable potential in modeling drug-target interactions. These models can effectively represent the molecular structure of drugs and proteins as graphs, capturing important topological information. (Lim et al., 2019) developed a GNN-based approach that could predict drug-target interactions across multiple species, showcasing the model's ability to generalize across diverse biological contexts.

The integration of multi-modal data sources has further enhanced the predictive power of AI models in drug-target interaction prediction. By combining information from genomics, proteomics, and chemical databases, researchers have developed more comprehensive and accurate prediction models. For example, (Wan et al., 2019) presented a deep learning framework that integrated drug chemical structures, protein sequences, and known drug-target interaction networks to predict novel interactions, achieving state-of-the-art performance on multiple benchmark datasets.

Transfer learning techniques have also been applied to address the challenge of limited labeled data in drug discovery. These approaches allow models trained on large, general datasets to be fine-tuned for specific prediction tasks with smaller, specialized datasets. (Huang et al., 2020) demonstrated the effectiveness of transfer learning in predicting drug-target interactions for rare diseases, where experimental data is often scarce.

The application of AI in drug-target interaction prediction has led to several notable successes in drug repurposing efforts. For instance, (Beck et al., 2020) used a deep learning-based approach to identify potential drug candidates for COVID-19 treatment, leading to the identification of atazanavir as a promising repurposing candidate, which was subsequently validated in experimental studies.Despite these advancements, challenges remain in the field of AI-driven drug-target interaction prediction. One significant hurdle is the interpretability of complex deep learning models, which often function as "black boxes." Researchers are actively working on developing more transparent AI approaches that can provide insights into the underlying mechanisms of predicted interactions. For example, (Rodríguez-Pérez and Bajorath, 2020) proposed an interpretable machine learning framework that not only predicts drug-target interactions but also identifies key molecular features contributing to these interactions. Another challenge lies in addressing the inherent biases in existing datasets, which can lead to skewed predictions and limit the discovery of truly novel interactions. Ongoing efforts focus on developing more diverse and representative datasets, as well as designing AI models that can account for and mitigate these biases.As the field progresses, the integration of AI-driven drug-target interaction prediction with other emerging technologies, such as high-throughput screening and CRISPR-based target validation, promises to create more comprehensive and efficient drug discovery pipelines. The combination of in silico predictions with rapid experimental validation could significantly reduce the time and cost associated with bringing new drugs to market, potentially revolutionizing the pharmaceutical industry and accelerating the development of treatments for a wide range of diseases.

Design of Novel Drug Candidates

The application of artificial intelligence (AI) in the design of novel drug candidates has revolutionized the pharmaceutical industry, offering unprecedented capabilities to explore vast chemical spaces and accelerate the drug discovery process. This innovative approach combines machine learning, deep learning, and generative models with computational chemistry and bioinformatics to create and optimize potential drug molecules with desired properties.One of the most significant advancements in AI-driven drug design is the development of generative models capable of creating entirely new molecular structures. Generative adversarial networks (GANs) and variational autoencoders (VAEs) have been particularly successful in this domain. For instance, (Zhavoronkov et al., 2019) demonstrated the power of deep generative models in designing novel inhibitors for discoidin domain receptor 1 (DDR1) kinase, a promising target for fibrosis and other diseases. Their AI system, utilizing a combination of generative tensorial reinforcement learning and predictive models, was able to design, synthesize, and experimentally validate new DDR1 inhibitors in just 21 days, a process that traditionally takes years. Another key area of progress is the use of AI to optimize existing lead compounds for improved efficacy and reduced side effects. Reinforcement learning techniques have been applied to guide the iterative modification of molecular structures towards desired properties.(Jin et al., 2020) developed a reinforcement learning framework that could optimize molecules for multiple objectives simultaneously, such as potency, selectivity, and synthesizability, demonstrating its effectiveness in designing novel checkpoint inhibitors for cancer immunotherapy.

The integration of AI with physics-based simulations has further enhanced the ability to predict drug-target interactions and design molecules with specific binding properties. (Staker et al., 2020) presented a deep learning approach that combined molecular docking simulations with generative models to design novel ligands for G-protein-coupled receptors (GPCRs), a major class of drug targets. This hybrid approach allowed for the generation of molecules with improved predicted binding affinities while maintaining drug-like properties.

AI has also been instrumental in addressing the challenge of de novo drug design for difficult targets, such as protein-protein interactions (PPIs). Traditional small molecule approaches often struggle with these targets due to their large, flat interaction surfaces. However, AI-driven methods have shown promise in designing novel PPI inhibitors. For example, (Gorgulla et al., 2020) used a combination of physics-based modeling and machine learning to design small molecule inhibitors of the PD-1/PD-L1 interaction, a key target in cancer immunotherapy.

The application of AI in designing multi-target drugs has gained traction, recognizing the complex nature of many diseases. Polypharmacology, where a single drug interacts with multiple targets, can potentially lead to more effective treatments with fewer side effects. (Merk et al., 2018) developed a deep learning model that could generate molecules with desired multi-target profiles, demonstrating its potential in designing drugs for complex disorders like neurodegenerative diseases.

Despite these impressive advancements, challenges remain in the field of AI-driven drug design. One significant hurdle is the synthesizability of AI-generated molecules. While AI can create novel structures, not all of these are readily synthesizable using current chemical methods. Efforts are underway to incorporate synthetic accessibility scores and retrosynthesis prediction into generative models to address this issue. (Gao and Coley, 2020) proposed a graph-based generative model that explicitly considers synthetic accessibility during the molecule generation process.

Another challenge lies in the interpretability of AI models used in drug design. As these models become more complex, understanding the rationale behind their decisions becomes increasingly difficult. This lack of interpretability can be a significant barrier in regulatory approval processes. Ongoing research focuses on developing more transparent AI approaches that can provide insights into the design process and the predicted properties of generated molecules.As the field progresses, the integration of AI-driven drug design with other cutting-edge technologies, such as high-throughput screening and rapid synthesis platforms, promises to create more efficient and comprehensive drug discovery pipelines. The combination of *in silico* design with automated synthesis and testing could significantly reduce the time and cost associated with bringing new drugs to market, potentially revolutionizing the pharmaceutical industry and accelerating the development of treatments for a wide range of diseases.

Optimization of Clinical Trial Design And Patient Selection

Optimization of clinical trial design and patient selection is crucial for improving the efficiency, cost-effectiveness, and success rates of drug development. Key strategies include adaptive trial designs, which allow modifications based on interim data analysis, potentially reducing sample sizes and trial duration (Pallmann et al., 2018, Das et al.,2024). Biomarker-guided patient selection can enhance treatment effects by identifying subgroups most likely to respond, as demonstrated in oncology trials using molecular profiling (Renfro & Sargent, 2017). Innovative recruitment methods, such as using electronic health records and social media, can accelerate enrollment and improve participant diversity (Köpcke& Prokosch, 2014). Master protocols, including basket, umbrella, and platform trials, enable the evaluation of multiple treatments or patient subgroups simultaneously, increasing efficiency and flexibility (Woodcock &LaVange, 2017). Bayesian statistical approaches offer advantages in decision-making and sample size optimization, particularly in rare disease trials with limited patient populations (Berry, 2015). Patient-centric trial designs, incorporating patient-reported outcomes and preferences, can improve retention and the relevance of study endpoints (Kost et al., 2015). Synthetic control arms, leveraging historical data or real-world evidence, may reduce the need for placebo groups in certain contexts, potentially accelerating trial timelines (Thorlund et al., 2020). The use of wearable devices and digital health technologies enables continuous, remote monitoring of patients, providing richer data sets and potentially reducing site visits (Perry et al., 2018). Artificial intelligence and machine learning algorithms can optimize protocol design, predict enrollment rates, and identify potential safety signals earlier in the development process (Harrer et al., 2019). Importantly, early engagement with regulatory agencies and incorporation of their feedback can help ensure that innovative trial designs meet regulatory requirements and generate sufficient evidence for approval (Proponents of this approach argue that it can lead to more efficient drug development and better patient outcomes, while critics caution that careful validation and standardization are necessary to maintain scientific rigor and regulatory acceptance (Elsäßer et al., 2014). As the field evolves, continued collaboration among stakeholders, including researchers, clinicians, patients, regulators, and industry partners, will be essential to refine and implement these optimization strategies effectively, ultimately accelerating the delivery of safe and effective therapies to patients in need.

Emerging trends

Use of Generative Models To Create New Molecular Structures

The use of generative models to create new molecular structures represents a paradigm shift in drug discovery and materials science, leveraging artificial intelligence to explore vast chemical spaces efficiently. Deep learning architectures, particularly generative adversarial networks (GANs) and variational autoencoders (VAEs), have shown remarkable success in generating novel, yet chemically valid and potentially bioactive molecules (Elton et al., 2019). These models learn the underlying distribution of known chemical structures and can generate new ones with desired properties, significantly accelerating the hit discovery process. Reinforcement learning approaches have been integrated with these generative models to optimize for specific molecular properties, such as drug-likeness, synthetic accessibility, and target affinity (Olivecrona et al., 2017). Graph-based models, which explicitly represent molecules as graphs, have proven particularly effective in capturing structural information and generating chemically feasible compounds (Li et al., 2018). The application of transformer architectures, originally developed for natural language processing, to molecular generation tasks has yielded impressive results in terms of chemical diversity and validity of generated structures (Grisoni et al., 2020). Conditional generative models allow for the targeted generation of molecules with specific properties or structural features, enabling focused library design for medicinal chemistry campaigns (Jin et al., 2018). Multi-objective optimization techniques have been developed to balance multiple, often competing, molecular properties simultaneously, better mimicking the complex decision-making process in drug design (Zhou et al., 2019). The integration of these generative models with high-throughput virtual screening and molecular docking tools has created powerful workflows for in silico drug discovery (Zhavoronkov et al., 2019). Moreover, generative models have been applied beyond small molecules to design peptides, proteins, and other macromolecules, expanding the toolkit for biological therapeutics (Anand & Huang, 2018). Recent advancements include the development of models that incorporate synthetic accessibility and retrosynthetic analysis, ensuring that generated molecules are not only theoretically interesting but also practically synthesizable (Bradshaw et al., 2019). The use of transfer learning techniques has enabled the application of generative models trained on large chemical databases to specific medicinal chemistry problems with limited data, enhancing their utility in real-world drug discovery projects (Gao & Coley, 2020). Despite these advances, challenges remain in ensuring the reliability, interpretability, and experimental validation of AI-generated molecules. Concerns about the potential for these models to generate toxic or controlled substances have led to discussions about ethical guidelines and regulatory frameworks for their use (Urbina et al., 2021). As the field progresses, the integration of generative models with experimental validation pipelines, including rapid synthesis and testing methodologies, will be crucial to realizing their full potential in accelerating drug discovery and materials development. The ongoing refinement of these models, coupled with increasing computational power and expanding chemical databases, promises to revolutionize the way we explore chemical space and discover new therapeutic agents and functional materials.

Integration of Multi-Omics Data For More Comprehensive Drug Response Prediction

The integration of multi-omics data for more comprehensive drug response prediction represents a significant advancement in personalized medicine and pharmacogenomics, offering a holistic approach to understanding the complex biological mechanisms underlying drug efficacy and toxicity. This approach combines diverse molecular data types, including genomics, transcriptomics, proteomics, metabolomics, and epigenomics, to create a more complete picture of cellular processes and their interactions with pharmaceutical compounds (Hasin et al., 2017). Machine learning and artificial intelligence techniques have been pivotal in handling the high-dimensional, heterogeneous nature of multi-omics datasets, enabling the discovery of intricate patterns and relationships that are not apparent when analyzing single omics layers in isolation (Chaudhary et al., 2018, Shakil et al.,2024). Network-based methods have proven particularly effective in integrating multi-omics data, capturing the complex interactions between different molecular entities and providing insights into the systemic effects of drugs (Yan et al., 2018). Deep learning architectures, such as multi-modal deep neural networks and autoencoders, have demonstrated superior performance in integrating diverse data types and predicting drug responses across various cancer types and other diseases (Sharifi-Noghabi et al., 2019). The incorporation of single-cell multi-omics data has further refined drug response predictions, accounting for intratumoral heterogeneity and enabling more precise targeting of specific cell populations (Pratapa et al., 2021). Pathway-based approaches to multi-omics integration have provided mechanistic insights into drug action and resistance, facilitating the identification of novel drug targets and combination therapies (Huang et al., 2019). The integration of pharmacological data with patient-derived multi-omics profiles has enhanced the ability to predict individual drug responses, supporting the development of personalized treatment regimens in oncology and other therapeutic areas (Paré et al., 2018). Moreover, the inclusion of microbiome data in multi-omics integration has shed light on the role of host-microbiome interactions in drug metabolism and efficacy, opening new avenues for improving drug response predictions (Wilmanski et al., 2019). Time-series multi-omics data have enabled the study of dynamic drug responses, providing insights into the temporal aspects of drug action and resistance development (Banaei-Esfahani et al., 2020). The integration of imaging data with molecular multi-omics has further enhanced drug response predictions by incorporating spatial information and tissue-specific effects (Perlasca et al., 2019). Despite these advancements, challenges remain in harmonizing diverse data types, managing batch effects, and developing robust statistical methods for high-dimensional data integration (Rappoport & Shamir, 2018). Efforts to standardize multi-omics data collection and analysis protocols are ongoing, aiming to improve reproducibility and facilitate cross-study comparisons (Suhl et al., 2019). As the field progresses, the integration of multi-omics data with electronic health records and real-world evidence is expected to bridge the gap between molecular-level predictions and clinical outcomes, further refining drug response models (Karczewski & Snyder, 2018). The ethical implications of using comprehensive molecular profiles for drug response prediction, including issues of data privacy and potential discrimination, are also being actively discussed (Townend, 2018). Looking forward, the continued development of advanced computational methods, including quantum computing approaches, promises to further enhance our ability to integrate and interpret complex multi-omics datasets, ultimately leading to more accurate and personalized drug response predictions that could significantly improve patient outcomes and revolutionize drug development processes.

While AI Shows Great Promise In Medicine, Several Challenges And Ethical Considerations Must Be Addressed:

While artificial intelligence (AI) shows great promise in medicine, several challenges and ethical considerations must be addressed to ensure its responsible and effective implementation. Data privacy and security concerns are paramount, as AI systems require vast amounts of sensitive patient data for training and operation. The risk of data breaches, unauthorized access, and potential misuse of personal health information pose significant threats to patient confidentiality and trust in healthcare systems (Cohen et al., 2018). Robust data protection measures, including encryption, anonymization, and secure data storage protocols, are essential to mitigate these risks. Additionally, the development of privacy-preserving AI techniques, such as federated learning and differential privacy, offers promising solutions for maintaining data confidentiality while enabling collaborative AI model development across multiple institutions (Rieke et al., 2020). Algorithmic bias and fairness in AI models represent another critical challenge, as biased datasets or algorithms can perpetuate or exacerbate existing health disparities. AI models trained on non-representative data may perform poorly for underrepresented populations, potentially leading to misdiagnoses or inappropriate treatment recommendations (Gianfrancesco et al., 2018). Efforts to address this issue include developing diverse and inclusive datasets, implementing fairness-aware machine learning algorithms, and conducting rigorous bias audits of AI systems before deployment (Rajkomar et al., 2018). Regulatory challenges in approving AI-based medical devices pose significant hurdles to the widespread adoption of AI in healthcare. The rapid pace of AI development often outstrips the ability of regulatory bodies to establish appropriate guidelines and approval processes. The FDA's efforts to create a regulatory framework for AI/ML-based Software as a Medical Device (SaMD) represent a step towards addressing this challenge, but ongoing collaboration between regulators, industry stakeholders, and healthcare providers is necessary to ensure that AI technologies are safe, effective, and continuously monitored post-market (Gerke et al., 2020). The integration of AI systems with existing healthcare workflows presents both technical and cultural challenges. Healthcare organizations must invest in infrastructure upgrades, data interoperability solutions, and staff training to effectively incorporate AI tools into clinical practice. Resistance to change among healthcare professionals and concerns about AI replacing human judgment must be addressed through education, clear communication of AI's role as a supportive tool, and the development of human-AI collaboration frameworks (Topol, 2019). Liability and responsibility in AI-assisted medical decisions raise complex legal and ethical questions. As AI systems become more involved in diagnosis and treatment recommendations, determining accountability in cases of medical errors or adverse outcomes becomes increasingly complicated. Clear guidelines for the appropriate use of AI in clinical decision-making, ongoing monitoring of AI system performance, and the development of legal frameworks that address the unique challenges posed by AI in healthcare are necessary to navigate this evolving landscape (Price et al., 2019). Ensuring transparency and explainability of AI models in healthcare is crucial for building trust among patients, healthcare providers, and regulatory bodies. The "black box" nature of many advanced AI algorithms, particularly deep learning models, can make it difficult to understand how decisions are made, potentially leading to skepticism and reluctance to adopt AI technologies. Developing interpretable AI models, implementing techniques for post-hoc explanations of AI decisions, and establishing standards for AI transparency in healthcare are essential steps in addressing this challenge (Holzinger et al., 2019). The potential for AI to exacerbate health inequities must also be carefully considered and mitigated. AI systems that rely on data from predominantly affluent or urban populations may not generalize well to underserved communities, potentially widening existing health disparities. Efforts to collect diverse, representative data and to develop AI models that explicitly account for social determinants of health are crucial for ensuring equitable access to the benefits of AI in medicine (Obermeyer et al., 2019). The ethical implications of AI in healthcare extend beyond technical considerations to fundamental questions about the nature of the patient-provider relationship and the role of human judgment in medicine. As AI systems become more sophisticated, there is a risk of over-reliance on automated recommendations, potentially eroding the human elements of care and empathy that are central to the practice of medicine. Developing frameworks for the ethical use of AI that prioritize human values, patient autonomy, and shared decision-making is essential for maintaining the integrity of healthcare practice (Char et al., 2018). The rapid pace of AI development in healthcare also raises concerns about the potential for premature adoption of unproven technologies. The pressure to implement cutting-edge AI solutions must be balanced against the need for rigorous validation and evidence of clinical benefit. Establishing standards for the evaluation of AI technologies in healthcare, including requirements for prospective clinical trials and real-world performance monitoring, is crucial for ensuring that AI truly improves patient outcomes (Liu et al., 2019). The global nature of AI development in healthcare presents challenges related to data sharing, cross-border collaborations, and the harmonization of regulatory approaches. Differences in data protection laws, ethical standards, and healthcare systems across countries can hinder the development and deployment of AI solutions on a global scale. International cooperation and the development of global governance frameworks for AI in healthcare are necessary to address these challenges and ensure that the benefits of AI are equitably distributed worldwide (Cath et al., 2018). As AI continues to evolve and permeate various aspects of healthcare, ongoing ethical deliberation and public engagement are essential. The societal implications of AI in medicine extend beyond technical and regulatory considerations to fundamental questions about the future of healthcare, the nature of medical expertise, and the values we prioritize in our health systems. Fostering interdisciplinary dialogue among AI researchers, healthcare professionals, ethicists, policymakers, and patient advocates is crucial for navigating the complex landscape of AI in medicine and ensuring that its development aligns with societal values and priorities (Vayena et al., 2018). Addressing these challenges and ethical considerations will require sustained effort, collaboration, and innovation from all stakeholders in the healthcare ecosystem. By proactively engaging with these issues, we can harness the transformative potential of AI in medicine while safeguarding patient rights, promoting equity, and maintaining the human-centric nature of healthcare.

5. FUTURE OUTLOOK

The future of AI in medicine is poised for transformative growth, with increased integration across the entire healthcare ecosystem expected to revolutionize patient care, research, and health system management. This integration will likely extend beyond clinical applications to encompass areas such as supply chain management, resource allocation, and public health surveillance, creating a more interconnected and efficient healthcare landscape (Topol, 2019). As AI systems become more deeply embedded in healthcare processes, we can anticipate the emergence of "learning health systems" that continuously improve based on real-world data and outcomes, enabling more agile and responsive healthcare delivery (Rajkomar et al., 2019). The development of more sophisticated, multi-modal AI models represents another key trend, with future systems capable of integrating diverse data types such as genomics, imaging, electronic health records, and wearable device data to provide more comprehensive and nuanced insights (Xu et al., 2020). These advanced models will likely leverage techniques such as transfer learning and multi-task learning to improve performance across a wide range of medical tasks, potentially leading to more generalizable and robust AI systems in healthcare (He et al., 2019). The integration of natural language processing with computer vision and other AI modalities may enable more human-like interactions between AI systems and healthcare providers, facilitating smoother adoption and more intuitive use of AI tools in clinical settings (Esteva et al., 2021). As AI becomes more pervasive in healthcare decision-making, there will be a greater emphasis on explainable and trustworthy AI. The development of interpretable AI models and advanced techniques for post-hoc explanations will be crucial for building trust among patients, healthcare providers, and regulatory bodies (Holzinger et al., 2019). This focus on explainability will likely extend beyond technical solutions to encompass new frameworks for AI governance in healthcare, including standards for model transparency, auditability, and continuous monitoring of AI system performance (Amann et al., 2020). The concept of "algorithmic stewardship" may emerge as a key principle in healthcare organizations, with dedicated teams responsible for overseeing the ethical and responsible use of AI across various clinical and operational contexts (Char et al., 2018). The expansion of AI applications in personalized and precision medicine is expected to accelerate, driven by advances in genomics, proteomics, and other -omics technologies. AI-powered systems will likely play an increasingly important role in interpreting complex molecular data, identifying novel biomarkers, and predicting individual patient responses to treatments (Würstle et al., 2021). This may lead to more tailored therapeutic approaches, optimized drug dosing regimens, and early detection of diseases based on subtle molecular signatures (Schork, 2019). The integration of AI with emerging technologies such as CRISPR gene editing and synthetic biology could open new frontiers in personalized medicine, potentially enabling the design of bespoke cellular therapies and targeted genetic interventions (Fellmann et al., 2017). As AI continues to demonstrate its potential in drug discovery and development, we can expect to see increased adoption of AI-driven approaches throughout the pharmaceutical R&D pipeline, from target identification to clinical trial design and post-market surveillance (Vamathevan et al., 2019).

The continued evolution of regulatory frameworks to keep pace with AI advancements will be crucial for ensuring the safe and effective deployment of AI in healthcare. Regulatory bodies such as the FDA are likely to develop more sophisticated approaches to evaluating AI/ML-based medical devices, potentially including real-time monitoring of AI performance and frameworks for regulating continuously learning systems (Babic et al., 2019). International collaboration on AI governance in healthcare may increase, aimed at harmonizing regulatory approaches and facilitating global development and deployment of AI technologies (Cath et al., 2018). The concept of "regulatory sandboxes" for AI in healthcare may gain traction, allowing for controlled testing of innovative AI applications in real-world settings while managing risks and gathering evidence on their impact (Ginsberg et al., 2021). The future of AI in medicine will likely see a greater focus on addressing health disparities and ensuring equitable access to AI-driven healthcare innovations. This may involve the development of AI models specifically designed to account for diverse populations and social determinants of health, as well as initiatives to improve data representation and reduce algorithmic bias (Obermeyer et al., 2019). The potential for AI to extend high-quality healthcare to underserved areas through telemedicine and mobile health applications may help bridge gaps in healthcare access, particularly in low- and middle-income countries (Wahl et al., 2018). As AI systems become more advanced, the nature of medical education and clinical practice is likely to evolve. Future healthcare professionals may need to develop new skills in data science, AI interpretation, and human-AI collaboration to effectively leverage these technologies in patient care (Kolachalama& Garg, 2018). The role of healthcare providers may shift towards more complex decision-making, emotional support, and oversight of AI systems, potentially leading to new specialties focused on the intersection of medicine and AI (Topol, 2019). The integration of AI in medical education, including AI-powered simulation and training tools, may enhance the learning experience and better prepare future healthcare professionals for a technology-driven healthcare landscape (Chan &Zary, 2019). The future of AI in medicine is also likely to see increased convergence with other emerging technologies, such as the Internet of Things (IoT), 5G networks, and quantum computing. This convergence may enable real-time, continuous health monitoring and interventions, more sophisticated predictive modeling of disease outbreaks, and the ability to process and analyze vastly larger and more complex datasets (Deo, 2015). The development of edge computing and AI-enabled medical devices may allow for more distributed and responsive healthcare delivery, reducing latency and improving the ability to provide care in remote or resource-limited settings (Azam et al., 2022). As these technologies mature, we may see the emergence of highly integrated, AI-driven health ecosystems that seamlessly connect various aspects of individual and population health management. While the potential benefits of AI in medicine are immense, the future will also bring new ethical challenges and societal implications that will require ongoing dialogue and careful consideration. Issues such as AI's impact on human autonomy in healthcare decisions, the potential for AI to exacerbate or create new forms of healthcare inequities, and the long-term effects of AI on the healthcare workforce will need to be addressed (Vayena et al., 2018). As AI becomes more deeply integrated into healthcare systems, ensuring the resilience and security of these systems against potential cyber threats or AI failures will be paramount (Rigby, 2019). The future of AI in medicine holds great promise for improving patient outcomes, increasing healthcare efficiency, and advancing medical knowledge. However, realizing this potential will require sustained collaboration among stakeholders, ongoing innovation in technology and governance, and a commitment to ethical and equitable deployment of AI in healthcare.

6. CONCLUSION

AI is set to revolutionize medical practice by enabling more accurate diagnoses, personalized treatments, and improved patient outcomes. From early disease detection to drug discovery, AI holds the potential to transform every aspect of healthcare. However, this power comes with significant challenges. Safeguarding patient data, addressing algorithmic bias, and ensuring fairness are critical concerns that need careful management. Building trust through explainable AI models and transparent decision-making processes will be key to integrating AI into healthcare effectively. As AI systems advance, the balance between human judgment and machine recommendations will require ongoing ethical consideration. Regulatory frameworks must evolve to keep pace with technological advancements, ensuring both safety and innovation. Furthermore, the role of healthcare professionals will shift, with greater emphasis on human-AI collaboration, necessitating new skills in data interpretation and AI oversight. Medical education will need to adapt to prepare future professionals for this tech-driven landscape. To ensure equitable benefits across all populations, especially in resource-limited settings, AI must be developed and deployed thoughtfully. As AI converges with other emerging technologies like genomics and the Internet of Things, it will likely drive new advancements in personalized and predictive medicine. Realizing AI's full potential in healthcare will require a commitment to responsible innovation, interdisciplinary collaboration, and an ongoing focus on ethical reflection to ensure that AI aligns with human values and benefits society as a whole.

REFERENCES

Aamir, M., Bazai, S., Bhatti, U. A., Dayo, Z. A., Liu, J., & Zhang, K. (2023, January). Applications of machine learning in medicine: Current trends and prospects. In *2023 Global Conference on Wireless and Optical Technologies (GCWOT)* (pp. 1-4). IEEE. DOI: 10.1109/GCWOT57803.2023.10064665

Aamir, M., Rahman, Z., Abro, W. A., Bhatti, U. A., Dayo, Z. A., & Ishfaq, M. (2023). Brain tumor classification utilizing deep features derived from high-quality regions in MRI images. *Biomedical Signal Processing and Control*, *85*, 104988. DOI: 10.1016/j.bspc.2023.104988

Aamir, M., Rahman, Z., Abro, W. A., Tahir, M., & Ahmed, S. M. (2019). An optimized architecture of image classification using convolutional neural network. International Journal of Image. *Graphics and Signal Processing*, *11*(10), 30–39. DOI: 10.5815/ijigsp.2019.10.05

Aamir, M., Rahman, Z., Dayo, Z. A., Abro, W. A., Uddin, M. I., Khan, I., Imran, A. S., Ali, Z., Ishfaq, M., Guan, Y., & Hu, Z. (2022). A deep learning approach for brain tumor classification using MRI images. *Computers & Electrical Engineering*, *101*, 108105. DOI: 10.1016/j.compeleceng.2022.108105

Abràmoff, M. D., Lavin, P. T., Birch, M., Shah, N., & Folk, J. C. (2018). Pivotal trial of an autonomous AI-based diagnostic system for detection of diabetic retinopathy in primary care offices. *NPJ Digital Medicine*, *1*(1), 1–8. DOI: 10.1038/s41746-018-0040-6 PMID: 31304320

Adamson, A. S., & Smith, A. (2018). Machine learning and health care disparities in dermatology. *JAMA Dermatology*, *154*(11), 1247–1248. DOI: 10.1001/jamadermatol.2018.2348 PMID: 30073260

Aerts, H. J., Velazquez, E. R., Leijenaar, R. T., Parmar, C., Grossmann, P., Carvalho, S., Bussink, J., Monshouwer, R., Haibe-Kains, B., Rietveld, D., Hoebers, F., Rietbergen, M. M., Leemans, C. R., Dekker, A., Quackenbush, J., Gillies, R. J., & Lambin, P. (2014). Decoding tumour phenotype by noninvasive imaging using a quantitative radiomics approach. *Nature Communications*, *5*(1), 1–9. DOI: 10.1038/ncomms5006 PMID: 24892406

Ahmad, M. A., Eckert, C., & Teredesai, A. (2018). Interpretable machine learning in healthcare. In *Proceedings of the 2018 ACM International Conference on Bioinformatics, Computational Biology, and Health Informatics* (pp. 559-560).

Alotaibi, Y. K., & Federico, F. (2017). The impact of health information technology on patient safety. *Saudi Medical Journal*, *38*(12), 1173–1180. DOI: 10.15537/smj.2017.12.20631 PMID: 29209664

Alsentzer, E., Murphy, J. R., Boag, W., Weng, W. H., Jin, D., Naumann, T., & McDermott, M. (2019). Publicly available clinical BERT embeddings. arXiv preprint arXiv:1904.03323.

Amann, J., Blasimme, A., Vayena, E., Frey, D., & Madai, V. I. (2020). Explainability for artificial intelligence in healthcare: A multidisciplinary perspective. *BMC Medical Informatics and Decision Making*, *20*(1), 1–9. DOI: 10.1186/s12911-020-01332-6 PMID: 33256715

Anand, N., & Huang, P. (2018). Generative modeling for protein structures. *Advances in Neural Information Processing Systems*, •••, 31.

Antropova, N., Huynh, B. Q., & Giger, M. L. (2017). A deep feature fusion methodology for breast cancer diagnosis demonstrated on three imaging modality datasets. *Medical Physics*, *44*(10), 5162–5171. DOI: 10.1002/mp.12453 PMID: 28681390

Ardila, D., Kiraly, A. P., Bharadwaj, S., Choi, B., Reicher, J. J., Peng, L., Tse, D., Etemadi, M., Ye, W., Corrado, G., Naidich, D. P., & Shetty, S. (2019). End-to-end lung cancer screening with three-dimensional deep learning on low-dose chest computed tomography. *Nature Medicine*, *25*(6), 954–961. DOI: 10.1038/s41591-019-0447-x PMID: 31110349

Artificial Intelligence in Drug Discovery Market. (2021). *Global Industry Analysis, Size, Share, Growth, Trends, and Forecast 2021-2028*. Retrieved from. [Market Research Report]

Ashley, E. A. (2016). Towards precision medicine. *Nature Reviews. Genetics*, *17*(9), 507–522. DOI: 10.1038/nrg.2016.86 PMID: 27528417

Attanasio, A., Scaglioni, B., De Momi, E., Fiorini, P., & Valdastri, P. (2020). Autonomy in surgical robotics. *Annual Review of Control, Robotics, and Autonomous Systems*, *3*, 651–676.

Azam, S., Amin, S. U., Hong, C. S., & Rahman, M. A. (2022). Edge AI for healthcare: Deep learning approaches, challenges, and future trends. *IEEE Access : Practical Innovations, Open Solutions*, *10*, 97457–97489.

Babic, B., Gerke, S., Evgeniou, T., & Cohen, I. G. (2019). Algorithms on regulatory lockdown in medicine. *Science*, *366*(6470), 1202–1204. DOI: 10.1126/science.aay9547 PMID: 31806804

Balagopal, A., Kazemifar, S., & Nguyen, D.. (2021). Fully automated organ segmentation in male pelvic CT images. *Physics in Medicine and Biology*, *66*(16), 163001. PMID: 30523973

Ballinger, B.. (2018). *DeepHeart: Semi-Supervised Sequence Learning for Cardiovascular Risk Prediction*. AAAI.

Banaei-Esfahani, A., Nicod, C., Aebersold, R., & Collins, B. C. (2020). Systems proteomics approaches to study bacterial pathogens: Application to Mycobacterium tuberculosis. *Current Opinion in Microbiology*, *55*, 17–23. PMID: 29032348

Banda, J. M., Seneviratne, M., Hernandez-Boussard, T., & Shah, N. H. (2018). Advances in Electronic Phenotyping: From Rule-Based Definitions to Machine Learning Models. *Annual Review of Biomedical Data Science*, *1*(1), 53–68. DOI: 10.1146/annurev-biodatasci-080917-013315 PMID: 31218278

Bates, D. W., Saria, S., Ohno-Machado, L., Shah, A., & Escobar, G. (2014). Big Data In Health Care: Using Analytics To Identify And Manage High-Risk And High-Cost Patients. *Health Affairs*, *33*(7), 1123–1131. DOI: 10.1377/hlthaff.2014.0041 PMID: 25006137

Bauman, K. (2018). Predicting Hospital Staffing Needs With Time Series Analysis. *Global Journal of Medical Research*, *18*(1).

Bayer, S., Maier, A., Ostermeier, M., & Fahrig, R. (2017). Intraoperative imaging modalities and compensation for brain shift in tumor resection surgery. *International Journal of Biomedical Imaging*, *2017*, 2017. DOI: 10.1155/2017/6028645 PMID: 28676821

Beam, A. L., & Kohane, I. S. (2018). Big data and machine learning in health care. *Journal of the American Medical Association, 319*(13), 1317–1318. DOI: 10.1001/jama.2017.18391 PMID: 29532063

Beck, B. R., Shin, B., Choi, Y., Park, S., & Kang, K. (2020). Predicting commercially available antiviral drugs that may act on the novel coronavirus (SARS-CoV-2) through a drug-target interaction deep learning model. *Computational and Structural Biotechnology Journal, 18*, 784–790. DOI: 10.1016/j.csbj.2020.03.025 PMID: 32280433

Becker, H., & Gartner, M. (2019). Machine Learning Approach for Automated Coding of Clinical Notes. *Studies in Health Technology and Informatics, 264*, 590–594.

Bernhardt, S., Nicolau, S. A., Soler, L., & Doignon, C. (2017). The status of augmented reality in laparoscopic surgery as of 2016. *Medical Image Analysis, 37*, 66–90. DOI: 10.1016/j.media.2017.01.007 PMID: 28160692

Berry, D. A. (2015). Bayesian clinical trials. *Nature Reviews. Drug Discovery, 14*(1), 27–36. DOI: 10.1038/nrd1927 PMID: 16485344

Berthet-Rayne, P., Gras, G., Leibrandt, K., Wisanuvej, P., Schmitz, A., Seneci, C. A., & Yang, G. Z. (2018). The i2Snake robotic platform for endoscopic surgery. *Annals of Biomedical Engineering, 46*(10), 1663–1675. DOI: 10.1007/s10439-018-2066-y PMID: 29948372

Bi, W. L., Hosny, A., Schabath, M. B., Giger, M. L., Birkbak, N. J., Mehrtash, A., Allison, T., Arnaout, O., Abbosh, C., Dunn, I. F., Mak, R. H., Tamimi, R. M., Tempany, C. M., Swanton, C., Hoffmann, U., Schwartz, L. H., Gillies, R. J., Huang, R. Y., & Aerts, H. J. W. L. (2019). Artificial intelligence in cancer imaging: Clinical challenges and applications. *CA: a Cancer Journal for Clinicians, 69*(2), 127–157. DOI: 10.3322/caac.21552 PMID: 30720861

Bradshaw, J., Paige, B., Kusner, M. J., Segler, M., & Hernández-Lobato, J. M. (2019). A model to search for synthesizable molecules. *Advances in Neural Information Processing Systems*, •••, 32.

Brinker, T. J., Hekler, A., Enk, A. H., Klode, J., Hauschild, A., Berking, C., Schilling, B., Haferkamp, S., Schadendorf, D., Holland-Letz, T., Utikal, J. S., von Kalle, C., Ludwig-Peitsch, W., Sirokay, J., Heinzerling, L., Albrecht, M., Baratella, K., Bischof, L., Chorti, E., & Schrüfer, P. (2019). Deep learning outperformed 136 of 157 dermatologists in a head-to-head dermoscopic melanoma image classification task. *European Journal of Cancer, 113*, 47–54. DOI: 10.1016/j.ejca.2019.04.001 PMID: 30981091

Brisimi, T. S., Chen, R., Mela, T., Olshevsky, A., Paschalidis, I. C., & Shi, W. (2018). Federated learning of predictive models from federated electronic health records. *International Journal of Medical Informatics, 112*, 59–67. DOI: 10.1016/j.ijmedinf.2018.01.007 PMID: 29500022

Bullock, J., Luccioni, A., & Pham, K. H.. (2020). Mapping the landscape of artificial intelligence applications against COVID-19. *Journal of Artificial Intelligence Research, 69*, 807–845. DOI: 10.1613/jair.1.12162

Burlina, P. M., Joshi, N., Pekala, M., Pacheco, K. D., Freund, D. E., & Bressler, N. M. (2017). Automated grading of age-related macular degeneration from color fundus images using deep convolutional neural networks. *JAMA Ophthalmology, 135*(11), 1170–1176. DOI: 10.1001/jamaophthalmol.2017.3782 PMID: 28973096

Callahan, T. J., Tripodi, I. J., Pielke-Lombardo, H., & Hunter, L. E. (2020). Knowledge-based Biomedical Data Science. *Annual Review of Biomedical Data Science*, *3*(1), 23–41. DOI: 10.1146/annurev-biodatasci-010820-091627 PMID: 33954284

Campanella, G., Hanna, M. G., Geneslaw, L., Miraflor, A., Werneck Krauss Silva, V., Busam, K. J., Brogi, E., Reuter, V. E., Klimstra, D. S., & Fuchs, T. J. (2019). Clinical-grade computational pathology using weakly supervised deep learning on whole slide images. *Nature Medicine*, *25*(8), 1301–1309. DOI: 10.1038/s41591-019-0508-1 PMID: 31308507

Cath, C., Wachter, S., Mittelstadt, B., Taddeo, M., & Floridi, L. (2018). Artificial intelligence and the 'good society': The US, EU, and UK approach. *Science and Engineering Ethics*, *24*(2), 505–528. PMID: 28353045

Chakraborty, B., & Murphy, S. A. (2014). Dynamic treatment regimes. *Annual Review of Statistics and Its Application*, *1*(1), 447–464. DOI: 10.1146/annurev-statistics-022513-115553 PMID: 25401119

Chan, K. S., & Zary, N. (2019). Applications and challenges of implementing artificial intelligence in medical education: Integrative review. *JMIR Medical Education*, *5*(1), e13930. DOI: 10.2196/13930 PMID: 31199295

Char, D. S., Shah, N. H., & Magnus, D. (2018). Implementing machine learning in health care—Addressing ethical challenges. *The New England Journal of Medicine*, *378*(11), 981–983. DOI: 10.1056/NEJMp1714229 PMID: 29539284

Chaudhary, K., Poirion, O. B., Lu, L., & Garmire, L. X. (2018). Deep learning–based multi-omics integration robustly predicts survival in liver cancer. *Clinical Cancer Research*, *24*(6), 1248–1259. DOI: 10.1158/1078-0432.CCR-17-0853 PMID: 28982688

Chen, R.. (2021). Deep Learning for 30-Day All-Cause Readmission Prediction Using Electronic Health Record and Temporal Data. *Journal of Biomedical Informatics.*

Chen, Y., Argentinis, J. D. E., & Weber, G. (2016). IBM Watson: How Cognitive Computing Can Be Applied to Big Data Challenges in Life Sciences Research. *Clinical Therapeutics*, *38*(4), 688–701. DOI: 10.1016/j.clinthera.2015.12.001 PMID: 27130797

Chen, Y., Elenee Argentinis, J. D., & Weber, G. (2016). IBM Watson: How Cognitive Computing Can Be Applied to Big Data Challenges in Life Sciences Research. *Clinical Therapeutics*, *38*(4), 688–701. DOI: 10.1016/j.clinthera.2015.12.001 PMID: 27130797

Chiu, C. C., Tripathi, A., Chou, K., Co, C., Jaitly, N., Jaunzeikare, D., . . . Zhang, X. (2017). Speech recognition for medical conversations. arXiv preprint arXiv:1711.07274.

Chuchu, N., Takwoingi, Y., Dinnes, J., Matin, R. N., Bassett, O., Moreau, J. F., Bayliss, S. E., Davenport, C., Godfrey, K., O'Connell, S., Jain, A., Walter, F. M., Deeks, J. J., & Williams, H. C. (2018). Smartphone applications for triaging adults with skin lesions that are suspicious for melanoma. *Cochrane Database of Systematic Reviews*, *2018*(12), 12. DOI: 10.1002/14651858.CD013192 PMID: 30521685

Codella, N., Rotemberg, V., Tschandl, P., ... (2019). Skin lesion analysis toward melanoma detection 2018: A challenge hosted by the international skin imaging collaboration (ISIC). arXiv preprint arXiv:1902.03368.

Codella, N. C., Gutman, D., Celebi, M. E., ... (2018). Skin lesion analysis toward melanoma detection: A challenge at the 2017 International symposium on biomedical imaging (ISBI), hosted by the international skin imaging collaboration (ISIC). In 2018 IEEE 15th International Symposium on Biomedical Imaging (ISBI 2018) (pp. 168-172). IEEE.

Cohen, I. G., Evgeniou, T., Gerke, S., & Minssen, T. (2020). The European artificial intelligence strategy: Implications and challenges for digital health. *The Lancet. Digital Health*, *2*(7), e376–e379. DOI: 10.1016/S2589-7500(20)30112-6 PMID: 33328096

Coravos, A., Khozin, S., & Mandl, K. D. (2019). Developing and adopting safe and effective digital biomarkers to improve patient outcomes. *NPJ Digital Medicine*, *2*(1), 1–5. DOI: 10.1038/s41746-019-0090-4 PMID: 30868107

Das, P., Banka, R., Ghosh, J., Singh, K., Choudhury, S. R., & Koner, S. (2024). Synergism of diet, genetics, and microbiome on health. In *Nutrition controversies and advances in autoimmune disease* (pp. 131–189). IGI Global. DOI: 10.4018/979-8-3693-5528-2.ch006

Davenport, T., & Kalakota, R. (2019). The potential for artificial intelligence in healthcare. *Future Healthcare Journal*, *6*(2), 94–98. DOI: 10.7861/futurehosp.6-2-94 PMID: 31363513

Dayan, I., Roth, H. R., Zhong, A., Harouni, A., Gentili, A., Abidin, A. Z., & Xu, Z. (2021). Federated learning for predicting clinical outcomes in patients with COVID-19. *Nature Medicine*, *27*(10), 1735–1743. DOI: 10.1038/s41591-021-01506-3 PMID: 34526699

De Fauw, J., Ledsam, J. R., Romera-Paredes, B., Nikolov, S., Tomasev, N., Blackwell, S., Askham, H., Glorot, X., O'Donoghue, B., Visentin, D., van den Driessche, G., Lakshminarayanan, B., Meyer, C., Mackinder, F., Bouton, S., Ayoub, K., Chopra, R., King, D., Karthikesalingam, A., & Ronneberger, O. (2018). Clinically applicable deep learning for diagnosis and referral in retinal disease. *Nature Medicine*, *24*(9), 1342–1350. DOI: 10.1038/s41591-018-0107-6 PMID: 30104768

Demner-Fushman, D., ... NLP for supporting eHealth interventions. In: Natural Language Processing for Social Media. 2017.

Demner-Fushman, D., Chapman, W. W., & McDonald, C. J. (2009). What can natural language processing do for clinical decision support? *Journal of Biomedical Informatics*, *42*(5), 760–772. DOI: 10.1016/j.jbi.2009.08.007 PMID: 19683066

Demner-Fushman, D., Chapman, W. W., & McDonald, C. J. (2009). What can natural language processing do for clinical decision support? *Journal of Biomedical Informatics*, *42*(5), 760–772. DOI: 10.1016/j.jbi.2009.08.007 PMID: 19683066

Deo, R. C. (2015). Machine learning in medicine. *Circulation*, *132*(20), 1920–1930. DOI: 10.1161/CIRCULATIONAHA.115.001593 PMID: 26572668

Dernoncourt, F., Lee, J. Y., Uzuner, O., & Szolovits, P. (2017). De-identification of patient notes with recurrent neural networks. *Journal of the American Medical Informatics Association : JAMIA*, *24*(3), 596–606. DOI: 10.1093/jamia/ocw156 PMID: 28040687

Došilović, F. K., Brčić, M., & Hlupić, N. (2018). Explainable artificial intelligence: A survey. In 2018 41st International convention on information and communication technology, electronics and microelectronics (MIPRO) (pp. 0210-0215). IEEE. DOI: 10.23919/MIPRO.2018.8400040

Elsäßer, A., Regnstrom, J., Vetter, T., Koenig, F., Hemmings, R. J., Greco, M., Papaluca-Amati, M., & Posch, M. (2014). Adaptive clinical trial designs for European marketing authorization: A survey of scientific advice letters from the European Medicines Agency. *Trials*, *15*(1), 383. DOI: 10.1186/1745-6215-15-383 PMID: 25278265

Elton, D. C., Boukouvalas, Z., Fuge, M. D., & Chung, P. W. (2019). Deep learning for molecular design—A review of the state of the art. *Molecular Systems Design & Engineering*, *4*(4), 828–849. DOI: 10.1039/C9ME00039A

Esteva, A., Chou, K., Yeung, S., Naik, N., Madani, A., Mottaghi, A., Liu, Y., Topol, E., Dean, J., & Socher, R. (2021). Deep learning-enabled medical computer vision. *NPJ Digital Medicine*, *4*(1), 5. DOI: 10.1038/s41746-020-00376-2 PMID: 33420381

Esteva, A., Chou, K., Yeung, S., Naik, N., Madani, A., Mottaghi, A., Liu, Y., Topol, E., Dean, J., & Socher, R. (2021). Deep learning-enabled medical computer vision. *NPJ Digital Medicine*, *4*(1), 1–9. DOI: 10.1038/s41746-020-00376-2 PMID: 33420381

Esteva, A., Kuprel, B., Novoa, R. A., Ko, J., Swetter, S. M., Blau, H. M., & Thrun, S. (2017). Dermatologist-level classification of skin cancer with deep neural networks. *Nature*, *542*(7639), 115–118. DOI: 10.1038/nature21056 PMID: 28117445

Fellmann, C., Gowen, B. G., Lin, P. C., Doudna, J. A., & Corn, J. E. (2017). Cornerstones of CRISPR–Cas in drug discovery and therapy. *Nature Reviews. Drug Discovery*, *16*(2), 89–100. DOI: 10.1038/nrd.2016.238 PMID: 28008168

Gao, J., Zhang, T., & Yang, X.. (2019). Graph neural network-based multi-modal fusion model for brain network analysis. In *International Conference on Medical Image Computing and Computer-Assisted Intervention* (pp. 475-483). Springer, Cham.

Gao, S.. (2020). Predicting Hospital Readmission using Clinical Text and Machine Learning Techniques. *AMIA ... Annual Symposium Proceedings - AMIA Symposium. AMIA Symposium.*

Gao, W., & Coley, C. W. (2020). The synthesizability of molecules proposed by generative models. *Journal of Chemical Information and Modeling*, *60*(12), 5714–5723. DOI: 10.1021/acs.jcim.0c00174 PMID: 32250616

Gareau, D. S., Browning, J., & Da Rosa, J. C.. (2020). Deep learning-level melanoma detection by interpretable machine learning and imaging biomarker cues. *Journal of Biomedical Optics*, *25*(11), 112906. DOI: 10.1117/1.JBO.25.11.112906 PMID: 33247560

Gerke, S., Babic, B., Evgeniou, T., & Cohen, I. G. (2020). The need for a system view to regulate artificial intelligence/machine learning-based software as medical device. *NPJ Digital Medicine*, *3*(1), 1–4. DOI: 10.1038/s41746-020-0262-2 PMID: 32285013

Ghosh, J. (2023). A review on understanding the risk factors for coronary heart disease in Indian college students. *International Journal of Noncommunicable Diseases*, *8*(2), 117–128. DOI: 10.4103/jncd.jncd_68_23

Ghosh, J. (2024a). Leveraging data science for personalized nutrition. In *Nutrition controversies and advances in autoimmune disease*. IGI Global., DOI: 10.4018/979-8-3693-5528-2.ch022

Ghosh, J. (2024b). Recognizing and predicting the risk of malnutrition in the elderly using artificial intelligence: A systematic review. *International Journal of Advancement in Life Sciences Research*, *7*(3), 01–14. Advance online publication. DOI: 10.31632/ijalsr.2024.v07i03.001

Ghosh, J., Choudhury, S. R., Singh, K., & Koner, S. (2024b). Application of machine learning algorithm and artificial intelligence in improving metabolic syndrome related complications: A review. *International Journal of Advancement in Life Sciences Research*, *7*(2), 41–67. DOI: 10.31632/ijalsr.2024.v07i02.004

Ghosh, J., & Sanyal, P. (2024). Development and evaluation of machine learning models for predicting constipation and its risk factors among college-aged females. *Nutrition & Food Science*, *12*(3). https://bit.ly/3MPo6eH

Ghosh, J., Shakil, S., Singh, K., & Mandal, S. (2024a). Depression and cognitive function in accordance with the nutritional status of elderly women residing in Rajarhat-Newtown area of Kolkata, India. *Medical Journal of Dr. D.Y. Patil Vidyapeeth*, *17*(5), 951–956. DOI: 10.4103/mjdrdypu.mjdrdypu_423_23

Gianfrancesco, M. A., Tamang, S., Yazdany, J., & Schmajuk, G. (2018). Potential Biases in Machine Learning Algorithms Using Electronic Health Record Data. *JAMA Internal Medicine*, *178*(11), 1544. DOI: 10.1001/jamainternmed.2018.3763 PMID: 30128552

Ginsberg, J., Mohebbi, M. H., Patel, R. S., Brammer, L., Smolinski, M. S., & Brilliant, L. (2021). Regulatory sandboxes: A cure for mHealth pilotitis? *Journal of Medical Internet Research*, *23*(3), e24838.

Gorgulla, C., Boeszoermenyi, A., Wang, Z. F., Fischer, P. D., Coote, P. W., Padmanabha Das, K. M., Malets, Y. S., Radchenko, D. S., Moroz, Y. S., Scott, D. A., Fackeldey, K., Hoffmann, M., Iavniuk, I., Wagner, G., & Arthanari, H. (2020). An open-source drug discovery platform enables ultra-large virtual screens. *Nature*, *580*(7805), 663–668. DOI: 10.1038/s41586-020-2117-z PMID: 32152607

Grisoni, F., Moret, M., Lingwood, R., & Schneider, G. (2020). Bidirectional molecule generation with recurrent neural networks. *Journal of Chemical Information and Modeling*, *60*(3), 1175–1183. DOI: 10.1021/acs.jcim.9b00943 PMID: 31904964

Guan, Y., Aamir, M., Rahman, Z., Ali, A., Abro, W. A., Dayo, Z. A., ... & Hu, Z. (2021). A framework for efficient brain tumor classification using MRI images.

Gulshan, V., Peng, L., Coram, M., Stumpe, M. C., Wu, D., Narayanaswamy, A., Venugopalan, S., Widner, K., Madams, T., Cuadros, J., Kim, R., Raman, R., Nelson, P. C., Mega, J. L., & Webster, D. R. (2016). Development and validation of a deep learning algorithm for detection of diabetic retinopathy in retinal fundus photographs. *Journal of the American Medical Association*, *316*(22), 2402–2410. DOI: 10.1001/jama.2016.17216 PMID: 27898976

Haenssle, H. A., Fink, C., Schneiderbauer, R., Toberer, F., Buhl, T., Blum, A., Kalloo, A., Hassen, A. B. H., Thomas, L., Enk, A., Uhlmann, L., Alt, C., Arenbergerova, M., Bakos, R., Baltzer, A., Bertlich, I., Blum, A., Bokor-Billmann, T., Bowling, J., & Zalaudek, I. (2018). Man against machine: Diagnostic performance of a deep learning convolutional neural network for dermoscopic melanoma recognition in comparison to 58 dermatologists. *Annals of Oncology : Official Journal of the European Society for Medical Oncology*, *29*(8), 1836–1842. DOI: 10.1093/annonc/mdy166 PMID: 29846502

Hafez, M. A., Chelule, K. L., Seedhom, B. B., & Sherman, K. P. (2016). Computer-assisted total knee arthroplasty using patient-specific templating. *Clinical Orthopaedics and Related Research*, *444*, 184–192. DOI: 10.1097/01.blo.0000201148.06454.ef PMID: 16446589

Han, S. S., Kim, M. S., Lim, W., Park, G. H., Park, I., & Chang, S. E. (2018). Classification of the clinical images for benign and malignant cutaneous tumors using a deep learning algorithm. *The Journal of Investigative Dermatology*, *138*(7), 1529–1538. DOI: 10.1016/j.jid.2018.01.028 PMID: 29428356

Harrer, S., Shah, P., Antony, B., & Hu, J. (2019). Artificial intelligence for clinical trial design. *Trends in Pharmacological Sciences*, *40*(8), 577–591. DOI: 10.1016/j.tips.2019.05.005 PMID: 31326235

Hashimoto, D. A., Rosman, G., Rus, D., & Meireles, O. R. (2020). Artificial intelligence in surgery: Promises and perils. *Annals of Surgery*, *268*(1), 70–76. DOI: 10.1097/SLA.0000000000002693 PMID: 29389679

Hasin, Y., Seldin, M., & Lusis, A. (2017). Multi-omics approaches to disease. *Genome Biology*, *18*(1), 83. DOI: 10.1186/s13059-017-1215-1 PMID: 28476144

Hatib, F., Jian, Z., Buddi, S., Lee, C., Settels, J., Sibert, K., Rinehart, J., & Cannesson, M. (2018). Machine-learning algorithm to predict hypotension based on high-fidelity arterial pressure waveform analysis. *Anesthesiology*, *129*(4), 663–674. DOI: 10.1097/ALN.0000000000002300 PMID: 29894315

He, J., Baxter, S. L., Xu, J., Xu, J., Zhou, X., & Zhang, K. (2019). The practical implementation of artificial intelligence technologies in medicine. *Nature Medicine*, *25*(1), 30–36. DOI: 10.1038/s41591-018-0307-0 PMID: 30617336

Holmer, A., Lehmann, K. S., Wanken, J., Reissfelder, C., Roggan, A., Mueller, G., & Ritz, J. P. (2018). Optical properties of thyroid tissue and the development of a thyroid tissue phantom. *Lasers in Surgery and Medicine*, *50*(10), 1027–1033.

Holzinger, A., Biemann, C., Pattichis, C. S., & Kell, D. B. (2017). What do we need to build explainable AI systems for the medical domain? arXiv preprint arXiv:1712.09923.

Holzinger, A., Langs, G., Denk, H., Zatloukal, K., & Müller, H. (2019). Causability and explainability of artificial intelligence in medicine. *Wiley Interdisciplinary Reviews. Data Mining and Knowledge Discovery*, *9*(4), e1312. DOI: 10.1002/widm.1312 PMID: 32089788

Hosny, A., Parmar, C., Quackenbush, J., Schwartz, L. H., & Aerts, H. J. W. L. (2018). Artificial intelligence in radiology. *Nature Reviews. Cancer*, *18*(8), 500–510. DOI: 10.1038/s41568-018-0016-5 PMID: 29777175

Huang, K., Altosaar, J., & Ranganath, R. (2019). Clinicalbert: Modeling clinical notes and predicting hospital readmission. arXiv preprint arXiv:1904.05342.

Huang, K., Fu, T., Glass, L. M., Zitnik, M., Xiao, C., & Sun, J. (2020). DeepPurpose: A deep learning library for drug–target interaction prediction. *Bioinformatics (Oxford, England)*, *36*(22-23), 5545–5547. DOI: 10.1093/bioinformatics/btaa1005 PMID: 33275143

Huang, S., Chaudhary, K., & Garmire, L. X. (2017). More is better: Recent progress in multi-omics data integration methods. *Frontiers in Genetics*, *8*, 84. DOI: 10.3389/fgene.2017.00084 PMID: 28670325

Hung, A. J., Chen, J., & Gill, I. S. (2018). Automated Performance Metrics and Machine Learning Algorithms to Measure Surgeon Performance and Anticipate Clinical Outcomes in Robotic Surgery. *JAMA Surgery*, *153*(8), 770–771. DOI: 10.1001/jamasurg.2018.1512 PMID: 29926095

Jiang, F., Jiang, Y., Zhi, H., Dong, Y., Li, H., Ma, S., Wang, Y., Dong, Q., Shen, H., & Wang, Y. (2017). Artificial intelligence in healthcare: Past, present and future. *Stroke and Vascular Neurology*, *2*(4), 230–243. DOI: 10.1136/svn-2017-000101 PMID: 29507784

Jin, W., Barzilay, R., & Jaakkola, T. (2018). Junction tree variational autoencoder for molecular graph generation. *International Conference on Machine Learning*, 2323-2332.

Jin, W., Barzilay, R., & Jaakkola, T. (2020). Multi-objective molecule generation using interpretable substructures. In *International Conference on Machine Learning* (pp. 4849-4859). PMLR.

Johnson, A. E. W.. (2021). Artificial Intelligence in Cardiology: The Time Is Now. *JAMA Cardiology*.

Jud, L., Fotouhi, J., Andronic, O., Aichmair, A., Osgood, G., Navab, N., & Farshad, M. (2020). Applicability of augmented reality in orthopedic surgery–A systematic review. *BMC Musculoskeletal Disorders*, *21*(1), 1–13. DOI: 10.1186/s12891-020-3110-2 PMID: 32061248

Jumper, J., Evans, R., Pritzel, A., Green, T., Figurnov, M., Ronneberger, O., Tunyasuvunakool, K., Bates, R., Žídek, A., Potapenko, A., Bridgland, A., Meyer, C., Kohl, S. A. A., Ballard, A. J., Cowie, A., Romera-Paredes, B., Nikolov, S., Jain, R., Adler, J., & Hassabis, D. (2021). Highly accurate protein structure prediction with AlphaFold. *Nature*, *596*(7873), 583–589. DOI: 10.1038/s41586-021-03819-2 PMID: 34265844

Kaissis, G. A., Makowski, M. R., Rückert, D., & Braren, R. F. (2020). Secure, privacy-preserving and federated machine learning in medical imaging. *Nature Machine Intelligence*, *2*(6), 305–311. DOI: 10.1038/s42256-020-0186-1

Kang, J.. (2022). Prediction of Drug-Drug Interactions Using Deep Learning Models with Various Feature Vectors. *International Journal of Molecular Sciences*.

Kang, Y.. (2021). Natural Language Processing for Patient-Reported Outcomes: Transforming Cancer Care. *JCO Clinical Cancer Informatics*.

Karczewski, K. J., & Snyder, M. P. (2018). Integrative omics for health and disease. *Nature Reviews. Genetics*, *19*(5), 299–310. DOI: 10.1038/nrg.2018.4 PMID: 29479082

Khera, A. V., Chaffin, M., Aragam, K. G., Haas, M. E., Roselli, C., Choi, S. H., Natarajan, P., Lander, E. S., Lubitz, S. A., Ellinor, P. T., & Kathiresan, S. (2018). Genome-wide polygenic scores for common diseases identify individuals with risk equivalent to monogenic mutations. *Nature Genetics*, *50*(9), 1219–1224. DOI: 10.1038/s41588-018-0183-z PMID: 30104762

Kickingereder, P., Bonekamp, D., Nowosielski, M., Kratz, A., Sill, M., Burth, S., Wick, A., Eidel, O., Schlemmer, H.-P., Radbruch, A., Debus, J., Herold-Mende, C., Unterberg, A., Jones, D., Pfister, S., Wick, W., von Deimling, A., Bendszus, M., & Capper, D. (2018). Radiogenomics of glioblastoma: Machine learning–based classification of molecular characteristics by using multiparametric and multiregional MR imaging features. *Radiology*, *281*(3), 907–918. DOI: 10.1148/radiol.2016161382 PMID: 27636026

Kittler, H., Marghoob, A. A., Argenziano, G., Carrera, C., Curiel-Lewandrowski, C., Hofmann-Wellenhof, R., Malvehy, J., Menzies, S., Puig, S., Rabinovitz, H., Stolz, W., Saida, T., Soyer, H. P., Siegel, E., Stoecker, W. V., Scope, A., Tanaka, M., Thomas, L., Tschandl, P., & Halpern, A. (2019). Standardization of terminology in dermoscopy/dermatoscopy: Results of the third consensus conference of the International Society of Dermoscopy. *Journal of the American Academy of Dermatology*, *74*(6), 1093–1106. DOI: 10.1016/j.jaad.2015.12.038 PMID: 26896294

Klann, J. G.. (2021). Taking advantage of continuity of care documents to populate a research information model: Integrating data from diverse sources. *Journal of Biomedical Informatics*.

Koike, R.. (2023). Development and Validation of Clinical Notes–Based Analysis for Heart Failure Detection in Emergency Department Using Large Language Models. *JAMA Network Open*.

Kolachalama, V. B., & Garg, P. S. (2018). Machine learning and medical education. *NPJ Digital Medicine*, *1*(1), 1–3. DOI: 10.1038/s41746-018-0061-1 PMID: 31304333

Köpcke, F., & Prokosch, H. U. (2014). Employing computers for the recruitment into clinical trials: A comprehensive systematic review. *Journal of Medical Internet Research*, *16*(7), e161. DOI: 10.2196/jmir.3446 PMID: 24985568

Koshima, I., Yamamoto, T., Narushima, M., Mihara, M., & Iida, T. (2017). Perforator flaps and supermicrosurgery. *Clinics in Plastic Surgery*, *44*(3), 683–693. PMID: 20816523

Kost, R. G., Mervin-Blake, S., Hallarn, R., Rathmann, C., Kolb, H. R., Himmelfarb, C. D., D'Agostino, T., Rubinstein, E. P., Dozier, A. M., & Schuff, K. G. (2015). Accrual and recruitment practices at Clinical and Translational Science Award (CTSA) institutions: A call for expectations, expertise, and evaluation. *Academic Medicine*, *89*(8), 1180–1189. DOI: 10.1097/ACM.0000000000000308 PMID: 24826854

Kreimeyer, K., Foster, M., Pandey, A., Arya, N., Halford, G., Jones, S. F., Forshee, R., Walderhaug, M., & Botsis, T. (2017). Natural language processing systems for capturing and standardizing unstructured clinical information: A systematic review. *Journal of Biomedical Informatics*, *73*, 14–29. DOI: 10.1016/j.jbi.2017.07.012 PMID: 28729030

Lai, S.. (2019). Forecasting dengue fever in Malaysia: A deep learning approach. *IEEE Access : Practical Innovations, Open Solutions*.

Lakkaraju, H., Bach, S. H., & Leskovec, J. (2016). Interpretable decision sets: A joint framework for description and prediction. In *Proceedings of the 22nd ACM SIGKDD international conference on knowledge discovery and data mining* (pp. 1675-1684). DOI: 10.1145/2939672.2939874

LeCun, Y., Bengio, Y., & Hinton, G. (2015). Deep learning. *Nature*, *521*(7553), 436–444. DOI: 10.1038/nature14539 PMID: 26017442

Lee, J., Yoon, W., Kim, S., Kim, D., Kim, S., So, C. H., & Kang, J. (2020). BioBERT: A pre-trained biomedical language representation model for biomedical text mining. *Bioinformatics (Oxford, England)*, *36*(4), 1234–1240. DOI: 10.1093/bioinformatics/btz682 PMID: 31501885

Leonard, S., Wu, K. L., Kim, Y., Krieger, A., & Kim, P. C. (2014). Smart tissue anastomosis robot (STAR): A vision-guided robotics system for laparoscopic suturing. *IEEE Transactions on Biomedical Engineering*, *61*(4), 1305–1317. DOI: 10.1109/TBME.2014.2302385 PMID: 24658254

Levin, S., Toerper, M., Hamrock, E., Hinson, J. S., Barnes, S., Gardner, H., Dugas, A., Linton, B., Kirsch, T., & Kelen, G. (2018). Machine-Learning-Based Electronic Triage More Accurately Differentiates Patients With Respect to Clinical Outcomes Compared With the Emergency Severity Index. *Annals of Emergency Medicine*, *71*(5), 565–574.e2. DOI: 10.1016/j.annemergmed.2017.08.005 PMID: 28888332

Li, Y., Zhang, L., & Liu, Z. (2018). Multi-objective de novo drug design with conditional graph generative model. *Journal of Cheminformatics*, *10*(1), 33. DOI: 10.1186/s13321-018-0287-6 PMID: 30043127

Li, Z., He, Y., Keel, S., Meng, W., Chang, R. T., & He, M. (2018). Efficacy of a deep learning system for detecting glaucomatous optic neuropathy based on color fundus photographs. *Ophthalmology*, *125*(8), 1199–1206. DOI: 10.1016/j.ophtha.2018.01.023 PMID: 29506863

Lim, J., Ryu, S., Park, K., Choe, Y. J., Ham, J., & Kim, W. Y. (2019). Predicting drug–target interaction using a novel graph neural network with 3D structure-embedded graph representation. *Journal of Chemical Information and Modeling*, *59*(9), 3981–3988. DOI: 10.1021/acs.jcim.9b00387 PMID: 31443612

Linte, C. A., Davenport, K. P., Cleary, K., Peters, C., Vosburgh, K. G., Navab, N., & Peters, T. M. (2019). On mixed reality environments for minimally invasive therapy guidance: Systems architecture, successes and challenges in their implementation from laboratory to clinic. *Computerized Medical Imaging and Graphics*, *54*, 45–68. PMID: 23632059

Litjens, G., Kooi, T., Bejnordi, B. E., Setio, A. A. A., Ciompi, F., Ghafoorian, M., van der Laak, J. A. W. M., van Ginneken, B., & Sánchez, C. I. (2017). A survey on deep learning in medical image analysis. *Medical Image Analysis*, *42*, 60–88. DOI: 10.1016/j.media.2017.07.005 PMID: 28778026

Littlejohns, T. J., Holliday, J., Gibson, L. M., Garratt, S., Oesingmann, N., Alfaro-Almagro, F., Bell, J. D., Boultwood, C., Collins, R., Conroy, M. C., Crabtree, N., Doherty, N., Frangi, A. F., Harvey, N. C., Leeson, P., Miller, K. L., Neubauer, S., Petersen, S. E., Sellors, J., & Allen, N. E. (2020). The UK Biobank imaging enhancement of 100,000 participants: Rationale, data collection, management and future directions. *Nature Communications*, *11*(1), 1–12. DOI: 10.1038/s41467-020-15948-9 PMID: 32457287

Liu, F.. (2021). Self-supervised learning for medical image analysis using image context restoration. *Medical Image Analysis*.

Liu, J., Jung, H., Dubra, A., & Tam, J. (2017). Automated photoreceptor cell identification on nonconfocal adaptive optics images using multiscale circular voting. *Investigative Ophthalmology & Visual Science, 58*(11), 4477–4489. DOI: 10.1167/iovs.16-21003 PMID: 28873173

Liu, X.. (2021). Generating Personalized Discharge Instructions using Natural Language Processing and Clinical Guidelines. *Journal of Biomedical Informatics.*

Liu, X., Faes, L., Kale, A. U., Wagner, S. K., Fu, D. J., Bruynseels, A., Mahendiran, T., Moraes, G., Shamdas, M., Kern, C., Ledsam, J. R., Schmid, M. K., Balaskas, K., Topol, E. J., Bachmann, L. M., Keane, P. A., & Denniston, A. K. (2019). A comparison of deep learning performance against health-care professionals in detecting diseases from medical imaging: A systematic review and meta-analysis. *The Lancet. Digital Health, 1*(6), e271–e297. DOI: 10.1016/S2589-7500(19)30123-2 PMID: 33323251

Liu, X., Faes, L., Kale, A. U., Wagner, S. K., Fu, D. J., Bruynseels, A., Mahendiran, T., Moraes, G., Shamdas, M., Kern, C., Ledsam, J. R., Schmid, M. K., Balaskas, K., Topol, E. J., Bachmann, L. M., Keane, P. A., & Denniston, A. K. (2019). A comparison of deep learning performance against health-care professionals in detecting diseases from medical imaging: A systematic review and meta-analysis. *The Lancet. Digital Health, 1*(6), e271–e297. DOI: 10.1016/S2589-7500(19)30123-2 PMID: 33323251

Liu, Y., & Lapata, M. Text summarization with pretrained encoders. In *Proceedings of the 2019 Conference on Empirical Methods in Natural Language Processing*. 2019.

Lundberg, S. M., Erion, G., Chen, H., DeGrave, A., Prutkin, J. M., Nair, B., Katz, R., Himmelfarb, J., Bansal, N., & Lee, S.-I. (2020). From local explanations to global understanding with explainable AI for trees. *Nature Machine Intelligence, 2*(1), 56–67. DOI: 10.1038/s42256-019-0138-9 PMID: 32607472

Lundberg, S. M., & Lee, S. I. (2017). A unified approach to interpreting model predictions. In Advances in neural information processing systems (pp. 4765-4774).

Lundberg, S. M., Nair, B., Vavilala, M. S., Horibe, M., Eisses, M. J., Adams, T., Liston, D. E., Low, D. K.-W., Newman, S.-F., Kim, J., & Lee, S. I. (2018). Explainable machine-learning predictions for the prevention of hypoxaemia during surgery. *Nature Biomedical Engineering, 2*(10), 749–760. DOI: 10.1038/s41551-018-0304-0 PMID: 31001455

Maier-Hein, L., Vedula, S. S., Speidel, S., Navab, N., Kikinis, R., Park, A., Eisenmann, M., Feussner, H., Forestier, G., Giannarou, S., Hashizume, M., Katic, D., Kenngott, H., Kranzfelder, M., Malpani, A., März, K., Neumuth, T., Padoy, N., Pugh, C., & Jannin, P. (2017). Surgical data science for next-generation interventions. *Nature Biomedical Engineering, 1*(9), 691–696. DOI: 10.1038/s41551-017-0132-7 PMID: 31015666

Martí-Bonmatí, L., Sopena, R., Bartumeus, P., & Sopena, P. (2010). Multimodality imaging techniques. *Contrast Media & Molecular Imaging, 5*(4), 180–189. DOI: 10.1002/cmmi.393 PMID: 20812286

McKinney, S. M., Sieniek, M., Godbole, V., Godwin, J., Antropova, N., Ashrafian, H., Back, T., Chesus, M., Corrado, G. S., Darzi, A., Etemadi, M., Garcia-Vicente, F., Gilbert, F. J., Halling-Brown, M., Hassabis, D., Jansen, S., Karthikesalingam, A., Kelly, C. J., King, D., & Shetty, S. (2020). International evaluation of an AI system for breast cancer screening. *Nature, 577*(7788), 89–94. DOI: 10.1038/s41586-019-1799-6 PMID: 31894144

Mei, X., Lee, H. C., Diao, K. Y., Huang, M., Lin, B., Liu, C., Xie, Z., Ma, Y., Robson, P. M., Chung, M., Bernheim, A., Mani, V., Calcagno, C., Li, K., Li, S., Shan, H., Lv, J., Zhao, T., Xia, J., & Yang, Y. (2020). Artificial intelligence-enabled rapid diagnosis of patients with COVID-19. *Nature Medicine*, *26*(8), 1224–1228. DOI: 10.1038/s41591-020-0931-3 PMID: 32427924

Menze, B. H., Jakab, A., Bauer, S., Kalpathy-Cramer, J., Farahani, K., Kirby, J., Burren, Y., Porz, N., Slotboom, J., Wiest, R., Lanczi, L., Gerstner, E., Weber, M.-A., Arbel, T., Avants, B. B., Ayache, N., Buendia, P., Collins, D. L., Cordier, N., & Van Leemput, K. (2015). The multimodal brain tumor image segmentation benchmark (BRATS). *IEEE Transactions on Medical Imaging*, *34*(10), 1993–2024. DOI: 10.1109/TMI.2014.2377694 PMID: 25494501

Meola, A., Cutolo, F., Carbone, M., Cagnazzo, F., Ferrari, M., & Ferrari, V. (2017). Augmented reality in neurosurgery: A systematic review. *Neurosurgical Review*, *40*(4), 537–548. DOI: 10.1007/s10143-016-0732-9 PMID: 27154018

Merk, D., Friedrich, L., Grisoni, F., & Schneider, G. (2018). De novo design of bioactive small molecules by artificial intelligence. *Molecular Informatics*, *37*(1-2), 1700153. DOI: 10.1002/minf.201700153 PMID: 29319225

Meystre, S. M., Lovis, C., Bürkle, T., Tognola, G., Budrionis, A., & Lehmann, C. U. (2017). Clinical data reuse or secondary use: Current status and potential future progress. *Yearbook of Medical Informatics*, *26*(1), 38–52. DOI: 10.15265/IY-2017-007 PMID: 28480475

Miotto, R., Li, L., Kidd, B. A., & Dudley, J. T. (2016). Deep Patient: An Unsupervised Representation to Predict the Future of Patients from the Electronic Health Records. *Scientific Reports*, *6*(1), 26094. DOI: 10.1038/srep26094 PMID: 27185194

Miotto, R., Wang, F., Wang, S., Jiang, X., & Dudley, J. T. (2018). Deep learning for healthcare: Review, opportunities and challenges. *Briefings in Bioinformatics*, *19*(6), 1236–1246. DOI: 10.1093/bib/bbx044 PMID: 28481991

Mullenbach, J., Wiegreffe, S., Duke, J., Sun, J., & Eisenstein, J. (2018). Explainable prediction of medical codes from clinical text. arXiv preprint arXiv:1802.05695. DOI: 10.18653/v1/N18-1100

Müller, M., Salathé, M., & Kummervold, P. E. (2023). Covid-twitter-bert: A natural language processing model to analyse covid-19 content on twitter. *Frontiers in Artificial Intelligence*, *6*, 1023281.

Murdoch, T. B., & Detsky, A. S. (2013). The inevitable application of big data to health care. *Journal of the American Medical Association*, *309*(13), 1351–1352. DOI: 10.1001/jama.2013.393 PMID: 23549579

Najafi, M., Abolmaesumi, P., & Rohling, R. (2019). Single-camera closed-form real-time needle tracking for ultrasound-guided needle insertion. *Ultrasound in Medicine & Biology*, *45*(6), 1429–1443. PMID: 26215491

Nemati, S., Holder, A., Razmi, F., Stanley, M. D., Clifford, G. D., & Buchman, T. G. (2018). An Interpretable Machine Learning Model for Accurate Prediction of Sepsis in the ICU. *Critical Care Medicine*, *46*(4), 547–553. DOI: 10.1097/CCM.0000000000002936 PMID: 29286945

Norgeot, B., Glicksberg, B. S., & Butte, A. J. (2019). A call for deep-learning healthcare. *Nature Medicine, 25*(1), 14–15. DOI: 10.1038/s41591-018-0320-3 PMID: 30617337

Obermeyer, Z., Powers, B., Vogeli, C., & Mullainathan, S. (2019). Dissecting racial bias in an algorithm used to manage the health of populations. *Science, 366*(6464), 447–453. DOI: 10.1126/science.aax2342 PMID: 31649194

Olivecrona, M., Blaschke, T., Engkvist, O., & Chen, H. (2017). Molecular de-novo design through deep reinforcement learning. *Journal of Cheminformatics, 9*(1), 48. DOI: 10.1186/s13321-017-0235-x PMID: 29086083

Orlando, J. I., Fu, H., & Breda, J. B.. (2020). REFUGE Challenge: A unified framework for evaluating automated methods for glaucoma assessment from fundus photographs. *Medical Image Analysis, 59*, 101570. DOI: 10.1016/j.media.2019.101570 PMID: 31630011

Osheroff, J. A., Teich, J. M., Middleton, B., Steen, E. B., Wright, A., & Detmer, D. E. (2007). A roadmap for national action on clinical decision support. *Journal of the American Medical Informatics Association : JAMIA, 14*(2), 141–145. DOI: 10.1197/jamia.M2334 PMID: 17213487

Öztürk, H., Özgür, A., & Ozkirimli, E. (2018). DeepDTA: Deep drug–target binding affinity prediction. *Bioinformatics (Oxford, England), 34*(17), i821–i829. DOI: 10.1093/bioinformatics/bty593 PMID: 30423097

Palanica, A., Flaschner, P., Thommandram, A., Li, M., & Fossat, Y. (2019). Physicians' Perceptions of Chatbots in Health Care: Cross-Sectional Web-Based Survey. *Journal of Medical Internet Research, 21*(4), e12887. DOI: 10.2196/12887 PMID: 30950796

Pallmann, P., Bedding, A. W., Choodari-Oskooei, B., Dimairo, M., Flight, L., Hampson, L. V., Holmes, J., Mander, A. P., Odondi, L., Sydes, M. R., Villar, S. S., Wason, J. M. S., Weir, C. J., Wheeler, G. M., Yap, C., & Jaki, T. (2018). Adaptive designs in clinical trials: Why use them, and how to run and report them. *BMC Medicine, 16*(1), 29. DOI: 10.1186/s12916-018-1017-7 PMID: 29490655

Paré, G., Mao, S., & Deng, W. Q. (2017). A machine-learning heuristic to improve gene score prediction of polygenic traits. *Scientific Reports, 7*(1), 12665. DOI: 10.1038/s41598-017-13056-1 PMID: 28979001

Patel, M. I.. (2020). Using Natural Language Processing to Extract Structured Epilepsy Data From Unstructured Clinic Letters: Development and Validation of an Open-Source Tool. *JMIR Medical Informatics.*

Pauws, S.. (2019). Personalized health communication: A novel approach for effective promotion of health and well-being. *Journal of Biomedical Informatics.*

Payrovnaziri, S. N., Chen, Z., Rengifo-Moreno, P., Miller, T., Bian, J., Chen, J. H., Liu, X., & He, Z. (2020). Explainable artificial intelligence models using real-world electronic health record data: A systematic scoping review. *Journal of the American Medical Informatics Association : JAMIA, 27*(7), 1173–1185. DOI: 10.1093/jamia/ocaa053 PMID: 32417928

Pena, M., & Duran, A. (2020). Artificial Intelligence in Supply Chain Management in Health. *Studies in Health Technology and Informatics, 270*, 56–60.

Perlasca, P., Farina, G., Allen, F., Manzoni, M., Liò, P., & Gnocchi, M. (2019). Integrating multi-omics data with graph convolutional networks to identify new cancer genes and their associated molecular mechanisms. *Nature Machine Intelligence*, *1*(8), 375–384.

Perry, B., Herrington, W., Goldsack, J. C., Grandinetti, C. A., Vasisht, K. P., Landray, M. J., & Moline, M. (2018). Use of mobile devices to measure outcomes in clinical research, 2010–2016: A systematic literature review. *Digital Biomarkers*, *2*(1), 11–30. DOI: 10.1159/000486347 PMID: 29938250

Phillips, M., Marsden, H., Jaffe, W., Matin, R. N., Wali, G. N., Greenhalgh, J., McGrath, E., James, R., Ladoyanni, E., Bewley, A., Argenziano, G., & Palamaras, I. (2019). Assessment of accuracy of an artificial intelligence algorithm to detect melanoma in images of skin lesions. *JAMA Network Open*, *2*(10), e1913436. DOI: 10.1001/jamanetworkopen.2019.13436 PMID: 31617929

Plis, S. M., Hjelm, D. R., & Salakhutdinov, R.. (2018). Deep learning for neuroimaging: A validation study. *Frontiers in Neuroscience*, *8*, 229. PMID: 25191215

Poplin, R., Varadarajan, A. V., Blumer, K., Liu, Y., McConnell, M. V., Corrado, G. S., Peng, L., & Webster, D. R. (2018). Prediction of cardiovascular risk factors from retinal fundus photographs via deep learning. *Nature Biomedical Engineering*, *2*(3), 158–164. DOI: 10.1038/s41551-018-0195-0 PMID: 31015713

Pratapa, A., Jalihal, A. P., Law, J. N., Bharadwaj, A., & Murali, T. M. (2021). Benchmarking algorithms for gene regulatory network inference from single-cell transcriptomic data. *Nature Methods*, *18*(3), 321–332. PMID: 33526888

Price, W. N.II, & Cohen, I. G. (2019). Privacy in the age of medical big data. *Nature Medicine*, *25*(1), 37–43. DOI: 10.1038/s41591-018-0272-7 PMID: 30617331

Price, W. N.II, Gerke, S., & Cohen, I. G. (2019). Potential liability for physicians using artificial intelligence. *Journal of the American Medical Association*, *322*(18), 1765–1766. DOI: 10.1001/jama.2019.15064 PMID: 31584609

Pushpakom, S., Iorio, F., Eyers, P. A., Escott, K. J., Hopper, S., Wells, A., Doig, A., Guilliams, T., Latimer, J., McNamee, C., Norris, A., Sanseau, P., Cavalla, D., & Pirmohamed, M. (2019). Drug repurposing: Progress, challenges and recommendations. *Nature Reviews. Drug Discovery*, *18*(1), 41–58. DOI: 10.1038/nrd.2018.168 PMID: 30310233

Qian, L., Barthel, A., Johnson, A., Osgood, G., Kazanzides, P., Navab, N., & Fuerst, B. (2018). Comparison of optical see-through head-mounted displays for surgical interventions with object-anchored 2D-display. *International Journal of Computer Assisted Radiology and Surgery*, *13*(6), 881–890. PMID: 28343301

Quer, G., Radin, J. M., Gadaleta, M., Baca-Motes, K., Ariniello, L., Ramos, E., Kheterpal, V., Topol, E. J., & Steinhubl, S. R. (2021). Wearable sensor data and self-reported symptoms for COVID-19 detection. *Nature Medicine*, *27*(1), 73–77. DOI: 10.1038/s41591-020-1123-x PMID: 33122860

Quiroz, J. C., Laranjo, L., Kocaballi, A. B., Berkovsky, S., Rezazadegan, D., & Coiera, E. (2019). Challenges of developing a digital scribe to reduce clinical documentation burden. *NPJ Digital Medicine*, *2*(1), 114. DOI: 10.1038/s41746-019-0190-1 PMID: 31799422

Raghavan, P.. (2014). Temporal Information Extraction from Clinical Text. *Journal of the American Medical Informatics Association : JAMIA*.

Rajkomar, A., Dean, J., & Kohane, I. (2019). Machine learning in medicine. *The New England Journal of Medicine*, *380*(14), 1347–1358. DOI: 10.1056/NEJMra1814259 PMID: 30943338

Rajkomar, A., Hardt, M., Howell, M. D., Corrado, G., & Chin, M. H. (2018). Ensuring fairness in machine learning to advance health equity. *Annals of Internal Medicine*, *169*(12), 866–872. DOI: 10.7326/M18-1990 PMID: 30508424

Rajkomar, A., Oren, E., Chen, K., Dai, A. M., Hajaj, N., Hardt, M., Liu, P. J., Liu, X., Marcus, J., Sun, M., Sundberg, P., Yee, H., Zhang, K., Zhang, Y., Flores, G., Duggan, G. E., Irvine, J., Le, Q., Litsch, K., & Dean, J. (2018). Scalable and accurate deep learning with electronic health records. *NPJ Digital Medicine*, *1*(1), 18. DOI: 10.1038/s41746-018-0029-1 PMID: 31304302

Rajpurkar, P., Irvin, J., Zhu, K., Yang, B., Mehta, H., Duan, T., . . . Ng, A. Y. (2017). Chexnet: Radiologist-level pneumonia detection on chest x-rays with deep learning. arXiv preprint arXiv:1711.05225.

Rappoport, N., & Shamir, R. (2018). Multi-omic and multi-view clustering algorithms: Review and cancer benchmark. *Nucleic Acids Research*, *46*(20), 10546–10562. DOI: 10.1093/nar/gky889 PMID: 30295871

Raumviboonsuk, P., Krause, J., & Chotcomwongse, P.. (2019). Deep learning versus human graders for classifying diabetic retinopathy severity in a nationwide screening program. *NPJ Digital Medicine*, *2*(1), 1–9. PMID: 31304372

Ravì, D.. (2019). Deep Learning for Health Informatics. *IEEE Journal of Biomedical and Health Informatics*. PMID: 28055930

Relling, M. V., & Evans, W. E. (2015). Pharmacogenomics in the clinic. *Nature*, *526*(7573), 343–350. DOI: 10.1038/nature15817 PMID: 26469045

Renfro, L. A., & Sargent, D. J. (2017). Statistical controversies in clinical research: basket trials, umbrella trials, and other master protocols: a review and examples. *Annals of Oncology : Official Journal of the European Society for Medical Oncology*, *28*(1), 34–43. DOI: 10.1093/annonc/mdw413 PMID: 28177494

Ribeiro, M. T., Singh, S., & Guestrin, C. (2016). "Why should I trust you?" Explaining the predictions of any classifier. In Proceedings of the 22nd ACM SIGKDD International Conference on Knowledge Discovery and Data Mining (pp. 1135-1144).

Rieke, N., Hancox, J., Li, W., Milletarì, F., Roth, H. R., Albarqouni, S., Bakas, S., Galtier, M. N., Landman, B. A., Maier-Hein, K., Ourselin, S., Sheller, M., Summers, R. M., Trask, A., Xu, D., Baust, M., & Cardoso, M. J. (2020). The future of digital health with federated learning. *NPJ Digital Medicine*, *3*(1), 119. DOI: 10.1038/s41746-020-00323-1 PMID: 33015372

Riga, C. V., Bicknell, C. D., Rolls, A., Cheshire, N. J., & Hamady, M. S. (2012). Robot-assisted fenestrated endovascular aneurysm repair (FEVAR) using the Magellan system. *Journal of Vascular and Interventional Radiology*, *23*(10), 1365–1367. PMID: 22920731

Rigby, M. J. (2019). Ethical dimensions of using artificial intelligence in health care. *AMA Journal of Ethics*, *21*(2), 121–124. DOI: 10.1001/amajethics.2019.121

Rodríguez-Pérez, R., & Bajorath, J. (2020). Interpretation of compound activity predictions from complex machine learning models using local approximations and shapley values. *Journal of Medicinal Chemistry*, *63*(16), 8761–8777. DOI: 10.1021/acs.jmedchem.9b01101 PMID: 31512867

Rotmensch, M., Halpern, Y., Tlimat, A., Horng, S., & Sontag, D. (2017). Learning a health knowledge graph from electronic medical records. *Scientific Reports*, *7*(1), 1–11. DOI: 10.1038/s41598-017-05778-z PMID: 28729710

Russell, S., & Norvig, P. (2020). *Artificial Intelligence: A Modern Approach* (4th ed.). Pearson.

Santillana, M., Nguyen, A. T., Dredze, M., Paul, M. J., Nsoesie, E. O., & Brownstein, J. S. (2015). Combining Search, Social Media, and Traditional Data Sources to Improve Influenza Surveillance. *PLoS Computational Biology*, *11*(10), e1004513. DOI: 10.1371/journal.pcbi.1004513 PMID: 26513245

Sayres, R., Taly, A., Rahimy, E., Blumer, K., Coz, D., Hammel, N., Krause, J., Narayanaswamy, A., Rastegar, Z., Wu, D., Xu, S., Barb, S., Joseph, A., Shumski, M., Smith, J., Sood, A. B., Corrado, G. S., Peng, L., & Webster, D. R. (2019). Using a deep learning algorithm and integrated gradients explanation to assist grading for diabetic retinopathy. *Ophthalmology*, *126*(4), 552–564. DOI: 10.1016/j.ophtha.2018.11.016 PMID: 30553900

Schmidt-Erfurth, U., Sadeghipour, A., Gerendas, B. S., Waldstein, S. M., & Bogunović, H. (2018). Artificial intelligence in retina. *Progress in Retinal and Eye Research*, *67*, 1–29. DOI: 10.1016/j.preteyeres.2018.07.004 PMID: 30076935

Schneider, G. (2018). Automating drug discovery. *Nature Reviews. Drug Discovery*, *17*(2), 97–113. DOI: 10.1038/nrd.2017.232 PMID: 29242609

Schork, N. J. (2015). Personalized medicine: Time for one-person trials. *Nature*, *520*(7549), 609–611. DOI: 10.1038/520609a PMID: 25925459

Schork, N. J. (2019). Artificial Intelligence and Personalized Medicine. *Cancer Treatment and Research*, *178*, 265–283. DOI: 10.1007/978-3-030-16391-4_11 PMID: 31209850

Shademan, A., Decker, R. S., Opfermann, J. D., Leonard, S., Krieger, A., & Kim, P. C. (2016). Supervised autonomous robotic soft tissue surgery. *Science Translational Medicine*, *8*(337), 337ra64. DOI: 10.1126/scitranslmed.aad9398 PMID: 27147588

Shakil, S., Ghosh, J., Singh, K., & Roy Choudhury, S. (2024). *Comparative analysis of nutritional status among institutionalized and community-dwelling elderly women and its* association with mental health status and cognitive function. *Journal of Family Medicine and Primary Care*, *13*(8), 3078–3083. Advance online publication. DOI: 10.4103/jfmpc.jfmpc_1932_23 PMID: 39228576

Shanafelt, T. D., Dyrbye, L. N., Sinsky, C., Hasan, O., Satele, D., Sloan, J., & West, C. P. (2016). Relationship between clerical burden and characteristics of the electronic environment with physician burnout and professional satisfaction. *Mayo Clinic Proceedings*, *91*(7), 836–848. DOI: 10.1016/j.mayocp.2016.05.007 PMID: 27313121

Sharifi-Noghabi, H., Zolotareva, O., Collins, C. C., & Ester, M. (2019). MOLI: Multi-omics late integration with deep neural networks for drug response prediction. *Bioinformatics (Oxford, England)*, *35*(14), i501–i509. DOI: 10.1093/bioinformatics/btz318 PMID: 31510700

Sheikhalishahi, S., Miotto, R., & Dudley, J. T.. (2019). Natural Language Processing for Clinical Applications: A State of the Art Review. *JMIR Medical Informatics*, *7*(2), e11879. DOI: 10.2196/12239 PMID: 31066697

Sheikhalishahi, S., Miotto, R., Dudley, J. T., Lavelli, A., Rinaldi, F., & Osmani, V. (2019). Natural Language Processing of Clinical Notes on Chronic Diseases: Systematic Review. *JMIR Medical Informatics*, *7*(2), e12239. DOI: 10.2196/12239 PMID: 31066697

Sheller, M. J., Reina, G. A., Edwards, B., Martin, J., & Bakas, S. (2018). Multi-institutional deep learning modeling without sharing patient data: A feasibility study on brain tumor segmentation. In *International MICCAI Brainlesion Workshop* (pp. 92-104). Springer, Cham.

Shen, F., Zhao, Y., & Wang, L.. (2019). Rare disease diagnosis as an information retrieval task. *Journal of Biomedical Informatics*, *94*, 103109.

Sherman, R. E., Anderson, S. A., Dal Pan, G. J., Gray, G. W., Gross, T., Hunter, N. L., LaVange, L., Marinac-Dabic, D., Marks, P. W., Robb, M. A., Shuren, J., Temple, R., Woodcock, J., Yue, L. Q., & Califf, R. M. (2016). Real-world evidence—What is it and what can it tell us? *The New England Journal of Medicine*, *375*(23), 2293–2297. DOI: 10.1056/NEJMsb1609216 PMID: 27959688

Shickel, B.. (2021). DeepSOFA: A Continuous Acuity Score for Critically Ill Patients using Clinically Interpretable Deep Learning. *Scientific Reports*. PMID: 30755689

Shin, H. C., Roth, H. R., Gao, M., Lu, L., Xu, Z., Nogues, I., Yao, J., Mollura, D., & Summers, R. M. (2016). Deep convolutional neural networks for computer-aided detection: CNN architectures, dataset characteristics and transfer learning. *IEEE Transactions on Medical Imaging*, *35*(5), 1285–1298. DOI: 10.1109/TMI.2016.2528162 PMID: 26886976

Shin, S. Y., Seo, D.-W., An, J., Kwak, H., Kim, S.-H., Gwack, J., & Jo, M.-W. (2016). High correlation of Middle East respiratory syndrome spread with Google search and Twitter trends in Korea. *Scientific Reports*, *6*(1), 32920. DOI: 10.1038/srep32920 PMID: 27595921

Shortliffe, E. H., & Sepúlveda, M. J. (2018). Clinical Decision Support in the Era of Artificial Intelligence. *Journal of the American Medical Association*, *320*(21), 2199–2200. DOI: 10.1001/jama.2018.17163 PMID: 30398550

Shrestha, P., Shrestha, S., & Phuyal, R. (2020). Artificial Intelligence in Medical Billing and Coding: A Systematic Review. *Studies in Health Technology and Informatics*, *272*, 245–248.

Siegel, R. L., Miller, K. D., Fuchs, H. E., & Jemal, A. (2021). Cancer statistics, 2021. *CA: a Cancer Journal for Clinicians*, *71*(1), 7–33. DOI: 10.3322/caac.21654 PMID: 33433946

Singh, H., Meyer, A. N., & Thomas, E. J. (2014). The frequency of diagnostic errors in outpatient care: Estimations from three large observational studies involving US adult populations. *BMJ Quality & Safety*, *23*(9), 727–731. DOI: 10.1136/bmjqs-2013-002627 PMID: 24742777

Staker, J., Marshall, G. R., Suffian, D. J., & Parrill-Baker, A. L. (2020). Molecular design via deep learning: A large-scale study on therapeutic antibody binding affinity prediction. *Journal of Chemical Information and Modeling*, *60*(10), 4487–4503. PMID: 32697578

Suhl, J. A., Markunas, C. A., Greer, C. B., Szatkiewicz, J. P., & Zhu, H. (2019). Genomic-epigenomic integration to detect DNAm-SNP association. *Bioinformatics (Oxford, England)*, *35*(14), i481–i489.

Thorlund, K., Dron, L., Park, J. J., & Mills, E. J. (2020). Synthetic and external controls in clinical trials–a primer for researchers. *Clinical Epidemiology*, *12*, 457–467. DOI: 10.2147/CLEP.S242097 PMID: 32440224

Ting, D. S. W., Pasquale, L. R., Peng, L., Campbell, J. P., Lee, A. Y., Raman, R., Tan, G. S. W., Schmetterer, L., Keane, P. A., & Wong, T. Y. (2019). Artificial intelligence and deep learning in ophthalmology. *The British Journal of Ophthalmology*, *103*(2), 167–175. DOI: 10.1136/bjophthalmol-2018-313173 PMID: 30361278

Tison, G. H.. (2020). Cardiovascular Risk Stratification Using Off-the-Shelf Wearables and a Multi-Task Deep Learning Algorithm. *Circulation*.

Tiwana, M. I., Redmond, S. J., & Lovell, N. H. (2012). A review of tactile sensing technologies with applications in biomedical engineering. *Sensors and Actuators. A, Physical*, *179*, 17–31. DOI: 10.1016/j.sna.2012.02.051

Tonekaboni, S., Joshi, S., McCradden, M. D., & Goldenberg, A. (2019). What clinicians want: contextualizing explainable machine learning for clinical end use. arXiv preprint arXiv:1905.05134.

Topol, E. J. (2019). High-performance medicine: The convergence of human and artificial intelligence. *Nature Medicine*, *25*(1), 44–56. DOI: 10.1038/s41591-018-0300-7 PMID: 30617339

Townend, D. (2018). Conclusion: harmonisation in genomic and health data sharing for research: an impossible dream? Human Genetics, 137(8), 657-664.4. Challenges and Ethical Considerations

Tsafnat, G.. (2013). Computerized clinical decision support systems for therapeutic drug monitoring and dosing: A decision-maker-researcher partnership systematic review. *PLoS One*.

Urbina, F., Lentzos, F., Invernizzi, C., & Ekins, S. (2021). Dual use of artificial-intelligence-powered drug discovery. *Nature Machine Intelligence*, *3*(12), 1021–1025. PMID: 36211133

U.S. Food and Drug Administration. (2021). *Artificial Intelligence/Machine Learning (AI/ML)-Based Software as a Medical Device (SaMD)*. Action Plan. FDA.

U.S. Food and Drug Administration. (2021). Artificial Intelligence/Machine Learning (AI/ML)-Based Software as a Medical Device (SaMD) Action Plan. Retrieved from https://www.fda.gov/media/145022/download

Vamathevan, J., Clark, D., Czodrowski, P., Dunham, I., Ferran, E., Lee, G., Li, B., Madabhushi, A., Shah, P., Spitzer, M., & Zhao, S. (2019). Applications of machine learning in drug discovery and development. *Nature Reviews. Drug Discovery*, *18*(6), 463–477. DOI: 10.1038/s41573-019-0024-5 PMID: 30976107

Vayena, E., Blasimme, A., & Cohen, I. G. (2018). Machine learning in medicine: Addressing ethical challenges. *PLoS Medicine, 15*(11), e1002689. DOI: 10.1371/journal.pmed.1002689 PMID: 30399149

Venkatraghavan, V., Bron, E. E., Niessen, W. J., & Klein, S. (2019). Disease progression timeline estimation for Alzheimer's disease using discriminative event based modeling. *NeuroImage, 186*, 518–532. DOI: 10.1016/j.neuroimage.2018.11.024 PMID: 30471388

Wahl, B., Cossy-Gantner, A., Germann, S., & Schwalbe, N. R. (2018). Artificial intelligence (AI) and global health: How can AI contribute to health in resource-poor settings? *BMJ Global Health, 3*(4), e000798. DOI: 10.1136/bmjgh-2018-000798 PMID: 30233828

Wan, F., Hong, L., Xiao, A., Jiang, T., & Zeng, J. (2019). NeoDTI: Neural integration of neighbor information from a heterogeneous network for discovering new drug–target interactions. *Bioinformatics (Oxford, England), 35*(1), 104–111. DOI: 10.1093/bioinformatics/bty543 PMID: 30561548

Willemink, M. J., Koszek, W. A., Hardell, C., Wu, J., Fleischmann, D., Harvey, H., Folio, L. R., Summers, R. M., Rubin, D. L., & Lungren, M. P. (2020). Preparing medical imaging data for machine learning. *Radiology, 295*(1), 4–15. DOI: 10.1148/radiol.2020192224 PMID: 32068507

Wilmanski, T., Rappaport, N., Earls, J. C., Magis, A. T., Manor, O., Lovejoy, J., Omenn, G. S., Hood, L., Gibbons, S. M., & Price, N. D. (2019). Blood metabolome predicts gut microbiome α-diversity in humans. *Nature Biotechnology, 37*(10), 1217–1228. DOI: 10.1038/s41587-019-0233-9 PMID: 31477923

Winkler, J. K., Fink, C., Toberer, F., Enk, A., Deinlein, T., Hofmann-Wellenhof, R., Thomas, L., Lallas, A., Blum, A., Stolz, W., & Haenssle, H. A. (2020). Association between surgical skin markings in dermoscopic images and diagnostic performance of a deep learning convolutional neural network for melanoma recognition. *JAMA Dermatology, 155*(10), 1135–1141. DOI: 10.1001/jamadermatol.2019.1735 PMID: 31411641

Wong, T. Y., Bressler, N. M., & Ahmed, I. I. K. (2016). Optical coherence tomography angiography. *Nature Reviews. Disease Primers, 2*(1), 1–18.

Woodcock, J., & LaVange, L. M. (2017). Master protocols to study multiple therapies, multiple diseases, or both. *The New England Journal of Medicine, 377*(1), 62–70. DOI: 10.1056/NEJMra1510062 PMID: 28679092

Wu, S., Roberts, K., Datta, S., Du, J., Ji, Z., Si, Y., Soni, S., Wang, Q., Wei, Q., Xiang, Y., Zhao, B., & Xu, H. (2020). Deep learning in clinical natural language processing: A methodical review. *Journal of the American Medical Informatics Association : JAMIA, 27*(3), 457–470. DOI: 10.1093/jamia/ocz200 PMID: 31794016

Würstle, M. L., Petzold, E., Becker, A., & Müller, O. J. (2021). Artificial intelligence in clinical decision support: A focused literature survey. *Artificial Intelligence in Medicine, 121*, 102199.

Xu, J., Yang, P., Xue, S., Sharma, B., Sanchez-Martin, M., Wang, F., Beaty, K. A., Dehan, E., & Parikh, B. (2019). Translating cancer genomics into precision medicine with artificial intelligence: Applications, challenges and future perspectives. *Human Genetics, 138*(2), 109–124. DOI: 10.1007/s00439-019-01970-5 PMID: 30671672

Xu, J., Yang, P., Xue, S., Sharma, B., Sanchez-Martin, M., Wang, F., & Parikh, B. (2020). Translating cancer genomics into precision medicine with artificial intelligence: Applications, challenges and future perspectives. *Human Genetics*, *139*(6), 803–818. PMID: 30671672

Xu, Y., Hosny, A., Zeleznik, R., Parmar, C., Coroller, T., Franco, I., Mak, R. H., & Aerts, H. J. W. L. (2019). Deep learning predicts lung cancer treatment response from serial medical imaging. *Clinical Cancer Research*, *25*(11), 3266–3275. DOI: 10.1158/1078-0432.CCR-18-2495 PMID: 31010833

Yala, A., Lehman, C., Schuster, T., Portnoi, T., & Barzilay, R. (2019). A deep learning mammography-based model for improved breast cancer risk prediction. *Radiology*, *292*(1), 60–66. DOI: 10.1148/radiol.2019182716 PMID: 31063083

Yan, A., McAuley, J., Lu, X., Du, J., Chang, E. Y., Gentili, A., & Hsu, C. N. (2022). RadBERT: Adapting transformer-based language models to radiology. *Radiology. Artificial Intelligence*, *4*(4), e210258.

Yan, J., Risacher, S. L., Shen, L., & Saykin, A. J. (2018). Network approaches to systems biology analysis of complex disease: Integrative methods for multi-omics data. *Briefings in Bioinformatics*, *19*(6), 1370–1381. PMID: 28679163

Yang, Z., Zeng, Z., Wang, K., Wong, S.-S., Liang, W., Zanin, M., Liu, P., Cao, X., Gao, Z., Mai, Z., Liang, J., Liu, X., Li, S., Li, Y., Ye, F., Guan, W., Yang, Y., Li, F., Luo, S., & He, J. (2020). Modified SEIR and AI prediction of the epidemics trend of COVID-19 in China under public health interventions. *Journal of Thoracic Disease*, *12*(3), 165–174. DOI: 10.21037/jtd.2020.02.64 PMID: 32274081

Yim, J., Chopra, R., Spitz, T., Winkens, J., Obika, A., Kelly, C., Askham, H., Lukic, M., Huemer, J., Fasler, K., Moraes, G., Meyer, C., Wilson, M., Dixon, J., Hughes, C., Rees, G., Khaw, P. T., Karthikesalingam, A., King, D., & De Fauw, J. (2020). Predicting conversion to wet age-related macular degeneration using deep learning. *Nature Medicine*, *26*(6), 892–899. DOI: 10.1038/s41591-020-0867-7 PMID: 32424211

Young, A. T., Xiong, M., & Pfau, J.. (2019). Artificial intelligence in dermatology: A primer. *The Journal of Investigative Dermatology*, *139*(8), 1617–1628. PMID: 32229141

Young, A. T., Xiong, M., Pfau, J., Keiser, M. J., & Wei, M. L. (2019). Artificial intelligence in dermatology: A primer. *The Journal of Investigative Dermatology*, *139*(8), 1617–1628. PMID: 32229141

Yu, K. H., Beam, A. L., & Kohane, I. S. (2018). Artificial intelligence in healthcare. *Nature Biomedical Engineering*, *2*(10), 719–731. DOI: 10.1038/s41551-018-0305-z PMID: 31015651

Zhan, C.. (2022). Medical Knowledge Graph Enhancement by Concept-based Explanations of Language Models. arXiv:2205.06958.

Zhang, Y.. (2022). Federated Learning for Healthcare: Systematic Review and Open Challenges. *ACM Computing Surveys*.

Zhang, Z.. Optimizing the factual correctness of a summary: A study of summarizing radiology reports. In *Proceedings of the 58th Annual Meeting of the Association for Computational Linguistics*. 2020. DOI: 10.18653/v1/2020.acl-main.458

Zhao, L., Zhao, Y., Deng, M., Song, Z., Xiao, Y., Li, X., & Qiu, B. (2020). A machine learning-based method for preoperative prediction of postoperative liver dysfunction after hepatectomy. *Frontiers in Oncology*, *10*, 1420.

Zhao, P., Yoo, I., Lavoie, J., Lavoie, B. J., & Simoes, E. (2017). Web-Based Medical Appointment Systems: A Systematic Review. *Journal of Medical Internet Research*, *19*(4), e134. DOI: 10.2196/jmir.6747 PMID: 28446422

Zhavoronkov, A., Ivanenkov, Y. A., Aliper, A., Veselov, M. S., Aladinskiy, V. A., Aladinskaya, A. V., Terentiev, V. A., Polykovskiy, D. A., Kuznetsov, M. D., Asadulaev, A., Volkov, Y., Zholus, A., Shayakhmetov, R. R., Zhebrak, A., Minaeva, L. I., Zagribelnyy, B. A., Lee, L. H., Soll, R., Madge, D., & Aspuru-Guzik, A. (2019). Deep learning enables rapid identification of potent DDR1 kinase inhibitors. *Nature Biotechnology*, *37*(9), 1038–1040. DOI: 10.1038/s41587-019-0224-x PMID: 31477924

Zhavoronkov, A., Ivanenkov, Y. A., Aliper, A., Veselov, M. S., Aladinskiy, V. A., Aladinskaya, A. V., Terentiev, V. A., Polykovskiy, D. A., Kuznetsov, M. D., Asadulaev, A., Volkov, Y., Zholus, A., Shayakhmetov, R. R., Zhebrak, A., Minaeva, L. I., Zagribelnyy, B. A., Lee, L. H., Soll, R., Madge, D., & Aspuru-Guzik, A. (2019). Deep learning enables rapid identification of potent DDR1 kinase inhibitors. *Nature Biotechnology*, *37*(9), 1038–1040. DOI: 10.1038/s41587-019-0224-x PMID: 31477924

Zhou, Z., Kearnes, S., Li, L., Zare, R. N., & Riley, P. (2019). Optimization of molecules via deep reinforcement learning. *Scientific Reports*, *9*(1), 10752. DOI: 10.1038/s41598-019-47148-x PMID: 31341196

Zou, J., Huss, M., Abid, A., Mohammadi, P., Torkamani, A., & Telenti, A. (2019). A primer on deep learning in genomics. *Nature Genetics*, *51*(1), 12–18. DOI: 10.1038/s41588-018-0295-5 PMID: 30478442

Chapter 21
Brain Tumor-Level Detection in 3D MRI Images:
An Advanced Approach for Analyzing and Classifying Tumor Severity Using Volumetric MRI Data

Muhammmad Sajid Khan
https://orcid.org/0000-0001-6413-5324
Wales Institute of Digital Information, UK

Andrew Ware
http://orcid.org/0000-0001-8596-2601
University of South Wales, UK

Fizza Asif
University of Engineering and Technology, Pakistan

Muhammad Usman Sharif
University of Engineering and Technology, Pakistan

Attia
University of Engineering and Technology, Pakistan

ABSTRACT

The field of neuroradiology has advanced significantly with the implementation of 3D Magnetic Resonance Imaging (MRI) technology. This imaging modality enables early-stage tumor diagnosis by detecting minute tumors and subtle abnormalities with high precision. Brain tumors are classified into three primary categories: benign, premalignant, and malignant. A brain tumor is defined as an abnormal proliferation of cells and tissues, with malignant tumors being characterized by rapid growth, irregular surfaces, lack of encapsulation, and deep attachments to surrounding structures. These tumors can exert substantial pressure on adjacent tissues and spread rapidly. The proposed method leverages 3D MRI scans for precise brain tumor detection. Users can choose between two advanced classification approaches: the Support Vector Machine (SVM) or Adaptive Neuro-Fuzzy Inference System (ANFIS) classifiers. The

DOI: 10.4018/979-8-3693-9816-6.ch021

preprocessing phase, which includes contrast enhancement, noise reduction, and grayscale conversion, optimizes image quality. Segmentation techniques are then applied to isolate the tumor region, followed by feature extraction to identify vector-based characteristics. These features are input into the classifier to accurately determine the tumor type. Tumor-affected MRI images are visualized through various graphs generated by a Self-Organizing Map (SOM), enhancing interpretability and aiding in diagnostic decision-making.Keywords: 3D brain Model, Detection, Tumour Stages, 3D MRI, segmentation.

1. INTRODUCTION

Magnetic Resonance Imaging (MRI) is a technology that uses magnetism, radio waves, and a sophisticated system to produce detailed images of internal body parts that are not visible to the naked eye. MRI images are highly detailed and can detect subtle changes in the body's internal structures. In some cases, specialized algorithms are applied to enhance the quality of MRI images. An MRI scanner operates based on the principles of electromagnetic waves and consists of two primary magnets that generate the required magnetic fields (DeAngelis, 2001).

The initial giant circular magnet aligns water molecules in the body to orient them in the same direction. The second magnet causes each hydrogen atom (H-atom) in the body to adjust its alignment under the influence of the magnetic field. When the magnetic field is removed, sensors detect the energy released as protons return to their original alignment. The patient is positioned inside the scanner using a sliding bed. After the entire process, the internal MRI mechanism processes the data, and an image is constructed (Liang & Lauterbur, 2000).

MRI images can be viewed on a computer screen and transmitted electronically. There are several reasons why MRI scans are performed. In addition to brain imaging, neurosurgeons use them to assess the spinal cord after trauma and to examine the vertebrae or intervertebral discs of the spine. MRI provides valuable information about the entire body and is also used to evaluate the structure of the heart. The precise results of an MRI scan can often help improve the accuracy of surgical procedures (Gordillo et al., 2013).

Magnetic Resonance Imaging (MRI) is an advanced method for detecting brain malignancies. A brain tumor is any intracranial tumor caused by abnormal cells, typically located inside or near the brain. Automated brain tumor identification is one of the most challenging tasks in modern medical imaging. It requires image segmentation, a process that divides an image into distinct regions based on specific characteristics. However, removing noise from MR images without compromising fine anatomical details is a complex task. These challenges make obtaining accurate MRI images difficult, yet precise tumor detection relies heavily on accurate brain image segmentation (Gondal & Khan, 2013).

Various algorithms are available for brain image segmentation, which is crucial for tasks such as surgical planning and post-surgical evaluation. Despite the availability of numerous automated methods, many of them fail due to challenges such as noise and low contrast in the images (Borole et al., 2015).

A brain tumor refers to any intracranial tumor caused by abnormal cell and tissue proliferation. In the human body, cells and tissues function as fundamental building blocks. Normally, cells proliferate and then die in an orderly manner as part of their life cycle. However, tumors form when these cells fail to undergo programmed cell death (apoptosis) and instead grow uncontrollably, replicate excessively, form blood vessels, and invade surrounding tissues in an unnatural manner.

The size, shape, and other physical characteristics of cancerous cells differ significantly from those of normal cells. For example, their nuclei are often larger and darker than those of normal cells. Cancerous cells may also form clusters without a defined cell wall or outer boundary, and they exhibit an abnormally high number of disorganized chromosomes compared to normal cells. Cancerous tumors are typically classified into benign and malignant .

A benign tumor is a slow-growing primary tumor that is unlikely to spread because it does not invade surrounding tissues or metastasize to other parts of the body. It is typically small, has a regular surface, is encapsulated, and may be attached to deeper structures. While it may exert slight pressure on nearby organs, it is generally not serious unless it transitions to a malignant state or reproduces secondary (malignant) tumor cells. However, there is a potential for recurrence of the tumor after surgery.

On the other hand, malignant tumors (secondary tumors) are fast-growing, large, cancerous cells that can spread easily. They are life-threatening, have irregular surfaces, are non-encapsulated, and are attached to deep structures, exerting significant pressure on neighboring tissues. These tumors can also reproduce after surgery. Tumors that originate in other parts of the body and spread to the brain via the bloodstream are known as secondary tumors or metastases (Pereira et al., 2016).

According to a recent research, the survival rate for individuals with brain cancer is 36% for women and 34% for males (Pereira et al., 2016). The type of cancer and the stage at which it was diagnosed are two of the many variables that may affect the survival rate.Our researchs goal are to promptly diagnose tumours and categorise them into two groups: benign (primary) and malignant (secondary) in three dimensions. The object can be seen in detail in the 3D perspective.

Using 3D MRI scans as input; our algorithm performs key tasks such as segmentation and feature extraction before identifying the tumor and its stage. This approach could potentially improve the survival rates of future brain tumor patients by enabling timely and appropriate treatment.

The structure of this document is as follows: Section 2 presents a literature review on brain tumor detection, Section 3 outlines our proposed method and classifier, and Section 4 provides an analysis of the results and discussion. The paper concludes with a summary of our research and findings in Section 5, followed by the conclusions in Section 6.

2. LITERATURE REVIEW

The identification of brain tumors using MRI scans is a crucial task in medical imaging, aimed at improving diagnostic precision and ensuring timely treatment. As medical imaging technology advances, researchers have developed various techniques to enhance the detection and classification of brain tumors.Various algorithms have been proposed by researchers to detect tumors. In 2020, some researchers developed algorithms that use an adaptive K-means clustering approach to enhance contrast and fill in gaps in MRI brain images. After receiving an MRI scan as input, the algorithm applies a threshold to eliminate undesirable pixels. The left portion of the processed image is then overlaid onto the original image to detect tumors.The left region is then mapped onto the original image for tumor detection. Tumor detection is performed in two stages: first, segmentation, and second, mapping onto the original image. After detection, classification is carried out using a Support Vector Machine (SVM). The tumor-detected image is input into a Discrete Wavelet Transform (DWT), which decomposes the image into four components: Low-Low (LL), Low-High (LH), High-Low (HL), and High-High (HH).

The Low-Low (LL) coefficient is further processed through Principal Component Analysis (PCA) to extract stronger features (Zulpe & Pawar, 2012).

The features are further characterized using the Gray Level Co-occurrence Matrix (GLCM). Finally, a Support Vector Machine (SVM) is trained on the dataset, using a linear kernel for classification and Gray Level Co-occurrence Matrix (GLCM)-derived features for tumor type determination. By doing so, they achieved an accuracy rate of 93% (Zulpe & Pawar, 2012).

The preprocessing techniques applied to an image in their study include various methods collectively referred to as convolution filtering. These methods encompass RGB to grayscale conversion, edge detection, and 2D convolution masking. The images are utilized to train the system, during which their features are systematically extracted. Morphological techniques are applied to remove unwanted pixels, enhancing image quality for further processing. Segmentation is performed by generating a Signed Distance Map (SDM), which aids in accurately delineating regions of interest. For the final classification, MATLAB's Classification Learner application is utilized, resulting in an achieved accuracy rate of 80% (Chander et al., 2020).

In this paper an automated technique was proposed to detect brain tumours using 3d MRI images. This technique involves around preprocessing of 3d MRI images using Bias field correction. The N4ITK (N4ITK Bias Field Correction) technique is used and Histogram matching in which histogram of each image is adjusted with image means histogram. After the preprocessing Otsu algorithm is applied for extracting the desired region of brain tumour cells. For classification or identification feature extraction is an important step, so they extracted Local Binary Patterns (LBP) features and Histogram Orientation Gradient (HOG) features of thebrain's MRI image. Inthe end, classification is carried out with the help of the random forest algorithm with the help of that proposed methodology; they got maximum accuracy of 83% (Abbasi & Tajeripour, 2017).

In this paper (Sharmila et al., 2019), the researchers proposed a technique for classifying brain tumors using a Support Vector Machine (SVM). Images from the dataset are input into the system, which begins by extracting features. First, the system uses the Wavelet-based Fractal Texture Analysis (WSFTA) technique, which includes Discrete Wavelet Transform (DWT) and Segmentation-Based Fractal Texture Analysis (SFTA). Second, Dimensionality Reduction is applied using Principal Component Analysis (PCA).

The system is then trained using the Support Vector Machine (SVM) algorithm, and two images are mapped for similarity checking. With this approach, they achieved an accuracy of 90.67%. In this methodology proposed in paper (Sharma et al., 2018), preprocessing techniques including grayscale conversion, binary thresholding, morphological operations, contour tumor region identification, and watershed segmentation are applied. Features are then extracted using the Gray Level Co-occurrence Matrix (GLCM). Finally, classification is performed using K-means clustering and an Artificial Neural Network (ANN). For this purpose, a neuro-fuzzy system is utilized. The proposed algorithm was compared with a single K-means clustering and neuro-fuzzy system.

In a separate study, researchers focused on extracting and identifying gliomas from MRI images. In their work (Selvapandian & Manivannan, 2018), they first applied preprocessing techniques to prepare the images. Afterward, features were extracted using the Gray Level Co-occurrence Matrix (GLCM) method. The four extracted features were then input into an Adaptive Neuro-Fuzzy Inference System (ANFIS) classifier to determine whether the tumor was glioma.

Kapoor and Thakur (2017) compared various image segmentation techniques, including threshold-based segmentation, region-based segmentation, and unsupervised learning algorithms (such as fuzzy clustering, C-means, and k-means). They assessed the advantages and disadvantages of each technique, highlighting that threshold segmentation is the easiest to implement, but it fails to provide all the necessary information and cannot be applied to images with low contrast. Although fuzzy clustering, C-means, and k-means are learning-based techniques, they do not produce accurate results when applied to noisy images. In contrast, region-based segmentation is more accurate, though slightly slower than the other methods.

In their 2018 study, S.M. Kamrul Hassan and Mohiuddin Ahmad et al. implemented a two-step verification process for brain tumor segmentation and brain status evaluation. The image datasets were sourced from the BRATS 2012 dataset, containing MRI scans from 30 patients with gliomas—20 with high-grade gliomas and 10 with low-grade gliomas. The segmented regions were then matched with the ground truth images using a watershed algorithm (Hasan & Ahmad, 2018).

Recent studies highlight the growing role of machine learning in brain tumor classification and medical imaging. Aamir et al. (2023) developed a method for classifying brain tumors by utilizing deep features derived from high-quality regions of MRI images, improving accuracy in detecting tumors.

In a previous study, Aamir et al. (2022) proposed a deep learning approach for brain tumor classification using MRI images, focusing on improving classification performance. The hybrid approach for object proposal generation by Aamir et al. (2017) also contributes to the field of medical imaging by enhancing image analysis techniques. Additionally, a framework developed by Guan et al. (2023) offers an efficient method for classifying brain tumors using MRI data. Finally, Aamir et al. (2023) explored the broader applications of machine learning in medicine, emphasizing current trends and future prospects in the context of medical technologies like MRI-based tumor classification.

Recent studies have demonstrated significant advancements in brain tumor detection using deep learning and machine learning techniques applied to MRI images (Zulpe & Pawar, 2012). Abdusalomov et al. (2023) explored deep learning approaches, emphasizing their ability to improve tumor detection through the use of convolutional neural networks (CNNs) and magnetic resonance imaging (Chander et al., 2020).

Anantharajan et al. (2024) further enhanced MRI-based brain tumor detection by integrating both deep learning and machine learning approaches, resulting in more robust tumor classification and detection. In 2021, Brindha et al. applied deep learning techniques, specifically CNNs, for automatic brain tumor detection from MRI scans, showcasing their capability to effectively analyze medical images. Ahmed et al. (2024) proposed a hybrid model combining Vision Transformer (ViT) and Gated Recurrent Unit (GRU) with explainable AI to improve classification performance and provide transparency in the decision-making process for tumor classification.

Martínez-Del-Río-Ortega et al. (2024) contributed to the field by utilizing CNNs for brain tumor detection, demonstrating their potential in enhancing MRI analysis for precise diagnosis. Lastly, Khaliki and Başarslan (2024) compared transfer learning techniques with traditional 3-layer CNN models, offering insights into their comparative efficacy in tumor detection. These studies collectively highlight the progressive shift towards AI-driven methods in brain tumor detection, promising more accurate, reliable, and efficient diagnostic tools for clinical applications.

The state-of-arts have demonstrated significant advancements in brain tumor detection using deep learning and machine learning techniques applied to MRI images. Abdusalomov et al. (2023) explored deep learning approaches, emphasizing their ability to improve tumor detection through the use of convolutional neural networks (CNNs) and magnetic resonance imaging.

3. METHODOLOGY

3D MRI brain tumour scans acquired from BRATS (2015-2019) are sliced into (150) slices inside a volume. The 3D slice is preprocessed using contrast enhancement to make the contrast of the image bright and bring visibility to scan and highlight the regions in the image. Now the scan is segmented using K-means for tumour detection and then self-organizing map representation is drawn for 3D MRI scan. Feature extraction is performed and the appropriate feature set is chosen using PCA that maximizes the accuracy result, at last, the tumour is classified into high-grade glioma and low-grade glioma, and the user is given an option that the user can choose either SVM for tumour classification or ANFIS.

The 3D MRI BRATS (2015 and 2019) brain tumor datasets are utilized, with each 3D volume containing approximately 150-155 slices. From these slices, only the key slices are extracted for further processing. These key slices include the full brain along with the tumor regions, which are then fed into the preprocessing step for the subsequent detection of brain tumors.

After slicing the 3D volume, the next step is improving and eliminating extra information from the data. 3D MRI brain tumor datasets (BRATS) are used for training as well as testing of data as the datasets choose are standard datasets that are already processed for noise removal so only contrast enhancement technique is applied on the 3D volumes. Contrast enhancement is useful here and when it is applied to each 3D slice, we get a balanced image in which the input pixel intensities are mapped to new values such that 1% of the values are saturated at low and high-intensity values resulting in increasing the contrast of the image. As the data is standard dataset, so no noise removal step is performed, see Figure 1.

Figure 1. Original image (left side), enhanced image (right side image)

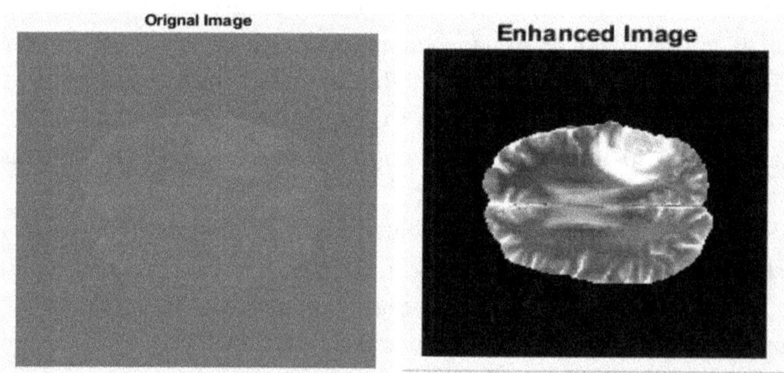

The key task is to segment the image in order to extract the desired region from the entire 3D slice. For this purpose, the K-means algorithm is employed with three clusters. The K-means algorithm initially assigns random positions to the cluster centers in a multidimensional feature space. Each point is then assigned to the cluster whose center is closest. This process continues iteratively until there is no significant change in the location of the class mean vectors between successive iterations. The segmentation is performed using three clusters: one for the brain region without the tumor, one for the non-brain area, and one for the tumor. Each pixel is assigned to the cluster it belongs to (See Figure 2).

Figure 2. Showing cluster formed in the image

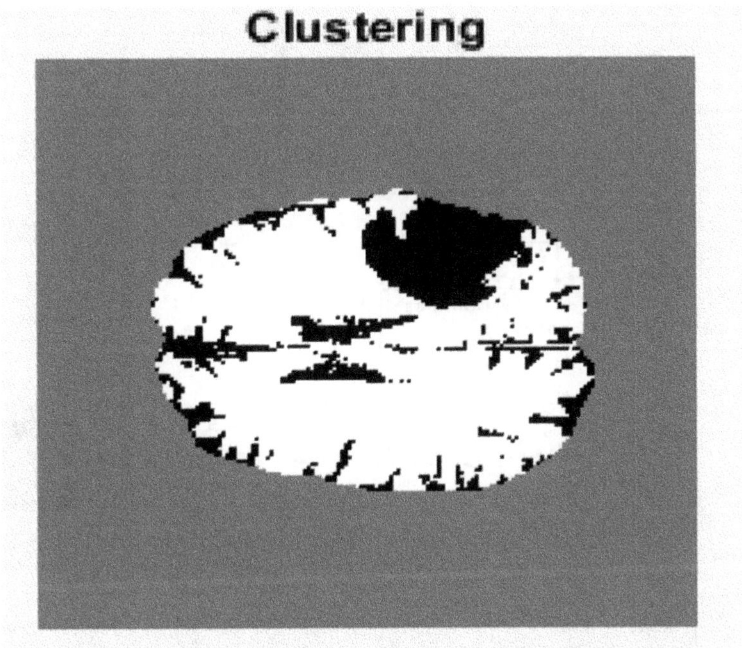

K-Means [29] clustering is applied to separate different clusters in the brain. For this purpose, three clusters are used that is one for one cluster is for the non-brain part, one for the brain with no tumour, and one for tumour. The steps of this method are described below in the algorithm:

Let suppose an image (x * y) having coordinates as 'x' and 'y' and the image will be divided into 'L' clusters and k(x, y) illustrate all the disorganized pixels and 'CL'is the cluster formed.Divide the image into 'l' no of clusters Then Estimate the Euclidean distance of each pixel from the cluster in equation (1)

$$Distance = \|k(x, y) - C_L\| \tag{1}$$

Assign the pixel to the cluster having minimum distance from that cluster.After grouping every pixel recalculate centroid by calculating data mean given by equation (2) (Guan et al., n.d.).

$$C_L = \frac{1}{L}\sum_{x \in C_L}\sum_{y \in C_L} k(x,y) \tag{2}$$

Repeat all the above steps until the centroids values stop changing.Now map the remolded clusters picture element on the image.

Figure 3 will show the detailed working of the K-Means Algorithm.

Figure 3. K-Means Algorithms

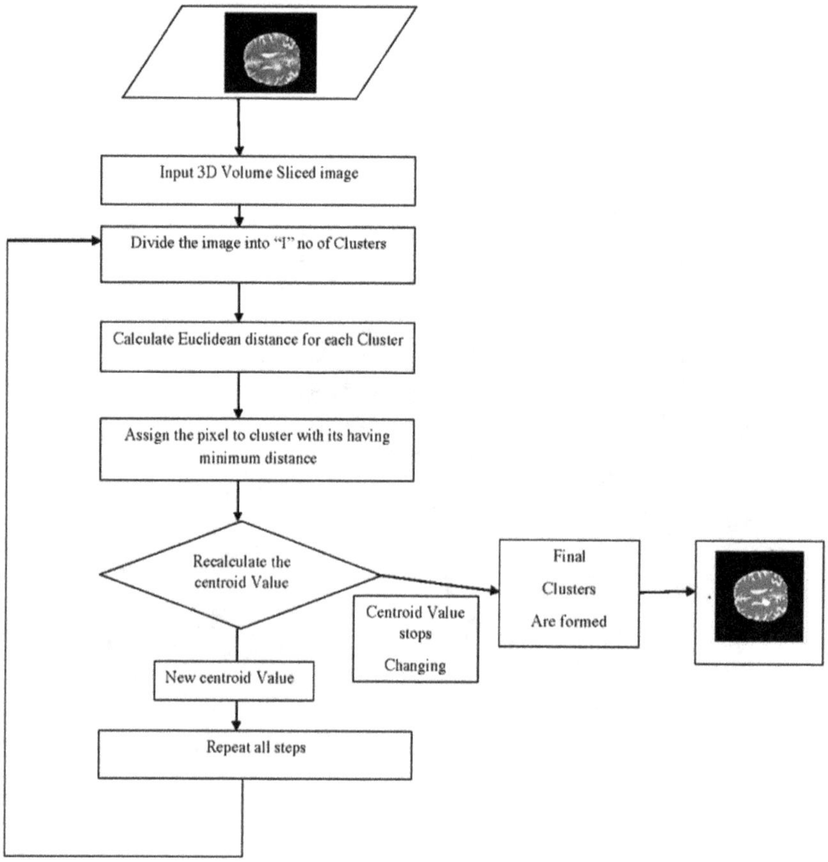

Morphological operations are carried out when the input pixel in the input image is compared to its neighbourhood for acquiring desired output results in the output image. Irrespective of the other types here in the proposed system opening is chosen according to the scenario. The morphological opening is useful when the objective is to eliminate the small objects carrying unnecessary information while preserving the shape and causing no disturbance to its size. The opening involves erosion and dilation that are the key types of morphological operations, erosion shrinks the region and dilation dilate it, so opening operation is a combination of erosion and dilation, same structuring element is utilized in both operations.

4.1 Self-Organizing Map (SOM)

Self-organizing maps are neural networks that are trained purely to perform the clustering of data. The structure included in a network so that the net is forced to decide as to which one unit will respond and learn to classify input vectors according to how they are grouped in the input space. In our case, an image size of 10*10 is used, having a neuron value of 25*25. Different graphs are given as an output by the system after the SOM training, which shows the position of different neurons at different locations. Self-organizing feature map network identifies a winning neuron i^* using the same procedure as employed by a competitive layer. However, instead of updating only the winning neuron, all neurons within a certain neighbourhood N_{i*} (d) of the winning neuron are updated, using the Kohonen rule. Specifically, all such neurons $i \in N_{i*}$ (d) are adjusted as follows:

$$iw(q) = iw(q-1) + \alpha(\mathrm{p(q)} - iw(q-1)) \tag{3}$$

Or

$$iw(q) = (1-\alpha)iw(q-1) + \alpha\mathrm{p}(q) \tag{4}$$

Here the *neighborhood* N_{i*} (d) contains the indices for all of the neurons that lie within a radius d of the winning neuron i^*.

$$Ni(d) = \{j, dij \leq \mathrm{d}\} \tag{5}$$

Thus, when a vector **p** is presented, the weights of the winning neuron *and* its close neighbors move toward **p**. Consequently, after many presentations, neighboring neurons have learned vectors similar to each other.

In every representation of SOM, the dimensions are

% Create a Self-Organizing Map

dimension1 = 25;

dimension2 = 25;

Which shows that the neurons are taken as 25*25.

While training the batch weight algorithm is used with the iterations of 200. Each graph shows the taken dimension of the neuron on the x-axis and y-axis describing the position of the first neuron to the last neuron.

Figure 4. SOM topology

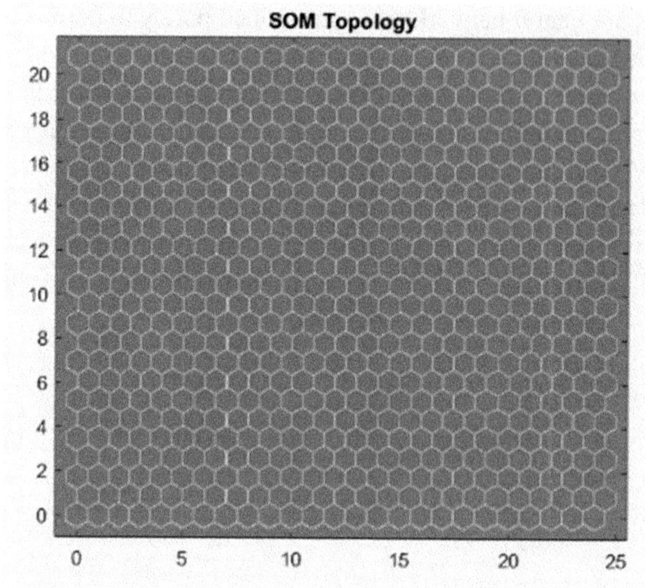

Figure 5. SOM neighbor connections

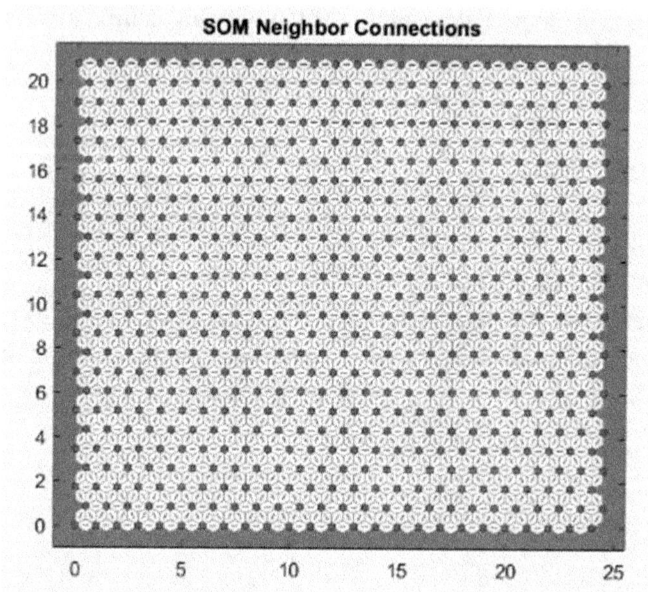

Figure 6. SOM neighbor weight distances

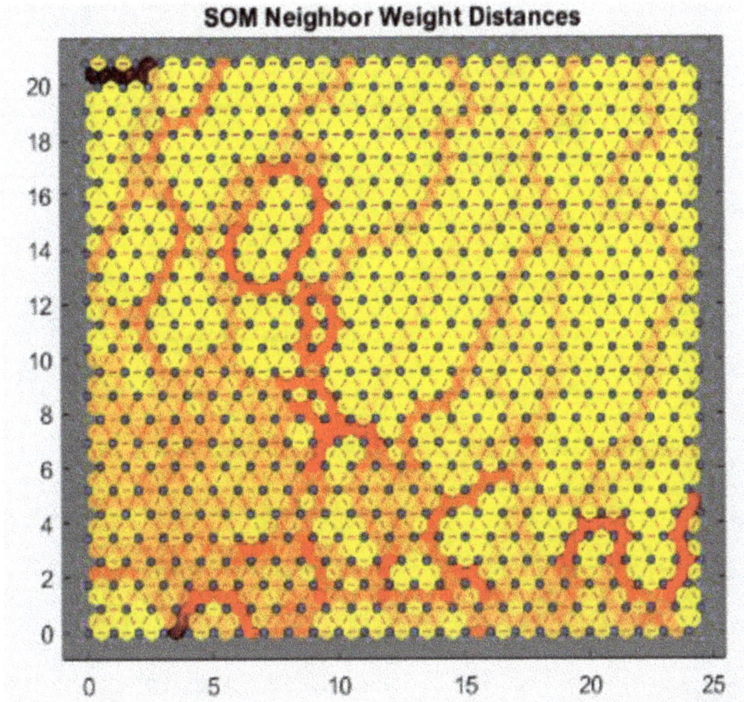

Figure 7. SOM hits

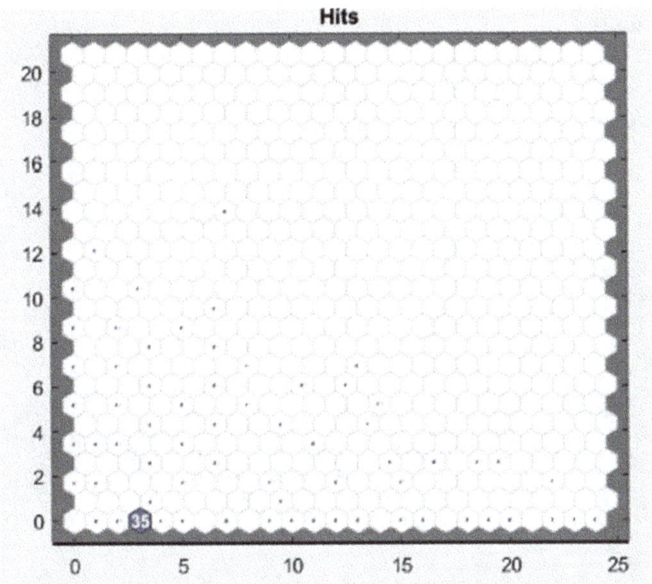

Figure 8. SOM input planes

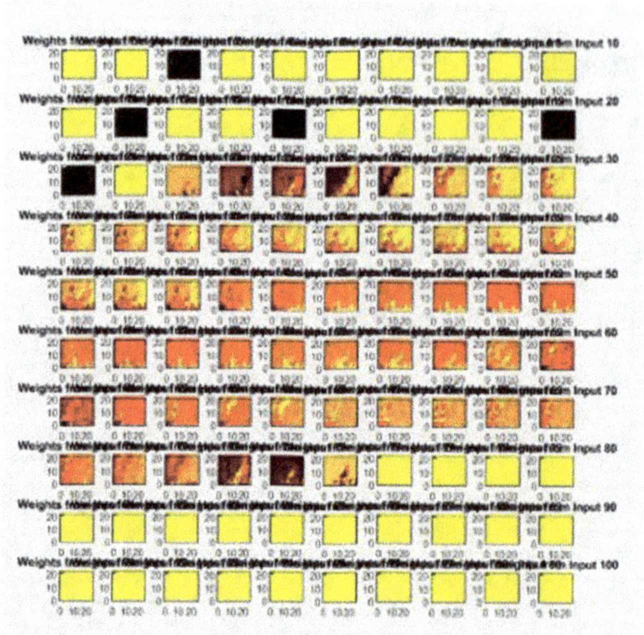

.The blue hexagons represent the neurons, while the red lines connect neighboring neurons. The colors within the regions containing the red lines indicate the distances between neurons. Darker colors represent larger distances, while lighter colors represent smaller distances. The Self-Organizing Map (SOM) hit tells us how many data points are associated with each neuron. The SOM neighbor weight distance grouping suggests that the network has clustered the data into two groups based on the proximity of the neurons, see Figure 9.

Figure 9. SOM weight positions

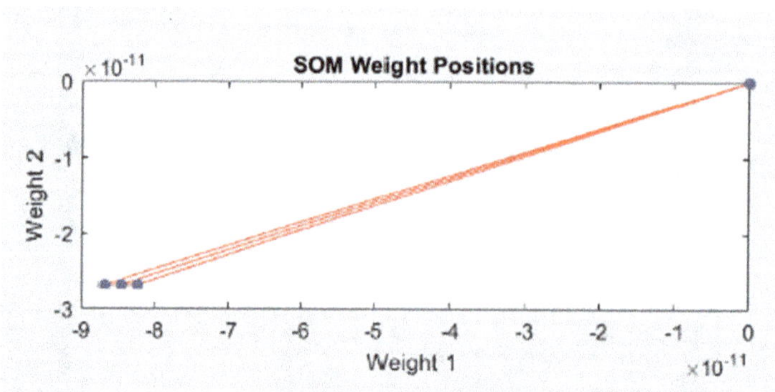

There is a weight plane for each element of the input vector (two, in this case). They are visualizations of the weights that connect each input to each of the neurons. If the connection patterns of the two inputs are very similar, you can assume that the inputs were highly correlated.

4.2 Feature Extraction

The figure below is giving a complete understanding of the feature extraction techniques used and what features are being extracted by using these techniques.

Figure 10. Feature extraction methods and feature labels

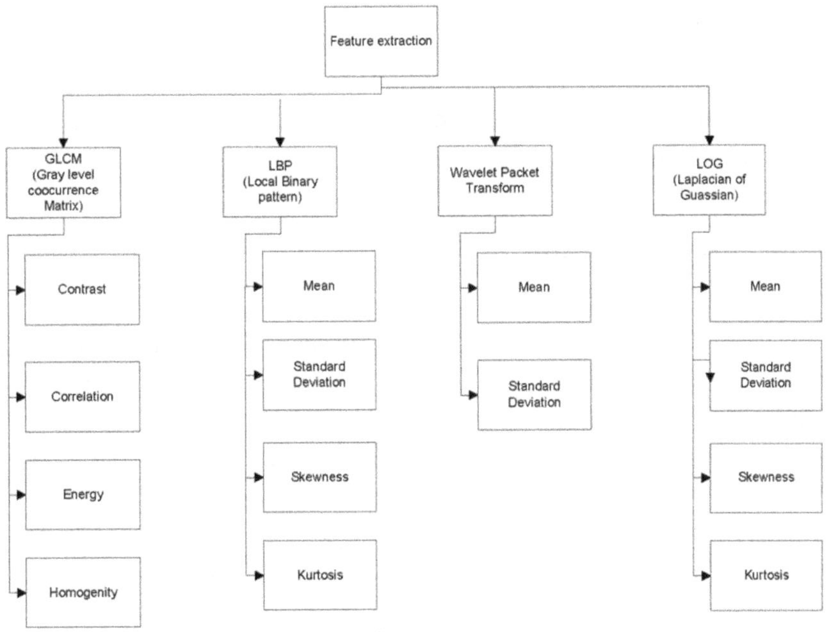

GLCM (Martínez-Del-Río-Ortega et al., 2024) is used to obtain the statistical textural second-order features (these features are generated using first-order statistics and provide information on the distribution of gray level in an image). The GLCM function is used to outline the texture (information of color arrangements in the picture) of the image to measure repeatedly certain pixels are appearing in a pair and distinct relationship for this purpose GLCM is created and then required texture features are extracted by utilizing the statistical calculations from the GLCM matrix.GLCM is a 2D histogram in which *(m,n)*th element s are the frequency of how usually an event *m* occurs with *n*. It is a function of distance D =1, calculated at four different angles that are 0, 45, 90 and 135 degrees resulting in values calculated from four different orientation for each of the below, and also calculate how regularly a pixel having intensity value *m* occurs in relation with another pixel *n* at a specific distance D and on these orientation.

Contrast: Measure the contrast between a pixel and its neighbor in equation (6)

$$Contrast = \sum_{a=0}^{p-1}\sum_{b=0}^{q-1}(a-b)^2 f(a,b) \quad (6)$$

Correlation: Measure of how much a pixel is dependent or associated to its neighbor pixel in the entire equation (7)

$$Correlation = \frac{\sum_{m=0}^{p-1}\sum_{n=0}^{q-1}(m \cdot n)f(m,n) - P_m P_n}{\sigma_m \sigma_n} \quad (7)$$

Energy: It is the squared sum of all reoccurring pixel pairs in GLCM equation (8)

$$Energy = \sqrt{\sum_{m=0}^{p-1}\sum_{n=0}^{q-1} f^2(m,n)} \quad (8)$$

Homogeneity: It measures the proximity of the element scattered in GLCM matrix to that of present in diagonal in GLCM equation (9)

$$Homogeneity = \sum_{m=0}^{p-1}\sum_{n=0}^{q-1}\frac{1}{1+(m-n)^2}f(m,n) \quad (9)$$

Laplacian of Gaussian is applied, and four features are obtained mean, standard deviation, skewness,kurtosis where p is length and q is width and C(x,y) is log value at the location stated by a and y, sigma (σ) is the variance, and Mu (μ) is average.

Mean: The mean calculate the part of each pixel intensity value in the whole image

$$\mu_x = \frac{1}{p \cdot q}\sum_{x=0}^{p-1}\sum_{y=0}^{q-1} C(x,y) \quad (10)$$

Standard deviation: It is the measure of how much the data is dispersed from its mean value

Skewness: It is the measure of lack of balance of inequality equation (11)

$$Skewness = \frac{1}{p \cdot q}\frac{\sum_{x=0}^{p-1}\sum_{y=0}^{q-1}\left(C(x,y) - \mu_x\right)^3}{\sigma_x^3} \quad (11)$$

Kurtosis: Kurtosis is the term used to describe the circulation of data equation (12)

$$Kurtosis = \frac{1}{p \cdot q}\frac{\sum_{x=0}^{p-1}\sum_{y=0}^{q-1}\left(C(x,y) - \mu_x\right)^4}{\sigma_x^4} \quad (12)$$

Local binary patterns are feature descriptors used to the texture properties of the surface. It is a mixture of earlier used divergent statistical features and structural models to examine and investigate the texture properties of the surface. These feature descriptors are prioritized due to its stiffness power to confront the monotonic grayscale images and its computational efficiency. Its algorithm threshold the adjoining neighborhood pixels on the ground of existing value. They mainly store grayscale contrast information and image patterns spatially. The following is description of features calculation procedure. Initially, several pixels are selected in the neighborhood of every pixel in radius R' then Intensity difference is calculated for the selected current pixel and its neighboring pixels .Now all the differences that have negative values will become 0, and all others are set to 1 by applying thresholding. At last the vector acquired will be changed into decimal value and is assumed as new intensity value for that current pixel

The following is the equation that calculates LBP for each pixel in equation (13)

$$LBP_{(A,R')} = \sum_{a=1}^{A} s(g_A - g_B) \cdot 2^{(a-1)} \tag{13}$$

And

$$s(x) = \{1, x \geq 00, x < 0 \tag{14}$$

Where A represents the number of neighboring pixels and R' shows the radius respectively. While g_A and g_B are intensity values of the present and neighborhood pixels respectively

Wavelet packet transform Image is decomposed using the wavelet packet transform by using different frequencies of the pixels range in the image. Here 2D-DWT is used that is truly constructive in defining and evaluating the features and the DB5 wavelet is used. By using region of interest four Sub bands that are HH(high-high), LL(low-low),HL (high-low) and LH (low-high) are achieved that will output 40 features having 20 values of mean and 20 values of standard deviationMean is the average of each decomposed level. It shows the data distribution in each decomposed level. Different features are extracted that is contrast, energy, correlation, and homogeneity from four different angles 0, 45,90, and 135, also the mean, standard deviation, skewness, and kurtosis is calculated, these features are called as Local Binary Patterns.

The second 40 features are extracted from Wavelet Based Features and their mean, standard deviation, skewness, and kurtosis are also calculated. LOG based features are 40 because images are decomposed to 40 levels so from every level one feature is extracted. Feature reduction is the process of reducing features to desired use from obtained features so for better accuracy; a matrix is formed of these features to be given as an input to classifiers for the process of classification. This step is performed using Principal Component Analysis Algorithm.

4.3 Classification

This research focuses on the classification of tumors into two categories: benign and malignant. For this purpose selected algorithms are SVM or ANFIS (Khaliki & Başarslan, 2024) and their results are compared SVM after applying PCA accuracy reached from 83% to 80% and for ANFIS accuracy reached from 92% to 97.76%. In this step the feature vector containing 64 features is ready to be input in the PCA algorithm, PCA will give 64 features as output as the same that is fed as input to the system but a new feature vector containing eigenvalues of the input feature vector.

The property of that feature vector will be, that its starting features will help in achieving high accuracy as compared to the last features they will reduce the accuracy, The modified ANFIS training dataset will be applied on ANFIS model and trained model of the system is achieved and then testing is done on that model to calculate the accuracy, the option is provided to the user between two classifiers either SVM or ANFI (See Figure 11 and 12).

Figure 11. Flow chart of contribution in modified ANFI

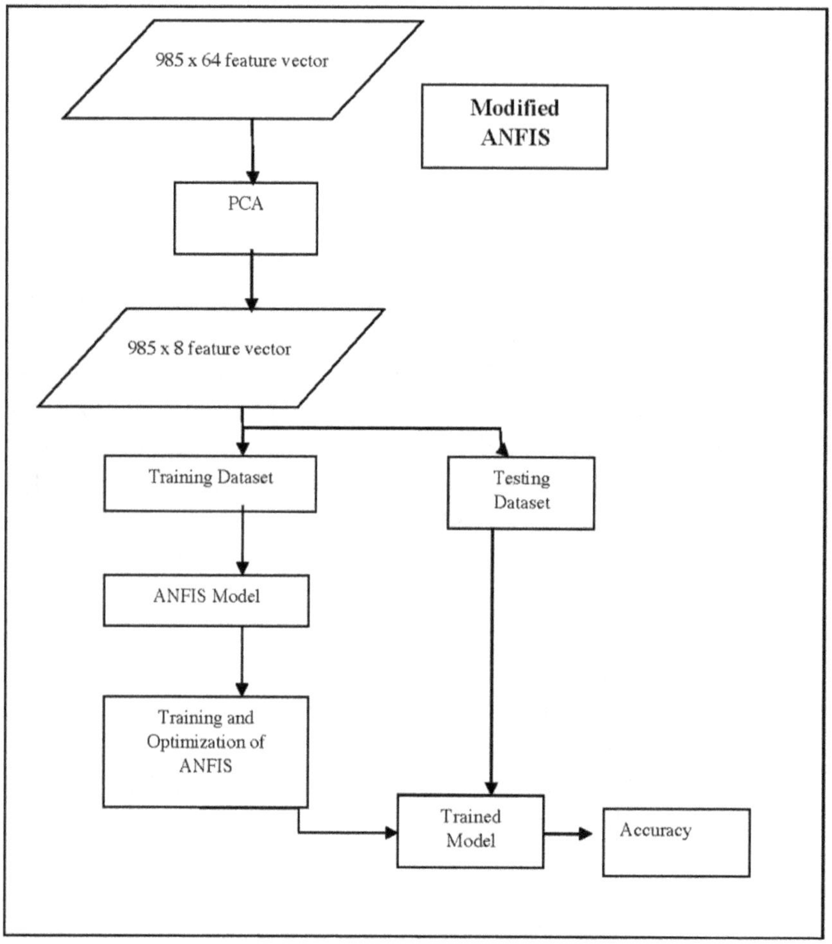

Figure 12. Block diagram of testing and training phase of SVM

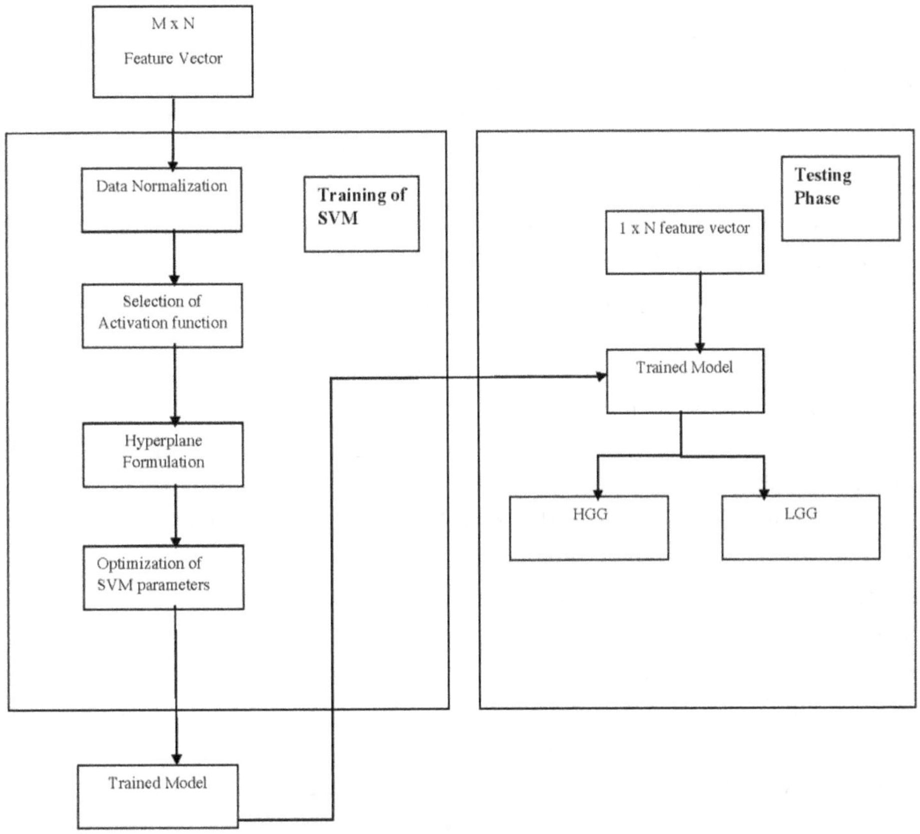

4.4 Implementation and Result Analysis

Training time usually requires 20-30% of development time it can be longer up to months and as low as days or weeks, depending on the datasets we train the system on.The Computation time and response time could not be predicted as early yet complete implementation is not done but definitely, the aim of the system will be increase performance and enhance results by increasing efficiency and decreasing time.The previous systems developed were not able to describe the tumor stage they only focused on the tumor extraction from the image, its detection and some were also discussing the tumor location. The classifier implemented will be able to specify tumor stage that whether its malicious or not. An error always affects the system results and usability of the system. They had a bad impact that the actual requirement is not fulfilled, As errors will be reduced, there will be better results which also affect the quality of the system and better performance directly.

It consist of at first 3D standard dataset containing brain tumor, magnetic resonance images are found and then downloaded from brats (brats2015). These images were present in **.mha**format that is not visible; a special code is needed in Matlab to read these images. Further, the image is processed using different noise removal and image quality improving functions and techniques as these are standard datasets so they are already processed for noise removal and also image quality is much better but to increase contrast, contrast adjustment is applied. The key 3D slice obtained from 3D MRI is the input to the proposed method.

Further, it is processed using contrast adjustment; it increases the pixel values difference by improving the contrast of the image, it applied for stretching the pixels gathered at the middle of the image, then to diagnose the tumor region and extract it from the required image, k-means clustering is applied making 3 clusters for the data one for the non-brain part, one for the brain with no tumor and last for tumor.

K-means estimates the Euclidean distance of each point or pixel from its centroid. It then assigns the pixel to the centroid with the smallest distance. This process continues for all points. After assigning each cluster to its respective points, the centroids are re-calculated by taking the mean of the data in each cluster. This iterative process is repeated until the stopping criteria are met, i.e., when the centroids' values no longer change.

Once the clustering is finalized, the clusters are mapped onto the image, resulting in a binary image as the output of the K-means algorithm.

Next, a morphological opening operation is applied to the binary image. This involves first eroding the image and then dilating it using the same structuring element. The opening operation smooths the object and removes small unwanted details that could interfere with the results.

After the opening operation, objects smaller than 200 pixels are removed from the image to eliminate any remaining noise or irrelevant objects. The final output is the segmented image, with unwanted objects successfully removed.

Feature extraction involves retrieving useful quantitative information from the image. A total of 64 features are obtained in this process. Several techniques are applied for feature extraction: GLCM, LBP, Discrete Wavelet Transform (DWT), and Laplacian of Gaussian (LoG).

In GLCM, four features are extracted from four different orientations (0°, 45°, 90°, and 135°). These features include contrast, correlation, energy, and homogeneity, each with four corresponding values.

Laplacian of Gaussian (LoG) is applied to calculate the mean, standard deviation, skewness, and kurtosis. LBP is used to extract mean, standard deviation, skewness, and kurtosis as well.

Finally, Discrete Wavelet Transform (DWT) is applied, and the mean and standard deviation are calculated. Each of these values has twenty different measurements, providing a comprehensive set of features for analysis.

The principal component analysis is applied for feature reduction to have the most relevant data from the given data, after using PCA when a tumor is classified using SVM its accuracy decreased from 83% to 80% and when PCA applied features are used in classification using ANFIS its accuracy increased from 92% to 97.76% then their results are compared and resulted as ANFIS with higher accuracy and som weight positions are presented in Table 1 (See Figures 13-16).

Figure 13. Clustered image

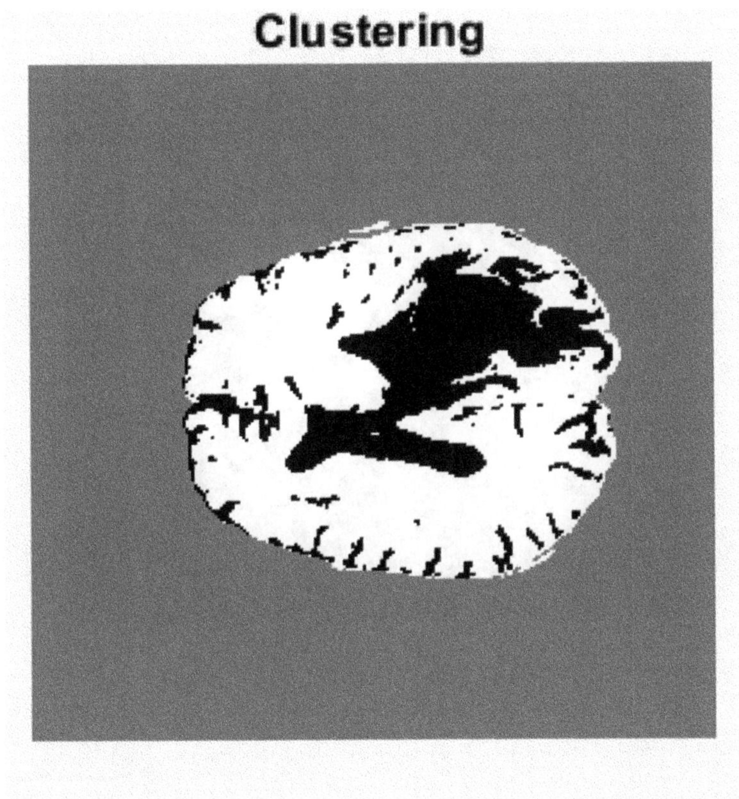

Figure 14. Binary image

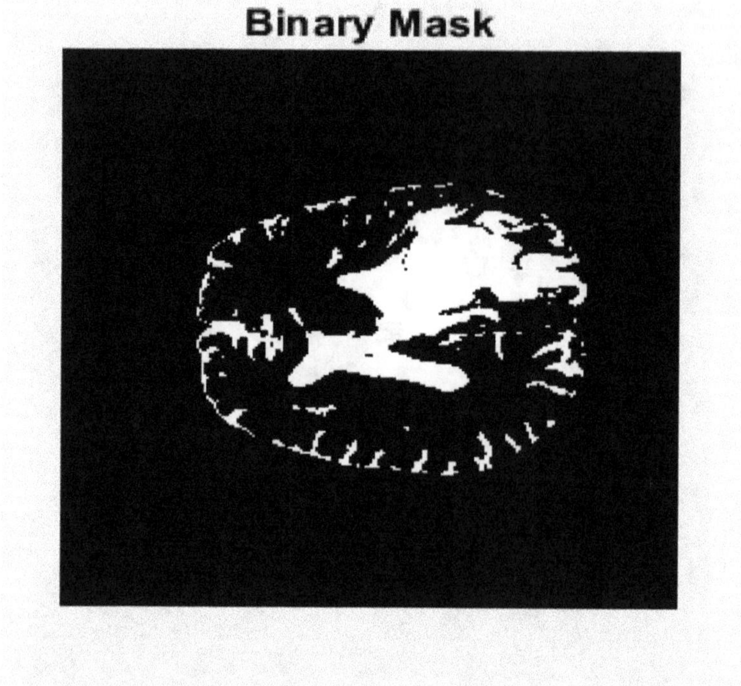

Figure 15. Segmented image

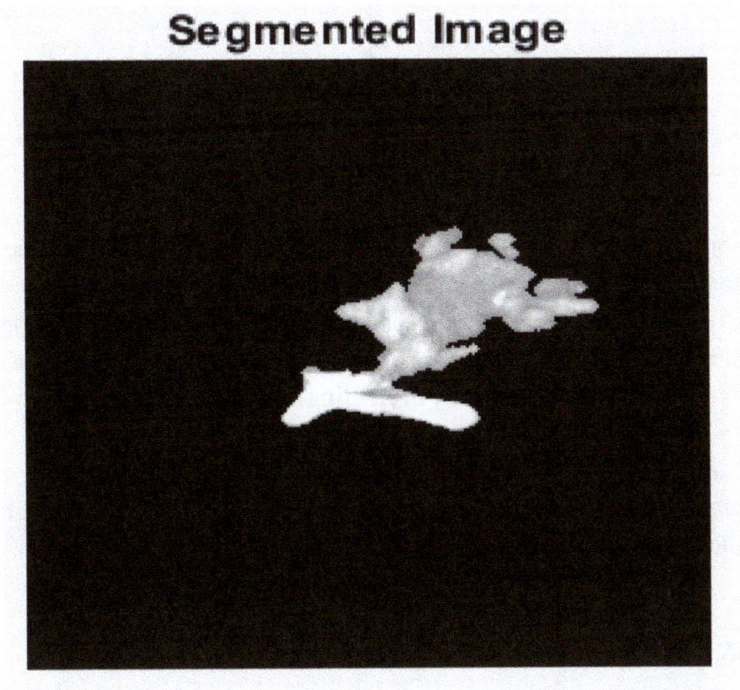

Figure 16. SOM weight positions

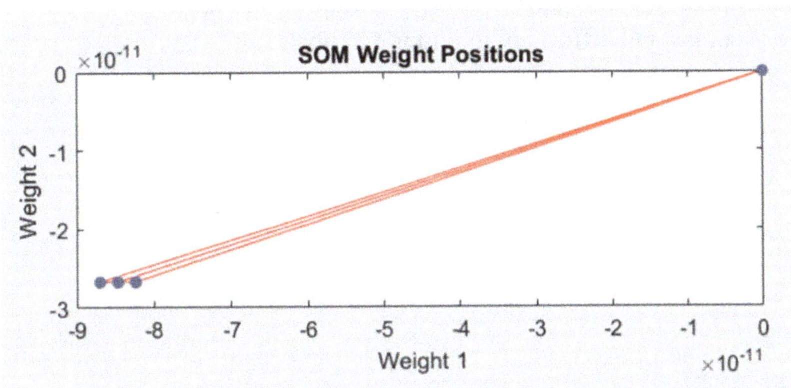

The existing system performs processing operation on the image then tumor detection is implemented using histogram equalization and clustering technique after this tumor classification is attained using type –II fuzzy inference system and ANFIS by using these they operated by using two datasets that is brats 2012 and brats 2013 by using brats12 accomplished accuracy was 91.2 and by brats13 it was 85.71 (Chander et al., 2020) and see Table 1.

Table 1. "comparison of previous work accuracy parameters with proposed work

Datasets	Models	Accuracy	Precision	Recall
Brats 12 (Khaliki & Başarslan, 2024)	Existing work (Chander et al., 2020)	91.2%	94%	93.3%
Brats 13 (Khaliki & Başarslan, 2024)	Existing work (Chander et al., 2020)	85.71%	100%	83.3%
Brats 15	Proposed work	97.76%	99.03%	97.19%

Perform validation using external datasets from different sources to ensure the model can handle diverse patient demographics, tumor types, and clinical conditions. This demonstrates the model's applicability across different clinical environments and enhances its clinical utility.Apply cross-validation techniques using independent subsets of the BraTS 2015 dataset or other datasets to check the model's performance consistency. This helps us identify overfitting or biases towards specific data characteristics, ensuring the model's robustness.

Finally, test the model in clinical environments with real-world MRI scans, which may contain artifacts, noise, or other variations not present in training data. This provides insights into the model's performance and reliability in routine clinical use.

5. CONCLUSION

In conclusion, MRI remains a vital tool for the identification of abnormalities and diseases across various organs. The proposed brain tumor identification model, evaluated on BraTS 2015, demonstrates significant improvements in accuracy, precision, and recall compared to earlier models on BraTS 2012 and 2013. These advancements highlight its potential for reliable tumor classification and clinical applications. Future work could integrate advanced deep learning techniques and real-time implementation to further enhance accuracy and efficiency in tumor diagnosis.

ACKNOWLEDGMENT

We would like to sincerely thank to everyone for their invaluable collaboration and support throughout the completion of this research project. This work, which began during the challenging times of the COVID-19 pandemic, is now ready for publication thanks to their continued dedication and support.

CONFLICT OF INTEREST

The authors declare that there is no conflict of interest.

REFERENCES

Aamir, M., Bazai, S., Bhatti, U. A., Dayo, Z. A., Liu, J., & Zhang, K. (2023). Applications of machine learning in medicine: Current trends and prospects. In *2023 Global Conference on Wireless and Optical Technologies (GCWOT)* (pp. 1–4). IEEE. https://doi.org/DOI: 10.1109/GCWOT57803.2023.10064665

Aamir, M., Pu, Y. F., Abro, W. A., Naeem, H., & Rahman, Z. (2017). A hybrid approach for object proposal generation. In *International Conference on Sensing and Imaging* (pp. 251–259). Springer. https://doi.org/DOI: 10.1007/978-3-319-60234-9_27

Aamir, M., Rahman, Z., Abro, W. A., Bhatti, U. A., Dayo, Z. A., & Ishfaq, M. (2023). Brain tumor classification utilizing deep features derived from high-quality regions in MRI images. *Biomedical Signal Processing and Control, 85*, 104988. DOI: 10.1016/j.bspc.2023.104988

Aamir, M., Rahman, Z., Dayo, Z. A., Abro, W. A., Uddin, M. I., Khan, I., Imran, A. S., Ali, Z., Ishfaq, M., Guan, Y., & Hu, Z. (2022). A deep learning approach for brain tumor classification using MRI images. *Computers & Electrical Engineering, 101*, 108105. DOI: 10.1016/j.compeleceng.2022.108105

Abbasi, S., & Tajeripour, F. (2017). Detection of brain tumor in 3D MRI images using local binary patterns and histogram orientation gradient. *Neurocomputing, 219*, 526–535. DOI: 10.1016/j.neucom.2016.09.051

Abdusalomov, A. B., Mukhiddinov, M., & Whangbo, T. K. (2023). Brain tumor detection based on deep learning approaches and magnetic resonance imaging. *Cancers (Basel), 15*(16), 4172. DOI: 10.3390/cancers15164172 PMID: 37627200

Ahmed, M. M., Hossain, M. M., Islam, M. R., Ali, M. S., Nafi, A. A. N., Ahmed, M. F., Ahmed, K. M., Miah, M. S., Rahman, M. M., Niu, M., & Islam, M. K. (2024). Brain tumor detection and classification in MRI using hybrid ViT and GRU model with explainable AI in Southern Bangladesh. *Scientific Reports, 14*(1), 22797. DOI: 10.1038/s41598-024-71893-3 PMID: 39354009

Anantharajan, S., Gunasekaran, S., Subramanian, T., & Venkatesh, R. (2024). MRI brain tumor detection using deep learning and machine learning approaches. *Measurement. Sensors, 31*, 101026. DOI: 10.1016/j.measen.2024.101026

Borole, V. Y., Nimbhore, S. S., & Kawthekar, S. S. (2015). Image processing techniques for brain tumor detection: A review. [IJETTCS]. *International Journal of Emerging Trends & Technology in Computer Science, 4*(5), 2.

Brindha, P. G., Kavinraj, M., Manivasakam, P., & Prasanth, P. (2021, February). Brain tumor detection from MRI images using deep learning techniques. In *IOP Conference Series: Materials Science and Engineering, 1055*(1), 012115. IOP Publishing. https://doi.org/DOI: 10.1088/1757-899X/1055/1/012115

Chander, P. S., Soundarya, J., & Priyadharsini, R. (2020). Brain tumour detection and classification using K-means clustering and SVM classifier. In *RITA 2018* (pp. 49–63). Springer., DOI: 10.1007/978-981-13-8323-6_5

Chatterjee, S., & Das, A. (2019). A novel systematic approach to diagnose brain tumor using integrated type-II fuzzy logic and ANFIS (adaptive neuro-fuzzy inference system) model. *Soft Computing*, 1–24. DOI: 10.1007/s00500-019-04553-7

Chaudhary, A., & Bhattacharjee, V. (2020). An efficient method for brain tumor detection and categorization using MRI images by K-means clustering & DWT. *International Journal of Information Technology: an Official Journal of Bharati Vidyapeeth's Institute of Computer Applications and Management, 12*(1), 141–148. DOI: 10.1007/s41870-018-0255-4

DeAngelis, L. M. (2001). Brain tumors. *The New England Journal of Medicine, 344*(2), 114–123. DOI: 10.1056/NEJM200101113440207 PMID: 11150363

Gondal, A. H., & Khan, M. N. A. (2013). A review of fully automated techniques for brain tumor detection from MR images. *International Journal of Modern Education and Computer Science, 5*(2), 55–61. DOI: 10.5815/ijmecs.2013.02.08

Gordillo, N., Montseny, E., & Sobrevilla, P. (2013). State of the art survey on MRI brain tumor segmentation. *Magnetic Resonance Imaging, 31*(8), 1426–1438. DOI: 10.1016/j.mri.2013.05.002 PMID: 23790354

Guan, Y., Aamir, M., Rahman, Z., Ali, A., Abro, W. A., Dayo, Z. A., Bhutta, M. S., & Hu, Z. (n.d.). A framework for efficient brain tumor classification using MRI images. *[Details incomplete – publication info or journal required]*

Hasan, S. M. K., & Ahmad, M. (2018). Two-step verification of brain tumor segmentation using watershed-matching algorithm. *Brain Informatics, 5*(2), 8. Advance online publication. DOI: 10.1186/s40708-018-0086-x

Khaliki, M. Z., & Başarslan, M. S. (2024). Brain tumor detection from images and comparison with transfer learning methods and 3-layer CNN. *Scientific Reports, 14*(1), 2664. DOI: 10.1038/s41598-024-52823-9 PMID: 38302604

Liang, Z.-P., & Lauterbur, P. C. (2000). *Principles of magnetic resonance imaging: A signal processing perspective*. SPIE Optical Engineering Press.

Martínez-Del-Río-Ortega, R., Civit-Masot, J., Luna-Perejón, F., & Domínguez-Morales, M. (2024). Brain tumor detection using magnetic resonance imaging and convolutional neural networks. *Big Data and Cognitive Computing, 8*(9), 123. DOI: 10.3390/bdcc8090123

Pereira, S., Pinto, A., Alves, V., & Silva, C. A. (2016). Brain tumor segmentation using convolutional neural networks in MRI images. *IEEE Transactions on Medical Imaging*, *35*(5), 1240–1251. DOI: 10.1109/TMI.2016.2538465 PMID: 26960222

Selvapandian, A., & Manivannan, K. (2018). Fusion-based glioma brain tumor detection and segmentation using ANFIS classification. *Computer Methods and Programs in Biomedicine*, *166*, 33–38. DOI: 10.1016/j.cmpb.2018.09.006 PMID: 30415716

Sharma, M., Purohit, G. N., & Mukherjee, S. (2018). Information retrieved from brain MRI images for tumor detection using hybrid technique K-means and artificial neural network (KMANN). In *Networking Communication and Data Knowledge Engineering* (pp. 145–157). Springer. DOI: 10.1007/978-981-10-8657-1_14

Sharmila, G., Karthika, S., & Vithiya, R. (2019, March). An hybrid wavelet-based SFTA technique for content-based MRI brain image retrieval. In *2019 IEEE International Conference on System, Computation, Automation and Networking (ICSCAN)* (pp. 1–7). IEEE. DOI: 10.1109/ICSCAN.2019.8878760

Zulpe, N., & Pawar, V. (2012). GLCM textural features for brain tumor classification. [IJCSI]. *International Journal of Computer Science Issues*, *9*(3), 354.

Zulpe, N., & Pawar, V. (2012). GLCM textural features for brain tumor classification. [IJCSI]. *International Journal of Computer Science Issues*, *9*(3), 354–359.

About the Contributors

Muhammad Aamir received his Bachelor of Engineering degree in Computer Systems Engineering from Mehran University of Engineering & Technology, Jamshoro, Sindh, Pakistan, in 2008. He went on to earn a Master of Engineering degree in Software Engineering from Chongqing University, China, in 2014, and later completed his PhD in Computer Science and Technology from Sichuan University, Chengdu, China, in 2019. Currently, he is an Associate Professor in the College of Computer Science at Huanggang Normal University, China. With extensive research experience and a prolific publication record, Dr. Aamir has made significant contributions to various fields including pattern recognition, computer vision, medical image processing, deep learning, and fractional calculus. His expertise and dedication to advancing these areas have earned him recognition as a peer reviewer for numerous prestigious journals and as an organizing committee member for several international conferences.

Uzair Aslam Bhatti is mostly active in the application and development of machine learning in signal processing problems, especially to the application of artificial intelligence in other fields. During his PhD studies at Hainan University, he won 2 Best Research Paper Awards and a Chinese Government Scholarship to pursue a doctorate. During his Post Doc at the School of Geography (Remote Sensing and Signal Processing) of Nanjing Normal University, he published 11 research papers as the first author in two years as the first author, 2 of which were published in the top SCI journals Transactions in Geoscience and Remote Sensing and Chemosphere. Due to the publication of 2 conference papers at CCF B-level conferences and 10 SCI papers as the first author, he was declared an excellent postdoctoral candidate by Nanjing Normal University. He has participated in many projects such as the National Natural Science Foundation of China, the National Key R&D Program, and the Hainan Provincial Major Science and Technology Program.

Ziaur Rahman obtained his B.S. degree in Computer Science from the University of Peshawar, Pakistan, in 2012, followed by an M.S. degree in Software Engineering from Chongqing University, China, in 2017. He completed his Ph.D. in Computer Science at Sichuan University, Chengdu, China, in 2021. Dr. Rahman is currently serving as an Associate Professor in the College of Computer Science at Huanggang Normal University, Huanggang, China. He has contributed significantly to the academic community by authoring or co-authoring over 29 research articles published in high-impact SCI journals and conferences. His primary research areas encompass image processing, computer vision, and deep learning. Additionally, he serves as a Reviewer for several esteemed journals, including IEEE Transactions on Image Processing, Future Generation Computer Systems, Signal Processing: Image Communication, IEEE Access, KSII Transactions on Internet and Information Systems, Mobile Information Systems, Applied Soft Computing, Alexandria Engineering Journal, and IET Image Processing.

Jameel Ahmed Bhutto received his Bachelor of Engineering in Telecommunication Engineering from Mehran University of Engineering and Technology, Pakistan in 2010. He received his Master of Engineering degree in Communication Systems and Networking from Mehran University of Engineering and Technology, Pakistan in 2016. He has completed his PhD degree from South China University of Technology, China in 2022. He is working as a distinguished associate professor at the Department of Computer Science, Huanggang Normal University, China. His major research interests include pattern recognition, deep learning, computer vision, image fusion, image enhancement and digital image processing.

Waheed Ahmed completed his joint Ph.D. in Computer Science from Southeast University, China, and Ulm University, Germany. Currently, he is a Postdoctoral Researcher at the Responsible AI Chair, Faculty of Sciences Jean Perrin, LENS, France. Prior to this, he served as an Assistant Professor at the National University of Computer and Emerging Sciences (FAST-NUCES), Pakistan. He earned his Bachelor's degree in Computer Systems Engineering from Mehran University of Engineering and Technology, Pakistan, and his Master's degree in Computer Science from the National University of Computer and Emerging Sciences (FAST-NUCES), Pakistan. His research interests include Artificial Intelligence, specifically in Natural language processing and large language models.

***

A. V. Kalpana is an accomplished academician and researcher, currently serving as an Assistant Professor in the Department of Data Science and Business Systems at the School of Computing, SRM Institute of Science & Technology, Kattankulathur, Chennai. She completed her Bachelor's degree in Computer Science and Engineering in 2004 from the University of Madras, showcasing her foundational understanding of computer science. Further enhancing her expertise, she pursued a Master's degree in Computer Science and Engineering from Anna University. She holds a Ph.D. degree from Anna University, Chennai, reflecting her dedication to advancing knowledge in her field. Her research contributions are evident through numerous publications in reputable journals and international conference proceedings. Driven by a passion for knowledge, her research interests span across Machine Learning, Deep Learning, Wireless Sensor Networks, and the Internet of Things (IoT).

Adeyinka Kehinde Iyioluwa is a dedicated student pursuing a degree in Information and Communication Engineering. With a strong passion for artificial intelligence and technology, Adeyinka has authored several academic papers, focusing on topics such as AI applications and data security. Currently, Adeyinka is actively involved in research related to privacy and security management practices in computer science

Adeyinka Taye Iyinoluwa is a passionate researcher and academic with a strong background in Information and Communication Engineering. Known for a deep interest in technology and its transformative impact, Adeyinka is driven by a commitment to advancing innovative solutions in the field of education and beyond.

Keerthi AJ I am an Integrated MTech Software Engineering student at Vellore Institute of Technology passionate about Machine Learning, Blockchain, Azure and App Development. Adept at both research and mentorship, I have worked on innovative projects and continually strive to create impactful solutions through technology.

Fikriye Ataman received a Computer Engineering degree from the Mersin University, Mersin, Turkey, a Master of Science Degree in Computer Engineering from Atatürk University, Erzurum, Turkey, and a PhD degree from the Van Yuzuncu Yıl University, Van. She is a full assistant professor of Computer Engineering at Van Yuzuncu Yıl University, Van, Turkey. Her research interests include cloud computing, high-performance computing, and applied ML/AI.

B. Bharathi, working as an Assistant Professor in RMK Engineering College. I have completed my B.E degree in Computer Science and Engineering in VEL TECH and M.E degree in Computer Science and Engineering in RMK Engineering College. Currently I am pursuing Ph.D Anna University. My area of research includes Artificial Intelligene, Cloud Computing.

B.Bhaskar Reddy working as professor in ECE department,St.Peter's Engineering college, Hyderabad. He graduated in Electronics and Communication Engineering at KSRMCE,S.V.University,Tirupathi. He secured M.E. Degree from TCE,Madurai,Madurai kamaraj University,Madurai.He secured PhD degree from S.K.University,Anantapur. He is in the teaching profession for more than two decades. He has presented number of papers in national and international symposiums and journals. His main areas of interest includes communication, signal processing, image processing and Internet of Things.

Lakshmi D is presently designated as a Senior Associate Professor in the School of Computing Science and Engineering (SCSE) & Assistant Director, at the Centre for Innovation in Teaching & Learning (CITL) at VIT Bhopal. She has 17 international conference presentations, and 21 international journal papers inclusive of SCOPUS & SCI (cumulative impact factor 31). 3 SCOPUS inee book chapters. A total of 24 patents are in various states and 18 patents have been granted at both national and international levels. One Edited book with Taylor & Francis (SCOPUS Indexed). She has won two Best Paper awards at international conferences, one at the IEEE conference and another one at EAMMIS 2021. She received two awards in the year 2022. She received two awards in the year 2022. She has addressed innumerable guest lectures, acted as a session chair, and was invited as a keynote speaker at several international conferences. She has conducted FDPs that cover approximately ~80,000 plus faculty members including JNTU, TEQIP, SERB, SWAYAM, DST, AICTE, MHRD, ATAL, ISTE, Madhya Pradesh Government-sponsored, and self-financed workshops across India on various titles.

Joyeta Ghosh is a dedicated faculty member and researcher with a passion for exploring diverse aspects of Nutrition and Dietetics. Her expertise spans areas including Metabolic Syndrome, Cancer Biology, Genomics, Neurophysiology, and Stress Physiology. With a Ph.D. in Nutritional Biochemistry from the University of Calcutta (DST-INSPIRE Fellow)(2021), a Masters in Applied Nutrition from AIIPH, Kolkata, and a Bachelor's in Food and Nutrition (Honors) from the University of Calcutta, Dr. Ghosh has built a strong academic foundation. She further expanded her skillset with an M.Sc. in Data Science from Liverpool John Moores University, UK. Her core skills encompass experimental design with human subjects, fieldwork, statistical data analysis, and a wide range of laboratory techniques. As a consultant and data scientist in Nutrition Artificial Intelligence, Dr. Ghosh continues to push the boundaries of innovation in the field. Her commitment to excellence in teaching and research, coupled with a relentless pursuit of knowledge, drives her contributions to the advancement of science and nutrition.

Shaik Hedayath Basha Working as Assoc. Professor in RMK College of Engineering and Technology, department of Electronics and Communication Engineering, Chennai, having 16 years of teaching Experience. Completed Bachelor Degree under Madras University, Chennai. Bagged two Master degress, one in Applied Electronics from Satyabama University, Chennai and the other from JNTU, Anantapuramu, Anantapur, Andhra Pradesh. Completed Ph.D from Anna University, Chennai. Published 10 International Journal papers, 5 International, and 3 Indian Conference. Area of interest is Image and Video Watermarking, Image Encryption, Image Analysis, Image Processing, and IoT.

Yuvan Shankar Baabu K is an M.Tech Integrated CSE student specializing in Business Analytics. I enjoy working on innovative projects, writing about emerging technologies, and simplifying complex ideas to create impactful solutions.

A.V.Senthil Kumar is working as a Professor and Director, PG and Research Department of Computer Applications, Hindusthan College of Arts & Science, Coimbatore, Tamilnadu. To his credit he has industrial experience for five years and teaching experience of 27 years. He has also received his Doctor of Science (D.Sc in Computer Science). He has to his credit 50 Book Chapters, 225 papers in International and National Journals 64 papers in International Conferences in International and National Conferences, and edited 14 books and 2 Text books. He is as Associate Editor of IEEE Access. He is an Editor-in-Chief for many journals and Key Member for India, Machine Intelligence Research Lab (MIR Labs). He is an Editorial Board Member and Reviewer for various International Journals. He is also a Committee member for various International Conferences.

Palak Mangal is a second-year student pursuing a Bachelor of Technology in Electronics and Communication Engineering at VIT Bhopal University. With a keen interest in electronics and communications, Palak has demonstrated strong academic performance and a passion for technology innovation. During their time at VIT Bhopal, Palak has engaged in various technical projects and extracurricular activities, further honing their skills and knowledge in the field.

T.C. Manjunath is a distinguished Professor in the Department of Computer Science & Engineering at Rajarajeswari College of Engineering, Bangalore, India. With expertise in IoT Cybersecurity and Blockchain Technology, he serves as the Dean of Research (R&D) at the institution. Dr. Manjunath's academic and research interests focus on emerging technologies in the fields of cybersecurity and blockchain, contributing to the development and advancement of innovative solutions. He is committed to fostering research initiatives and promoting technological growth at the college, located in Kumbalgodu, Bangalore.

Firas Mahmood Mustafa holds a Ph.D. in Computer Engineering from Mosul University, Iraq. His academic journey began with a B.Sc. in Electrical Engineering (Electronics and Communication), graduating in the top quarter of his class. He earned an M.Sc. in Computer Engineering from Mosul University in 2000. Mustafa joined the Computer Science Department at AlHadba University in 2003 and completed his Ph.D. in 2007. From 2013 to 2017, he was with DPU University, and from 2017 to

2020, he chaired the CCE Department at Nawroz University. An active participant in Erasmus+ and IREX programs, he now teaches at DPU University, shaping future computer engineering professionals.

Kamlesh Narwani is a PhD scholar at the school of Information and Communication Engineering, South China University of Technology. He research interests include cyber security in 5G and beyond networks and Computer Vision. He received his masters degree from University of Science and Technology Beijing and he is also associated with DHA SUFFA University, Karachi Pakistan as a senior lecturer.

Abdul Haseeb Nizamani, currently pursuing Ph.D in Computer Science and Engineering from School of Computer Science and Engineering at Central South University. Received his B.S degree from Sindh University Jamshoro and M.S degree from Shandong University, Jinan, China in 2013 and 2019 respectively. He has published research papers as a 1st and co-author in international journals and conferences. His research interests include deep learning, medical image analysis, medical image segmentation and classification, object detection, and feature fusion models.

P. Mercy is a dedicated faculty member in the Department of Computer Science and Business Systems at Anand Institute of Higher Technology, located in Chennai, Tamil Nadu. With a strong focus on integrating technology and business principles, she plays an instrumental role in shaping the academic and professional journeys of students. Her expertise lies in areas of computer science, information systems, and their application in modern business contexts. At the college, she is committed to fostering innovation, encouraging practical learning, and ensuring that students are equipped to succeed in the ever-evolving tech-driven business world.

P. Selvakumar is currently an Associate Professor in the Department of Science and Humanities at Nehru Institute of Technology, Coimbatore, Tamil Nadu, India. Since 2023, he has served as the Department IQAC Coordinator at the institute. Prior to joining Nehru Institute of Technology, he held positions as an Assistant Professor in the Department of Science and Humanities various engineering colleges in Coimbatore, Tamil Nadu, India, spanning from 2011 to 2023. Dr.P. Selvakumar's academic and research interests lie primarily in the field of phytochemistry. He has made significant contributions to his field, with an impressive record that includes 30 journal publications, 12 patents, and 20 conference papers. Additionally, he has organized 5 seminars and conferences, further demonstrating his commitment to academic and scientific exchange. Throughout his career, Dr. P.Selvakumar has been recognized for his dedication and excellence in teaching, having been honored with several awards, including the Best Teacher Awards. He holds a prominent position in the academic community, contributing actively to research.

Sathish Jackson P V is an experienced IT professional with over 15 years of expertise in the field. He is currently serving as an Assistant Professor in the Department of Computer Science and Engineering at Sathyabama Institute of Science and Technology, Chennai, Tamil Nadu, since 2023. Sathish is passionate about teaching and is dedicated to shaping the future of technology professionals. His versatile and customer-centric approach has been a hallmark throughout his career, delivering results in the IT industry before transitioning to academia.

Hari Shankar Punna is working as Assistant Professor, Department of CSE(Data Sceince), CVR College of Engineering (An Autonomous Institution), Affiliated to JNTUH, Vastunagar, Mangalpalli, Ibrahimpatnam, Telangana and Pursuing PH.D. from GITAM (Deemed to be University), Hyderabad, Telangana. He has 13 years of experience in Teaching & Research in Computer Science and Engineering, Cloud Computing, Data Mining. Has guided many Mini & Major projects for B.Tech Students. Mr. Hari Shankar Punna has authored and Co- authored research publications in the field of Cloud Computing and Data Mining, Artificial Intelligence.

Ziaur Rahman has joined the Department of Computer Science, Huanggang Normal University, Hubei, China as a Distinguish Associate Professor in November 2021. Currently, he is an associate professor in Huanggang Normal University. Before that, he received Ph.D degree in Computer Science from Sichuan University, Chengdu, China in 2021 and a Master degree in Software Engineering from Chongqing University, Chongqing, China in 2017. His research interests cover image processing, computer vision, and deep learning, with a special emphasis on low-light image enhancement. Specifically, he is dedicated to designing learning frameworks by exploring the physical properties of various vision applications, including low-light image enhancement, dehazing, denoising, and underwater image enhancement. He is also interested in exploring learning algorithms for medical image analysis.

Shilpi Rana is a seasoned IT professional with over 15 years of experience in academics. Passionate about demystifying complex IT concepts, she is committed to empowering readers with the knowledge and skills they need to succeed in today's rapidly evolving tech landscape. Her academic qualifications include B.Tech in Information and Technology and Masters in IT & HR. She has conducted a number of Management Development and Faculty Development programs for various corporate professionals. She has publications in various esteemed journals and conference proceedings. She has reviewed a number of research papers and has published book chapters for renowned publications. She has conducted various guest and training sessions for Masters and Engineering students.

Anitha S, Professor in the ECE Department at Rajarajeswari College of Engineering, Bengaluru, brings 24 years of rich teaching experience. Her academic credentials are impressive, with over 40 research publications in national and international journals. She actively contributes to academic governance, serving on the Board of Studies and as an examiner for IT/ML/EI at VTU Belagavi. Dr. Anitha S has chaired sessions at numerous international and national conferences and serves as a reviewer for various international conferences. A dedicated researcher, she has guided two PhD scholars and is currently mentoring four. Her contributions are recognized through prestigious awards, including the Bharat Education Excellence Award 2024 and the GRABS Educational Charitable Trust awards. Dr. Anitha holds three patents and has authored five book chapters. Her research interests encompass Digital Image Processing, Medical Imaging, Instrumentation, and Artificial Intelligence. She is a lifetime member of ISTE.

Law Kumar Singh I am an Associate Professor, Amity School of Engineering and Technology, Amity University Punjab, Mohali, India, having more than 16+ years of expertise in academic research and teaching, specializing in cutting-edge fields such as medical image processing, computer vision, machine learning, and deep learning. My enthusiasm is for using sophisticated AI approaches to solve complex problems in the healthcare industry and beyond. I have a demonstrated track record of research quality, having published 43 Scopus-indexed documents, including 26 SCI publications. My study focuses on the use of computer vision and deep learning techniques to medical imaging, with the goal of improving patient outcomes and diagnostic accuracy.

Mansi Singh holds a Master's degree in Computer Application from Banasthali University and is currently pursuing a PhD specializing in IoT and Blockchain. With over a decade of experience in academics, she is a dedicated professional at the Institute of Technology & Science, Mohan Nagar. Her research interests lie in Information Technology and Blockchain, fields in which she has made significant contributions. Mansi has published four research papers in international journals and one paper in a Scopus-indexed journal, reflecting her commitment to advancing knowledge and innovation in her areas of expertise.

Pudi Sree Lakshmi is an Associate Professor in the Department of Electronics and Communication Engineering at Audisankara College of Engineering and Technology, Gudur, Andhra Pradesh, India. With over 15 years of academic and research experience, she has expertise in telecommunications and electronics and communication engineering. She earned her Ph.D. from Saveetha University in 2024, M.Tech from Sathyabama Institute of Science and Technology in 2011, and B.Tech from Narayana Engineering College in 2005. Dr. Sree Lakshmi has authored several publications, including journal articles, book chapters, and conference proceedings, and holds multiple patents in innovative engineering and technology solutions. Her research work has received significant citations and recognition for contributing to advanced wireless applications and deep learning-based systems. She is a life member of ISTE and continues to contribute to the academic and professional development of the field through her research and teaching. Her recent research focuses on ultra-wideband antennas, traffic flow prediction using deep learning, and driver assistance systems.

A. Swetha Rani completed B.TECH in ECE and MT.ECH with specialization in DECS from JNTU Anantapuram.Now pursuing Ph.D in JNTU Anantapuram and her area of interest is Image processing. Qualified UGC NET as assistant professor.Worked as assistant professor in BITS,ADONI.Present Working as assistant professor in Gpcet kurnool.

T. V. V. Satyanarayana is currently working as Professor in the Department of ECE, Mohan Babu University, Tirupati. He completed his Graduation and Post Graduation from Acharya Nagarjuna University in 2002 and 2007 respectively. In 2015, he obtained Ph.D from Jawaharlal Nehru Technological University, Hyderabad. His research contributions include development of novel techniques for Iris Recognition. He has improved the existing Iris Recognition System by improving the accuracy to 99.63% and reduced the time in recognition from 31 seconds to 3.1 seconds, which is a ten-fold improvement. One of his research papers entitled “Multilevel Network Security Based on Iris Biometric” is listed as Iris Image Quality reading materials by NIST Laboratory under U.S. Department of Commerce. His research interests include IoT, Machine Learning and allied fields. Currently he is the reviewer of various International Journals. He has 45 International publications and 4 patents to his credit.

Kalyanasundaram V is an Integrated MTech student in Computer Software Engineering at Vellore Institute of Technology, with a passion for exploring cutting-edge technologies and their real-world applications. In addition to my studies, I am actively engaged in research focused on artificial intelligence, machine learning, cloud computing, and blockchain. These pursuits aim to address complex challenges and drive innovation at the intersection of these transformative fields, shaping a future where technology empowers progress and growth.

Veena V.S., B.E., M.E., MBA, is an accomplished academic professional with extensive experience in electrical engineering education and administration. Holding degrees in Electrical and Electronics Engineering, Power System Engineering, and Human Resources Management, she serves as an Assistant Professor at St. Peter's College of Engineering and Technology. She specializes in power systems, renewable energy technologies, and instrumentation, with notable contributions including authoring a book, publishing papers in conferences, and holding leadership roles such as President of the Institution Innovation Council and AICTE Campus Ambassador. An Anna University rank holder and a life member of the International Association of Engineers (IAENG), she is dedicated to fostering academic excellence, mentoring students, and ensuring successful placements. Proficient in MATLAB and an advocate for continuous learning, she has completed many courses, attended faculty development programs, and actively promotes innovation and entrepreneurship in her field.

Aparna VB is an undergraduate neuroscience student at Yenepoya University, India, with a strong interest in research, particularly in brain-computer interfaces (BCIs) and neurological disorders.

Deepika Yadav is working with SRM University as an Assistant Professor in Electrical and Electronics Engineering since August 2017. She did her Master of Engineering from LIMAT (affiliated to M.D.U), Faridabad with specialization in Power electronics, Electrical Machines and Drives. She has been awarded doctorate degree on topic "Optimal Operation and Scheduling of Hydro Power Plant" by NIT Hamirpur (H.P) in 2014. She has presented her work at national and international levels. Her research work has been published in the form of papers in international journals and conferences and is duly recognized. She has reviewed various papers for International journals such as Elsevier Journal of Renewable and Sustainable Energy Reviews, Taylor and Francis and Springer plus. She is a Life Member of ISTE. She has more than 8.5 years of teaching experience in various institutes. Earlier, she has also worked at Adama Science and Technology University, Ethiopia in Electrical and Computer Science Department. Her research area is Soft Computing Techniques application in Power System and Renewable Energy.

Hewa Majeed Zangana is an Iraqi lecturer and assistant professor in computer science and information technology. He holds a Bachelor's degree from Nawroz University, a Master's degree from the International Islamic University Malaysia, and an Honorary Doctorate from the British Accreditation EB - JAS, and currently studying PhD of ITM at DPU. With expertise in network systems and teaching experience, Hewa has taught various subjects and held positions such as Curriculum Division Director and Head of the Computer Science Department at Nawroz University. He has also published research articles in prestigious journals and presented at conferences.

Index

Symbols

A

B

C

D

E

F

G

H

I

L

M

N

P

R

S

T

V

W

X

www.ingramcontent.com/pod-product-compliance
Lightning Source LLC
LaVergne TN
LVHW060252011026
849161LV00011B/2694